You Can Heal With Every Meal
When You Use Food As Your Pharmacy

Cooking For Healthy Healing

Book One
The Healing Diets

by

Linda Page, N.D., Ph.D.

Linda Page N.D. Ph.D.

Long before natural foods and herbal formulas became a "chic," widely accepted method for healing, Dr. Linda Page was sharing her extensive knowledge with those who dared to listen.

Through what some would call an accident of fate but she calls a blessing, she was compelled to research alternative avenues of healing. Sequestered in a hospital with a life-threatening illness, watching her 5-foot frame wither to 69 pounds, her hair drop out, and her skin peel off, doctors told her they had no cure. With only a cursory knowledge of herbs, she began a frantic research process of test-combinations on herself. She read voraciously about herbal healing. Good friends shopped for herbs and she began to formulate the many compounds which would eventually save her life, revitalize her health and restore beautiful new hair and skin. It was that incident that led her to seek her degrees in Naturopathy and Nutrition.

A prolific author and educator, Dr. Page has sold over a million books including **Healthy Healing, Cooking For Healthy Healing, How To Be Your Own Herbal Pharmacist, Party Lights, Detoxification** and a popular series of books which address specific healing therapies for topics like menopause, male and female energy, colds and flu and cancer. **Healthy Healing** is a textbook for course work at UCLA, The Institute of Educational Therapy, and Clayton College of Natural Health. Dr. Page also formulated over 250 herbal formulas for Crystal Star Herbal Nutrition. She received one of the first herbal patents in the United States for her formulas that help balance hormones to ease menopausal symptoms.

Dr. Page is an Adjunct Professor at Clayton College of Natural Health. She has appeared weekly on a CBS television station with a report on natural healing; she has been featured on national CBS television; she is a principle speaker at national health symposiums and conventions; she is featured regularly in national magazines; she appears on hundreds of radio and television programs, and websites like WebMD. Dr. Page also leads educational healing tours around the world.

Today, Dr. Page delights in having come full circle. "I feel I am living my dream. I am so grateful that knowledge of healing through herbal formulas and good foods is becoming so widespread. I see it as an opportunity for people to seize the power to heal themselves. Knowledge is power. Whether one chooses conventional medicine, alternative healing avenues, or combines them both in a complementary process, the real prescription for healing is knowledge."

Dr. Page is a member of The American Naturopathic Medical Association, The California Naturopathic Association, The American Herbalists Guild, The American Botanical Council and The Herb Research Foundation.

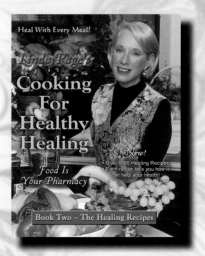
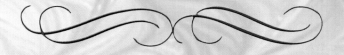
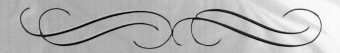

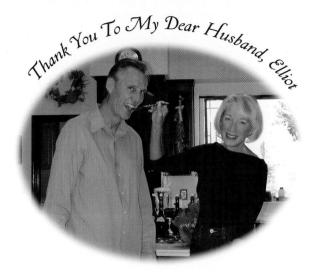

Thank You To My Dear Husband, Elliot

For being the loving life partner that he is.
For all the lively comments, and all the hours of proofreading and analysis.
For taste-testing his way through the recipes,
and never getting to have the same thing twice....even when he liked it!

Thanks also to:
Barbara Howard - Marketing Director, Cover Design, Graphic Design, Editor
Sarah Abernathy - Editor, Research, Prepress Director, Graphics
Kim Tunella - Research, Drafting
Jim Rector - In-house Sales Processing, Customer Service

Publisher's Cataloging-in-Publication
  (Provided by Quality Books, Inc.)

Rector-Page, Linda G.
    Linda Page's cooking for healthy healing. Book one,
The healing diets : food is your pharmacy.
    p. cm.
    Includes bibliographical references and index.
    ISBN: 1884334814

    1. Diet therapy--Popular works. 2. Nutrition--
Popular works. I. Title. II. Title: Cooking for
healthy healing III. Title: Healing diets

RM217.R43 2002   615.8´54
                              QB101-201460

For a free Healthy House catalog,
call 1-888-447-2939

Visit
Linda Page's World of Healthy Healing
on the web for the latest,
updated information on natural
healing techniques,
herbal remedies, and more!

www.healthyhealing.com

Cooking For Healthy Healing - Book One - The Healing Diets
Copyright © April 2002

Traditional
Inc.
Wisdom

Published by Traditional Wisdom, Inc.
Printed in the United States of America

Testimonials

Read what other people say about Linda Page!

Dear Linda,

I have worked with <u>Cooking For Healthy Healing,</u> with good results. It is a wonderfully helpful book! I have found your book extraordinarily helpful and the menus and recipes are delicious! Thank you!

Sincerely,
Ms. Anne L.
Sarasota, FL

Dear Linda,

I believe everyone can benefit from periodic detoxification, but it must be done with care. In your book, <u>Detoxification,</u> you bring together comprehensive individualized detox programs that are safe and effective.

Sincerely,
Randy Ruben Baker, M.D.
Soquel, CA

Dear Linda,

Your video, "Unleashing The Healing Power of Herbs," is a joy to watch.
It is visually beautiful, well organized and very informative! Thank you for your important work and for keeping us all educated about natural healing!

Sincerely, Mrs. M. Engles, Charleston, SC

Dear Linda,

Almost three years ago <u>Healthy Healing</u> became my "bible" and most frequently given gift. There is no need for trips to the drugstore in this household!

Sincerely,
C.M.
San Francisco, CA

Dear Linda,

Your book, <u>How To Be Your Own Herbal Pharmacist</u> is an excellent resource on how herbal nutrition can enhance your health. Thank you for this book that can empower people and help them to live healthier lives.

Sincerely,
Bernie Seigel, M.D.
Author - Love, Medicine & Miracles

A personal letter to my readers.....

Before our "modern age," food was pretty wholesome. People were close to their gardens and farms, and animals and natural resources. Today, we live in a man-made jungle of food substances instead of foods - many of them highly processed, devoid of nutrients, full of hidden fat, chemical-laced, and sugar-drenched.

It doesn't stop there. The hottest topic in the food industry today is functional foods. Manufacturers are creating new "pharmafoods" (often low-nutrient foods like margarine or pastries) by packing them with a slew of vitamins, minerals, herbs and isolated plant essences. In the first half of 1999 alone, functional foods were a $62 billion industry!

It's all in the name of health. The claims are exuberant.... the new foods can fight heart disease, stress, weight gain, even cancer. But, is this stuff really good for you? Make no mistake about it. These aren't Nature-made foods. They're man-made foods.

By stuffing these foods with substances - even natural ones - that aren't a normal part of the food, are we making our foods into drugs? The food is being sold as, say, a muffin. But is it a real muffin, or a medicated muffin?

What's the difference? An essential nutrient is something your body needs but cannot make for itself. Nutrition, like foods and herbs, provides your body with essential nutrients, elements it needs and can use to heal. There is no such thing as an essential drug. A drug can't combine with your body to restore and revitalize.

Nature's whole, ready-to-use medicines are often the only "prescription" your body needs to get better. Nature is, after all, the perfect pharmacy. Many foods and herbs are such highly complex medicines that they are almost micro-pharmacies in themselves.

Still, the world has changed! The explosion of enthusiasm and interest in plant medicine means everybody wants to get on the bandwagon. The sales of herbal products alone increased by more than 100% since 1994. Yet just a few short years ago, practically every medical expert was calling food and herbal healing worthless, demonizing herbalists, calling all naturopaths quacks.

The American public has changed this view from the grass roots up. The rise of individual, personal health care has begun. Clearly, Americans want to take more responsibility for their health and that of their families. But that means lots of answers to thousands of questions are going to be needed.
We don't completely understand exactly how foods and herbs work. They are foods. They are medicines. We may never fathom their intricacies.

We feel uncomfortable when something isn't logical. But Nature isn't logical. The way natural healing works isn't logical either. It just doesn't "fit" into the way western Science sees and understands things. Science breaks things down and takes them apart in order to measure and understand them. There's nothing wrong with that, as long as we realize it isn't the only way... especially when we're dealing with an incredible, whole human person who is so much more than a lab test or a blood panel.

The truth is, people aren't logical either.... healers need to pay much more attention to the whole person for healing to be long-lasting.

If we can't understand it, can it work to heal us? Our scientific culture relies totally on things like lab tests and substances that are man-made because they fit into our ability to understand. "Scientific" medicine attacks anything that can't be specifically isolated, broken down, peeled apart or synthesized. It discounts the value of something it can't understand, believing that something can't possibly work if we can't understand it.

It doesn't even matter if the natural, whole substance works. A "silver bullet" must be identified so that it can be synthesized and manufactured. Even advanced medical techniques, like genetic science, work this way.

I believe only the whole food can give the whole benefit. Many plants can only work in their whole form. While single plant elements can be tested and measured, a lab can only give a partial answer about a highly complex living thing. When we take one out of the literally hundreds of elements in a plant and say, "That's it, that's what this plant is good for," we lose. It's never the whole story. Healing foods and herbs are never just one plant for one problem.

If we make our foods and herbs into drugs, will we get unwanted side effects, adverse reactions, drug interactions, even addictions that are the downside of drugs?

I had to learn the hard way, but it made me a firm believer in the old way, in the traditional way of herbal healing. Isolating constituents or boosting certain plant elements changes the balance of the plant and the protective factors it has built in.

But foods and herbs are so much more than a test or a scientific measurement. Plants are the only medicines I know of that treat the whole person, not just their symptoms... I believe God shows his face to us in natural healers.

I say, let foods and herbs do what they do so well.... heal and balance from the inside out, naturally and safely. Use them in their whole form as medicinal foods.

Health for each of us is personal. To approach it impersonally, only through big business, science and government means that your health is bound to lose.

Linda

About this Book....

Food is potent medicine. Your diet can literally transform your body.

Wholesome food not only fuels your body, eating wholesome foods can also help solve your health problems. Your diet can keep your energy levels up and stress levels down, your skin, hair, and nails healthy, your complexion glowing, your eyes bright, and your bones and muscles strong. It can fine-tune mental awareness and prevent disease from taking hold. A poor diet and junk foods produce lethargy, illness, and indifference.

Good food is good medicine. It is the prime factor for changing your body chemically and psychologically. A good diet is even a key to higher consciousness. A well-nourished system opens body receivers and transmitters for higher energies. By creating new balance in a body where there was imbalance, a clean healthy body allows the beauty of the spirit to shine through.

The food you eat changes your weight, your mood, the texture and look of your body, your outlook on life, indeed the entire universe for you.... and therefore your future. Eating right is the first step to the health and balance of your universe. This book is about getting back to the basics... because basics are basics, like classics are classics, for a reason.

The book you hold in your hands took me seventeen years to write. It's the result of an enormous amount of work in using foods as medicine. All the recipes and diet plans were tested again and again, first through the Rainbow Kitchen restaurant and juice bar I owned in the early eighties, to the diet programs I developed for Country Store Natural Foods and Crystal Star Herbal Nutrition, to the highly focused healing diets of today using foods as Nature's Pharmacy.

Through all this time, the results were clear and undeniable..... Foods and herbs (we have to remind ourselves that herbs are foods) can indeed heal — even serious diseases — sometimes dramatically. Foods and herbs can prevent some health problems from happening at all and many illnesses from developing further. The secret is using foods and herbs to change body chemistry. Drugs can't do it. Only foods and herbs can do it. This two book set tells you how.

The history of the world would be entirely different if the human diet had been different. Our children are literally formed from, and become, the nutrients (or poisons) within us. Not only are we what we eat, our children are as well, before and after birth. The pattern for the immune system and inherited health of your children and grandchildren is laid down by you.

Healthy parents = healthy children.
Healthy grandparents = healthy grandchildren.
and thus the world.
That's how important diet is!

How to Use this Book....

Good food can be great medicine!

All the advances made by modern medicine still don't address chronic diseases very well; they don't address disease prevention at all.

Sometimes food can be your best medicine... even for serious diseases. We tend to think that the healing powers of foods are subtle or mild, without the overwhelming potency of drugs. Yet healing doesn't always need to deal a hammer blow.... even for serious problems.

As new research advances the science of nutrition, there's an enormous thirst for information about how to use it. Most people are actively trying to eat better. Organic foods are mainstream today. But most people don't know HOW to use foods as medicine. This two book set can help you navigate the healing path easily and effectively. It's all a matter of the way you direct what you eat.

You'll have everything you need to do it yourself, day by day, and succeed.
—Detailed **STEP-BY-STEP DIETS** for a wide range of illnesses and health problems.
—A large **FOOD and NUTRIENT DIGEST,** with the important elements and healing
    properties of hundreds of foods and herbs so you can build your own target diet.
—**RECIPES and MENU PLANS** for every health problem in the book.
—Over **1000 RECIPES** to choose from to keep your diet interesting and focused on healing.

In the 1930's, at the height of the scientific love affair with orthodox medicine, the Nobel prize winning doctor, Albert Schweitzer said, *"the doctor of the future will be oneself."* He already saw the limitations of drugs and surgery-based healing. He knew that immune strength was the only real way to prevent disease.

In fact, the immune system of each one of us is so entirely unique to us, that it may be impossible for a laboratory to ever develop a drug to activate immunity. Only foods or herbs, that combine with each person individually, and work with each person's distinctive enzymes at the deepest levels of each person's body, can do the job for immune response.

Medicines from foods and herbs work just the opposite from drugs. They nourish the body and enhance the immune system. Drugs function outside the system, usually operating to overwhelm a harmful organism. Today's orthodox medicine is "heroic medicine," largely developed in wartime for emergency wartime requirements. It's a patching up system. It isn't supportive or nourishing; it's often risky over the long term; and it doesn't stimulate immune response.

Yet, I feel we need both types of medicine. Drugs can stop an emergency and stabilize your body to give your immune system a chance to take over.

Clearly, orthodox medicine has saved many lives. Just as clearly, alternative medicine has prevented much illness. Use the healing diets in this book to put yourself on the path to the best health you've ever had!

Table of Contents

Section Two: **The Healing Diet Programs**   **Pg. 139**

Detoxification: Body System Cleansing   Pg. 142
• **About Detoxification:** Body signs you need to detoxify; Steps in a detox program.
• **Diets:** 1} Colon-Bowel Elimination 2} Lung Cleanse 3} Bladder- Kidney Cleanse 4} Liver Cleanse 5} Blood Cleanse 6} Lymph Cleanse 7} Skin Cleanse

Allergy-Asthma Control and Management   Pg. 174
• **Diets:** 1} Mucous Purging Diet 2} Asthma Diet 3} Allergy Control Diet: Seasonal Allergies 4} Allergy Control Diet: Chemical-Contaminant Allergies
• **Health Conditions Effective For:** *Allergies; Sinusitis; Adrenal Exhaustion; Asthma; Headaches.*

Arthritis: Changing Your Body Chemistry   Pg. 187
• **Diets:** 1} Arthritis Cleansing Diet 2} Arthritis Control Diet
• **Health Conditions Effective For:** *Arthritis; Fibromyalgia; Bursitis; Lupus; Bone Spurs and Corns; Gum Disease; Gout; Prostate Inflammation; Osteoporosis; Post-Menopausal Bone Loss; Shingles.*

Bone Building with High Mineral Building Blocks   Pg. 191
• **Diets:** 1} Osteoporosis Intervention Diet 2} Strong Bones Diet
• **Health Conditions Effective For:** *Osteoporosis; Back, Nerve, Muscle Pain; Thyroid Health; Easy Bruising; Hair and Nail Health; Indigestion; Bad Breath; Low Attention Span; Memory; Emotional Health.*

Cancer: Controlling and Rebuilding Health   Pg. 200
• **Diets:** 1} Intensive Macrobiotic Diet 2} Cancer Control Die 3} Normalizing after Chemotherapy or Radiation
• **Health Conditions Effective For:** *Systemic Cancer (Colon, Stomach, Organ, Lung); Melanoma; Malignant Tumors; Leukemia; Pernicious Anemia; M.S.; Muscular Dystrophy.*

Immune Power: Building a Strong Defense System   Pg. 213
• **Diets:** 1} Chemical, Metal, Pollutant Cleanse 2} Immune Stimulation Diet
• **Health Conditions Effective For:** *Infections of all kinds; Herpes; Poisoning; Parasites; Cysts.*

Immune Breakdown Diseases   Pg. 223
• **Diets:** 1} HIV-AIDS Infection Diet 2} Lupus-M.S. Diet 3} Herpes and STD's Healing Diet 4} Parasite Infection Cleanse
• **Health Conditions Effective For:** *HIV Infection and AIDS Syndromes; Lupus; M.S.; Muscular Dystrophy; Herpes; HPV- Viral Warts Infection; Hepatitis; Parasite Infections; Environmental Pollutants.*

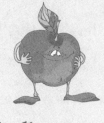

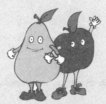

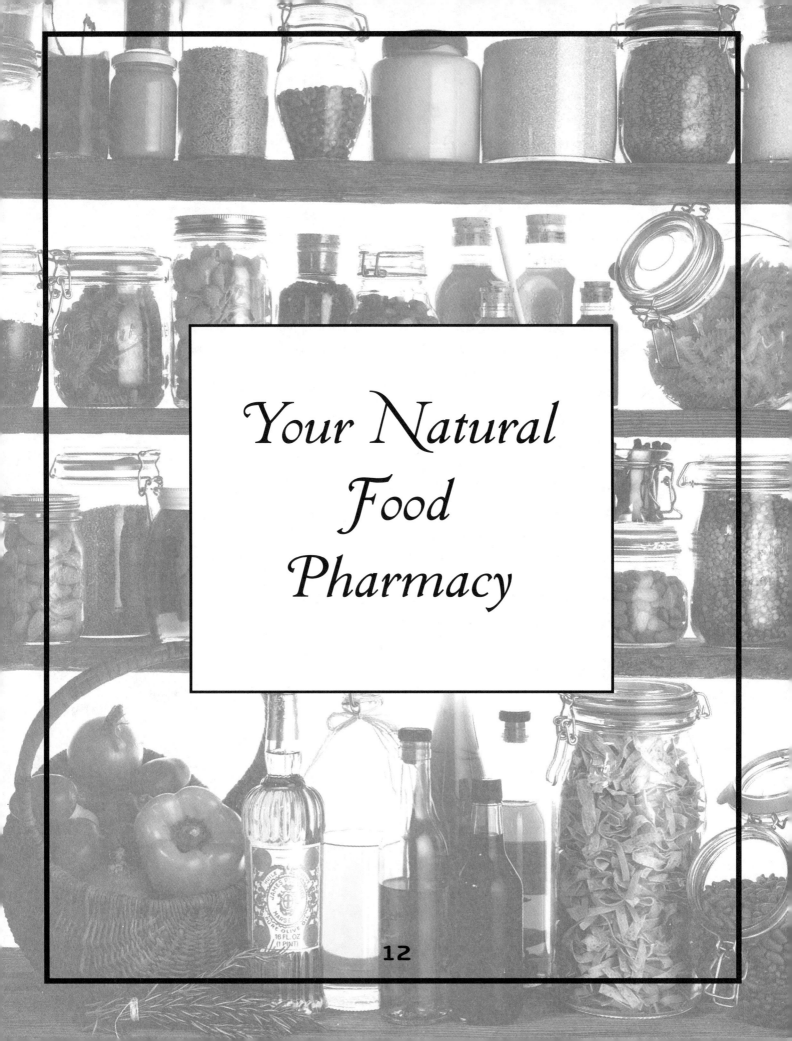

Your Natural Food Pharmacy

The Food Pharmacy

What is a food pharmacy? Your diet is one of the most powerful tools you have for your health. All the advances made by modern medicine still don't address chronic diseases very well. They don't address disease prevention at all.

Food is powerful medicine. Sometimes it's your best medicine.... even for difficult diseases. We think of foods as very gentle, without the overwhelming potency of drugs. Yet healing doesn't always need to deal a hammer blow.... even for serious problems.

It's all a matter of how you direct what you eat. As research advances nutritional science, everybody understands that foods and herbs can heal. But most people don't know HOW to use them as medicine. That's where this book comes in. Its information can help you navigate the healing path easily and effectively.

You're the Doctor — Food Is Your Pharmacy, the book you hold in your hands, took me seventeen years to write. It's the result of an enormous amount of work in using foods as medicine. The recipes and diet plans were tested again and again, first through my Rainbow Kitchen restaurant and juice bar in the early eighties, then in the diet programs I developed for Country Store Natural Foods and Crystal Star Herbal Nutrition, then by using highly focused healing diets that treat foods as natural medicines.

Through all this time, the results were clear and undeniable..... foods and herbs (sometimes we have to remind ourselves that herbs are foods) can indeed heal disease - sometimes dramatically. Beyond healing, I saw that foods and herbs prevented many health problems from occurring in the first place, and some illnesses from developing further.

The secret is using foods and herbs to change body chemistry. Drugs can't do it. Only foods and herbs can do it.

Here's why: each one of us is entirely individual; our immune systems are individual to each of us. It would be impossible for a laboratory to <u>ever</u> develop a drug to activate immunity for everyone. Only something like foods or herbs, which are able to combine with each of us individually, operate at the deepest levels of our bodies, and work with our own enzyme activity, can do the job.

Nature is after all, the perfect pharmacy. I think it's time to return to Mother Nature.....

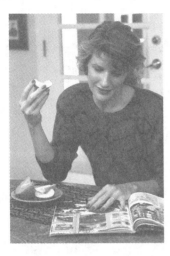

How can you get the most from your food pharmacy?

The foods you eat can accomplish almost every health and healing need. Medicines from foods and herbs work just the opposite from drugs. They nourish the body and enhance the immune system. The essence of human health is body balance, establishing body chemistry that resists disease, and encourages energy and well-being. Drugs don't work with your body systems; they usually operate by checking an infection or overwhelming a harmful organism. I call today's orthodox medicine "heroic medicine" because it was developed largely in wartime for emergency needs, arresting death in a normally healthy body until immune response could take over. But for chronic or degenerative diseases, this type of medicine hits the body with a drug punch that isn't supportive, and doesn't stimulate immune response.

Medicines from foods and herbs should be taken differently than drugs. Ordinarily, you have to take more and more of a drug to get the same effect.... in some cases creating dependency or tolerance. With herbal medicines, instead, you might start with a larger amount to stimulate your body's vital healing force, then reduce the amount you take as your healing program goes on and your body picks up its own work from the nutrients you have been giving it.

I feel we need both types of medicine. Clearly, orthodox medicine has saved many lives. Just as clearly, alternative medicine has prevented much illness.

Today we're flooded with information (and misinformation) about nutrition. Yet, there's still a real need for people to learn what a healthy diet is and what it is not. Nutrition is both a science and an art of nourishing yourself. Sound nutritional knowledge can help people navigate through all the unhealthy foods and eating habits they're faced with today.

America's food marketing methods operate for business success rather than for health, especially for kids. Highly visible, star-endorsed advertising pressures young people to eat foods that are often unhealthy junk foods - with high amounts of sugar, meat and dairy products that can cause mucous build-up. These foods are clearly big contributors to the skyrocketing rise in degenerative disease and overweight problems in children, who under normal conditions, are naturally immune-protected, and youthfully fit.

Even the government knows our diets are letting us down. Population studies and recent clinical data have linked the "Western diet" to many common diseases.

A 1997 Surgeon General's report notes that "diet-related diseases account for 68% of all deaths in America!" The study goes on to say that "a diet rich in plant foods protects against many common diseases in Western society," and that "a diet with low intake of plant foods contributes to the development of common modern diseases, encouraging conditions under which disease factors can become active."

It seems that we've all been talking about diet and nutrition forever. Everyone's aware of the need to keep a clean, well-nourished body.... right? This is simply not the case.

The general diet today in our society still consists mainly of meat, dairy products, highly processed foods, and **only occasional fresh foods**. Instead of a diet that easily supports us, our bodies are forced into stress procedures in order to process an overload of concentrated proteins, refined food substances and chemicals.

Diet overload means our bodies don't work very efficiently, and digestive organs and glands work overtime. Here are some of the diseases we get when we overload:

• diabetes and hypoglycemia (overload from carbohydrates)
• hardening of the arteries (overload from fat)
• degenerative problems and premature aging (overload from proteins)
• poor digestion (overload of chemicalized foods, alcohol, drugs and sugars)
• obesity (overload from all of the above)

How can we remind ourselves in a positive way that we really are what we eat?
It's hard for anybody to make major diet changes with a "cold turkey approach." Weight loss dieters know too well that "all or nothing" plans don't work. Overnight changes are just too difficult to maintain. A gradual re-education program works best. Keep yourself motivated with small improvements that show initial positive results and provide a framework for more changes.
You'll be delighted when you start to see your energy level change, when you feel the first golden suffusion of well being as your body chemistry balances, and when you get a taste of physical power you haven't experienced in years.

1: **Simplify your diet** — reduce fried foods, meat and dairy, foods with chemicals.

2: **Buy the highest quality foods you can find** — organically grown when you can.

3: **Read food product labels before you buy** — your food decisions will be better.

4: **Eat more foods that don't have ANY labels** — like fresh fruit and vegetables.

5: **Eat a variety of foods.** Some drastic detox or weight loss diets limit you to only one or two types of foods. These diets provide limited nutrition; they wreak havoc on your body chemistry and lead to immune compromised disorders. I have tried diets like this. They can be devastating to your health. The greater the variety of foods you eat, the less likely you are to develop either a deficiency or an excess of any single nutrient. The healthiest people eat a wide variety of low fat, fresh foods.

6: **A food reward program works.** Eat a super healthy diet Monday through Friday, then relax your diet on weekends to eat some of your old favorite foods.

7: **Be gentle with yourself.** Mark Twain said that a habit can't simply be tossed out the window. Escort it like an old friend, down the stairs one at a time, then out the door.

Your Diet Can Literally Transform Your Body

The latest research validates the ancient wisdom..... we literally are what we eat. Every time you eat you can do something good for your health. You can <u>always</u> use your food as medicine.

What you eat is your best protection against disease. Foods and herbs have powerful medicinal properties. The latest studies confirm it. You can work on your health problems every day as you choose your foods.

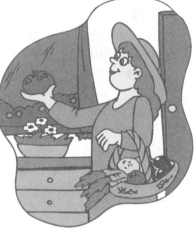

It's getting easier to eat better. Organic foods are mainstream today. Food regulations are changing, too. In 1998, the FDA allowed Kellogg to claim psyllium fiber's link to reduced heart disease on a product label, a monumental step for them.

Entire departments in universities are being developed to research the power of foods and food chemicals on the human body and for human health. Test results are coming in at an ever increasing pace. Foods are finally starting to be seen for what they really are.... a reliable way to deliver healing and support nutrients to our bodies.

I've been an advocate for using food as medicine for decades.
—In the early eighties, I talked about healthy foods tasting good, because in those days most people thought health food tasted like cardboard.... (a lot of it did).
—But, we all got more educated, so in the late eighties, I talked about diets, and how to integrate a good diet into your everyday life.
—In the early nineties, I talked about the dangers of adding chemicals to foods, microwaving food and altering foods by hydrogenating fats.
—In the mid-nineties, I talked about tailoring specific foods with specific constituents to solve your health problems.
—Today, functional foods are the darling of science and gourmet food producers alike. Scientists and innovative food manufacturers combine foods with different constituents, making a "new" food to apply to a certain health problem. Sometimes they hybridize plants to form a more powerful, healing food.

The health food industry started the movement, but entire medicinal food lines are now being developed at the mainstream level. Every day new herbally-enriched foods and drinks are launched to recharge our energy, detox us, protect us against free radicals, or relax us. Intelligent Cuisine, marketed by Campbell, has a line of "clinically proven" meals for diabetics and for people with high blood pressure and high cholesterol.

Immune enhancing drinks, libido boosting lollipops, power bars to unclog arteries and cholesterol lowering spreads are widely available.

Functional foods are clearly booming.

They seem a perfect answer for health and a very efficient way to eat. People feel that they've got to eat anyway, so why not eat a medicinal, enhanced food rather than buying supplements or taking drugs. Even in its infancy, nutraceutical creations are a $62 billion industry! The idea sounds great. The splashy packaging make them appealing, but how good are these foods for our health?

Well, it all depends on what you're looking at. Let's not become beguiled by functional foods or genetically altered foods too quickly. Over and over again, we find that when we mess with Mother Nature at the basic level, we lose. I want to make a clear case in this book for whole foods. I believe whole foods and herbs are the real medicine.

What about adding synthetic vitamins to fortify foods?

Some food producers now add isolated vitamins and other supplemental nutrients to pastries, frozen foods and microwaved foods. Even though this may seem like a quick, easy way to pump up your nutrient intake, these creations are usually high calorie, chemicalized foods that aren't good for long term health.

In Nature's food pharmacy, vitamins are never isolated. Our bodies are uniquely designed to use nutrients as they naturally occur in foods.

While I still hear some scientists say that our bodies can't distinguish between synthesized vitamins and nutrients from whole foods, I know from my own experience, as well as from respected studies that food-source vitamins ARE superior to isolates or synthesized variations. For instance, if you've read the reports on vitamin E, the naturally-occurring form (D-alpha tocopherol) is twice as absorbable as the synthetic version (dl-alpha tocopherol)!

Here's one of the reasons why: Food complex vitamins have smaller, more bioavailable molecules. Your body can use them more efficiently for healing. Further, I've personally seen that even food source supplements aren't a substitute for the amazing power of whole foods.

Your body needs whole foods to heal, with all the enzymes and balanced nutrients built in. Food has essential nutrients, nutrients your body needs but can't make for itself.

Today we call herbs and vitamins the alternative medicine industry, but drugs are the real alternative medicine. Drugs don't nourish or normalize. There is no such thing as an essential drug. Drugs are powerful chemical compounds used best as short-term medical measures to arrest, overpower a harmful organism and stabilize your body so that your immune forces have a chance to rise to your defense.

Whole foods and herbs are at <u>their</u> best as body normalizers. Drugs can't do it. Only foods and herbs as foods can do it. I believe strongly in the power of herbs — they are the supreme healing foods. I saw it clearly in my own life-threatening illness. Herbs are a lot more than remedies for colds and flu. They can change your life.

Getting the most from your Natural Food Pharmacy

Food Pharmacy Details

Learn about your "food as medicine" choices for a healing diet.

- Fruits, vegetables and chlorophyll for plant enzyme therapy.

- Is a vegetarian diet better? The truth about red meat.

- Protein: How much do you need for healing?

- Green superfoods, healing mushrooms for fast healing.

- Macrobiotics balances body chemistry for serious healing.

- Soy foods and cultured foods provide natural probiotics.

- Water is essential for healing.

- Caffeine in a healing diet? Can green and black teas heal?

- Does wine fit into a healing program?

- Fats and oils: There's good news and bad news.

- Dairy foods in a healing diet? Are butter and eggs okay?

- Sugar and sweeteners: Are they all bad?

- Low salt or no salt? What's the best for long term health?

- Sea greens can help almost every health problem.

- Desert powerhouses: Healing bee superfoods and aloe vera.

- Foods are part of Nature's aromatherapy.

- Herbs and spices are medicinal foods.

Fresh Fruits, Vegetables & Juices

Fruits and vegetables top the list of healing foods! Massive research is validating what natural healers have known for decades. The more fruits and vegetables you eat, the more nutrition you get and the less your risk of disease.

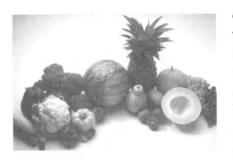

Fresh fruits and veg-cines do best..... work with in restorative abilities. Even against you, your diet still in your odds for better health and vegetables accelerate malize body chemistry. I em-juice diet as part of almost ev- etables do what natural medi-your body so it can use its built-if your genetics and lifestyle are makes a tremendous difference and fast healing. Fresh fruits body cleansing, and help nor-phasize a detoxification fresh ery healing program.

Fruits and vegetables are full of nutraceuticals, the natural chemicals in plants that have pharmacologic action. Today, scientists are enthusiastically embracing the healing possibilities of the plant nutrients in "garden variety" foods.

Green leafy vegetables, for example, contain almost <u>20 times</u> more essential nutrients, ounce for ounce than any other foods. What's more, the nutrients in greens actually make the nutrients in other foods work better for our health.

The preventive medicine possibilities are astounding.

Studies show that people who eat plenty of vegetables have <u>over 50% less cancer risk</u> than people who eat few vegetables. Even moderate amounts of vegetables make a big difference. For instance, eating fresh vegetables twice a day, instead of twice a week, can cut the risk of lung cancer by 75%.... even for smokers. One National Cancer Institute spokesman said it is almost mind-boggling that common foods can be so effective against a potent carcinogen like tobacco!

There's more. Certain body chemicals must be "activated" before they can initiate cancer cell growth. Fresh foods are able to block the activation process, because food chemicals in cells can determine whether a cancer-causing virus, or a cancer promoter like excess estrogen, will turn tissue cancerous.

<u>Fruits and vegetables are able intervene even if you already have cancer</u>. When cells mass into tumors, food compounds can restrain further growth by flushing certain carcinogens out of the body (cruciferous vegetables), or shrinking patches of precancerous cells (sea greens). Antioxidant-rich foods can snuff out carcinogens, nip free radical cascades in the bud, even repair some cellular damage.

<u>Fresh foods help prolong your life even after cancer takes hold</u>, fostering an environment that deters wandering cancer cells from attaching to new tissue. The evidence is so overwhelming that researchers are starting to view fruits and vegetables as powerful preventive "drugs" that might wipe out cancer - **what an about-face for cancer study!**

Fresh fruits are Nature's smiles.

Fruits are wonderful for a quick system wash and cleanse. Their high natural water and sugar content speeds up metabolism to release wastes rapidly and accelerate calorie burning for quick energy. Fresh fruit has an alkalizing effect in the body.

But these advantages are only true of fresh fruits. The way that you eat fruit is as important as which fruit you eat. Fruits have their best healing and nutrition effects when eaten alone or with other fruits, as in a fruit salad, separately from grains and vegetables. With a few exceptions, both fruits and fruit juices should be taken before noon for best energy conversion and cleansing benefits.

The activity of fruit changes from alkalizing to acid-forming in our bodies when it's cooked. This is also true of sulphured, dried fruit, and combining fruits with vegetables or grains. When you eat fruit in these ways, digestion slows down because the fruits stay too long in the stomach; gas forms as the fruit sugars concentrate, and fermentation instead of assimilation results.

New studies on fruits show more amazing benefits. Citrus fruits possess fifty-eight known anti-cancer compounds, more than any other food! Some researchers call citrus fruits a total anti-cancer package because they have every class of nutrient - carotenoids, flavonoids, terpenes, limonoids, coumarins, and more - known to neutralize chemical carcinogens. Yet citrus fruits act more powerfully as a whole than any of the separate anti-cancer compounds they contain. One phytochemical for example, in oranges, is the powerful antioxidant glutathione, a confirmed disease combatant. When chemically extracted, however, orange juice loses its glutathione concentration. Oranges are also rich in beta-carotene and vitamin C, and the highest food in glucarate, a powerful cancer-inhibitor.

Eat organically grown fruits whenever possible. The pesticides from sprayed fruits can enter your body very rapidly because fruit sugar metabolism is so fast.

Fresh vegetables are Nature's "Superfoods."

The healing power of vegetables works both raw and lightly cooked. It is not always true that raw vegetables are better. Some fragile anticancer agents, like indoles and vitamin C, are indeed destroyed by heat, but a little heat makes beta carotene more easily absorbed. The action of lightly cooked vegetables is gentler, especially if your digestion is impaired.

What is a serving of fresh fruits or vegetables? One serving is about $1/2$ cup of cooked, chopped veggies; 1 cup of leafy vegetables; 1 medium piece of fruit, or 6-oz. of fruit or vegetable juice. Only 10 percent of Americans eat this much every day.

Take a look on the next few pages to see the astounding new studies on everyday foods. They show that the same phytochemicals that protect plants from pests, viruses and bacteria may also protect our bodies from cancers and heart disease.

• **ORGANIC SULPHUR COMPOUNDS, like allylic sulfides in garlic and onions,** contain more than 30 different anti-carcinogens - like quercetin and ajoene that can block the most feared cancer-causing agents like nitrosamines and aflatoxin, linked specifically to stomach, lung and liver cancer. In the county where Georgia's Vidalia onions are grown, for instance, the stomach cancer rate is only half that of other Georgia counties, and less than one-third that of the rest of the United States.

Allylic sulfides are both antimutagenic and anti-carcinogenic. **Ajoene in garlic is three times as toxic to malignant cells as to normal cells.** Interleukin in garlic boosts macrophages and T-lymphocytes, your immune agents responsible for destroying tumor cells. Harvard scientists protect mice against some cancers by putting onions in their drinking water. Their tests show mice who eat garlic have 75% fewer colon tumors than those who don't. Even mice given breast cancer causing agents are protected.... not a single one in recent tests who ate garlic got cancer.

A new German study shows that garlic compounds destroy malignant cells in the same way chemotherapy does. Garlic also discourages colon cancer by working as an antibiotic against the bacteria identified with colon cancer.

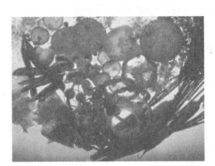

Garlic's allylic sulfides also provide cardiovascular protection, suppressing cholesterol synthesis in the liver, lowering serum cholesterol by reducing LDL cholesterol (while maintaining high density lipoprotein, HDL, at normal levels. Garlic reduces heart attack risk by 1) lowering triglyceride blood fats associated with heart attack; 2) lowering blood pressure by decreasing peripheral vascular resistance; 3) reducing the tendency of blood to clot, and helping to dissolve existing clots. It may even reverse atherosclerosis blockages.

—**Sulforaphane, a sulphur compound in cruciferous vegetables,** mustard and horse-radish, induces protective, phase II enzymes, which detoxify carcinogens. Sulforaphane delays onset of cancer, and inhibits the size and number of tumors.

• **ANTIOXIDANTS** in foods like wheat germ, soy foods, yellow, orange and green vegetables, green tea, citrus fruits and olive oil help normalize pre-cancerous cells, by snuffing out carcinogens, nipping free radical cascades in the bud, and repairing cellular damage.

—**Allylic sulfides** (see above) are also powerful antioxidants, defending cells against damage by oxidizing toxins. Allylic sulfides in garlic and onions inhibit the growth of a wide spectrum of bacteria and viruses, including staphylococcus, streptococcus and salmonella. Garlic particularly fights funguses and parasites, making it a specific for candida albicans yeast overgrowth and HIV-related conditions.

—**Green leafy vegetables** show extraordinarily broad cancer protective powers, largely because they are so rich in antioxidants. Recent studies reveal many different antioxidants — alpha, beta and other carotenes, folic acid, zeaxanthin, and lutein a little-known antioxidant that scientists think is more potent than beta carotene against cancer. The darker green the vegetables, the more cancer-inhibiting carotenoids they have. Eat a green salad every day!

• **ORGANIC ACIDS,** metabolic compounds with significant antioxidant activity, are being tested for their potential anti-cancer effects which experts think is far-reaching.

—**Phytic acid,** an antioxidant compound from rye, wheat, rice, lima beans, sesame seeds, peanuts and soybeans, appears to prevent colon cancer and enhance immune killer cell activity. It may be a better antioxidant than vitamin C, because it naturally chelates both iron and zinc to help prevent heart disease. Too much stored iron in the body (especially as we age) increases oxidative damage and the risk for heart disease.

—**Folic acid,** a B vitamin in wheat, wheat germ, leafy vegetables, beets, asparagus, fish, sunflower seeds, and citrus fruits is critical to normal DNA synthesis - so healthy cells stay healthy. Folic acid reduces the risk of two birth defects, lowers the risk of atherosclerosis and, potentially cancer. Yet, while folic acid is seen as a cancer protector after menopause, excess folate can be tumor promoting. **The key is getting plenty of folic acid from your food instead of just taking supplements.** For example, people who eat lots of leafy greens have a low incidence of lung cancer. People who merely take folic acid supplements but do not eat leafy greens still lack protective folic acid in their lungs.

Folic acid is also a weapon against heart disease because it reduces homocysteine levels. **New research implicates homocysteine levels in Down's syndrome and Alzheimer's deterioration, too.** When methylation, your body's chief mechanism for protecting your genes, isn't working well, toxins like homocysteine build up, generating a cascade reaction that sets the stage for degenerative diseases like heart disease and cancer. Folic acid and vitamin B-12 help methylation to lower homocysteine levels. Vitamin B-6 helps convert homocysteine to cysteine, a safe amino acid. Foods like beans, garlic, sea foods and sea greens, nutritional yeast, brown rice and green vegetables are rich in vitamins B-6, B-12 and folic acid to keep homocysteine levels normal.

Note: Normal estrogen levels keep homocysteine levels down; but since estrogen production is reduced in postmenopausal women, I recommend a plant-estrogen herbal combination as part of a menopausal woman's heart-protecting program. Plant estrogens balance, rather than build up in her body.

—**Vitamin C,** an antioxidant in citrus fruits, cherries, tomatoes, green peppers, strawberries, leafy greens, hot red peppers and broccoli, is one of the most effective antioxidants in blood plasma. Vitamin C reduces both LDL cholesterol and triglyceride levels, and significantly lowers serum lead levels. Vitamin C's antioxidants also promote wound healing, and boost interferon for immune response and T-cell production.

Oxidative stressors, like ultraviolet light, play a central role in cataract development. Antioxidants like vitamin C, E and carotenoids (see next page), can lower this common cataract risk. Vitamin C's antioxidants also improve blood sugar levels in non-insulin dependent diabetics.

Vitamin C is the most abundant antioxidant in our lungs and a major factor in the body's low protection against asthma. Americans show increasingly less vitamin C in blood plasma as our exposure to smoke pollutants rises and as we eat less vitamin C rich foods. Some scientists believe that America's high rates of asthma are a direct result of our decrease in antioxidant consumption.

• **Bioflavonoids,** initially called vitamin P (for their rapid permeability), play a significant role for healing in the vitamin C complex. They are essential for absorption of vitamin C and prevent vitamin C from being destroyed by oxidation. Bioflavs help vitamin C keep your collagen (the body's intercellular "glue") healthy. One of the most vital benefits of bioflavonoids are their superb ability to strengthen capillaries, connective tissue and blood vessel walls. Boost your bioflavonoid intake to reduce hemorrhages and ruptures in the capillaries and connective tissues which lead to spider veins, varicose veins, and bruises. The first signs of deficiency in vitamin C and bioflavonoids is a tendency to bruise and bleed easily, the appearance of varicose veins, or noticeable purplish spots on the skin.

Find bioflavs in the skin and pulp of citrus fruits, grapes, cherries and many berries. Good herbal sources of bioflavonoids: *buckwheat greens, peppers, yellow dock, elder, hawthorn, horsetail, rose hips, shepherd's purse, sea plants,* and *nettle.*

Some of the benefits bioflavonoids have for you:
- Bioflavs help build a protective antibiotic barrier against infections.
- Bioflavs have potent anti inflammatory effect without the side effects of aspirin.
- Bioflavs boost immune response and recovery from infections.
- Bioflavs help prevent allergies and asthma.
- Bioflavs reduce internal bleeding and promote healing from injuries.
- Bioflavs help detoxify carcinogenic chemicals.
- Bioflavs assist in preventing cardiovascular disease.
- Bioflavs curtail menopausal symptoms (they act much like estrogens).
- Bioflavs help relieve pain and promote healing of ulcers.
- Bioflavs help prevent cataracts and other eye problems.

—**Genistein,** a flavonoid in soy and cruciferous vegetables like broccoli, impedes angiogenesis (the growth of blood vessels that feed tumors), and deters cancer cell development by inhibiting enzymes that promote tumor formation. New tests on genistein from soy show that it promotes the positive effects of estrogen while preventing many of estrogen's bad actions, especially its role in hormone-driven cancers like breast and ovarian cancers. Genistein offers menopausal women a good choice against menopause symptoms - it works much like the hormone replacement drug Premarin without the risks.

—**Quercetin,** a flavonoid in garlic, dark berries and supergreen foods like chlorella, is one of the strongest anti-cancer food agents known. Quercetin blocks cell changes that initiate cancer, and stops malignant cells from clumping together to become tumors. As an antioxidant, quercetin inhibits free radicals in the cardiovascular system and prevents free radicals from oxidizing LDL (bad cholesterol). Quercetin also controls sticky blood, a risk factor for arteriosclerosis and coronary artery disease, by preventing platelet build-up and removing excess iron in the blood.

A powerful natural antihistamine and anti-inflammatory, quercetin is one of nature's most valuable protectors against allergy attacks. It works best against allergies when a strong quercetin healing base is allowed to build up in the body.

• <u>**CAROTENOIDS,**</u> found mainly in fruits, vegetables and sea plants, are critical to any successful healing program. Carotenoids are present in virtually every cell of the human body, stored by lipoproteins in our fatty tissues. Most of us have heard of beta-carotene, but there are over 600 other carotenoids, some even more important against degenerative disease and boosting immune response. Research shows clear cancer-preventative influence from carotene-containing fruits and vegetables. New studies on carotenes like alpha-carotene, lycopene, lutein, zeaxanthin, and beta-cryptoxanthin show a 3 to 1 reduction in strokes and other heart risks when they're added to your diet.

Note: <u>**Carotenes are most effective when working together as they do in nature.**</u> Different body organs selectively store different carotenoids depending on their protective needs. There is mounting evidence that high doses of one carotenoid can result in depressed levels of other carotenoids. Excessively high supplementation of any one carotene may reduce the protective level of other carotenes. Plant carotenes, while effective in a raw foods cleansing diet, are fat-soluble, so they may be even more effective cooked for a healing diet.

New healing benefits attributed to carotenes:

1: <u>**Cataract protection**</u> -research shows that people who eat less than 3 servings of carotene-rich fruits and vegetables daily have an increased risk of developing cataracts.

2: <u>**Immune system**</u> -carotenes enhance both infection-fighting functions and immunity against tumors by increasing activity of the body's natural killer cells.

3: <u>**Heart disease protection**</u> -cardiovascular disease drops almost 50% in heart disease prone men who take beta-carotene every other day for five years.

—<u>**Lycopene,**</u> a carotene in tomatoes, red grapefruit, apricots and watermelon, protects plants from harmful UV rays. As our body's most common carotene, it protects humans in the same way. Lycopene is 56 percent more powerful than beta carotene and 100 times more efficient than vitamin E as a free radical scavenger. It is the most powerful carotene available against oxidative damage by free-radicals. Lycopene is concentrated in the prostate gland; naturopaths use it successfully as a prostate cancer preventive. Lycopene also protects against cancer of the mouth, lung, stomach, pancreas, bladder, colon and rectum. Lycopene is fat-soluble, so when lycopene-rich tomatoes are cooked with oil, as in spaghetti sauce, their bio-availability improves.

—<u>**Lutein**</u> is the most abundant carotenoid in fruits and vegetables, especially dark leafy greens like spinach, kale and broccoli, and in egg whites. Lutein is a potent antioxidant, especially concentrated in the macula of the eye, responsible for detailed vision. The macula is covered by a layer of two carotenes, lutein and zeaxanthin, natural sunscreens which selectively accumulate in the retina, where they filter out visible blue light. If blue light is allowed to reach the retina, it can cause photodamage that contributes over time to degeneration of the macula. When macular pigment becomes thin, macular degeneration is likely to develop. So, lutein and zeaxanthin help protect against photodamage to the retina, against oxidation of fatty acids in the photoreceptor membrane, and strengthen the tiny capillary blood vessels that supply the macular region.

—**Zeaxanthin,** found in dark leafy greens, broccoli and okra, is another potent antioxidant carotene, most important for its recent success against age-related macular degeneration, the leading cause of blindness in older adults. Other tests show benefits for decreased risk of lung cancer and protection against heart disease.

—**Beta carotene,** in red, yellow and dark green vegetables and fruits, and sea plants, protects against cancer, heart disease and cataracts, enhances immune response, and lowers cholesterol. Beta carotene reduces tumor cell proliferation and free-radical activity in the tumor. Even after they form, studies show tumors exposed to beta carotene are substantially smaller than tumors not exposed. Harvard studies say that beta carotene acts like a chemotherapy agent on squamous carcinoma tumor cells. Tufts University studies show that beta carotene changes into a substance called retinoic acid which can treat bladder cancer with significant success.

—**Alpha carotene,** found in apricots, carrots, peaches and yams, is even more powerful than its relative beta carotene. New alpha-carotene studies show it to be a stronger antioxidant than beta-carotene, where it is 30% more effective in inhibiting cancerous tumor formation.

—**Canthaxanthin,** a carotene found in mushrooms, long used as a natural cheese coloring, now shows that it can decrease the risk of skin cancers by inhibiting the growth of cancer cells and improving immune response.

• **PLANT POLYPHENOLS** are a form of bioflavonoids, especially active in grapes, pomegranates, raspberries, huckleberries, strawberries and green tea. Some experts credit polyphenols as the successful factors in the famous "Grape Cure" for cancer early in this century. Polyphenols inhibit the growth of cancerous tumors, and help remove carcinogens from the body. Polyphenols lower risk of heart attack by decreasing the likelihood of blood clots and cholesterol plaques.

—**Catechins,** the most abundant plant polyphenol, protects cells by breaking up free radical fat chains and preventing DNA damage from free radicals. Catechins help block carcinogens and UV rays from promoting cancer, and protect against digestive and respiratory infections.

—**Green Tea catechins** show excellent antioxidant effects, especially on fatty, oily foods. The antioxidant properties of green tea catechins are 30 times more powerful than vitamin E and 50 times more potent than those in vitamin C.

Don't miss out on these benefits from Green Tea:
- Free radical fighting capabilities of green tea strengthen immune response.
- Green tea protects against stomach and respiratory infections.
- Green tea helps block cancer promoting actions of some carcinogens and UV rays.
- Green tea helps reduce high total and LDL - cholesterol levels.
- Green tea helps block the attachment of cavity-forming bacteria to teeth.
- Green tea helps lower high blood pressure by suppressing angiotensin I enzyme.
- Green tea reduces platelet aggregation, a risk for arteriosclerosis and coronary disease.
- Green tea inhibits bacteria that cause food poisoning; helps promotes friendly bacteria.

—**Ellagic acid,** a plant phenol found in walnuts, berries, grapes, apples, tea and pomegranates, is effective as an anti-mutagen, inhibiting nicotine-induced lung tumors, and anti-carcinogen, especially for skin tumors. It shows high potential against chemically induced cancers.

• **SAPONINS** are abundant steroids in plants like beans, spinach, tomatoes, potatoes, oats, alfalfa and sea foods. They are significant in many herbs (the two most studied saponins are in panax ginseng and licorice root). Interest in saponins stems from their ability to fight infections by forming <u>disease-specific</u> antibodies. They effectively ward off microbial and fungal infections, even protect against viruses. Saponins biochemically stimulate the immune system to help the body protect itself from cancerous growths.

Saponins also lower cholesterol. Ginseng saponins for example, bind cholesterol in the gastrointestinal tract, making cholesterol unavailable for absorption by the bloodstream.

—**Glycyrrhizin,** a hormone-like saponin in licorice root, is an effective treatment for women trying to normalize menopausal hormone levels. Glycyrrhizin has anti-viral properties, especially in the treatment of HIV, where it is able to slow progression of the HIV virus by inhibiting cell infection and inducing interferon activity for immune response. Glycyrrhizin appears to deter hormone driven tumors (like those of breast cancer) by its action as a natural estrogen blocker. Glycyrrhizin encourages the production of hormones like hydrocortisone for anti-inflammatory properties. Like cortisone, but without the side effects, it can relieve arthritic and allergy symptoms, including those that accompany candida albicans yeast infections.

• **INDOLES,** like indole-3-carbinole from broccoli, cabbage, brussels sprouts, radishes, turnip or mustard greens, are natural antioxidants with tumor preventing activity.

Indole-3-carbinole also prevents cancer in two other amazing ways:

1: <u>**Indoles help the enzyme pathways through which our bodies get rid of carcinogens**</u>. Indole-3-carbinol changes the metabolism of carcinogenic toxins by producing phase 1 and phase 2 detoxification enzymes that make the toxins water soluble. But since oil and water don't mix, <u>water soluble</u> toxins can't be stored in fatty body tissues, so your body rids itself of them more easily, reducing the risk of cancer. The same detox enzymes produced by indole-3-carbinole also reduce the ability of certain carcinogenic material to bind with our DNA. When the material cannot attach to DNA, cancer can't get started. Nature is always amazing.

2: <u>**Indoles improve estrogen metabolism and our ability to eliminate excess estrogens**</u>, especially from exogenous estrogen sources like pesticides and synthetic hormones. Women who eat plenty of vegetables containing indole-3-carbinole lower their risk of breast cancer. Men who eat plenty of vegetables containing indole-3-carbinole have a substantially lower risk of colon cancer compared to men who eat little or none.

<u>**The benefits of indole-3-carbinol don't stop at cancer prevention.**</u>

—Vegetables that contain indole-3-carbinol can dramatically lower bad cholesterol, low density and very low density lipoproteins. In one of Nature's miracle pathways, the <u>by-products</u> formed when indole-3-carbinol reacts with stomach acids are more bio-active than indole-3-carbinol itself. It is the by-products that help clear the body of harmful cholesterol.

—Indole-3-carbinol shows dramatic results in a viral disease called recurring respiratory laryngyl papillomatosis (RRPL), which causes warts on the vocal chords. Symptoms range from hoarseness to complete stoppage of the airway. Suffering is often severe. Laser surgery can remove the warts, but they reappear if the virus remains active. Substantial doses of indole-3-carbinol impede or stop the growth of the warts.

—Recent studies show that indole-3-carbinol also alleviates many symptoms of fibromyalgia and similar symptoms in chronic fatigue syndrome.

• **ISOPRENOIDS** are active, fat soluble antioxidants that neutralize free radicals in a unique way. They anchor themselves to fatty membranes with a long carbon side chain. Free radicals trying to attach to the membranes are quickly grabbed and passed to other antioxidants.

—**Vitamin E,** from almonds, wheat germ, wheat germ oil, leafy veggies, salmon, soy foods and organ meats, is an antioxidant isoprenoid. There's clear correlation between vitamin E, a lower risk of heart disease and Alzheimer's, and better body balance for women during menopause or menstrual difficulties. I believe the best vitamin E comes from dietary sources - foods and herbs. Many doctors say synthetic vitamin E may increase hemorrhaging during surgery; they don't recommend it for a pre-op or post-op nutritional program. I have found this not to be a problem for dietary vitamin E, which is safe before and after surgery.

—**CoQ-10,** an isoprenoid also known as ubiquinone or ubiquinol, is available mainly through protein sources like fish, meats, sea vegetables and some of the green superfoods. CoQ-10 is an extremely important antioxidant enzyme that does a lot more than just protect us from free radical damage. It's part of our cell energy process, and actually targets particular diseases with its powerful brand of enzyme therapy. CoQ-10 is highly successful against heart disease, gum disease, ulcers, even effective against some AIDS-related diseases.

But the benefits don't stop there. CoQ-10 also:
—Strengthens your entire cardiovascular system against coronary artery disease, especially if you have had a previous heart attack. (I often recommend CoQ-10 to someone who might be planning a heart operation as a fortifying antioxidant.)
—Helps strengthen the heart muscle when there is mitral valve prolapse
—Helps lower high cholesterol levels
—Helps lower high blood pressure, reduces hypertension and overcomes fatigue
—Helps lower the risk of breast and prostate cancers; some studies show, and I have seen myself, that it can even reduce the rate of growth once the cancer has begun.
(For more about CoQ-10, see ENZYMES AND ENZYME THERAPY, page 31.)

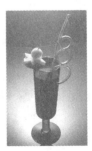

Don't forget fruit and vegetable juices. They offer quick absorption of protective antioxidants. Juices provide nutrition in the most easily digestible form for a healing diet. **See a complete discussion of fresh fruits, vegetables and juices on page 20-21.**

Chlorophyll is a Primary Key to Healing from Green Vegetables

Green foods are power plants for humans. Our best body chemistry comes from plant nutrients because plant chlorophyll (one of the most powerful nutrients on earth) transmits the energies of the sun and soil to our bodies. Eating plants is the most direct method of conserving the energy we receive from the sun, the earth's energy source. Fruits, vegetables, grains and grasses reach out to us on branches and stems, making themselves beautiful to attract us. Plants have no fear of being eaten as animals do. Plant energy simply transmutes into our human life form.

Chlorophyll offers amazing health benefits for humans:

The most therapeutic element of green foods is chlorophyll, the basic "blood" component of plants. Chlorophyll is the pigment that plants use to carry out the process of photosynthesis, absorbing light energy from the sun and converting it into plant energy. This energy is transferred into our cells and blood when we consume fresh greens. Chlorophyll is in all green plants, but is especially rich in green and blue-green algae, wheat grass, barley grass, parsley and alfalfa.

—**Chlorophyll has a unique affinity to our blood**. The chlorophyll molecule is remarkably similar to human hemoglobin in composition, except that it carries magnesium in its center instead of iron. Eating chlorophyll-rich foods helps our bodies build oxygen-carrying red blood cells. To me, eating green foods is almost like giving yourself a little transfusion to help treat illness and enhance immunity.

—**Chlorophyll is a better tonic than Geritol for tired blood**. It calms the nerves, so it's helpful for insomnia, exhaustion and nervous irritability. It's beneficial for skin disorders, helps you cope with deep infections, and dental problems like pyorrhea. Its anti-bacterial qualities are a proven remedy for colds, ear infections and chest inflammation.

—**Chlorophyll detoxifies your liver**. It helps neutralize and remove drug deposits and purifies the blood. Even the medical community sees chlorophyll as a means of removing heavy metal buildup, because it can bind with heavy metals to help remove them. A U.S. Army study reveals that a chlorophyll-rich diet doubles the lifespan of animals exposed to radiation. Chlorophyll is even being considered as protection against some chemical warfare weapons.

—**Chlorophyll is rich in vitamin K, necessary for blood clotting**. Naturopathic physicians use chlorophyll for women with heavy menstrual bleeding and anemia. Vitamin K helps form a compound in urine that inhibits growth of calcium oxalate crystals, so chlorophyll helps with kidney stones. Vitamin K also enhances adrenal activity, so chlorophyll-rich foods help maintain steroid hormone balance for a more youthful body.

Experience is a hard
teacher. She gives
the test first and the
lessons afterwards.

Plant Enzymes Offer Built-In Enzyme Therapy

Enzymes are the cornerstone of healing because they are the foundation elements of the immune system, providing active antioxidants that fight free-radical destruction.

Enzymes operate on both chemical and biological levels. Chemically, they are the workhorses that drive metabolism to use the nutrients we take in. Biologically, they are our life energy. Without enzyme energy, we would be a pile of lifeless chemicals.

Each of us is born with a battery charge of enzyme energy. As we age our internal enzyme stores are naturally depleted. A 60 year old has 50% fewer enzymes than a 30 year old. Enzyme depletion, lack of energy, disease and aging all go hand in hand. Unless we stop the one-way-flow out of the body of enzyme energy, our digestive-eliminative capacities weaken, obesity and chronic illness set in, lifespan shortens. The faster you use up your enzyme supply - the shorter your life. The first signs of low enzymes are fatigue, premature aging and weight gain.

Do you have enough enzymes?

Nature has designed an interlocking digestive system for us. Most nutrient deficiencies result not from a lack of the nutrients themselves, but from our lack of enzymes to absorb them.

When our foods don't have enough enzymes for us to digest them, enzymes reserved for metabolic processes get pulled from their normal work to digest food. Pancreas and liver enzymes are called in, too. But these substitute measures don't make up for the missing food enzymes because we still need those enzymes to break down and actually deliver the nutrients.

It doesn't stop there. Low enzymes mean we end up with undigested food in our blood. So, white blood cell immune defenses are pulled from their jobs to take care of the undigested food, and the immune system takes a dive, setting up a perfect environment for disease.

Enzyme-rich foods take care of this unhealthy cascade of reactions before it ever starts. Fresh foods have the most plant enzymes. When you eat more fresh foods, you add to your enzymatic activity. If you don't get enough fresh foods, or you need extra enzymes for healing, plant-based enzyme supplements are the next best choice, especially from herbs and superfoods. **If you can't make them, take them.**

How does enzyme therapy work to heal?

Enzyme therapy uses metabolic enzymes to stimulate immune response through lymphocytes, or white blood cells. Immune organs, like the thymus and lymph nodes keep a constant level of white blood cells circulating through the body to attack foreign invader cells. When toxins are detected, white blood cells attack them, digesting them by secreting enzymes on their surfaces. Some diseases, like cancer, leukemia, anemia and heart disease can even be diagnosed by measuring the amount and activity of certain enzymes in the blood and body fluids.

Proteolytic enzymes may be used as anti-inflammatories for injuries like sprains and strains, for respiratory problems to allow vessels to unclog, for degenerative diseases, and for recovery healing from surgery by reducing swelling and pain. Bromelain from pineapples is a good example of a rapid recovery proteolytic enzyme to use for these things.

Enzymes clean wounds, dissolve blood clots, and control allergic reactions to drugs. Enzyme therapy is most helpful for heart disease, tumors, skin problems, low and high blood sugar, stomach and colon pain, eye diseases and headaches.

There are three categories of enzymes:

1: Metabolic enzymes repair cells and stimulate enzymatic activity. Proteolytic enzymes (proteases), are metabolic enzymes that help us heal faster by reducing inflammation, and breaking up debris in the injured area. They stimulate without repressing immune response (unlike cortisone or hydro- cortisone drugs). *Note: How you take enzymes is important. Taking enzyme supplements between meals without food, allows them to absorb directly into your body and function as metabolic enzymes in the repair and healing process.*

2: Human digestive enzymes assimilate our food nutrients. In fact, digestive enzymes are stronger than any other enzymes in human beings, and more concentrated than any other enzyme combination in nature. A very good thing, since our processed, overcooked, nutrient-poor diets demand a great deal of enzymatic work!

3: Fresh plant enzymes start food digestion, and aid our own digestive enzymes. All foods contain the enzymes required to digest them. The best food sources of plant enzymes for humans are bananas, mangos, sprouts, papayas, avocados and pineapples.

What about Co-enzyme Q_{10}?

Co-enzymes work as catalysts in biochemical reactions. I call CoQ_{10} the "holistic enzyme," because it's found in every cell, especially the heart, brain, liver and kidneys. All live foods contain a form of Co-enzyme Q_1 to Q_{10}.

CoQ_{10} is one of the most powerful antioxidants known. It boosts immune response and cardiac strength, reverses high blood pressure, promotes weight loss, slows aging, and heals gum disease. Specific CoQ_{10} enzyme therapy treatments include congestive heart failure, angina, ischemic heart disease, cardio-myopathy, mitral valve prolapse, diabetes, tumors and candidiasis. CoQ_{10} can alleviate toxic effects of drugs commonly used to treat cancer and hypertension.

Like other anti-oxidant co-enzymes, glutathione peroxidase, and superoxide dismutase, (SOD) for example, CoQ_{10} scavenges and neutralizes free radicals by turning them into stable oxygen and H_2O_2, and then into oxygen and water.

How much CoQ_{10} should you take? As little as 30mg a day of CoQ_{10} is an effective dose. Some cancer patients take up to 400mg a day. CoQ_{10} is a fat soluble nutrient, so your body assimilates it better if taken in conjunction with fatty acids like Omega-3 oils or evening primrose oil. CoQ_{10} is only effective as long as it is taken; once discontinued, the illness may return. This is especially true in cancer treatment. After 35, the ability to synthesize CoQ_{10} declines. Take $CoQ_{10,}$ for one to three months to saturate deficient tissues.

What reduces healthy CoQ_{10} levels? An overactive thyroid, aging, some cholesterol lowering drugs, some antidepressants and beta blockers.

Can we maximize daily enzyme benefits?

Enzymes are extremely sensitive to heat. Heat above 120° F. completely destroys them. Even low degrees of heat greatly reduce digestive ability. Enzymes are also affected by tobacco, alcohol, caffeine, fluorides, chlorine in drinking water, air pollution, chemical additives and many drugs. Enzyme protection and enzyme therapy are dramatically reduced by the use of a microwave oven.

Is a Vegetarian Diet Better?

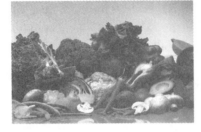

Vegetarian eating today is a social expression by a newly conscious, planet-saving community of people that sees itself as the first world-wide culture to try and understand the Earth and it's inhabitants as equal players in a greater whole. It is seen as a practice of enlightenment, of increased understanding, of responsibility for mankind's place on the Earth, perhaps even of higher consciousness.

The horrors on our daily news make us shrink from violence. Killing should be reserved for our "enemies." But as our world grows smaller, and we see people just like us everywhere, who is our enemy? Certainly not the Earth's animals. Even our view of our ancient ancestors is changing as our view of ourselves changes. The stereotype of early humans as "Man the hunter" is now more accurately seen as "Man the gatherer" rather than hunter.

Today's vegetarian culture is not the first. Vegetarianism was widely practiced by the ancient Greeks. Pythagoras was a vegetarian. He and many others believed that both animals and humans had souls, that all souls had equal worth, and that after death, animals might be reincarnated as humans and vice versa. Plato, in *The Republic*, depicts a vegetarian diet as ideal for an ideal society, because plant foods promote health and require less land to produce than animal foods.

The Romans included vegetarianism in the ideas they borrowed from the Greeks. But, the fall of Rome and the spread of other cultures across Europe led to "dark ages" in vegetarian thought as it did in the arts. From medieval times on, intellectual rationale dominated western thought. Animals were killed, eaten, and exploited under the argument that animals were placed on earth for the convenience and use of humans.

After the Roman Empire, vegetarianism was lost to the Dark Ages in Europe for over 1500 years. Leonardo da Vinci stood almost alone as a confirmed vegetarian, predicting accurately that "the time would come when men would look upon the murder of animals as they look upon the murder of men." The Christian abbeys however, kept vegetarian diet principles alive. The powerful monastic orders of the Benedictines, Trappists and Cistercians all abstained from eating meat to suppress animal passions that hindered spiritual progress.

Darwin began the vegetarian "renaissance" of the late 18th and 19th centuries. His theory of evolution challenged the justification for eating animals. He believed that humans and other animals were part of a continuum of life, only separated in degree, not in kind.

What is a vegetarian?

It's a legitimate question. When we try to apply different social foundations and ideas from around the world to vegetarianism, an easy definition becomes incredibly confusing. Food and diet are inextricably intertwined in both the religion and culture to which they belong. So different kinds of foods are seen differently by different peoples. Beyond religion or culture, people choose a vegetarian diet for animal welfare, environmental ecology, finances and personal health.

<u>**Here are the ways vegetarians are classified today.**</u>
- Semi vegetarian: eats poultry, fish, eggs and dairy foods, but not red meats or pork
- Pesco vegetarian: eats fish, eggs and dairy foods, but not poultry, red meats or pork
- Lacto ovo vegetarian: eats eggs and dairy foods, but no animal food that "has eyes"
- Ovo vegetarian: eats eggs, but no other animal food product
- Vegan: excludes all animal derived foods.

<u>What are the benefits of a vegetarian diet?</u>

Becoming a vegetarian has long term effects on both body and mind. As their diet changes, people find their point of view about life changes, too. Nutrition awareness and knowledge about foods increases. Most vegetarians support a "green" lifestyle as their consciousness of animal welfare and environmental issues heightens.

Further:

—A vegetarian diet is low fat, so it's heart smart. Vegetarians have a well documented history of lower risk for high blood pressure, heartburn, obesity, diabetes, osteoporosis, even cancer.

—Most vegetarians are energetic. Energy comes from carbohydrates and fats, which abound in the natural starches and oils of grains, legumes, fruits and vegetables. Energy also comes from vitamins, minerals, and amino acids, plentiful in plant foods.

—Vegetarians report better body balance, especially in terms of their protein intake. Vegetable protein abounds in whole grains, legumes like soy foods, beans and lentils, potatoes, green vegetables, nuts and seeds, pasta, and corn.

—Vegetarians are better hydrated from the high water content of fresh foods.

—Being a vegetarian is easy on your pocket book. It takes only a fraction of the land, water and money to grow fruits, vegetables and grains than to produce animal crops.

<u>**Make the transition easy.**</u> Some new vegetarians say they lack knowledge of vegetarian cooking and familiarity with many of its non-traditional foods. I say this "drawback" is a new adventure in eating. Vegetarian cuisine is incredibly diverse and interesting. Get a new cookbook or two and tantalize your taste buds!

<u>**Does it take long to become a vegetarian if you've been a lifelong meat-eater?**</u> Transition time varies widely. Only 30% of newly converted vegetarians stop eating meat immediately; 70% eliminate meat from their diets over months or even years.

<u>**Do vegetarians still crave meat?**</u> Almost half of new vegetarians experience cravings for meat. Women are as likely as men to report meat cravings as men. Ethical vegetarians are as likely as health vegetarians to crave meat (it is easier to change our minds than to change our taste buds).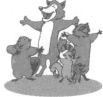

If you eat no animal foods at all, you need to be more aware of nutrients and their sources. Vitamin B-12 is at the center of the vegetarian diet debate. B-12 is responsible for the growth and repair of body cells. A deficiency can take a long time to notice and can cause serious health problems. The most reliable dietary sources are meat, eggs and dairy foods. Pay special attention to your protein, calcum, iron and zinc intake.

<u>Non-animal sources of hard-to-find nutrients in the vegetarian diet:</u>
—Vitamin B-12 is in sea vegetables, soy foods, cereals and supergreens like chlorella, spirulina and barley grass.
—Vitamin D is in sea greens, soy foods and sunshine.
—Calcium is in root vegetables, broccoli, nuts and seeds, leafy greens, legumes like peas and beans, soy foods, whole grains, and supergreens like chlorella and spirulina.
—Iron is in legumes, soy foods, leafy greens, dried fruit, whole grain breads and cereals. Iron absorption is enhanced by vitamin C (citrus fruits, tomatoes, strawberries, broccoli, peppers, sea greens, leafy vegetables, and potatoes with skins).
—Zinc is in whole grains, legumes, seeds, nuts, sea vegetables and soy foods.

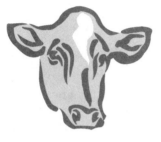

What's the Truth about Red Meat?

I believe eating red meats puts us a step away from environmental harmony. Animals are closer to us on the bio-scale of life. They experience fear when killed. They don't want to be eaten. When we eat plants, there is an uplifting transmutation of energy. The human digestive system is not easily carnivorous. Our bodies have to struggle to use red meat energy. When we eat red meats our bodies become denser, with more internal fermentation and body odor. Eating red meat is a lot like extracting oil out of the ground; it may cost more to get the oil out than it's worth on the market. Meat protein, which the body can use, is often cancelled out by lengthy digestion time and after-dinner lethargy, because a disproportionate amount of energy goes to the task of assimilation. Heavy red meat eaters have far more kidney stones, caused by toxicity from an overload of unused nitrogens from the highly concentrated proteins in red meat.

Further, most red meat available today are shot through with hormones and slow-release antibiotics (stockyard animals are often sick and over-medicated), and preserved with nitrates or nitrites. These substances are passed into us at the dinner table.

On the health side, red meat is our biggest diet contributor to excess protein and saturated fat levels. No one argues that less dietary fat is healthier, or that saturated fats are the most harmful. Even the livestock industry has made some changes. Beef now has 27%, and pork 43% less trimmable fat than supermarket cuts sold in the 1970s and 1980s. (There's still a lot of saturated fat in the meat marbling, however.)

When red meat is cooked all the way to well-done or charred on a BBQ grill, carcinogenic chemical compounds are created that are capable of causing many diseases.

Finally, meat eating promotes more aggressive, arrogant behavior - a lack of gentleness in personality. From a spiritual point of view, red meat eating encourages ties to life's material things, expansion of territory, and the self-righteous intolerance that makes adversaries.

Most of us eat more meat than we really need. A 100 gram serving of meat is the size of a deck of cards, smaller than your computer mouse. A small can of salmon or tuna is two servings. Half a chicken breast or a small hamburger patty is one serving. A small boneless roast weighing a kilogram (just over 2 pounds) provides 10 servings.

About Red Meat and A Healing Diet

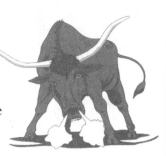

Recent scientific studies find that eating red meat increases the risk of degenerative diseases like heart disease, stroke and cancer. The American Heart Association, American Cancer Society, National Academy of Sciences, and American Academy of Pediatrics are just a few of the medical and scientific organizations recommending less red meat and other animal foods, and a shift to a more vegetarian diet.

Here's why I don't believe red meat should be part of a healing diet:

—Health implications begin when meat is killed because it immediately starts to decompose. Although salt preservation and refrigeration retard spoilage, even slight putrefaction produces toxins and amines that accumulate in your liver, kidneys, and intestines, destroy friendly bacteria cultures (especially those that synthesize B vitamins), and degrade small intestine villi where food is absorbed into the blood. Saturated fats from animal foods accumulate around organs and blood vessels, leading to cysts, tumors, cholesterol build-up and clogged arteries. Experts say that too much meat protein may **overstimulate** immune response, resulting in immune tolerance.

—Meat is significantly harder to digest than plant foods, taking over 4 hours to be absorbed in the intestines versus 2 to 2 $\frac{1}{2}$ hours for grains and vegetables.

—Beef contains the highest concentration of herbicides of any food in America. The National Research Council (NRC) of the National Academy of Sciences cites **pesticide-tainted beef as nearly 11 percent of the total cancer risk to consumers from pesticides.** Eighty percent of all herbicides used in the U.S. are sprayed on corn and soybeans, used primarily as feed for cattle. The chemicals accumulate in the cattle and are passed onto consumers in finished cuts of beef.

There's even more recent bad news about red meat.

1) Tainted meats are becoming so widespread in America, the FDA has approved irradiation of red meat to destroy deadly bacteria like e-coli. Proponents of the move say that for a few cents a pound, hamburger or sausage can be zapped with radiation that kills pathogens by altering the genetic makeup of the harmful bacteria.

The problem? Irradiated meat is exposed to the equivalent of 10 to 70 million chest X-rays, and there are no long term studies to prove that food irradiation is safe. Benzene, a potent carcinogen, is created when red meat is exposed to irradiation. Just one molecule of benzene absorbed into the body is enough to cause cancer.

2) More than 95 percent of all feedlot-raised cattle in the U.S. currently receive growth hormones, antibiotics or other drugs; residues are usually present in finished cuts of beef. In order to speed weight gain and time-to-market, cattle hormone levels are increased two to five times with anabolic steroids. Time-released synthetic estradiol, testosterone and progesterone slowly seep into the animal's blood. These hormones then become part of the hormone assault on people, now implicated in increased cancer risk and other hormone-driven diseases.

In 1992, more than 15 million pounds of antibiotics were given to U.S. livestock to fight diseases which were running rampant in cramped feedlots and contaminated pens. Today, the beef industry says it has discontinued automatic use of antibiotics in beef cattle, but still give antibiotics to dairy cows, which account for 15% of the beef eaten in the America. Antibiotic residues still show up in our meat with virulent strains of disease-causing bacteria.

Veal calves become so sick in their tiny pens that antibiotics are routinely used to keep them alive until slaughter. Contrary to veal industry claims, no drugs have been approved by the U.S. FDA for formula-fed veal calves. Some of the drugs used routinely, like sulfamethazine, are carcinogenic and residues may be present in consumer veal.

3) Since 1985, the National Academy of Sciences has reported that federal meat inspections are inadequate to protect the public from meat-borne diseases. Recommended corrective steps were never adopted; instead, an inspection system to increase online meat production by 40 percent was developed. It virtually eliminated the federal meat inspector and placed responsibility for carcass inspection on packing house employees. Under the system, thousands of carcasses pass through inspection with pneumonia, measles, peritonitis, abcesses, fecal or insect contamination, and contaminated heads (called "puke heads"), on their way to American dinner tables.

4) There appears to be a new link between cattle diseases and disease in humans. Bovine leukemia virus (BLV), an insect-borne retrovirus that causes malignancy in cattle, is found in 20% of cattle and 60% of U.S. herds. BLV antibodies have been found in leukemia patients.
Bovine immunodeficiency virus (BIV), widespread in American cattle herds since the 1980s, genetically resembles the human HIV virus, and like HIV in humans, appears to suppress the immune systems in cattle, making them susceptible to a wide range of infections. At least one study suggests that BIV "plays a role in either malignant or slow viruses in humans."

We've seen the down side of a meat-based diet, especially for a healing diet. Are there enough benefits in red meat to add it back to your diet after healing?

—Red meat has complete protein and all the amino acids. In order to build human protein, we need 22 amino acids. Our bodies make amino acids, except for the eight essential amino acids that can only be obtained from our foods. Plant proteins contain some amino acids, but no plant on its own has enough of the essential amino acids.
Can vegetarians get enough amino acids for protein building? Plant protein combinations are good choices - like beans with rice or corn; tofu with whole grains; and legumes like peanuts and beans with whole wheat or corn. Bee pollen and sea plants contain all the amino acids and are considered complete foods by many vegetarians.

—Red meat is the best source of food iron. Hemoglobin, the plasma of red blood formation, is part of red meat tissue, and delivers from 2 to 10 times more iron than any other source. Yet research shows that body absorption of red meat iron may not be very efficient, because vegetarians have almost the same levels of iron in their blood as people who eat meat daily.
Can vegetarians get enough absorbable iron? Legumes, whole grains, nuts, spinach, clams, asparagus, poultry, prunes, raisins, pumpkin seeds, beets and soy foods all provide easy-to-use iron. Food sources of iron are better absorbed than most iron supplements which are often constipating, especially for children and pregnant women. Herbal source iron is best in combinations that include *yellow dock root, dandelion, alfalfa, sea plants* and *nettles.*
—Red meat is a good source of zinc needed for growth and immunity.
Can vegetarians get enough zinc for proper growth? Food sources include chicken, seafood, whole wheat and wheat germ, lima beans, legumes, nuts, milk, and eggs.

—Red meat is a good source of B vitamins like riboflavin, thiamine and niacin. B vitamins help muscles use food energy, so it's not surprising that animal muscle is a good source.

Do vegetarians get enough B vitamins? Whole grains are important sources of B vitamins. But how about vitamin B-12? Its role is essential for our body cell growth, particularly for new red blood cells. **Can vegetarians get B-12 from their diet?** Sea greens, bee pollen and royal jelly are the best non-meat sources of vitamin B-12. If you aren't including these foods in your vegetarian diet, take a vitamin B-12 supplement.

Note: If you decide to include red meat in your diet, consider ostrich meat as a healthier red meat in America. Ostrich meat tastes, looks and feels like beef. It is comparable to beef in iron and protein content. But ostrich meat has less than half the fat of chicken and two-thirds less fat and calories than beef and pork.

Realities of the 2000's

"The diet of North Americans has changed significantly since 1900, when most meals were based on whole grain products, potatoes, fresh seasonal vegetables and fruits - with meats consumed only occasionally. In recent years we have replaced this way of eating, rich in complex carbohydrates and fiber, low in fats and cholesterol, with a high-fat, low-fiber diet - largely based on meats and pasteurized dairy foods. By the 1980s, consumption of grains and potatoes had fallen to half of their 1900 levels, while the amount of fats has more than doubled. Such drastic dietary changes cannot occur without significant consequences - for public health, the economy, and the environment." –*John Robbins, author of The Food Revolution.*

- *Number of underfed and malnourished people in the world:* 1.2 billion
    Children in Bangaladesh who are so underfed and underweight that their health is diminished: 56 percent
- *Number of overfed and overweight people in the world:* 1.2 billion
    Adults in the United States who are so overfed and overweight that their health is diminished: 55 percent.
- *Shared by the hungry and the overweight:* high levels of sickness, shorter life expectancy, low productivity.
- *Cattle alive today on the Earth:* More than 1 billion.
- *Weight of the world's cattle compared to weight of the world's people:* Almost double.
- *Area of Earth's land mass used as pasture for cattle and other livestock:* One-half.
- *Grassland needed to support one cow under optimal conditions:* 2.5 acres.
- *Grassland needed to support one cow under far more common marginal conditions:* 50 acres.
- *U.S. farmland producing vegetables:* 4 million acres.
- *U.S. farmland producing hay for livestack:* 56 million acres.
- *U.S. grain and cereals fed to livestack:* 70%.
- *Human beings who could be fed by the grain and soybeans eaten by U.S. livestock:* over 1,400,000,000.
- *Number of people whose food energy needs can be met by the food produced on 2.5 acres of land:*
    If the land is producing cabbage: 23 people.
    If the land is producing potatoes: 22 people.
    If the land is producing rice: 19 people.
- *If the land is producing corn:* 17 people.
- *If the land is producing wheat:* 15 pople.
- *If the land is producing chicken:* 2 people.
- *If the land is producing milk:* 2 people.
- *If the land is producing beef:* 1 person.

- *World's population living in the United States:* 4%.
- *World's beef eaten in the United States:* 23%.
- *Grain needed to adequately feed every person on the planet who dies of hunger and hunger disease:* 12 million tons.
- *Amount Ameicans would have to reduce their beef consumption to save 12 million tons of grain:* 10%.

• • • • •

- *Gallons of oil spilled by the Exxon Valdez:* 12 million.
- *Gallons of excrement spilled into the New River in N.C. when an 8-acre "lagoon" of hog waste burst:* 25 million.
- *Fish killed as an immediate result:* 10-14 million
- *Fish breeding area decimated by this disaster:* Half of all mid-east coast fish species.
- *Acres of coastal wetlands closed to shell fishing as a result:* 364,000.
- *Amount of waste N.C.'s 7-million factory-raised hogs produce compared to the state's 6.5 million people:* 4 to 1
- *Concentration of pathogens in hog waste compared to human sewage:* 10 to 100 times greater.

• • • • •

- *Leading cause of food-borne illness in the United States:* Campylobacter.
- *Americans who become ill with Campylobacter poisoning every day:* 5,000.
- *Campylobacter-related fatalities annually in the U.S.:* more than 750.
- *Primary source of Campylobacter bacteria:* Contaminated poultry meat.
- *American chickens sufficiently contaminated with Campylobacter to cause illness:* 70 percent.
- *American turkeys sufficiently contaminated with Campylobacter to cause illness:* 90 percent.
- *Number of hens screened in 3 separate flocks for Campylobacter by U. of Wisconsin researchers:* 2,300.
- *Number of screeened hens that were not infected with Campylobacter:* 8.
- *Chickens infected with Campylobacter in the U.S.:* 70 percent compared to Norway (10%).
- *Annual Salmonella cases in the U.S.:* more than a million compared to Sweden (800).
- *Americans sickened from eating Salmonella-tainted eggs every year* 650,000.
- *Increase in Salmonella poisoning from raw or uncooked eggs:* 600 percent.

• • • • •

- *Death rate from breast cancer in the U.S.* 22.4 per 100,000.
- *Death rate for breast cancer in Japan:* 6.3 per 100,000.
- *Death rate for breast cancer in China::* 4.6 per 100,000.
- *Primary reasons for difference:* Asians eat more vegetables, less animal foods, weigh less, get more exercise.
- *Breast cancer rate for meat eating Japanese women compared to vegetarian Japanese women:* 8.5 times greater.
- *Impact on breast cancer for U.S. women who are 45 pounds overweight:* double.

• • • • •

- *Risk of colon cancer for women who eat red meat daily compared to those who eat it once a month:* 250% more.
- *Risk of colon cancer for people who eat red meat once a week compared to those who abstain:* 38% greater.
- *Risk of colon cancer for people who eat poultry 4 times a week compared to those who abstain:* 200% greater.
- *Risk of colon cancer for people who eat peas, lentils and beans twice a week compared to peole who don't:* 50% lower.
- *Impact on colon cancer risk when diets are rich in the B-vitamin folic acid:* 75% lower.
- *Primary food sources of folic acid:* Green leafy vegetables, peas and beans.

• • • • •

- *Drop in heart disease risk for every 1 percent decrease in blood cholesterol:* 3 to 4 percent
- *Blood cholesterol levels of vegetarians compared to non-vegetarians:* 14 perent lower.
- *Risk of death by heart disease for vegetarians compared to non-vegetarians* half.
- *Cholesterol intake of non-vegetarians:* 300-500milligrams/day.
- *Cholesterol intake of lacto-ovo-vegetarians:* 150-300milligrams/day.
- *Cholesterol intake of vegans:* zero.
- *Average cholesterol level of people eating a meat-centered diet:* 210.
- *Average cholesterol level of U.S.vegetarians:* 161.

• • • • •

- *Antibiotics allowed in U.S. cow's milk:* 80.
- *Antibiotics found in soy milk:* none

- *Children with chronic constipation so intractable that it can't be treated by laxatives, but who are cured by switching from cow's milk to soy milk:* 44 percent.
- *Countries with highest consumption of dairy products:* Finland, Sweden, United States, England.
- *Countries with highest rates of osteoporosis:* Finland, Sweden, United States, England
- *Foods that produce the most calcium loss through urinary excretion:* Animal protein and coffee.
- *Amount of calcium lost in the urine after eating a hamburger:* 28 milligrams.
- *Amount of calcium lost in the urine after drinking a cup of coffee:* 2 milligrams.
- *Avergae calcium absorption rates of green leafy vegetavbles:* 56% compared to cow's miilk 32%.

• • • • •

- *Water required to produce 1-lb. of U.S. beef according to the National Cattleman's Beef Association:* 441 gallons.
- *Water required to produce 1-lb. of U.S. beef according to the Ag College of Michigan State Univ.:* 2,500 gallons.
- *Water required to produce 1-lb. of other foods according to the UC Ag Extension department of livestock advisors:*
  For 1-lb. tomatoes: 23 gallons.
  For 1-lb. lettuce: 23 gallons.
  For 1-lb. wheat: 25 gallons.
  For 1-lb. carrots: 33 gallons.
  For 1-lb. apples: 49 gallons.
  For 1-lb. chicken: 815 gallons.
  For 1-lb. pork: 1,630 gallons.
  For 1-lb. beef: 5,214 gallons.

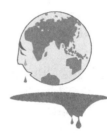

• • • • •

- *Number of species of birds in one square mile of Amazon Rainforest:* more than exist in all of North America.
- *Life forms destroyed producing each fast food hamburger made from rainforest beef:* 20 to 30 different plant species, 100 different insect species, dozens of bird, mammal and reptile species.
- *Length of time before all 280 million acres of Indonesian forests would be completely gone if they were cleared to produce as much beef for Indonesians, per person, to eat as Americans do:* 3.5 years.
- *Length of time before all 280 million acres of Costa Rica forests would be completely gone if they were cleared to produce as much beef for Costa Ricans, per person, to eat as Americans do:* 1 year.
- *Cost of a hamburger produced by clearing forests in India if real costs were included rather than subsidized:* $200.
- *Earth's mammal species curently threatened with extinction:* 25%.
- *Leasding cause of species extinction in tropical rainforests:* Livestock grazing.
- *Leading cause of species being threatened or eliminated in the U.S.:* Livestock grazing.

• • • • •

- *Calories of fossil fuel used to produce 1 calorie of protein from soybeans:* 2.
- *Calories of fossil fuel used to produce 1 calorie of protein from corn and wheat:* 3.
- *Calories of fossil fuel used to produce 1 calorie of protein from beef:* 78.
- *Amount of greenhouse carbon gas released by a typical American car in one day:* 1 kilogram.
- *Amount released by clearing and burning enough Costa Rican rainforest to produce beef for 1 hamburger:* 75 kilograms.

• • • • •

- *Number of cows and calves slaughtered every 24 hours in the United States:* 90,000.
- *Number of chickens slaughtered every minute in the United States:* 14,000.
- *Food Animals not counting ocean animals slaughtered every year in the U. S.:* 10 billion.
- *Only entities producing more chicken than Tyson Foods:* The countries of China and Brazil.
- *Year John Robbins' Diet For A New America was published with its exposé of veal calf treatment:* 1987.
- *Years Humane Farming Association launched anti-veal campaign:* 1986 and 1987.
- *Veal calves raised in the Unites States in 1987:* 3.2 million.
- *Veal calves raised in the Unites States in 1999:* 1.2 million.

• • • • •

Quoted with permission from John Robbins' new book, *The Food Revolution*. Avoiding red meats, and conserving precious water and energy resources wasted by an animal-based diet may be one of the most important things you can do for your own health and that of the planet.

Protein: How Much do you Need?

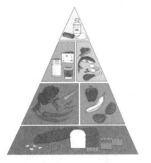

You must have protein to heal. Next to water, protein is the body's most plentiful substance, the primary source of building material for muscles, blood, skin, hair, nails, and organs like the heart and brain. All body tissues depend on protein. Blood can't clot without protein. Protein and its precursors, amino acids, work at hormonal levels to control elemental body functions like growth, sexual development and metabolism. The most basic enzymes, those for immune function and antibody response, are formed from protein.

We've seen the advantages of a vegetarian diet, and the problems with a meat-based diet on the preceeding pages. The heart of the debate is protein.

<u>**How much protein do you really need?**</u> People are so individual that experts can't agree on how much protein is best. Protein requirements differ according to your health, body size and activity level. The official RDA for adult men and women is 0.8g for each kg of body weight per day, about 55 grams of protein for 150 pound person. *American Journal of Clinical Nutrition* says adults need 2.5% of calorie intake in protein. The World Health Organization sets adult protein needs at 4.5% of calorie intake. The National Acadamy of Sciences recommends 6%. The National Research Council says 8%. The FDA says protein should make up 10% of your total daily calories.

The rule of thumb is to divide your body weight by 2; the result is the approximate number of grams of protein you need each day. An easy way to translate protein grams into your diet is to eat an amount of protein food that covers the palm of your hand at each meal; vegetarians should double the amount to two palmfuls. A 2,000-calorie diet allows for 50 grams of protein. America's average consumption of protein is about 90 grams daily.

The human body cannot make protein, it must be obtained through diet. But since protein is available from a wide range of foods, usually only people with severe malnutrition are protein deficient. The protein deficiency health threat is over-stated in wealthy countries. The only people who <u>might</u> have trouble getting enough protein are vegans who eat <u>no</u> animal foods. Eating protein-rich plant foods like lentils, tofu, nuts, peas, seeds and grains as healthy people do in less industrialized countries, should provide plenty of protein. Signs that you might be protein deficient are low stamina, mental depression, low resistance to infection and slow wound healing. (In children, extremely low protein means higher disease risk, stunted mental and physical growth, and inflamed joints.) Surgery, wounds, or prolonged illness use up protein stores fast. At times of high stress, you may want to take in extra protein to rebuild worn-out tissues.

<u>**For Americans, the problem is normally too much protein.**</u>
Experts say that Americans eat too much protein for good health. Unlike carnivorous animals, whose body systems are adapted to a meat diet, humans who consume more than half their calories as meat are at risk for fatal protein poisoning (a serious watchword for dieters on the new extra high-protein "zone" diets). The National Academy of Sciences recommends that Americans reduce their protein intake by 12 to 15 percent and switch from animal to plant protein sources.

Of all the body's cellular engines (fats, carbohydrates and protein), protein is the least efficient. To burn it the body must boost its metabolic rate by 10%, straining the liver's ability to absorb oxygen. Protein does not burn cleanly either, leaving behind nitrogen waste that your body must eliminate, a taxing process on your kidneys. It's why excessive protein consumption is linked to urinary tract infections, (overworked kidneys have to expel excess nitrogen through urine). For diabetics, the extra workload increases the risk of serious diabetic kidney disease. John's Hopkins Hospital now treats and cures severe kidney disease with a very low protein diet and amino acid supplements. Their studies show that eating a moderate or vegetarian protein diet may prevent kidney disease, even renal cancer.

Too much protein is linked to high cholesterol levels, converted by the liver and stored as fat.
Too much protein irritates the immune system, keeping it in a state of overactivity.
Too much protein causes fluid imbalance, so calcium, other minerals are lost through urine.
Too much protein is linked to arteriosclerosis, cataracts, kidney stones, and arthritis.
Too much animal protein contributes to osteoporosis and some cancers through mineral loss.

Does your body know the difference between animal and vegetable protein? Does your body work differently for the type of protein you eat? Amazingly enough, it does.

Animal source proteins have been considered superior in the past because they are:
1: **high in protein.** *Actually they have too much protein, which is stored in the body as toxins or fat.*
2: **complete protein.** Nearly every animal food, including dairy products, contains all eight amino acids. *But they also include inorganic acids which are unhealthy for humans.*
3: **thought to supply larger, easier absorbed iron and zinc than plant foods.** *A benefit off-set by the cholesterol, fat and calories that meat also supplies.*

Yet, even medical opinion about protein is changing. An important study by Baylor College of Medicine showed that men on diets high in soy protein had a drop in cholesterol, compared to men on diets high in animal protein. The study concluded that we should replace up to 50% of meat protein with vegetable protein for health. Most nutrition researchers now recommend eating meat in 3-ounce low-fat servings.

Research shows that eating lots of high protein animal foods may cause the body to extract calcium from the blood and excrete it, which can cause osteoporosis. Further, excess protein may cause calcium to be transferred from the bones to the soft tissues of the body in an attempt to neutralize protein acids. A 1990 international study in China confirmed that osteoporosis is rare in Chinese people with a plant-based protein diet. It only appears in Chinese cities where people are living more western lifestyles. In contrast, Eskimos, who have a heavily meat-based protein diet, with twice the RDA of calcium, have the highest rate of osteoporosis in the world.

Chinese research also shows that as the amount of animal protein in the diet rises, so does coronary disease and cancer, even after accounting for the fat that accompanies the protein.

Women may need more protein than men per pound of body weight to attain the same level of health. Women's depression, PMS, menopause symptoms, and chronic fatigue often disappear when protein is increased. But protein from meat tends to be high in fat, so protein for women should lean in favor of seafoods, whole grains, beans and other legumes.

Can vegetable protein satisfy your body's needs?

Eating a wide variety of plant protein foods is the secret. While vegetarians typically eat less protein than non-vegetarians, most vegetables are over the recommended 8% protein, so their diets still meet or exceed the protein RDA.

Protein is formed from combinations of the 22 amino acids. Protein from food is slowly released into the bloodstream; it combines with the amino acid pool in our blood, allowing maximum use of amino acids. In the past, experts held that vegetable proteins had to be carefully combined so that all essential amino acids and proteins were available at each meal to create a complete protein. Today we know this is not necessary; since the body breaks proteins down into amino acids and redistributes them, food combinations with incomplete proteins have the same effect as a complete protein.

Plant foods easily team up to make complete proteins in a process called protein complementarity. Beans and rice are a good example. Soy foods provide protein complementarity with whole grains and legumes. Many beans contain equal or more protein than beef. Black beans are a good protein source that also alkalizes excess acid.

Vegetable protein sources are some of the healthiest foods you can eat:

Whole grains, nuts, seeds, sprouts, grains, legumes and soy foods are good sources of protein and essential fatty acids. Dark green, leafy vegetables, like kale and chard, and cruciferous vegetables like broccoli, cabbage and cauliflower, have easily absorbed protein content plus EFA's. Blue-green algae, spirulina and chlorella are also concentrated plant protein sources.

• **Nutritional yeast** is an excellent source of protein, B vitamins, amino acids and minerals, and one of the best immune-enhancing supplements available in food form. Chromium-rich, nutritional yeast is a key food for improving blood sugar metabolism, and for substantially reducing cholesterol. It helps speed wound healing by boosting production of collagen. Its antioxidant properties allow skin tissues to take up more oxygen for healing. Its B vitamin and mineral content improves both skin texture and blemishes. Nutritional yeast flakes and aloe vera gel make an effective cleansing facial mask.

• **Sprouts** are an ideal plant source of protein, rich in almost every nutrient, vitamins (especially fat soluble vitamins like A, K, D and E), enzymes, essential fatty acids, and minerals, (like iron, potassium, magnesium, phosphorus, calcium, zinc and chromium), and are all natural antioxidants that strengthen immune response and protect the body from toxic chemical buildup.

• **Flax, sesame, sunflower, pumpkin, almonds, and chia** are my favorite nuts and seeds for protein. Nuts and seeds contain enzyme inhibitors. It's why they last so long and can sprout after decades. But enzyme inhibitors make them harder to digest. Soaking nuts and seeds overnight and spilling off the water is a way to deactivate the enzyme inhibitors to make nuts and seeds easier to digest for healing. Roasting or heating also deactivates enzyme inhibitors.

Human health thrives on a balanced diet. Strict vegans who eat no eggs or dairy foods should eat plenty of legumes and grains to insure sufficient amino acids. People on very low calorie diets or those who exclude whole food groups should pay special attention to their protein content.

Nature's Superfoods Help You Heal Faster

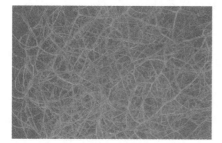

Green "superfoods" are superior sources of essential nutrients - nutrients we need but can't make ourselves. While we're adding more salads and vegetables to our diets, concern for the quality of foods grown on mineral-depleted soils makes green superfoods like chlorella, spirulina, barley and wheat grass popular. They are nutritionally more potent than regular foods, and wonderful food antioxidants for healthy healing.

<u>Green, and blue-green algae (phyto-plankton), are almost perfect superfoods</u>. They have rich high quality protein, fiber, chlorophyll, vitamins, minerals and enzymes. They can be used therapeutically to stimulate immune response, enhance tissue repair, accelerate healing, help prevent degenerative disease and promote longer life.

- **They are the most potent source of beta carotene available in the world today.**
- **They are the richest plant sources of vitamin B-12.**
- **Their amino acids are virtually identical to those needed by the human body.**
- **Their protein yield is greater than soy beans, corn or beef.**
- **They are superior food sources of DHA, (an EFA found in high amounts in breast milk).**
- **They are natural detoxifiers to protect against chemical pollutants and radiation.**

<u>Chlorella has a higher concentration of chlorophyll than any known plant</u>. It is a complete protein food, with all the B vitamins, vitamin C and E, and many minerals actually high enough to be considered supplemental amounts. The list of chlorella benefits is long and almost miraculous, from detoxification to energy enhancement, to immune system restoration through a unique molecular compound called Controlled Growth Factor.

- **Chlorella's cell wall material is especially beneficial for intestinal health, detoxifying the colon, stimulating peristaltic activity, and promoting friendly bacteria.**
- **Chlorella eliminates heavy metals, like lead, mercury, copper and cadmium.**
- **Chlorella is an important source of carotenes in healing tumors.**
- **Chlorella strengthens the liver, the body's major detoxifying organ, so that it can rid the body of infective agents that destroy immune defenses.**
- **Chlorella reduces arthritis stiffness.**
- **Chlorella normalizes blood pressure.**
- **Chlorella relieves indigestion, hiatal hernia, gastritis and ulcers.**
- **Chlorella is effective in weight loss programs. It cleanses, has rich nutrients that keep energy up during dieting, and maintains muscle during lower food intake.**

<u>Spirulina is the original green superfood</u>. It's an ecological wonder because it grows in both ocean and lake waters and can be cultivated in extreme environments useless for conventional agriculture. It grows in such a variety of climates and conditions that some consider it the nutrition answer for whole populations on the brink of starvation. Amazingly prolific, spirulina doubles its bio-mass every two to five days.

Big business isn't necessary for spirulina. Small scale community farms are spirulina's biggest producers. Researchers say that spirulina alone could double the protein available to people on a fraction of the world's land, while helping restore the environmental balance of the planet. (See Realities of The 90's, page 37) Acre for acre, spirulina yields 20 times more protein than soybeans, 40 times more protein than corn, and 400 times more protein than beef. It is a complete protein, with all 22 amino acids, the entire vitamin B-complex, including B-12, carotenes, minerals, and essential fatty acids. Digestibility is high, for both immediate and long range energy.

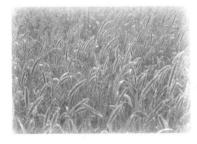

Green grasses are the only plants on earth that can give sole nutritional support to an animal throughout life. Grasses are some of the planet's, lowest-calorie, most nutrient-rich edibles, and some of the most underused. Grasses have the extraordinary ability to transform inanimate elements from soil, water and sunlight into living cells. Grasses contain all the known mineral and trace minerals, balanced vitamins and hundreds of enzymes. The molecular proteins and chlorophyllins in grasses are absorbed directly through our cell membranes. Their rich chlorophyll helps humans as it does plants, to resist the destructive effects of air pollution, carbon monoxide, X-rays and radiation. Studies on barley, wheatgrass and alfalfa show effects against a wide range of health problems: high blood pressure, diabetes, gastritis, ulcers, liver disease, asthma, eczema, hemorrhoids, skin infections, anemia, constipation, body odor, bleeding gums, burns, even cancer. Good sources of vitamin K, green grasses are also effective for bone strength.

Barley grass is loaded vitamins, minerals, enzymes, proteins and chlorophyllins. It has eleven times more calcium than cow's milk, 5 times more iron than spinach, and 7 times more vitamin C and bioflavonoids than orange juice. It helps a vegetarian diet with 80mcg of vitamin B-12 per 100 grams of powdered juice. Barley juice has anti-viral activity, shows results for DNA damage repair, and neutralizes heavy metals like mercury. It is an ideal anti-inflammatory for healing stomach ulcers and hemorrhoids. Dr. Kubota of Tokyo Pharmacy Science says, "Barley grass has effects measurably stronger than either steroid or non-steroid drugs, with few if any side effects."

Alfalfa is one of the world's richest mineral-source foods, pulling up earth minerals from root depths as great as 130 feet! Alfalfa's high chlorophyll content and rich plant fiber make it a good spring tonic, infection fighter and natural body deodorizer. It is a restorative in cases of narcotic and alcohol addiction, a recognized therapy for arthritis, colon and skin disorders, anemia and liver problems. Its high content of vitamin K helps herbalists use alfalfa to encourage blood-clotting. Alfalfa's recognized phytohormones are effective in normalizing estrogen levels.

Wheat grass liquid has curative powers for cancer growths, with success as rectal implants in colon cancer cases. Its ability to provide protection from carcinogens comes from chlorophyll's capacity to strengthen cells, detoxify the liver and blood, and biochemically neutralize pollutants. Wheat grass also normalizes the thyroid gland to stimulate metabolism which may be helpful in correcting obesity problems. Fifteen pounds of fresh wheat grass has the nutritional value of 350 pounds of vegetables with all their enzyme activity.

Medicinal mushrooms boost your resistance to toxic chemicals and pathogenic organisms.

Maitake mushrooms are the strongest tumor growth inhibitors of all the healing mushrooms. They are also highly effective against hormone-driven cancers like breast, prostate and endometrial cancer, even high mortality cancers like lung, liver, pancreas and brain cancer. Maitake has a most unusual synergistic effect with chemotherapy. Most natural therapies do not co-exist well with either chemotherapy or radiation, but patients taking maitake along with che-motherapy report a lessening of side effects such as loss of appetite and nausea. Maitake also appears to protect healthy cells from becoming cancerous, and may prevent the spread of cancer once it has taken hold.

Maitake's chemical structure stands apart from other mushrooms. Known as D-fraction, research-ers say it's Nature's most effective agent for stimulating cell immune response to target foreign substances. Researchers document anti-diabetes, anti-hypertension, anti-obesity and anti-hepati-tis activity, and success for Chronic Fatigue Syndrome, an immune deficiency disease.
Studies confirmed by the Japan National Institute for Health and the U.S. National Cancer Institute, show that maitake works rapidly to prevent the destruction of T-cells by HIV. Almost 40% of AIDS patients develop Kaposi's Sarcoma, a malignant skin cancer. Conventional medi-cine has not developed an effective treatment. Naturopaths report improvement in just a few days when maitake extract is applied topically to the KS lesions.
Maitake is effective taken orally, an advantage over other mushrooms where extracts often need to be injected, or where the therapeutic benefit is lost when taken orally.

Reishi mushrooms (ganoderma) have strong antioxidant protection and free radical scavenging activity for deep immune support. They are in the highest class of adaptogen

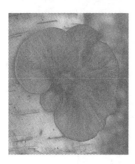

tonics for promoting longevity, especially effective for recovery from seri-ous illness. Science confirms what traditional healers have long known — reishi is an excellent cardiotonic, even significantly lowering blood pres-sure in those individuals with hypertension who were unresponsive to ACE inhibitors. Reishi may also be used therapeutically against fatigue, to re-lieve allergy symptoms, liver toxicity (especially hepatitis), bronchitis and carcinoma. New research shows success against chronic fatigue syndrome. Reishi may be used daily to lower cholesterol and triglycerides, induce sound sleep and increase resistance to infections.

Shiitake mushroom extracts are especially effective in treating systemic conditions related to early aging and sexual dysfunction. Renowned in Japan and China as both food and medicine for thousands of years, shiitake helps lower cholesterol levels, reduce blood pressure, and fight viruses and bacteria. Shiitakes stimulate immunity by producing a virus which stimu-lates our body's interferon. It can protect the body from cancer risk, even help shrink existing tumors. An immense amount of research has been done on two components of shiitake, *lentinan* and *lentinula edodes mycelium (LEM)* which show strong antitumor power. These constituents work by bolstering the body's own ability to eliminate the tumor rather than by attacking the tumor cells themselves. One Japanese study found that chemotherapy patients who received extra *lentinan* injections twice a week survived signifi- than patients who received chemo- results for hepatitis and chronic fa-

Studies with HIV patients show venting the spread of the HIV virus in monly prescribed drug in AIDS treat- blocking the initial stages of HIV infec- of the virus, and generally becomes less

cantly longer with less tumor regrowth, therapy alone. LEM also shows good tigue syndrome.

that LEM may be more effective at pre- the body than AZT, the most com- ment, possibly because LEM works by tion, while AZT merely slows replication effective over time.

Add shiitakes frequently to your diet, just a few each time. A little goes a long way.

Poria cocos is a mushroom amphoteric (with both alkaline and acidic properties) and has a unique ability to balance body chemistry, especially mineral balances. A Traditional Chinese Medicine herb, poria cocos works on the heart, spleen, and kidney meridians, and is used to remove spleen dampness when indicated by poor appetite, diarrhea and lethargy. TCM specialists believe that poria replenishes the spleen, thus strengthening the body against dizziness, and fluid elimination problems.

American naturopaths use poria to reduce water retention, balance body fluids and prevent toxic build-up. Poria cocos is used in herbal remedies for insomnia, restlessness, fatigue, sleep disorder, tension, and nervousness.

We get so caught up in our destination that we forget to appreciate our journey – especially the good people we meet along the way. Appreciation makes everybody feel good.

Macrobiotics: A Choice for Serious Healing

In America, macrobiotics has become a purification diet approach for serious, degenerative illness. It is an effective technique because it works to normalize body chemistry — not only to remove toxins, but also to rebuild healthy blood and cells.

Most notably, macrobiotics is seen as an effective method of improving body chemistry against cancer, and for most of this century has been part of the natural healing tradition for cancer. Macro-biotic (or long life), stems from the Oriental philosophy that considers the seasons, climate, traditional culture, and a person's health and activity level in determining the way to eat. A macrobiotic regimen encourages body harmony by teaching that vitality is achieved through living in harmony with the universe. A macrobiotic way of life requires the realization that we create our health through our lifestyle choices.

Macrobiotics adapts to individual needs. There is no single macrobiotic diet. Rather, it is a way of eating that is low in fat, non-mucous-forming, and rich in plant fiber and protein. It stimulates the heart and circulation by emphasizing Asian foods like miso, green tea and shiitake mushrooms. It alkalizes with foods like ume plums, sea vegetables and soy. It is nutrient rich - high in potassium, natural iodine, calcium and magnesium, and B-complex vitamins.

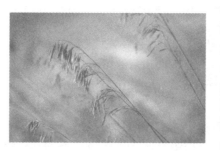

For most Americans, becoming macrobiotic requires a major shift in the way we look at life. It is usually a complete lifestyle change. I recommend changing to a macrobiotic diet slowly.

1: <u>The first diet change is to eat organically grown, whole foods whenever possible</u>. This is often a greater change than it might seem, because it means seeking these foods out, changing shopping habits and-or markets to find new sources. One of the cornerstones of macrobiotic body balancing is eating with the seasons. Yet, America's world access, market driven culture stands at the opposite end of this principle. We import all foods any time of the year without regard to our own seasons. Buying organically grown produce is good way to ensure this fundamental element of macrobiotics.

2: <u>The next change is to gradually eliminate foods not at ease in a macrobiotic diet</u>, like fried foods, highly processed, chemicalized foods, frozen, packaged and canned foods, and foods with colorants and preservers. Most animal protein and fat should be avoided, including dairy products (except fertile eggs). Eliminate white sugar foods. Use sweeteners like rice syrup and barley malt in small amounts instead. Refrain from sweet, tropical fruits, carbonated sodas and caffeine. Hot spices, artificial vinegar and strong alcoholic beverages should be avoided.

3: <u>The third change is learning to prepare foods in their whole form</u>, a change that takes some attention for people used to pre-prepared foods. It means buying fresh foods, and preparing them simply to keep the greatest value of the nutrients.

4: The fourth change is to include foods that are in harmony with macrobiotic principles, and to begin eating them in the macrobiotic way. The most apparent difference between macrobiotics and other diet approaches is its reliance on **whole grains.** In macrobiotics at least half of the daily food intake is whole grains - brown rice, whole wheat, oats, barley, millet, buckwheat, rye, amaranth, kamut and corn. Cooking grains with a little seasalt is recommended; my favorite way to season is with the mineral salts of sea vegetables. Don't use processed grains like pastas or non-yeasted breads.

–**Vegetables,** both raw and cooked, are the second most important foods for macrobiotics, comprising about 30% of the diet. Steam, sauté in olive or sesame oil, parboil or bake them. Healing vegetables to include: dark leafy greens, cruciferous vegetables, parsley, burdock root, carrots, squash and scallions. Potatoes, tomatoes, eggplant, peppers, spinach, beets and zucchini are not recommended for a serious healing diet because they may aggravate body acidity.

–**Beans and sea vegetables** are considered supplementary, rather than daily foods, comprising about 5 to 10 percent of a macrobiotic diet. Yet, for Americans used to more protein in their diets, I find that eating beans makes an easier change to macrobiotics. Aduki beans, chickpeas, soy and lentils are recommended. Sea greens such as kombu, dulse, kelp, sea palm, wakame, hijiki, arame and nori are excellent with grains, beans, and vegetables, especially in soups.

–**Soups** may make up 10 to 15% of the initial macrobiotic diet. I recommend a daily bowl of miso soup to get the alkalizing, immune-boosting process started.

Other foods in order of their importance in a macrobiotic diet are vegetable oils, nuts, fruits, fish and occasional fertile eggs. Although many people who follow a macrobiotic diet prefer to avoid all animal foods, macrobiotics is not a vegetarian system. White meat fish, like flounder, cod, sole and halibut are recommended 2 to 3 times a week. Fruits are considered pleasure foods, eaten only occasionally as desserts or snacks, generally 2 to 3 times a week. Nuts and seeds, like pumpkin, sesame and sunflower seeds are occasional snacks.

–Therapeutic foods, like green tea, shiitake, maitake and reishi mushrooms, raw sauerkraut, and umeboshi plums should be included regularly.

5: The fifth change is learning to chew food well - about 50 times per bite for the best absorption of nutrients. For Americans, who lead fast-paced, high stress lives, this change is sometimes the hardest to make. Yet, chewing is the cornerstone of a grain-based macrobiotic diet because grains are by nature acidic; saliva which is alkaline, counteracts the acid. The acid-alkaline balance of your body's blood is crucial to the health of your cells, tissues and organs, and to your body's healing ability. When your blood becomes overly acidic, all body functions, including mood and emotion, are adversely affected.

Once you've made the changes to eat macrobiotically, is there a way to tell if the diet is helping your healing program?

Here is a typical sequence for normalizing body chemistry: It usually takes 10 days for plasma to recycle, so improvements become noticeable after ten days. It takes 30 days for white blood cells to renew, so immune function begins to improve after a month. It takes 120 days for red blood cells to renew, so it is then that true healing begins. Most people say they notice results in healthier emotional and mental patterns around this time as well.

Even in its strict form a macrobiotic diet is nutritionally balanced with adequate protein and low fat. The majority of the foods are from the center of the food spectrum – vegetables and whole grains – with a minimum of foods from the extremes; fruits and sugars are more cooling, meat and dairy foods are more stimulating. Some herbs and spices, like garlic, onions, and cayenne are considered too stimulating.

Recently, Harvard's School of Public Health analyzed the "standard recommendations" of a macrobiotic diet. The results showed that the diet exceeded the recommended daily nutrient allowances of both the FDA and the World Health Organization, without having to take extra protein, vitamins or minerals. In fact, from a macrobiotic perspective, it is not desirable to take supplements other than whole herbs, since it is thought that they interfere with the nutrients in the whole foods themselves.

A macrobiotic diet's greatest benefit is that it is cleansing and strengthening at the same time. I view macrobiotics a little differently than the traditional Asian model. I see macrobiotics not as a "no deviation" regimen, but as a way of life based on a whole foods diet and an active lifestyle in harmony with nature.

Cautionary note: A strict macrobiotic diet used over a long period of time, can be too stringent for a person living a busy, stressful life in today's polluted environment. I normally recommend a strict macrobiotic diet for three to six months, then a gradual move to a modified macrobiotic diet which doesn't follow rigid rules, but rather emphasizes the principles of macrobiotics with the flexibility of each person's needs.

As we learn more about therapeutic ways of eating - such as macrobiotics, fruit fasting diets, mono diets, etc., I urge caution if you are not in a controlled clinical environment. In their strict cleansing-healing form, excessively limited diets should be used only as short term programs. Balance is the real key.

Is macrobiotics for you? Here's an easy way to get a taste of what macrobiotics might mean to your health. Check out the Food Pharmacy Digest, page 475, to find out what foods have the elements you need. Include them in your diet, regularly.

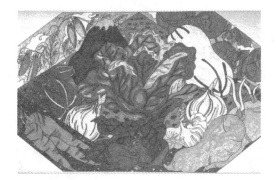

Cultured Foods Offer Healing Probiotics

What are probiotics? Why are they so important for your healing diet? Probiotics are beneficial microorganisms like *Lactobacillus, Bifidobacteria,* and *Streptococcus* in your intestinal tract. They manufacture vitamins, especially B vitamins like biotin, niacin, folic acid and B-6, that detoxify chemicals and metabolize hormones. They enable enzymes that maximize food assimilation and digestion.

Probiotics (as opposed to antibiotics), are an amazing fighting force that compete at a basic level with disease-causing microorganisms in your body. First, probiotics prevent the growth of undesirable bacteria by producing substances that deprive them of nourishment. Second, probiotics attack specific pathogens by changing the body's acid/alkaline balance to an *antibiotic* environment. (Probiotic activity against vaginal yeast infections is a good example of this.)
If you are taking long courses of drug antibiotics, remember that they kill <u>all</u> bacteria, both bad and good. All intestinal flora are severely diminished. For most people, poor digestion, diarrhea or constipation, flatulence, bad breath, bloating, tiredness, migraines, even acne are a result of long antibiotic treatment.

It doesn't matter how good your diet is if your body can't use it. Much in our modern lifestyle destroys normal body balance. Stress, alcohol, chemicalized foods, environmental pollutants, antibiotic and steroid drugs all have an adverse effect on our ability to use nourishment. When unfriendly bacteria get the upper hand in the balance, the door opens to infections and allergy reactions. Your body ecology must maintain a balance of bacteria that protects intestinal and immune function. Probiotic organisms prevent disease, even treat infections by restoring microorganism balance in the intestinal tract.

Why do you need plenty of probiotics?
—Probiotics boost immune response by inhibiting growth of pathogenic organisms.
—Probiotics detoxify the intestinal tract by protecting intestinal mucosa levels.
—Probiotics develop a barrier to food-borne allergies.
—Probiotics neutralize antibiotic-resistant strains of bacteria.
—Probiotics reduce cancer risk.
—Probiotics reduce the risk of inflammatory bowel disease (IBS) and diverticulosis.
—Probiotic synthesize needed vitamins for healing.
—Probiotics prevent diarrhea by improving digestion of proteins and fats.

What's the best way to get probiotics in your diet? Add them through foods like yogurt, miso, kefir, raw sauerkraut or vinegars.
I see probiotic supplements as a health insurance policy. Most supplements have *lactobacillus acidophilus,* (which attaches in the small intestine), *bifidobacterius* (which attaches in the large intestine), and *lactobacillus bulgaricus* (three protective strains of flora). Together they produce hydrogen peroxide, a by-product that helps maintain protective microbial balance and protects against pathogens.

There's more. Important new discoveries about probiotics:
Probiotics play a key role in the prevention of osteoporosis. Bone loss is an unfortunate result of a lack of friendly microorganisms in the gastrointestinal tract. Vitamin K, a vital building block to healthy bones, is a by-products of *lactobacilli*.

New research shows new benefits for acidophilus. *Lactobacilli acidophilus,* part of the normal flora in your urinary tract and vaginal tissue, helps you digest dairy foods, prevents most yeast infections and restores intestinal balance especially traveler's or antibiotic-induced diarrhea. Acidophilus is highly successful for children's diseases. Children have naturally strong immune systems and may only need the gentle body balancing of friendly flora instead of a harsh drug or chemical antibiotic.

Acidophilus:

—**helps synthesize essential B vitamins and produces essential enzyme stores.**
—**helps overcome lactose intolerance by digesting milk sugars.**
—**reduces blood fat and cholesterol levels.**
—**improves elimination - contributing to sweet breath and normal body odor.**
—**kills harmful bacteria that contribute to cancer; helps block tumor development.**
—**inactivates some harmful viruses.**
—**helps detoxify the G.I. tract and improves G.I. health.**
—**prevents yeast infections, and most urinary tract infections.**

Note: Acidophilus is effective as a healing medicine when it is sprinkled <u>directly on food</u>..... particularly for low immune response conditions, like candida albicans, eating disorders and HIV infection where nutrient assimilation is seriously compromised.

Can everyone use probiotics? Each person's digestive system is highly individual, like the immune system to which it is a gateway. No single bacteria strain is adequate, however friendly. Some probiotics strains are not able to survive in the intestinal tract. Some experts question whether any probiotic supplements survive the digestion process, because digestion itself, even though it protects against unfriendly bacteria, can't differentiate between good and bad bacteria.

*Prebiotics like FOS may be a more practical approach. Pre-biotics feed the beneficial bacteria you already have in your gastrointestinal tract. Fructo-oligo-saccharides (FOS) are naturally-occurring carbohydrates in fruits and vegetables like artichokes, bananas, onions, garlic, barley and tomatoes. The FOS saccharides are easily used by our intestinal flora. Our lower intestines house hundreds of microorganisms, both helpful and harmful. Competition for food and attachment sites is fierce. FOS supplements give your friendly bacteria a competitive edge and actually increase your body's population of beneficial bacteria.

<u>Cultured foods add natural friendly flora to your healing diet.</u>

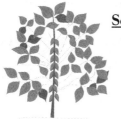

<u>Soyfoods are nutritional powerhouses.</u> Even if soy isn't a magic bullet for preventing heart disease or curing cancer, it has amazing health benefits. Soy protein compares in quality to animal protein — it's a good alternative to meat or dairy foods (see Protein, page 40). Soy foods are rich in other essential nutrients, too, like calcium, iron, zinc and B vitamins.

What do cultured soy foods do for your health?

1: **Soy protein helps lower blood cholesterol.** Numerous studies show that when animal protein in the diet is replaced by soy protein, there is significant reduction in both total blood cholesterol and LDL (bad) cholesterol. Adding 25 to 50 grams of soy protein daily to your diet for only a month can result in a cholesterol drop.

2: **Soy's amino acids help lower high insulin levels.** Low insulin levels mean that your liver manufactures less cholesterol, too.

3: **Soy's high antioxidant activity helps control atherosclerosis,** by preventing oxidative damage to LDL cholesterol - the main culprit in progressive blocking of arteries.

4: **Soy possesses rich diet sources of five known anticancer agents:**

a. protease inhibitors, which hinder the development of colon, oral, lung, liver, pancreatic and esophageal cancers.

b. antioxidants that block formation of nitrosamines leading to liver cancer.

c. phytosterols that inhibit cell division and proliferation in colon cancer.

d. saponins that slow the growth of cancerous skin cells.

e. isoflavones that slow osteoporosis and lower risk of hormone-related cancers, like breast and prostate cancer. (One study shows that pre-menopausal females who rarely eat soy foods have *twice the risk of breast cancer* as those who frequently eat soy foods. The study showed that just one serving a day of soy protein led to significant lengthening of the menstrual cycle, suppressing the midcycle surge of gonadotrophins, luteinizing and follicle-stimulating hormones - effects that decrease the risk of breast cancer. Not surprisingly, the Japanese, with low rates of hormone-driven cancers, eat five times more soy products than Americans. While the typical U.S. diet yields 80 milligrams of phytosterols per day, the Japanese typically eat 400 milligrams a day. Western vegetarians eat about 345 milligrams a day.

—Genistein - an abundant isoflavone in soy works much like human estrogen. Genistein helps balance the body's estrogen supply, acting both as an estrogen, and as an estrogen blocker, depending on the body's need. Like many phytohormone herbs, it promotes the positive actions of estrogen, while preventing many of its bad effects by competing for both estrogen and progesterone receptors to prevent their availability for tumor growth. Genistein also inhibits angiogenesis, the forming of new blood vessels necessary for the nourishment of a growing tumor.

Genistein's benefits for men's health show promise, too. Research on 8,000 Hawaiian men found that the men who ate the most tofu had the lowest rates of prostate cancer, as well as kidney disease and complications related to diabetes.

Common soy foods that benefit a healing diet:

• **Tofu**, made from cooked, curdled soybean milk, water and nigari (a mineral-rich seawater precipitate), is the soy food highest in both isoflavones and genistein. Ironically, nearly all the soybeans raised in the U.S. go into animal feed. Most of the rest is shipped to Japan. Tofu, combined with whole grains, yields a complete protein, providing dairy richness without the fat or cholesterol, yet with all the calcium and iron.

As tofu's popularity has risen in America, so have its culinary talents. Fresh tofu has a light, delicate character that can take on any flavor, from savory to sweet. It comes firm-pressed in cubes, in a soft, delicate form with a custard-like texture. It is smoked or pre-cooked in seasonings for more flavor. It comes in deep-fried pouches called age (pronounced "ah-gay") for stuffing. It is both aseptically packaged and freeze-dried to be stored at room temperature and reconstituted for later use, camping and travel. Tofu is a nutritionally balanced healing food. Cooked, it is easy to digest, full of fiber, and a non-mucous-forming way to add richness and creamy texture to recipes.

Tofu by the numbers:
—Tofu is low in calories. 8-oz. has only 164 calories.
—Tofu provides organic calcium. 8-oz. supplies the same amount of calcium as 8-oz. of milk, about 12% of the adult calcium RDA, with more absorbability.
—Tofu is high in iron. 8-oz. supplies the same amount of iron as 2-oz. of beef liver or 4 eggs; yet it is easily assimilated, suitable even for the elderly, or small children.
—Tofu has almost 8% quality protein, 65% of which is actually usable by the body. Eight ounces supplies the same amount of protein as $3\,{}^1/_4$ oz. of beef, $5\,{}^1/_2$ oz. of hamburger, $1\,{}^2/_3$ cups of milk, 2-oz. of cheese, or 2 eggs; but it is lower in fat than any of these. Unlike most animal protein, cooked tofu is easy to digest, with a digestion rate of 95%.
—Tofu contains all 8 essential amino acids.
—As little as 4-oz. of tofu a month offers women breast cancer prevention benefits.

• **Miso,** a tasty food made from fermented soybean paste, is body alkalizing, lowers cholesterol, represses carcinogens, helps neutralize allergens and pollutants, lessens the effects of smoking, and provides an immune-enhancing environment, even to the point of rejuvenating damaged cells. Miso also attracts and absorbs environmental toxins like radioactive elements in the body and helps to eliminate them.

—**Miso has even stronger antioxidant effects than soy itself.** As miso ages, its color turns deep brown from melanoidine. Melanoidine suppresses the production of fat peroxides in the body. Fat peroxides (oxidized fats) become free radicals, which destroy normal cell functions and accelerate aging. Miso helps preserve cell youthfulness through its unique antioxidant effects and its free-radical quenching saponins.

—**Miso is a healthy substitute for salt or soy sauce;** a tasty base for soups, sauces, dressings, dips, spreads and cooking stocks. There are many kinds, strengths and flavors of miso, from chickpea (light and mild) to hatcho (dark and strong). Natto miso is sweet, a mix of soybeans, barley and barley malt, kombu, ginger and sea salt.

A fatty acid in miso, *ethyl linoleate,* has an anti-mutagenic effect against carcinogens found in scorched foods like charcoal barbecued meats and French roasted coffee.

Another fatty acid in miso, *linoleic acid* (LA), stimulates sebaceous glands for baby soft skin texture. LA also significantly inhibits melanin production, the pigment that causes dark spots on the skin, by repressing synthesis of the enzyme tyrosinase that synthesizes melanin. Miso's linoleic acid works synergistically with its plant sterols and vitamin E to suppress cholesterol accumulation in the body, inhibiting cholesterol absorption in the small intestine and promoting excretion of serum cholesterol. Vitamin E, a component of HDL (good cholesterol), helps transport harmful cholesterol and increase HDL levels.

A few of miso's many health benefits:
—Controls cholesterol levels
—Helps preserve beautiful skin texture
—Antioxidant activity boosts immune response and slows the effects of aging
—Helps eliminate radioactive substances from the body
—A known preventive of some types of cancer - liver, stomach, breast, skin
—Helps maintain balanced body chemistry by alkalizing an over-acid system

Unpasteurized miso is preferred for a healing diet. Because it is naturally fermented, unpasteurized miso is still a living food, with its active enzymes and beneficial microorganisms intact to aid digestion in the intestines. Miso is highly concentrated; use $\frac{1}{2}$ to 1 teasp. of dark miso, or 1 to 2 teasp. of light miso per person. Dissolve in a small amount of water to activate the beneficial enzymes before adding to a recipe. Omit salt from the recipe if you are using miso.

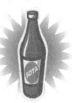

• **Tamari** is a wheat-free soy sauce, lower in sodium and richer in flavor than regular soy sauce. Bragg's LIQUID AMINOS, an energizing protein broth sold in health food stores, is of the tamari family, but unfermented, even lower in sodium, with all 8 essential amino acids.

• **Soy cheese,** made from soy milk, is lactose and cholesterol free. (A small amount of calcium caseinate, milk protein, is added to allow soy cheese to melt.) Mozzarella, cheddar, jack and cream cheese types are widely available. Use it cup for cup in place of any low-fat or regular cheese.

• **Soy mayonnaise** has the taste and consistency of regular mayonnaise.

• **Soy milk,** nutritious, smooth, delicious and versatile is made simply by pressing ground, cooked soybeans. It's lactose and cholesterol free, with less calcium and calories than cow's milk, but more protein and iron. Use it cup for cup like milk in cooking; it adds a slight rise to baked goods. Soy milk formulas are good for infants allergic to cow's milk. It's often used in treatment diets for diabetes, anemia and heart diseases.

• **Soy ice cream, frozen desserts and yogurt** are also widely available.

• **Tempeh,** a complete protein with all essential amino acids, is a meaty, Indonesian soy food with a robust texture and mushroom-like aroma. Tempeh is an enzyme-active, predigested culture, making it highly absorbable. It's rich in B vitamins (especially B-12), low in calories and fat, and cholesterol-free. Tempeh differs from tofu; it has a firmer texture, is denser, and higher in fiber. Fresh tempeh has the highest quality protein of any soyfood. It contains 19.5% protein (about as much as beef and chicken), and 50% more protein than ground beef.

• **Kombucha,** although known as a "mushroom," is not a mushroom at all, but a symbiotic culture of yeast and other microorganisms. Today, it is a popular natural tonic beverage of Russian origin, for lowering blood pressure, raising immune T-cell counts, and increasing vitality. It is noted for its dramatic antibiotic and detoxifying activity.

—To make kombucha tonic, place a small amount of kombucha culture into sweetened black or green tea. The culture feeds on the sugar and like a tiny biochemical factory, produces glucuronic acid, glucon acid, lactic acid, vitamins, amino acids, antibiotic substances, and more to make it a healthful cultured drink.

The benefits of kombucha culture tonic:

—helps the liver bind up toxic substances so they can be eliminated from the body
—cleanses the colon, relieves constipation and colitis, arrests simple diarrhea
—relieves arthritis pain and carpal tunnel syndrome
—helps return gray hair to its natural color; thickens hair and strengthens nails
—relieves bronchitis and asthma
—helps overcome candida albicans yeast infections
—reduces menopausal hot flashes, headaches and migraines
—reduces cravings for fatty foods
—improves eyesight, cataracts and floaters
—relieves acne, eczema and psoriasis
—vitalizes flagging libido and sexual energy

Note: I recommend buying Kombucha tea from the refrigerated section of your health food store. I have personally known several cases where making kombucha culture at home was unsuccessful, and the kombucha became contaminated with unsafe organisms.

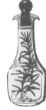

• **Vinegar** is an ancient cultured food that has been used all over the world for 5000 years as a health enhancer and food preserver. Vinegar is full of beneficial organisms that help digest heavy foods and high protein meals. Brown rice, balsamic, apple cider, herbal, raspberry, ume plum and wine vinegars are all popular today.

Healing benefits of vinegar include:

—Diluted vinegar eardrops can ward off and gently relieve children's ear infections.
—A vinegar footbath softens hard callouses; and because vinegar acids are anti-bacterial and anti-fungal, a footbath is an effective treatment for athlete's foot.
—Vinegar has remarkable effects for treating arthritis, osteoporosis and memory loss.
—Vinegar helps maintain healthy heart tissue. It's full of pectin and potassium which help smooth a healthy, relaxed heartbeat and blood pressure.
—Vinegar assists in killing infections, and helps fight environmental carcinogens.
—Vinegar is a powerful food remedy for resolving liver stagnation and indigestion. It's loaded with gallbladder enhancing enzymes and essential acids that aid digestion.
—Vinegar's high potassium helps balance body sodium, encourages bowel regularity and sustains nerve health.

A warm water vinegar drink has remarkable detoxifying effects.

Mix 1 tsp. apple cider vinegar, 1 tsp. honey or maple syrup, and warm water. Drink a half hour before each meal. A regular drink like this can help ease heartburn and chronic indigestion, soothe throat irritation, halt hiccups, and for many people, improve memory.

Egg vinegar is a popular high blood pressure remedy called Tamago-su in Japan. The Japanese warrior culture believes it is an important source of strength and power. (Roman soldiers also believed in the strengthening power of vinegar, too.)

Here's how to make this potent remedy: Place a whole raw egg (uncracked) in one cup of brown rice vinegar. Leave it undisturbed for one week. After the week, the shell dissolves and only the inner membrane of the egg remains. Remove the egg's membrane and mix its contents into the vinegar. Take three times a day with hot water.

The most nutritious vinegars are not overly filtered (they look slightly cloudy) and still contain the "mother" mixture of beneficial bacteria and enzymes in the bottle.

• **Yogurt** is a cultured, intestinal cleanser that helps balance and replace friendly flora in the G.I. tract. Yogurt is nutrient-dense, providing a wealth of proteins, with more protein and calcium than milk. The culturing process makes yogurt a living, healthy food. Most yogurt contains the beneficial bacteria *lactobacillus bulgaricus* and *streptococcus thermophilus*; some have extra *lactobacillus acidophilus* as well. Yogurt is dairy in origin, but is far better tolerated than regular dairy foods, even by those with lactase enzyme deficiency. Yogurt itself stimulates lactase activity; bio-fermentation elements in yogurt actually substitute for the missing lactase. *Note: Make sure you're buying naturally cultured yogurt for all the active probiotic benefits. Commercial brands often have gums and fillers.*

Yogurt has wide-ranging health benefits:
—helps lower bad cholesterol and raise protective lipoprotein levels (HDL's).
—boosts blood levels of gamma interferon, an immune component that rallies killer cells to fight infections, especially pathogens that cause ulcers and intestinal infections.
—enzymes in yogurt cultures help lessen intolerance for lactase-deficient people.
—a good source of absorbable calcium, yogurt strengthens against osteoporosis.
—helps decrease diarrhea in children, especially when exacerbated by antibiotics.
—Yogurt lactic acid bacteria lower enzymes responsible for developing colon cancer.
—Spoonable yogurt with fruit (or even veggies) is good for infants through toddlers after three months. Introduce it gradually into the diet when the child begins to eat solid foods.

• **Yogurt cheese** is delicious, creamy, meltable and widely available in health food and gourmet stores. It's easy to make from plain yogurt, is much lighter in fat and calories than sour cream or cream cheese, but has the same richness and consistency.
To make all natural yogurt cheese: Spoon 16-oz of plain yogurt onto a piece of cheesecloth or into a sieve-like plastic funnel (available from kitchen catalogs or hardware stores). Hang cheesecloth over a kitchen sink faucet, or put funnel over a large glass. Let drain for 14 to 16 hours for yogurt cheese (save the whey and use it as a tasty part of the liquid in soups and stews). Store in a covered container in the refrigerator; keeps well for 2 to 3 weeks.

• **Low-fat cottage cheese** is a cultured dairy food, but okay for those with slight lactose intolerance. A good alternate for ricotta, cream cheese or chemical-filled cottage cheese, mix with low-fat plain yogurt to add the richness of cream or sour cream to recipes without the fat.

• **Kefir,** is made from kefir grains or mother cultures prepared from grains. Kefir is a complete protein, essential to healing. It's full of biotin; B vitamins, especially B-12; calcium; magnesium; and the amino acid tryptophan, for natural calming benefits. In Russia, kefir is used medicinally as part of the treatment for metabolic and gastric disorders, tuberculosis, atherosclerosis, allergies, even cancer. Kefir replenishes beneficial intestinal bacteria, producing lactic acid which balances stomach pH. Kefir is easy to digest because its friendly bacteria contain partially digested proteins along with minerals which contribute to the assimilation of proteins.

—**Kefir cheese** is a delicious cultured food, low in fat and calories, similar to sour cream or cream cheese. It has a slightly tangy rich flavor that really enhances snack foods and raw vegetables. Use it cup for cup in place of sour cream, cottage cheese, cream cheese or ricotta.

• **Cultured vegetables,** or sauerkraut, from the Austrian words sauer (sour) and kraut (greens), are fresh veggies changed by fermentation into one of the richest food sources of lactobacilli and enzymes, loaded with vitamin C and minerals. Cultured vegetables improve digestion for animal proteins and grains, and re-establish your inner ecosystem for toxin elimination and immune response.

Raw cultured vegetables are pre-digested and alkaline-forming for better body balance. The lactobacilli in cultured veggies are star players in beating Candida albicans yeast overgrowth and controlling the cravings for sugar common in candidiasis. Sauerkraut is also effective for peptic ulcers, ulcerative colitis, colic, food allergies, cystitis, vaginal infections and constipation.

Important: the healing power of sauerkraut's probiotics and enzymes is only in unpasteurized sauerkraut. The sauerkraut on today's supermarket shelves is highly salted and pasteurized, with its lactobacilli and enzymes destroyed. Find effective cultured veggies instead at your health food store in the refrigerated section. Or call Rejuvenative Foods, P.O. Box 8464, Santa Cruz, CA 95061, 800-805-7957.

If you can't find cultured veggies, here's how to make your own:

Cabbage is the main element of unheated, fresh sauerkraut. You can use green cabbage alone, or make a half-and-half blend of green and red cabbage, and add mixed vegetables.

To make: shred a small head of green cabbage in a food processor and set aside. Chop a blend of other vegetables, like 1 beet, 2 carrots and 1 green bell pepper. Or make a Kim Chee blend of cabbage, carrots, onions, red or yellow bell pepper, some grated ginger and chili pepper. Place the veggies in a sanitary glass or stainless steel pot (never use plastic). *Note: you can promote the fermentation process by bringing some of the juices out of the vegetables. Pound the chopped or shredded vegetables with a wooden mallet in a big stainless steel bowl, or put the vegetables through a Champion Juicer using the plastic piece instead of the screen.* Cover the veggies with whole cabbage leaves. Put a large plate on top of the leaves - add a weight on top of the plate like a large stone or brick, to help the circulation of juice and enhance fermentation. Let sit for 5 to 7 days at moderate room temperature (60° to 72°). The naturally present enzymes, *lactobacillus acidophilus, lactobacillus plantarum* and *lactobacillus brevis* in the vegetables proliferate, transform the sugars and starches in the vegetables into lactic and acetic acids.

—After 7 days throw away the old cabbage leaves and moldy, discolored vegetables on top. Put remaining fermented vegetables in glass jars and refrigerate. They'll hold their flavor, enzymes and *lactobacillus* cultures for four to eight months if kept at 34° and opened minimally. Do not freeze. (*For more details, call Rejuvenative Foods for their Seven Step Cultured Vegetable Guidelines.*)

Water is Essential for Healing

Your body goes down fast without water. Water is second only to oxygen in importance for health; just a few short days without water can be fatal! Making up almost three-fourths of the body, every cell is regulated, monitored by, and dependent on an efficient flow of water. Messages in the brain cells are transported on "waterways" to the nerve endings. Water transports minerals, vitamins, proteins and sugars around the body for assimilation. Water maintains body equilibrium and temperature, lubricates tissues, flushes wastes and toxins, hydrates the skin, acts as a shock absorber for joints, bones and muscles, and adds needed minerals.

When your body gets enough water, it works at its peak. Fluid retention decreases, gland and hormone functions improve, the liver breaks down and releases more fat, hunger is curtailed. Dehydration plays a role in elimination ailments like chronic constipation and urinary tract infections, peripheral vascular problems like hemorrhoids and varicose veins, kidney stones, even many degenerative diseases like arthritis.

Experts tell us that thirst is an evocate severe dehydration. Drinking only keep your skin moist and supple, your regular. What's more, many Americans ing the good Omega-3 fats and other their bodies can't hold or use the water regularly recommend adding sea greens and lustrous hair.... a quality of sea

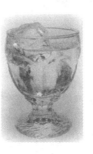

lutionary development designed to indi- if you're thirsty may not be enough to brain sharp or your elimination systems have reduced their intake of fats (including essential fatty acids) to the point that they do take in. It's one of the reasons I to your diet for moister skin, shining eyes plants known since ancient Greek times.

Water quality is poor in many areas of the U.S. Most tap water is chlorinated, fluoridated, and treated to the point where it can be an irritating, disagreeable fluid instead of a healthful drink. City tap water may contain as many as 500 different disease-causing bacteria, viruses and parasites. Fluoridated water increases absorption of aluminum from deodorants, pots and pans, etc. by 600%, a possible concern for Alzheimer's dementia. Chemicals used by industry and agriculture find their way into our ground water, adding more pollutants. Some tap water is so bad, that without the enormous effort our bodies exert to dispose of these chemicals, we would have ingested enough of them to turn us to stone by the time we were thirty! These concerns keep many people from drinking tap water. Keep plenty of bottled water at hand. Purifiers or a purifier hooked to your refrigerator are easy solutions for making your tap water more potable.

<u>Should you drink more water?</u> Here's how your body uses it up every day. Your kidneys receive and filter your entire blood supply 15 times each hour! If you become overheated, your 2 million sweat glands perspire to cool your skin and keep your internal organs at a constant temperature, using 99% water. You use a small amount of water during breathing and through tear ducts that lubricate the upper eyelids 25 times per minute. Crying and hearty laughter release water from your eyes and nose. Even normal activity uses up at least 3 quarts of replacement water each day. Strenuous activity, a hot climate or a high salt diet increases this requirement.

What happens when you don't get enough water? A chain reaction begins.
1: A water shortage message is sent from your brain;
2: Your kidneys conserve water by urinating less (constipation and bloating occur);
3: At 4 percent water depletion, muscle endurance diminishes - you start to get dizzy;
4: At 5 percent water loss, headaches from mild to quite severe begin — you get drowsy, lose the ability to concentrate and get unreasonably impatient;
5: At 6 percent water loss, body temperature is impaired — your heart begins to race;
6: At 7 percent body water depletion, there is a good possibility of collapse.

Other common signs that you might be dehydrated:
  —unexplained headaches (mild to severe), usually with some dizziness
  —unexplained irritability, impatience, restlessness and difficulty sleeping
  —unusually dry skin and loss of appetite along with constipation
  —dull back pain that is not relieved by rest
  —unexplained weight gain; swollen hands and-or feet (from water retention)

To tell whether or not you're drinking enough water, check your urine. The color should be a pale straw and you should urinate every few hours. If your urine color is dark yellow, start drinking more water!

Gradual loss of body water accelerates aging. It is also a major complication in illness. Dehydration is reportedly one of the top 10 causes of hospital stays among the elderly. Some studies show thirst-impaired seniors do not even seek water when they need it because their sense of thirst is so impaired. Fear of urinary incontinence makes some seniors drink less liquid — doubly unfortunate because hydration is important on many levels, from body cleansing to skin beauty.

Water is critical for an effective detoxification program. It dilutes and eliminates toxin accumulations in the bloodstream, and cleanses the kidneys. Add half a squeezed lemon to each glass of water for the best cleansing effects. The best time to detoxify is at night, while you sleep.

Water is the most important factor in losing weight and keeping it off. It suppresses appetite and helps your body flush stored fats. Low water intake causes fat deposits to increase — more water intake actually reduces fat deposits. If you are overweight, the more body fat you have, the less system water you have. Larger people have larger metabolic loads — they need more water.

Thirst is not a reliable signal that your body needs water.
By the time you feel thirsty, you're probably already suffering from some degree of dehydration. Thirst is an evolutionary effect, controlled by a part of the forebrain called the hypothalamus, (which also controls sleep, appetite, satiety and sexual response) designed to alert us to severe dehydration. You can easily lose a quart of water during activity before thirst is even recognized.

  —**Solving the dehydration problem:** Human bodies have some strange anomalies. We have to plan for our water supply. From an early adult age our thirst sensation begins to fail, putting us inexplicably at risk for dehydration. Even more strange, our thirst signal shuts off before we have had enough for well-being.

Where does your body get its replacement water? Cool water replaces body fluids best, but other healthy liquids count as water replenishment, like unsweetened fruit juices and vegetable juices. Fruits and vegetables themselves are more than 90% water, and provide up to $1^1/_2$ quarts a day. Even dry foods like bread are about 35% water. Digestion yields as much as a pint a day for metabolism.

—Alcohol and caffeine drinks are counter-productive because they are diuretic.
—Drinks loaded with sugars or milk increase water needs instead of satisfying them.
—Commercial sodas leach several important minerals from your body.

Can you drink too much water? Even though most of us don't get enough water today, drinking too much water can have some adverse health effects. It can severely depress electrolytes, imperative for energy, pH balance and mineral uptake. Purified water, such as distilled or reverse osmosis techniques may compound the problem.

It sounds like a lot, but eight to ten 8-ounce glasses of water daily is a sufficient amount. If you are physically active or working under hot weather conditions, you'll need more. Replace lost electrolytes with electrolyte drinks like Alacer EMERGEN-C, or supplement drinks like Nature's Path TRACE-LYTE.

Are you worried about retaining too much water, or getting water logged? Believe it or not, drinking more water is the best treatment <u>against</u> retaining water!

When you don't get the water you need, your body holds onto the water it has. Diuretics are only a temporary solution because you'll end up ravenously thirsty as your body tries to replace the water that the diuretics flush out. (See "What happens when you don't get enough water," previous page.) Diuretics also compromise important nutrients like potassium. Overcome a water retention problem by giving your body what it needs, <u>plenty of water</u>. When your body has the right amount, it will naturally release the excess.

Hydrate before, during and after exercise. You may not be pushing yourself to the brink of collapse, but even 30 minutes of exercise can put you at risk for dehydration. Humans sweat more than any mammal; normal exercise causes a loss of one to two quarts of fluid every hour of a workout. Sweat acts as your body's air conditioner, keeping your muscles (which generate 8 to 10 times more heat during exercise), cooled. Take in water, juice or an electrolyte drink during your workout to maintain fluid needs.

In hot weather, drink about 20-ounces of fluid two hours before your workout, even if you aren't thirsty. This gives your body time to absorb what it needs. Drink another 8-oz. about 15 minutes before you exercise. During exercise, drink 8-oz. of water or an electrolyte drink every 20 minutes. Don't wait until you feel thirsty. You may already be a quart or more low. When your workout is over, weigh yourself. The scale may show some weight loss, but it's not fat loss — it's water. Conditioned athletes drink a pint of water for every pound lost during a workout.

For a healing program, several types of water are worth consideration.

—**Mineral water** comes from springs with varying mineral content and widely varying taste. The natural minerals help digestion and regularity. In Europe, bottled mineral water has become a fine art, but in the U.S., it isn't tested for purity except in California and Florida.

—**Distilled water** can be from a spring or tap source; it is "de-mineralized" so that only oxygen and hydrogen remain. Distilling is accomplished by reverse osmosis, filtering or boiling, then converting to steam and recondensing. It is the purest water available.

—**Sparkling water** comes from natural carbonation in underground springs. Most bottles are also artificially infused with CO_2 to maintain a standard fizz. This water aids digestion, and is excellent in cooking to tenderize and give lightness to a recipe.

—**Artesian well water** is the Cadillac of waters. It always comes from a deep uncontaminated source, has a slight fizz from bubbling up under pressure, and is tapped by a drilled well.

Water Fluoridation's Tainted History

Historically, water fluoridation is mandated by governments but rejected by citizens. The controversy has raged since fluoride was introduced in 1945. Most developed countries have banned fluorides in their water. Japan has rejected fluoridation. Europe is 98% fluoridation-free, with active opposition in Britain, Australia and New Zealand.

The U.S. federal government continues to push for the mass fluoridation of the American water supply. Yet, even many in our government don't think it's a good idea. On July 2, 1997, the union representing all toxicologists, chemists, biologists and other professionals at the Environmental Protection Agency in Washington, D.C., went on record against the practice of adding fluoride to public drinking water, stating "As the professionals who are charged with assessing the safety of drinking water, we conclude that the health and welfare of the public is not served by the addition of fluoride to the public water supply."

The fluoridated water controversy affects every city and county in America.

If you're like most people, finding out the truth about our public water supply is a shock. After extensive research into the history of fluoride use and its results over the last two decades, as well as many conversations with scientists and knowledgeable, holistic dentists, I feel that no other substance added to food or water poses the health risks that fluoride does. Fluoride is in almost all commercial toothpastes and added to over 60% of public drinking water. Mandatory water fluoridation throughout the U.S. is either about to begin or has already been instituted.

We need to dispel the myths about fluoride. It could mean your health....

Fiction: Fluoride is safe for humans.

Fact 1: Fluoride is more toxic than lead, and even in minute doses, is damaging to brain/mind development of children. In areas where fluorosis (fluoride poisoning) is prevalent, a higher concentration of fluoride is found in fetal brain tissue of unborn children.

Fact 2: Postmenopausal women, people over 50, people with nutrient deficiencies and people with cardiovascular and kidney problems are especially affected by fluoride exposure. Our own U.S. Dept. of Health and Human Services stated in its Toxicological Profile (1993) that "postmenopausal women and elderly men in fluoridated communities may be at increased risk for bone fractures."

Fact 3: Some studies show that fluoride is linked to Alzheimer's and senile dementia. One link appears to come through a fluoride- aluminum combination in the brain. A new study shows fluoride increases the body's absorption of aluminum from deodorants, pots and pans by over 600%! The aluminum concentration in the brains of Alzheimer's patients is 15 times higher than in healthy people.

Fact 4: Hip fracture rates are much higher in people living in fluoridated communities. Fluoride's cumulative effect on bone density is devastating.

Fiction: <u>Calcium fluoride found naturally in water is safe.</u>

Fact 1: All forms of fluoride are poisonous. The most toxic forms are those with a higher solubility of free fluoride ions such as in hydrofluosilicic acid, a hazardous waste product of the phosphate fertilizer industry..... the substance routinely added to fluoridate water.

Fiction: <u>Fluoride reduces tooth decay.</u>

Fact 1: A survey by the National Institute of Dental Research shows that children who live in fluoridated areas have tooth decay rates almost identical with those who live in non-fluoridated areas. Even large-scale studies show no difference in decay rates of permanent teeth in fluoridated and non-fluoridated areas. In fact, in a recent study by the New York Department of Health, children who drank fluoridated water had <u>more</u> cavities and tooth discoloration than children who drank non-fluoridated water.

Fact 2: The U.S. National Research Council admits that dental fluorosis (fluoride poisoning causing teeth to become brittle and chip easily) affects from 8% to 51% of children drinking fluoridated water. Dental fluorosis has steadily increased since the introduction of fluoride to drinking water in 1945.

Fiction: <u>Mandatory water fluoridation is safe for the American population.</u>

Fact 1: Evidence from animal and human epidemiology studies links fluoride exposure to cancer, genetic damage, nervous system dysfunction and bone diseases. Fluoride exposure is also linked to low IQ in children.

Fiction: <u>Fluoride toothpaste is safe and prevents cavities.</u>

Fact 1: A University of Arizona study finds that the more fluoride a child drinks, the more cavities appear.

Fact 2: The poison control center receives over 11,000 calls a year for poisoning from ingesting fluoride toothpaste. In 1997, the FDA even mandated a poison warning label on fluoride toothpaste! Small children, who tend to swallow toothpaste are most at risk. Signs of fluoride poisoning include vomiting and muscle cramps.

Look for non-fluoridated toothpastes like Nature's Gate SPEARMINT or CINNAMON TOOTHPASTE at your health food store. Try Neem toothpaste, or Ayurvedic Peelu (literally "tree for tooth care"). Peelu is a natural antibacterial that removes tartar and has natural chlorine to help whiten teeth.

As we enter the new millennium our country's water supply is in a grave situation. Americans need to work hard to stop mandatory water fluoridation before it's too late. It isn't just the water we drink, it's the food we eat, too. Crops watered with fluoridated water mean fluoride is leeched into our fruits and vegetables. Not even organic produce is safe from fluoride in the water supply.

Some counties and cities are already winning the battle. After forced fluoridation by its public health service, the city of Natick, Mass mailed its water bills with a warning that pregnant women, parents of children under 3 years, and anyone with fluoride sensitivity should consult their physicians before drinking the Natick city water.

Santa Cruz, California became the first city in California (following the state fluoridation mandate of Oct. 1995) to pass an ordinance to prevent its waters from being fluoridated. Other California cities are jumping on the "no fluoridation" bandwagon as their citizens become aware and alarmed about water safety.

Massive fluoridation in our water, food, beverages, and dental products may cause massive fluoride poisoning in the U.S. population. I equate it to something like the widespread lead poisoning that decimated the health of Romans, especially the children, 2000 years ago.

If you want to help stop mandatory water fluoridation: *contact David C. Kennedy, D.D.S. @ Citizens for Safe Drinking Water 2425 3rd Ave, San Diego, CA 92101, 888-728-3833. or E-mail: davidkennedy-dds@home.com· jgreen@abac.com*
For more information about fluoride, check the internet: *www.sonic.net/~kryptox/fluoride.htm; or www.fluoridation.com.*

The beauty of self-healing is reconnecting with nature and letting your body take care of the rest.

Ann Wigmore

Caffeine in a Healing Diet?

Like most of mankind's other pleasures, there is good news and bad news about caffeine. Moderate use of caffeine has been hailed for centuries for its therapeutic benefits. Every major culture uses caffeine in some food form to overcome fatigue, handle pain, open breathways, control weight and jump-start circulation. Caffeine is a plant-derived nutraceutical - a food with medicinal attributes. Coffee, black tea, colas, sodas, chocolate and cocoa, analgesics like Excedrin, and over-the-counter stimulants like Vivarin, all have caffeine. Taking regular aspirin or an herbal pain reliever with a caffeine drink increases the pain relieving effects. Caffeine absorbs rapidly into the bloodstream. In just a few minutes, it enters all organs and tissues. Within an hour after ingestion it is distributed in body tissues in proportion to their water content. Caffeine remains in the body for only about three hours and is then excreted in the urine; it does not accumulate in body tissue.

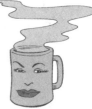

Caffeine is an effective short-term energy booster. It mobilizes fatty acids into the circulatory system, allowing greater energy production, endurance and work output. It has a direct potentiating effect on muscle contraction for both long and short-term sports and workout activity.

Caffeine has solid evidence of its effects on clearer mental performance and shortened reaction times. Caffeine stimulates serotonin, a brain neurotransmitter produced by tryptophan that increases the capacity for intellectual tasks and alertness by releasing adrenaline into the bloodstream. The net effect also decreases drowsiness and improves mood.

Caffeine promotes weight loss because it enhances thermogenesis, the conversion of stored body fat to energy. Overweight dieters don't burn enough calories during dieting. When they add caffeine, obese and post-obese people respond with greater thermogenesis. Even relatively small, commonly consumed doses of caffeine significantly influence calorie burning. Caffeine actually raises metabolic rate, and the rise lasts for several hours, far beyond its direct stimulation. One study shows that a single dose of 100mg of caffeine (the amount in a cup of coffee) increases metabolic rate 4% for up to three hours! When the same amount of caffeine was consumed at two-hour intervals for 12 hours, metabolic rate increased between 8 to 11%. These metabolic increases seem small, but over several months there is steady, substantial weight loss. Low doses of caffeine help weight control _even after_ initial weight loss because caffeine blocks appetite while keeping calorie-burning efficient.

Caffeine stimulates nerve and heart action, relaxes smooth muscles in the digestive tract and blood vessels, increases urine flow, enhances stomach acid secretion and boosts muscle strength. Research in India reports that caffeine, taken with antioxidant supplements, provides powerful protection against DNA damage by altering the behavior of a gene-damaging chemical. The DNA-protective effect was strongest with the combined coffee-antioxidant regimen than with either coffee or antioxidants alone.

Caffeine's health problems are also well known. *In excessive amounts,* caffeine has drug-like activity, causing jumpiness, nerves and heart palpitations. *In excessive amounts,* caffeine means too much oxalic acid in the system, causing health problems waiting to become diseases. It can lodge in the liver, restricting proper function, and constrict arterial blood flow. It leaches B vitamins from the body, particularly thiamine, which is needed for stress control. It depletes essential minerals, including calcium and potassium.

Like any addictive substance, caffeine is difficult to overcome, but if you have caffeine-related health problems, it is worth going through the temporary withdrawal symptoms. Improvement in the health condition is often noticed right away.

Decide for yourself. Here are the caffeine links to specific health concerns:
• **Caffeine and Bone Health:** excessive caffeine causes calcium depletion increasing risk of osteoporosis. *(Moderate amounts do not cause calcium depletion or contribute to bone loss.)*
• **Caffeine and Fertility:** caffeine seems to affect woman's health more than men's. Some experts say the more coffee a woman drinks the less likely she is to conceive, but new studies show there is no relationship between a morning cup of coffee and infertility.
• **Caffeine and Pregnancy:** avoid caffeine during pregnancy. It can affect the fetus' brain, central nervous system and circulation. High doses of caffeine can double a woman's risk of miscarriage.
• **Caffeine and PMS:** reduce, rather than avoid caffeine during menses. Caffeine causes congestion through cellular overproduction of fibrous tissue and cyst fluids. Yet low-dose caffeine intake improves memory and alertness during menses.
• **Caffeine and Breast Disease:** the link between caffeine and breast fibroids isn't official, but there is almost immediate improvement when caffeine is decreased or avoided.
• **Caffeine and Menopause:** caffeine is a trigger for hot flashes in menopausal women, and can provoke night time panic attacks in some women.
• **Caffeine and Sleep:** caffeine consumed late in the day or at night disrupts brain wave patterns. You'll take longer to get to sleep.
• **Caffeine and Severe Blood Sugar Swings:** caffeine causes the liver to release glycogen which triggers insulin release, and a sharp blood sugar drop within 1 to 2 hours.
• **Caffeine and Exhausted Adrenal Glands:** excessive caffeine exhausts the adrenals by releasing too much adrenaline; so you have less resistance to stress and are more vulnerable to hormone imbalances that affect health in both men and women.
• **Caffeine and Cancer:** studies on caffeine and cancer, particularly bladder and organ cancers, show a link but no definite causal relationship. Further, the carcinogenic effects blamed on caffeine are now thought to be caused by the hydrocarbon roasting process used in making coffee, since decaffeinated coffee is also implicated in some organ cancers. I believe the acidic body state promoted by caffeine is not beneficial to the healing process because it interferes with the way your body works to normalize its bio-chemistry during healing.
• **Caffeine and Heart Disease:** heavy coffee drinking (more than 4 cups a day), has been directly implicated in heart disease. New research shows caffeine may increase homocysteine, an amino acid whose high levels contribute to heart disease. Moderate caffeine does not appear to increase heart disease risk.

• **Caffeine and High Blood Pressure:** excessive caffeine can elevate blood pressure significantly and produce nervous anxiety. Watch out when caffeine is combined with phenyl-propanolamine, the appetite suppressant in most commercial diet pills.

• **Caffeine and Ulcers:** caffeine is not linked to gastric or duodenal ulcers, but it stimulates gastric secretions, sometimes leading to a nervous stomach or heartburn. On the good side, caffeine is a "bitter" food, stimulating bile secretion for good digestion.

• **Caffeine and Headaches:** caffeine causes headaches in some people — and withdrawal headaches when it's eliminated after regular use. Yet, strangely enough, coffee is a niacin-rich healing remedy for temporary <u>relief</u> of migraine headaches (the niacin content of coffee increases when the beans are roasted).

• **Caffeine and Asthma:** caffeine reduces asthma symptoms by dilating lung and nasal passages. Regular caffeine consumption reduces wheezing considerably. Some researchers believe this is why asthma symptoms decrease when children become adults.

• **Caffeine and Incontinence:** a 2000 study in the journal *Obsetrics and Gynecology* shows women who drink more than four cups of coffee daily double their risk of urinary incontinence. All caffeine-containing foods - coffee, tea, cola, or chocolate make urine control difficult.

Caffeine in common foods: (a pharmacologically active dose of caffeine is about 200 mg)

CAFFEINE FOOD	APPROXIMATE CAFFEINE
Coffee — 5-oz. cup Decaf	4mg
Coffee — 5-oz. cup Instant	65mg
Coffee — 5-oz. cup Percolated	110mg
Coffee — 5-oz. cup Drip	135mg
Tea — 5-oz. cup Bag, brewed 3 minutes	45mg
Tea — 5-oz. cup Loose, black, brewed 3 minutes	55mg
Tea — 5-oz. cup Loose, green, brewed 3 minutes	35mg
Tea — 5-oz. cup Iced	30mg
Cola — 12-oz. glass	45mg
Chocolate/Cocoa — 5-oz. cup	10mg
Milk chocolate — 1-oz	10mg
Bittersweet Chocolate — 1-oz	30mg

You can break the caffeine habit more easily with herb teas, caffeine-free coffee substitutes, and energy supportive herbal pick-me-ups with no harmful stimulants of any kind. Use green tea and kola nut as bio-active forms of caffeine for weight loss and mental clarity. Neither has the heated hydrocarbons of coffee.

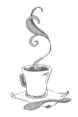

Tea and Your Healing Diet

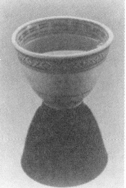

Black and green teas have caffeine. Is it different than the caffeine in coffee or chocolate? All black, green and Oolong teas come from one plant, *thea sinensis*, an incredibly productive shrub that ranges from the Mediterranean to the tropics. Tea leaves can be harvested every 6 to 14 days for 25 to 50 years! Tea is defined by the way its leaves are processed. For green tea, the first tender leaves of spring are picked, rolled, steamed, crushed and dried with hot air. Green tea leaves are not fermented. Oolong tea leaves are semi-fermented for one hour. Black tea is fermented for 3 hours, then often scented with spices to strengthen aroma and reduce bitterness.

How does tea fit into a healing diet? Both green tea and black tea have enzymes that promote digestion and help our bodies kill antibiotic-resistant bacteria like *Staphylococcus aureus*. High flavonoids in both teas reduce harmful blood clotting linked to heart attacks. Both contain polyphenols that bind to mouth bacteria as a shield to strengthen tooth enamel against plaque. Polyphenols (not tannins as commonly believed) act as antioxidants but don't interfere with iron or protein absorption. The natural, bioactive caffeine contained in both black tea (50 to 80mg per cup) and green tea (about 30mg per cup) helps combat mental fatigue.

Yet far more health benefits lie in green tea. It contains larger amounts of healing nutrients..... twice as much vitamin C, more than twice the amount of bioflavonoids and six times the antioxidant activity of black tea. Two cups a day of green tea can meet the body's daily requirements for bioactive bioflavonoids. Green tea is highly enzyme-active for weight loss. It is a good fasting tea, providing energy support and clearer thinking during cleansing. Green tea is a vasodilator and smooth muscle relaxer with theophylline for bronchial dilating help against asthma.

Should you be drinking a daily cup of green tea for better health? Modern science validates green tea's broad spectrum of traditional health benefits. Most studies center around the more than 200 different catechin polyphenol compounds that make up about 35% of green tea. The polyphenols lower cholesterol, and protect against cancer by thwarting nitrosamines that produce cancer-causing substances. Research at the American Health Foundation in New York shows that green tea's anticarcinogens are anti-mutant factors "preventing activation of carcinogens so that free radicals never even form."

One green tea compound, EECG (epigallocatechin-3 gallate), has formidably high levels of free-radical-scavenging activity. Green tea's EECG is 30 times more powerful than vitamin E against DNA-destroying attacks. Black tea loses its EECG and other beneficial polyphenols entirely during fermentation. Scientists also believe EECG is the substance that inhibits the enzyme urokinase, crucial for cancer growth and metastasis. EECG attaches to urokinase and prevents it from invading cells to form tumors. Some cancer tests show that EECG may even engender a process called apoptosis, in which cancer cells shrivel and die.

More amazing, research shows that green tea's caffeine is a delivery system for therapeutic catechins like EECG. A cup of green tea contains 100 to 200mg of EECG. Scientists believe <u>2 to to 4 cups per day may actually provide cancer protection.</u>

Green tea has an astounding catalog of curative applications.

—<u>**Green tea is antibacterial,**</u> a quality known for 5,000 years by the Chinese, who used it to purify water. Abundant polyphenol compounds in green tea provide antimicrobial action against a wide range of pathogens that cause food poisoning, and streptococcus mutans, a mouth bacterium that forms tooth decay and may cause serious illness if it establishes in sterile parts of the body like the heart valve. Green tea's antibacterial activity also provides protection against dental caries and strengthens tooth enamel against plaque.

Note: Don't add milk to green tea. Milk inhibits absorption of the protective polyphenols.

—<u>**Green tea provides protection against esophageal and oral cancers,**</u> according to the American National Cancer Institute. *Note: To fully benefit from green tea's anti-cancer properties, pour hot, not boiling water over the tea leaves.*

—<u>**Green tea reduces the risk for colon and pancreatic cancers,**</u> with benefits strongest for women who drink it once a week for six months. A dual study by the Shanghai Cancer Institute and the U.S. National Cancer Institute also shows that green tea increases female fertility through its body-balancing effects.

—<u>**Green tea reduces the risk of several environmentally induced cancers.**</u> Research in Japan on stomach, skin and lung cancers, where people drink large amounts of green tea shows a low incidence of these cancers. The large Japanese study showed that drinking several cups daily of green tea was effective in reducing lung cancer death rates even in men who smoked two packs of cigarettes a day. Smoking is far more prevalent in Japan than in the U.S., but the instance of lung cancer is much lower, indicating to researchers that green tea protects against lung cancer.

—<u>**Green tea may protect our skin against radiation damage.**</u> As the ozone layer thins and UV radiation increases, skin cancers have risen sharply throughout the world, in some continents reaching epidemic proportions. In a Rutgers University study, green tea showed good results against skin cancer when it was taken before and during exposure to UV rays.

—<u>**Green tea is an antimicrobial body freshener.**</u> Acne, cuts, sunburn and athlete's foot all benefit from a cool green tea bath.

—<u>**Green tea offers significant heart protection.**</u> Its catechins are potent inhibitors of blood clumping which leads to atherosclerosis. The catechins also suppress the formation of the angiotensin I conversion enzyme which contributes to high blood pressure.

—<u>**Green tea increases elimination of harmful blood lipids to prevent the oxidation of LDL cholesterol.**</u> University of Kansas research shows that green tea is over 100 times more effective than Vitamin C at protecting cells from heart disease damage, and 25 times more effective than Vitamin E as a heart protecting antioxidant.

—**<u>Green tea promotes fat burning</u>,** regulates blood sugar and insulin, and has a satiating and tension calming effect during dieting.

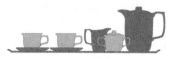

Tea nomenclature can be confusing. Names like oolong, black or jasmine tea refer to how the tea leaf is processed. Names like Assam, Darjeeling or Ceylon, etc., refer to region where the tea is grown. Names like pekoe, orange pekoe, etc., refer to leaf size.

• **Green tea (bancha)** - tender spring leaves of the Japanese tea plant. (See above.)
• **Green tea (kukicha)** - a Japanese tea, made from roasted twigs rather than the leaves of the tea plant. Kukicha is a favorite in macrobiotic diets for its blood cleansing qualities, high bioavailable calcium, and mellow, smooth flavor.
• **Darjeeling** - the finest, most delicately flavored of the black Indian teas.
• **Earl Grey** - a popular, hearty, aromatic black tea scented with bergamot oil.
• **English Breakfast** - a connoisseur's rich, mellow, fragrant black tea.
• **Ceylon** - a tea grown in Sri Lanka with a intense, flowery aroma and flavor.
• **Irish Breakfast** - a combination of Assam and Ceylon flowery orange pekoes.
• **Jasmine** - a black tea scented with white jasmine flowers during firing.
• **Lapsang Souchong** - a fine black tea with a strong, smoky flavor.
• **Oolong** - a complex, delicate tea, semi-fermented, fired in baskets over hot coals.

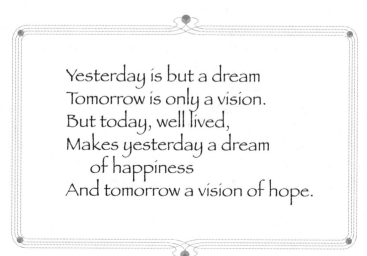

Yesterday is but a dream
Tomorrow is only a vision.
But today, well lived,
Makes yesterday a dream
    of happiness
And tomorrow a vision of hope.

Does Wine Fit into a Healing Diet?

Naturally fermented wine is still a living food. It is a complex biological fluid possessing definite physiological values. Records dating back 4,000 years refer to wine as a food, a medicine, a part of religious ceremonies and a pleasing element in social life.

Wine is much more than an alcoholic beverage - and vastly more complex than beer or spirits. It is never boiled, so its biologically active compounds are not destroyed or altered by heat. Many small, family owned wineries make chemical and additive-free wines that retain their nutrients, including B vitamins, and minerals like potassium, magnesium, calcium, organic sodium, iron and phosphorus.

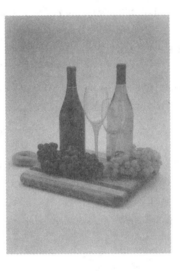

Wine has significant
is a mild tranquilizer for the
Davis research on wine tannins
may cut coronary heart disease
clot formation, and consider-
wine reduces blood platelet
lesterol levels, and lowers dan-
protect against heart disease
Wine is a cultured food,
zyme activity in the same way
do. Wine boosts circulation, re-
acid production. It is superior
nervous tension. It is important
glass of wine relaxes. When you

health benefits. In moderation, it
heart and blood pressure. U.C.
shows that two glasses of wine a day
risk by 50%, help prevent blood
ably reduce stress. Tannin-rich red
stickiness, increases good HDL cho-
gerous LDL cholesterol levels to
and atherosclerosis.
so it helps digestion by boosting en-
yogurt and other fermented foods
lieves pain and reduces excess body
to tranquilizers or drugs for easing
in a weight loss program, because a
are relaxed, you tend to eat less.

Wine is full of antioxidants. Recent studies at U.C. Berkeley show that red wine is rich in polyphenols, powerful antioxidants that help neutralize free radicals which damage DNA and alter body chemistry. Wine antioxidants, along with its carotenes like lutein and zeaxanthin, are significant protectors for the eyes. A new study reveals that just drinking 2 to 4 glasses of wine a month can cut the risk of macular degeneration (the leading cause of blindness in people over 60) by over 20 percent. A study of wine antioxidants by the *Epidemiology Journal*, shows that its polyphenols even help prevent hepatitis A virus replication.

Wine is a more powerful anti-microbial against common bacteria than some drugs. It can, for example, reduce the growth of some harmful stomach bacteria colonies within 20 minutes. Bismuth salicylate, a pharmaceutical remedy for traveller's diarrhea, takes two hours to do the same job. The latest research shows wine can successfully counter the food and water-borne micro-organisms that cause digestive havoc and upset tummies referred to as "Delhi belly," and "Montezuma's revenge".

There's much more......

—**Quercetin,** an antioxidant flavonoid in red wine may be one of the most powerful anticancer agents ever discovered. Early results show that quercetin reverses tumor development by blocking the conversion of normal body cells to cancer cells. Quercetin activity is boosted by the wine fermentation process and by friendly flora in our intestinal tracts. Quercetin also normalizes insulin release levels, so it prevents some complications of diabetes like cataracts, diabetic retinopathy (blindness), neuropathy (nerve damage) and nephropathy (kidney damage). Doctors use quercetin in wine as a potent free radical scavenger against HIV infection, because wine also relieves AIDS pain and stress.

Scientists believe that *resveratrol,* a compound in red grape skins, is a key to wine drinkers' healthy cholesterol levels. *Resveratrol* also seems to prevent blood platelet aggregation, and reduce blood clotting in arteries narrowed by years of heavy fat consumption. In nature, *resveratrol* fights off fungal disease for the grape plants. In animal tests, *resveratrol* stops production of abnormal cells, like cancer cells at three separate stages of development — inhibiting the enzyme cyclooxygenase that stimulates tumor growth.

Are sulfites in wine really a health hazard? Sulfur dioxide (SO_2) is a naturally occurring sulfite that protects the wine's character by inhibiting the growth of molds and bacteria. Wine yeasts naturally produce up to 20 parts per million of SO_2 during fermentation. (Human bodies produce about 1,000mg of sulfites a day in our normal biochemical processes.) Top European winemakers have counted on sulfur dioxide to prevent wine spoilage for centuries. In a method used since Roman, even Egyptian times, today's winemakers use mined SO_2 heated into a liquid, to protect wine from oxidizing.

What is organic wine? The health dangers of pesticides on grapes mean that wines made from organically grown grapes are increasingly popular in both Europe and California. To a purist organic wine means wine made from organically-grown grapes, without using sulfites, yeast, bentonite, egg whites, gasses like N_2 or CO_2 in the process. To most people an "organic" wine label signifies only whether sulfites have been added or not.

In 1988, following a food-borne sulfites scare, the U.S. ATF required alcoholic beverages of all kinds, both imported and domestic, to carry a "CONTAINS SULFITES" label if there were more than 10 parts per million sulfites in the beverage, regardless of whether sulfites had actually been added. This hasty ruling became, and still is, a major problem for winemakers, especially when wine has **naturally-occurring** sulfites at this level.

Are both red and white wines healthy? Research shows that phenol compounds in both red and white wine reduce LDL oxidation, platelet formation and the fat buildup in the arteries. Both white and red wines seem to be protective for women against heart disease.

Note: I don't recommend any alcoholic drinks other than wine during a healing program, even for cooking. Although most people can stand a little hard liquor without undue effect, and alcohol burns off in cooking, concentrated sugar residues won't help a recovering body.

Fats and Oils in a Healing Diet

The debate about fat has filled the American media for more than a decade, but much of the information is contradictory and inaccurate. Most people know today that there is a direct relationship between the quantity of fat we consume and the quality of health we can expect. **Yet, in the last half of the 20th century, Americans have increased their intake of fat calories by over 33%, especially omega-6 fats.**

The link between high salt and fat intake on health has also become clear. **Too much salt inhibits the body's capacity to clear fat from the blood.** Yet, in the last thirty years, Americans have consumed more salt than ever before, largely because we eat almost 50% more restaurant and pre-prepared foods than our parents did. Much of this food is fried and salty, or salt-preserved (animal foods), and full of spicy or salty condiments.

We need to clear up the confusion about fats and oils, so you can make the best choices for your healing diet. Regardless of its "bad press," our bodies need fat to keep warm, protect body tissues and organs and supply us with energy. Fat is the most concentrated source of energy in our diets, providing nine calories per gram of energy compared to four calories per gram from carbohydrates or protein. Fat even helps us use carbohydrates and proteins more efficiently by slowing down digestive processes.

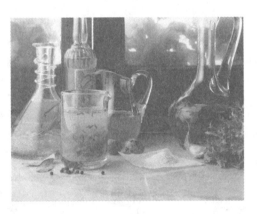

Fat supplies essential 74). We need fat for ing cholesterol and for mone-like body regulatory found effect on body in- releases a hormone in the nin that sends the brain a has been satisfied so that fat in order to absorb fat- K. Fats elevate our calcium for strong bones and elas- fatty acids, (see EFA's page healthy skin, for metaboliz- prostaglandin balance, (hor- substances that have a pro- flammatory processes). Fat stomach called cholecystoki- "full" message when hunger we don't overeat. We need soluble vitamins A, D, E and levels and transport calcium tic muscles.

But not all fats are alike. What is the difference between saturated, poly-unsaturated and mono-unsaturated fats?

The difference is in molecular structure. All fat molecules are composed of carbon and hydrogen atoms. A saturated fatty acid has the maximum possible number of hydrogen atoms attached to every carbon atom — hence the term "saturated." An unsaturated fatty acid is missing one pair of hydrogen atoms in the middle of the molecule — a gap called an "unsaturation." A fatty acid with one gap is said to be "monounsaturated." Fatty acids missing more than one pair of hydrogen atoms are called "polyunsaturated."

Animal foods have more saturated fat, and except for palm oil and coconut oil, plant foods have more unsaturated fats. Saturated fats, like butter, meat and dairy fats, shortening and lard, are solid at room temperature. They are the culprits that clog the arteries and lead to heart disease. Saturated fats tend to thicken the blood, causing blood pressure to rise and increasing the work load on your heart. They also promote blood stickiness, exaggerate plaque build-up on the arteries and reduce oxygen availability to your heart muscle. Unsaturated fats, both mono and polyunsaturated, like seafood, plant or nut oils, are liquid at room temperature. Although research supports unsaturated fats as helping to reduce cholesterol, just switching to unsaturated fats <u>without increasing dietary fiber</u> will not bring about health improvement. For the best benefits, eat moderate amounts of unsaturated fats along with a high fiber diet.

Is there a health difference between polyunsaturated and monounsaturated fats?

Monounsaturated fats, in seafoods, avocados, nuts, olive oil, canola and peanut oil, are considered the healthiest fats. Monounsaturated oils are rich in fatty acids and important for normalizing prostaglandin levels. Tests show that eating moderate amounts of unrefined, monounsaturated oils also significantly lower allergic reactions.

Polyunsaturated fats, in seafoods, walnuts and vegetable oils, are healthier than saturated fats, but not as healthy as monounsaturated fats. Polyunsaturated vegetable oils are good sources for "essential fatty acids" (linoleic, linolenic and arachidonic acids) necessary for cell membrane function, balanced prostaglandin production and metabolic processes. Good polyunsaturates include sunflower, safflower, sesame oil, and flax oil.

Are all plant oils unsaturated fats?

All plant oils are cholesterol-free, but commercial oils go through several processing stages to prevent rancidity. Refined oils are degummed, de-pigmented through charcoal or clay, clarified by deodorizing under high heat, and chemically preserved. Unfortunately, processing also destroys healthy antioxidants and forms hazardous free radicals. Refined oils are clear, odorless..... and almost totally devoid of nutrients.

—**Unrefined vegetable oils** are the least processed and most natural. They are mechanically pressed and filtered (cold pressing applies only to olive oil). They have small amounts of sediment, and taste and smell like the nut, seed or fruit they came from.

—**Solvent-extracted oil** is a second pressing from the first pressing residue. The petroleum chemical *hexane* is generally used to get the most efficient extraction; even though minute amounts of *hexane* remain, it is still considered an unrefined oil.

Note 1: **Vegetable oils are traditionally seen as top dietary sources of essential fatty acids. New research shows this to be true only of cold pressed olive oils. Commercial oils contain such a large number of contaminants and are so heavily processed that they can no longer be regarded as good sources of EFAs.**

Note 2: **Heat and air exposure easily cause unrefined oils to spoil, so store them in an air-tight container in a cool dark cupboard (65°F) or the fridge. Purchase small bottles if you don't use much oil in your cooking.**

What are hydrogenated fats?

All fats, especially unsaturated fats, tend to break down when exposed to air. To delay rancidity, hydrogenation bubbles hydrogen molecules through a polyunsaturated oil to reconstruct its chemical bonds for more stability. For example, hydrogenation converts liquid corn oil to a semi-solid form — margarine. Some tests show that these altered fats are comparable to animal fats in terms of saturation and effects by the body.

What are trans fats? Why are they such a problem for our health?

Trans fatty acids are byproducts of hydrogenation. When hydrogen molecules are added back to a polyunsaturated fatty acid, some of the hydrogenated fatty acids take on a "straight" structure, and become trans fatty acids. Originally only used for foods like shortening and margarine, today trans fats are now part of most snack foods, pastries and desserts. Some researchers think they may be real villains in America's health problems.

Here's why:

Trans fatty acids raise blood cholesterol almost as much as saturated fat. They may even be worse. Where saturated fats increase <u>both</u> LDL and HDL cholesterol levels, trans fats <u>increase</u> LDL cholesterol, and <u>decrease</u> HDL cholesterol, the good cholesterol which actually helps clear arteries. Trans fats have been linked to more cancer risk, premature skin aging and lowered immune response by impairing prostaglandin and cell functions. Most significant, they interfere with the metabolism of natural fats and with the body's ability to utilize essential fatty acids.

How do you know if trans fats are part of the foods you buy?

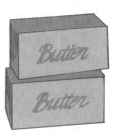

You don't. Trans fats are not saturated, monounsaturated, or polyunsaturated, so food labels don't have to disclose how much a food has. Foods with "partially hydrogenated oil" in their ingredient lists have trans fats, but some foods have only slightly hydrogenated oils with tiny amounts of trans fats. Other foods contain heavily hydrogenated oils. FDA limits the saturated fat in foods labeled "no-cholesterol" or "low-cholesterol." But there is no label requirement <u>or limit</u> on the trans fats allowed in those same foods.

What about margarine? We used to think it was healthier than butter. Is it?

Margarine products today are lower in calories, total fat, saturated fat and trans fats than ever before. Many are made from soy oil, so they are cholesterol-free and contain vitamin E. Most are sold in a squeeze tube, soft and liquid, meaning thay have low amounts of trans fatty acids.

Yet margarine manufacturerers are allowed to omit trans fats from their labels. Since margarine is a main source of polyunsaturated fats in the American diet, hopefully this consumer information problem can soon be solved. A good, low saturated fat alternative to margarine or shortening is a combination of equal amounts of warm butter and vegetable oil.

What are essential fatty acids?

Essential fatty acids (EFA's), are the healthy fats that do the job of protecting our bodies from degenerative disease and boosting our brain power. EFA's help us maintain energy, insulate our body, and protect our tissues and organs.

Essential fatty acids (EFAs) and the essential amino acids from which protein is made, are indispensable to each other and work synergistically in our bodies. Together they form lipoproteins, the organic compounds that make up our bodies.

Like other essential nutrients, fatty acids AA-arachidonic acid, ALA-omega 3, LA-omega 6, DHA-docosahexaenoic acid, EPA-eicosapentaenoic acid and GLA-gamma linolenic acid, are nutrients your body needs, but cannot make for itself. A healthy body can make GLA from linoleic acid (LA), the most common fatty acid in foods, but that ability is impaired if your body is deficient in zinc, magnesium and vitamins A, B_6, B_3 and C. Conversion is also blocked if the diet is high in saturated fats or hydrogenated oils.

—EFA's are major components of hemoglobin production and cell membranes; without them the membranes would become stiff and lose their ability to function.
—EFA's are significant components of nerve cells. They are central to the cascade that converts the cells into prostaglandins, hormone-like messengers that are instrumental in energy production, essential to circulatory health, and integral to good metabolism. Low EFA's disconnect the hormone-prostaglandin cascade.
—EFA's play an important role in regulating blood trigylceride levels.
—EFA's impact our growth, vitality, and mental state, by connecting oxygen, electron transport, and energy in the body's vital oxidation processes.

An amazing amount of scientific research has been done on the effects of essential fatty acids for specific ailments. Here are some of the positive results:

—EFA's make up over 60% of the brain's dry weight which supports the vital transmission of nerve impulses. A deficiency of EFA's rapidly leads to learning impairment and recall capacity. A severe EFA deficiency may lead to attention deficit disorder (ADD), violent behavior, memory loss, autism, mental retardation, anxiety-depression syndromes, senility or seizures.
—EFA's inhibit harmful blood clots in the arteries, and help prevent cardiovascular damage through significant antioxidant and anti-bacterial activity.
—EFA's reduce the risk of breast and colon cancer, and inhibit tumor growth.
—EFA's help reduce the inflammation of arthritis (rheumatoid and osteo), Parkinson's and MS.
—EFA's are significant for healthy skin and hair. In fact, EFA deficiency is involved in most serious skin diseases like eczema, dermatitis, psoriasis, acne and hair loss.
—EFA's reduce irritability and depression associated with PMS and menopause through their involvement in the hormone-prostaglandin cascade process.
—EFA's, especially linoleic acid, LNA and CLA (conjugated linoleic acid), fight fat. They protect against damage from hard fats, because they repel their stickiness and disperse them in the body. The more saturated fats you eat, the more EFA's you need.

Warning: If you're on a serious weight loss diet, you should know that a very low-fat diet may cause a deficiency in EFA's. The first sign of a deficiency may be dermatitis — red, dry, scaly skin that appears first on the face, clustered near the oil-secreting glands (in the folds of the nose, lips, forehead, eyes and cheeks). Dry, rough areas may also appear on the forearms, thighs and buttocks. A diet rich in plant foods results in low levels of saturated fat and relatively higher levels of essential fatty acids.

Scientific research continues. Here are recent successes for EFA treatment:
- Autoimmune disorders — chronic fatigue syndrome, Lupus (SLE) and fibromyalgia
- Hypertension and high blood pressure
- Certain cases of schizophrenia
- Childhood infections, especially recurrent respiratory problems like asthma
- Neurologic conditions - multiple sclerosis, Guillaume Barre syndrome
- Reynauds disease (unexplained cold hands and feet)
- Chronic headaches especially from drug, caffeine or alcohol withdrawal symptoms
- Lowered incidence of anaphylactic shock from allergic reactions
- Colon and bowel inflammatory conditions like Crohn's disease and I.B.S.
- Adult onset diabetes
- Scleroderma

We hear a lot about Omega-3 and Omega-6 health oils today. What are they?

Omega oils contain a family of fatty acids — EPA (eicosapentaenoic acid), DHA (docosahexaenoic acid), CLA (conjugated linoleic acid), LNA (alpha linolenic acid) and GLA (gamma linolenic acid). Omega oils are found in walnut, canola and wheat germ oil, dark greens like spinach, and herbs like evening primrose oil, ginger and flax, but the richest Omega oils come from the sea. Omega oils are synthesized by plankton at the base of the ocean food chain. They are in the tissues of all sea life, both plant and animal.

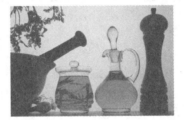

Omega-3 and Omega-6 fatty acids differ in chemical structure, but both are important in maintaining proper body fat balance. They are equally important in the development and levels of prostaglandins, the essential hormone-like substances that control reproduction and fertility, inflammation reactions, immunity and cell communications.

Clinical results show a long list of benefits for Omega oils - smoother skin, smoother muscle action, stronger cardiovascular performance and better digestion. Health problems like P.M.S., high blood pressure and rheumatoid arthritis all improve from treatment with omega fatty acids.

Omega oils effectively lower cholesterol for the 30% of America's population who need diet help to lower their cholesterol levels. Research shows that omega oils reduce excess blood fats of all kinds - slowing down the rate at which the liver produces harmful triglycerides.

Omega oils help prevent artery blood clots, by inhibiting excess production of thromboxane which promotes clotting. They improve circulation by vasodilation, allowing more blood to reach the muscles, relaxing blood vessels and increasing oxygen supply. Enhanced blood flow is important in lowering high blood pressure, may even repair some damage caused by clogged arteries, and relieve the chest pain of coronary heart disease.

Omega-3 oils are abundant in sea foods, sea greens, flaxseed oil, perilla oil and purslane (the dark green vegetable highest in omega 3's). Omega-3 fatty acids increase metabolism, rid your body of excess fluids, increase energy and reduce your risk of heart disease. If you're experiencing reduced vision and unexplained mood swings, you may have an omega-3 deficiency.

Omega-3 oils are precursors for series 3 prostaglandins (PGE 3), which help balance cholesterol by raising HDLs and decreasing triglycerides. PGE 3 prostaglandins also enhance lymph function for immune response, inhibit platelet aggregation to fight atherosclerosis and protect against cancer growth by suppressing malignant cell division.

Omega-6 fatty acids are found in plant oils like black currant seed, borage, flaxseed, walnut, chestnut, soy, hemp and primrose oil. Linoleic acid (LA), gamma-linolenic acid (GLA) and its derivative, conjugated linoleic acid (CLA) belong to the omega-6 family of oils. Alpha-linolenic acid (LNA), is the omega-6 essential fatty acid in flax oil. Omega-6 oils are precursors for series 1 prostaglandins (PGE1) needed for T-lymphocyte immune function, kidney health, protection against tumors, low cholesterol levels and inhibiting blood platelet stickiness.

A closer look at some of the beneficial fatty acids in omega oils.

Omega-3 fatty acids, **DHA and EPA**, are naturally found in fish, sea vegetables, marine algae and eggs; they are synthesized from LNA in the body. Experts have known for years that fish eaters suffer less heart disease, and have lower cholesterol and triglyceride levels than those who don't eat fish. Both DHA and EPA support coronary health. EPA, however, especially from salmon and herring is given the major credit for heart protection. Its primary medicinal uses today are to improve cholesterol levels, and to thin the blood to prevent re-clogging of arteries after balloon angioplasty (especially promising treatment for the elderly who regularly experience re-clogging).

Both EPA and DHA help overcome food allergies. Both help clear skin inflammatory diseases like eczema and psoriasis. Both benefit inflammatory rheumatoid arthritis. More studies are currently being done on the ability of EPA and DHA to eliminate binging and food addiction during dieting, help burn fats and increase stamina by supporting good liver function, and on their positive effects for kidney disease.

Does non-insulin dependent diabetes benefit from treatment with fish oil EPA?

There is conflicting information about EPA from fish oil for diabetics. Early 90's studies showed that fish oil supplements might raise blood sugar levels, a health risk for type II diabetes or clinical hypoglycemia. Newer data in the American Journal of Clinical Nutrition reports that fish oil supplements are <u>NOT</u> linked to higher blood sugar or insulin. Further, research from Mayo clinic reveals fish oil <u>REDUCES</u> high triglycerides in type 2 diabetics without affecting glucose levels. More information is needed. If you have blood sugar disturbances, use fish oil supplements under professional supervision.

<u>DHA is the most predominant EFA in our brain tissue.</u> Low levels of DHA are linked to mental problems like depression, memory loss, attention deficit disorders, hostility, Alzheimer's and senility. Both DHA and EPA help protect against Alzheimer's and promote clearer thinking.

—DHA significantly lowers blood fats, normalizing high cholesterol and triglyceride levels.

—DHA is a large part of the retina of the eye and is needed for good eye function.

—DHA is the most abundant fatty acid in breast milk. Recent studies show that American women have the lowest levels in the world of DHA and pregnancy depletes stores even further.

—DHA, like EPA, is a marine lipid from sea foods and sea plants. Since our body's ability to make these EFA's decreases as we age, eating more of these foods helps boost their levels.

CLA is a relatively new discovery getting a lot of media attention.

CLA *(conjugated linoleic acid)* occurs naturally in dairy products, especially cheese, lamb, sunflower oil and beef. (Its discovery occurred during scientific studies on the cancer-causing substances in beef where it was found to actually inhibit cancer growth.) CLA is popular among athletes for increasing muscle mass and burning fat because it plays a role in muscle growth and is able to convert the most energy from the least amount of food. Like other fatty acids, CLA has powerful antioxidants for immune health and shows remarkable results for lowering cholesterol.

CLA studies were the first to show that fats can help you lose fat. CLA especially inhibits the body's mechanism for storing *saturated* fat by boosting its ability to use fat reserves for energy. The more saturated fat you eat, the more CLA you need. Since Americans are eating more vegetable oils, chicken and fish, and reducing their dairy and meat intake, CLA has dropped in our diets over the last 20 years. Some researchers speculate that the marked increase in body fat in the American population may be due to CLA decrease.

Is GLA the most bioactive fatty acid? My healing observations show that it is.

GLA *(Gamma Linolenic Acid - an omega-6 fatty acid)* is made in the body from LA *(linoleic acid)*. LA itself is an omega-6 fatty acid found abundantly in most vegetable oils. GLA can also be obtained from evening primrose oil (the most bio-active), black currant or borage seed oil.

GLA is a source of cell energy and helps the body burn fat instead of storing it. It's part of the team of structural fats that form the brain, bone marrow, cell membranes and muscles. It acts as electrical insulation for nerve fibers, is an anti-coagulant and an anti-inflammatory. GLA is significant as a precursor of prostaglandins which regulate hormone and metabolic functions.

GLA is therapy for breast tenderness during PMS, for menopause symptoms like vaginal dryness, for better nerve transmission in M.S cases, for weight loss, for the swelling, pain and morning stiffness of arthritis, chronic fatigue syndrome, heart health, diabetes, eczema, hyperactivity in children, schizophrenia and skin or hair dryness.

What about hemp seed oil? Experts say it has the most broad spectrum, most remarkable fatty acid profile we know. It has GLA, absent from the fats we normally eat. Hemp contains a perfect balance of omega and gamma fatty acids — a ratio of 3:1.

Hemp has been used for thousands of years as a valuable resource of seeds, oil and medicine, and as fiber for clothes and rope. It's popularity is rising as people once again learn about its rich nutritional properties. Hemp seeds contain 25% high quality protein and 40% fat with high amounts of EFA's - Omega-6 *(Linoleic Acid- 58%)*, Omega-3 *(Alpha-Linolenic Acid-20%)*, Omega-9 *(Oleic Acid-11%)*, Saturated Fatty Acids- 9% and GLA *(Gamma Linolenic Acid- 2%)*.

Research shows that hemp oil has anti-inflammatory properties highly useful as a topical first aid for wounds and burns. It stimulates the growth and health of skin, hair and nails. Many cosmetic manufacturers are using hemp's rich EFA's as a primary ingredient in skin products.

Hemp oil is a light green color, has a distinct, nutty flavor and is good in salad dressings, spreads, dips and baked potato mixed with fresh herbs. Hemp oil is <u>not</u> good for cooking; it shouldn't be heated above 120°F/49°C. Keep hemp oil refrigerated. Buy unrefined, unfumigated, residue-free oil like Omega Nutrition Virgin Hemp Seed Oil.

**<u>Does hemp seed oil alter your consciousness?</u> *Hemp seed oil DOES NOT contain the psychoactive marijuana compound, THC (tetra-hydrocannabinol). THC exists in the resin produced by the flowering tops of female plants before the seeds mature. <u>Hemp seed oil</u> is perfectly legal and not psychoactive. Canada passed an Industrial Hemp Act in 1998 so that this remarkable plant could be used for its nutritional benefits. Unfortunately, hemp is still illegal to grow in the U.S.*

Are coconut oil, palm oil and other tropical oils healthy?

Coconut oil, maligned for decades in attacks by the American Soybean Association, is making a comeback for its taste and therapeutic value. The sponsored studies were used to promote polyunsaturated oils and replace the use of tropical oils. Coconut oil was falsely accused. Scientists now know that the studies were flawed and the conclusions of the studies were incorrect. The true villains were actually found to be hydrogenated oil products along with a lack of healthy EFA's in the diet. For more than forty years, however, the negative publicity caused a coconut oil scare and set fire to the foundation of its popularity.

What's the real picture on coconut oil?

You may be avoiding coconut oil because you've read that it's over 90% saturated fatty acids (SFA), and therefore unhealthy. The truth is there are two kinds of saturated fats - long chain and medium chain. Long chain saturated fats (LCT's) are associated with "bad" cholesterol, **medium chain saturates or triglycerides (MCT's)** like those in coconut oil provide energy and do not clog arteries like the long chain group. MCT's help your body metabolize fat efficiently, so that the fats provide energy instead of being stored.

MCT's are easily digested so coconut oil is useful for people who have trouble digesting fat. Natural practitioners use a formula with coconut oil MCT's for patients with malabsorption problems, like those with eating disorders who cannot digest conventional fats. Infant formula with coconut MCT's can be a lifesaver for premature babies.

Common misconceptions of coconut oil are that it raises blood cholesterol, causes heart disease and obesity. However, coconut oil does not cause heart disease nor raise blood cholesterol in a normal diet. Studies show coconut oil has a neutral effect on blood cholesterol. Polynesian islanders, who have gotten most of their fat calories from coconut oil for centuries *have an exceedingly low rate of heart disease.*

Coconut oil is actually a good choice if you are a dieter, body builder or athlete concerned about weight and body fat. Coconut oil is <u>less likely</u> than other oils to cause obesity, because the body easily converts its calories into energy rather than depositing them as body fat.

Coconut oil contains an antimicrobial element, *Lauric Acid* (almost 50% of its fatty acid content), a rare disease fighting fatty acid. It's also found in mother's milk and protects an infant from infections. Coconut oil is one of the few plant sources of *lauric acid*. It is excellent for immune-compromised conditions like HIV, fibromyalgia and lupus, respiratory infections like chronic bronchitis and pneumonia, and as an immune boosting agent. For example, natives who live in the tropics, an ideal environment for parasites, use coconut oil in their food and on their skin and hair to protect themselves from infections.

Coconut oil is a good cooking oil with a sweet, tropical flavor. Compared to flax oil, which has alpha-linolenic acid easily oxidized by heating, the SFA's of coconut oil are 300 times more resistant to oxidation. It is a healthy alternative to refined oils and hydrogenated vegetable oils, such as margarine. It may be used in place of butter - use three-quarters the amount of coconut butter to obtain the same baking results. Omega Nutrition COCONUT BUTTER is made from 100% organic, unrefined coconut oil.

Why is coconut oil hard to find? Unfortunately, more than forty years of false dietary information have taken their toll in the marketplace. Today, slowly the general public is catching on to the truth. Coconut oil is still one of the best kept nutritional secrets, but the new, more balanced information means that this healthy oil will finally rise out of the ashes of unfair publicity like a phoenix to take its place in our healing pantheon.

Is palm oil good for you? It's another tropical oil that's received a great deal of negative publicity. Palm oil was falsely accused under the same series of polyunsaturated oil tests. Once again, all the evidence wasn't taken into account. Like coconut oil, palm oil is high in saturated fats, but no discernment was made between the two kinds of saturated fats - long chain and medium chain. (See previous page.) Palm oil, too, was accused of hiking blood cholesterol levels and contributing to clogging of the arteries.

In fact, of all the commonly used vegetable oils, palm oil is the most versatile. Even after refining, palm oil keeps all the characteristics required for its wide variety of uses without needing hydrogenation - the big health culprit. As with coconut oil, several new studies show that even a diet high in palm oil doesn't boost cholesterol in people with normal levels. Palm oil is a rich source of beta carotene and vitamin E.

The main drawback to palm oil, as it is used today, is that it is usually heavily refined (coconut oil is not) which depletes its nutrient value and makes it harder for the body to digest. For this reason, I recommend avoiding palm oil in a healing diet.

How do you maintain the right balance of fats in your diet?

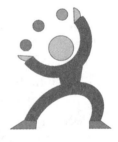

As we fight the battle of the bulge in America we have seriously disrupted our fat balance. We've cut back on saturated fat from meats and dairy foods and increased our intake of omega-6's from corn and soybean oils. In the U.S. we eat the highest amount of omega-6 fatty acids of any people on Earth! The animals we eat are fed a diet high in omega-6 oils, so we get even more omega 6's when we eat them.

A good ratio of omega 6 to omega 3 fatty acids may be about 1:1, (the ratio our primitive forebears lived on), but diet amounts for modern man are 10 to 20 parts Omega-6 oils to 1 part Omega-3's, a highly unbalanced ratio. Americans are eating 10:1, even 40:1! The result for health? Experts say that an overload of Omega-6 fatty acids leads to bio-chemistry changes that increase risk for heart disease. Further, an overload of Omega 6's causes the body to overproduce certain prostaglandins, hormone-like substances that have pro-inflammatory and pro-clotting effects!

Take a look at your diet. If you eat a lot of vegetable oils and animal foods, you may be getting too many Omega 6's. Reduce your ratio of these foods for better fat balance.

Here's an easy way to do it. Simply increase your intake of omega-3 fatty acid foods like fish, flaxseed and dark green vegetables. They help your body compete with the production of omega 6 prostaglandins, and reduce their adverse effects.

Why is Mother's milk the best for balancing your baby's fats? Breast milk contains the full range of EFA's needed for proper development of a child's central nervous system, brain and eyes. An 18 year study published in the journal of Pediatrics shows that breast-feeding your baby may make him or her smarter throughout life, giving your child an academic advantage! The determining factor seems to be the high content of DHA in breast milk, an essential fatty acid which comprises over 50% of the brain.

Cholesterol and Triglycerides

Cholesterol and triglycerides are part body lipids — the fats and fat-like substances essential to human health. Lipids are in every cell - integral to membrane, blood and tissue structure, hormone-prostaglandin production, and nervous system function. Lipids are dynamic in the body. A good example of a highly active fat is "brown fat" (brown adipose tissue or BAT), which has a very high metabolic rate capable of burning large amounts of calories, stimulating thermogenesis, and assisting weight control.

Triglycerides are dietary fats used by the body as fuel and as energy for metabolism.

Cholesterol is a phospholipid fat like lecithin, made by the liver for cell membranes, nerve fibers, brain tissue, bile salts and to produce sex hormones.

Facts about cholesterol:

—Vitamin D is synthesized from cholesterol for calcium metabolism.

—Lower than normal cholesterol levels may mean anemia, autoimmune disorders and excess thyroid function.

—About 10 percent of the dry weight of your brain is cholesterol. You don't need to eat dietary cholesterol because your liver and brain make about 1.5 gm. of cholesterol every day to insure your body has enough. Only animal foods have dietary cholesterol. If you eat a typical U.S. diet, high in animal foods, you probably get too much dietary cholesterol.

—Cholesterol travels in the blood bound to lipoproteins, molecules of fat and protein, LDL-cholesterol (bad) is carried in low-density lipoproteins (most cholesterol is this type). HDL-cholesterol (good) is carried in high-density lipoproteins. LDL cholesterol deposits fatty cholesterol on arterial walls, narrowing them, impeding blood flow from the heart, and increasing the risk of heart attack. High levels of LDL cause atherosclerosis, and accrue in the gall bladder causing gallstones. HDL-cholesterol protects your heart. HDL clears fat away from artery walls and returns it to the liver for excretion.

—Your cholesterol "number" refers to the total amount of cholesterol in your blood measured in milligrams per deciliter (mg/dl) of blood. Most experts recommend that total blood cholesterol be kept below 200 mg/dl to avoid risk of coronary heart disease.

81

—A low-cholesterol diet is not the same thing as a <u>cholesterol-lowering</u> diet. Foods that <u>have</u> cholesterol do not necessarily <u>raise</u> your cholesterol. Cholesterol levels are regulated by the body, which will produce less itself when more cholesterol is taken in through food. Conversely, reduced consumption of cholesterol spurs the body to increase its own production.

Saturated fat is the real culprit. Cholesterol-free foods may still be full of saturated fat. The best way to lower your cholesterol level is to attain the proper weight for your height, reduce your intake of saturated fat and eat plenty of fiber.

Facts about triglycerides:

Triglycerides consist of three fats (saturated, monounsaturated, and polyunsaturated fat) and a glyceride molecule. They make up 95% of our dietary fats. If you take in more calories than your body needs, the extra calories are converted by your liver to triglycerides, then transported to fat cells for storage. In fact, body fat is made up largely of stored triglycerides. Unlike cholesterol, triglycerides are used up when your body needs extra energy. Triglycerides increase with weight gain and decrease with physical activity.

Excess triglycerides develop into a fat stomach or fat thighs because they are stored in fat cells that can increase up to fifty times in size to handle them. New fat cells form when existing cells are full. By the time we see fatty bulges in these regions, the other storage areas are already full.

Between meals, and at night, the liver produces triglyceride-rich particles called very-low-density-lipoproteins (VLDLs). VLDLs distribute triglyceride particles into the blood to deliver their energy. But, as the triglycerides shed their buoyant fats they become LDLs, bad cholesterol.

Most people who have high LDL-cholesterol and low HDL-cholesterol have elevated triglycerides and are at more risk for heart disease. People with diabetes or kidney disease, conditions that increase risk of heart disease, are also prone to high triglycerides.

High sugar intake is implicated in high triglycerides. In fact, a low-fat, but high-carbohydrate diet (white flour, sugary foods, sodas, alcohol), raises triglycerides and lowers HDL's, a bad situation. **You can significantly reduce your triglycerides.** The first lines of defense against high triglycerides are weight loss by reducing saturated fat and sugary foods, regular exercise, stopping smoking, and a high fiber diet. A largely vegetarian diet can do wonders.

A normal triglyceride level should be below 200mg/dl. Borderline levels are 250 to 400mg/dl. High levels are 400 to 1000mg/dl. Very high triglycerides are over 1000mg/dl.

What about the new synthetic "designer fats?"

Fake fats have the potential of becoming a substantial portion of your diet if you substitute them for fat, (fat is 33 to 35% of the nutrients most Americans eat). Synthetic fats are formed by chemical combinations of sucrose (sugar) with fatty acids to give them properties similar to those of a naturally-occurring fat so they can pass through the digestive tract. But the synthetic substitutes are undigestible, provide no calories or nutrients and are not absorbed into the body.

What effect do fake fats have on your intestines if they are not absorbed? The composition of fake fat chemicals raises major health concerns. Even the FDA requires a warning about loose stools and abdominal cramping for synthetic fat foods.

Do fake fats interfere with absorption of other nutrients or with drugs? When a synthetic fat dissolves in natural fat, the fake fat carries the natural one out of the body. But during this process, the fake fat molecules also absorb and eliminate fat-soluble vitamins, like A, E, D and K, critical to your body's hormone and weight balance. Fake fat manufacturers know this and have temporarily curbed the unhealthy nutrient outflow by saturating the synthetic fat with fat-soluble vitamins. More worrying, fake fats also rob the body of carotenoids. Research from the Harvard School of Public Health shows that eating just one-ounce of olestra potato chips daily can reduce blood carotene levels by 50%! Some experts now believe the fats may increase the risk of cancer, heart disease and blindness, because they lower critical blood carotenes.

Synthetic fat causes immediate digestive problems when you eat a lot of it. As the fake fat works its way through the digestive tract, your body eliminates it as a greasy stool often accompanied by diarrhea. The yucky side effects and discomfort may be a good thing if it discourages people from eating the fake fat.

Even losing weight by eating fake fats instead of real fats is unlikely because fake fats fool only your tastebuds, not your stomach. In one study where synthetic fats were used in place of natural fat, people simply increased their intake of protein and carbohydrates to get needed nutrients. Total diet calories remained the same.

In another study, people who replaced 20% of their fat intake with fake fats were still hungry at the end of the day, even though they had eaten twice as much food as normal!

In a Netherlands study, fake fat (olestra) consumption reduced lutein levels 20% after only two weeks, increasing risk for macular degeneration, the leading cause of blindness in the elderly.

Can fake fats lower your fat intake enough to improve your heart health? I believe the body imbalancing, nutrient-robbing qualities of synthetic fats far outweigh any fat reduction benefits. Researchers say that the amount of dietary fat cut out by fake fats probably won't lower the risk of heart disease for most adults..... and might even increase the hazard for some. Fat makes up 34% of the American diet today, close to the 30% level recommended by heart organizations.

What's the verdict on fats? You need fat in your diet, but the right kind of fat is critical.

Some suggestions for healthy fat consumption:
• Avoid processed fats: refined oils, partially hydrogenated oils and foods that contain them. Buy unrefined oils instead, and keep them in dark containers, tightly covered and refrigerated. The more unsaturated a fat is the more sensitive it is to light and heat.
• Eat essential fatty acids every day: nuts, seeds, greens like spinach, sea vegetables and fish. If you don't eat many of these foods, or need more EFA's, get extra EFA's from herbal supplements.
• Buy organic oils, meats and dairy foods. Fats within foods store fat-soluble toxins.
•Avoid fat free, sugar-y, processed foods because sugar raises blood triglycerides.

In a nutshell, here are the best fats and oils for a healing diet.
(See previous pages for information about hemp, coconut and palm oils.)

—**Almond oil** is a 70% monounsaturated fat, with at least 39mg/100g of vitamin E. Almond oil is rich in vitamin A, a natural antioxidant, a specific for eye health and a lung cancer protector. While effective in treating gastric ulcers and as an intestinal cleanser, almond oil is most often used externally to soothe sunburned skin, and as a massage oil.

—**Apricot kernel oil,** largely composed of 74% oleic and linoleic fatty acids, is a primary source of laetrile (vitamin B-17), indicated by some studies as an effective cancer treatment, reducing tumor size as well as inhibiting further progression of tumorous growths. Other studies show B-17 is useful in treating hypertension and rheumatism. Using B-17 to treat any disease is illegal in the U.S., so here, its use is strictly cosmetic.

—**Canola oil** from rapeseeds, is full of healthy unsaturated fats and omega 3 fatty acids. Extensive research shows canola oil can be a key factor in reducing LDL cholesterol levels without disrupting HDL levels. Some tests show that adhesions to artery walls and blood clots can be prevented by consumption of canola oil. Canola inhibits tumor growth, aids asthmatic breathing difficulty, and helps maintain healthy skin. Current studies show canola oil may also be useful against breast and pancreatic cancers.

—**Castor oil** relieves constipation by stimulating intestinal contractions that cause bowels to move. As an external poultice, castor oil dissolves cysts, tumors and warts. As an emollient, it softens and dissolves scars. Nursing mothers rub castor oil on their nipples for soreness. *Caution: Prolonged use damages intestinal lining, and reduces absorption of minerals like sodium and potassium.*

—**Flax seed oil** is rich in omega 3 fatty acids, polyunsaturated and monounsaturated fats. Flax seed oil helps regulate blood pressure, lowers cholesterol, metabolizes calcium and boosts energy. It aids mood disorders, low vitality, liver and cancer conditions (increasing T-cell levels), and even renews radiation damaged cells. Used topically, flax seed oil helps prevent the development of stretch marks after childbirth.

—**Grapeseed oil,** made from grapeseeds after wine is pressed, is high in polyunsaturated fat (72%). Grapeseed oil is a strong antioxidant, helpful in preventing heart disease, clogged arteries and blood clots, and good for maintaining cholesterol balance. Its higher smoke point (485°F) is better tasting and a better choice than olive oil in the kitchen.

—**Olive oil,** a monounsaturated oil, is rich in essential fatty acids. Olive oil improves bile flow for gall bladder and liver, strengthens body tissue and acts as a nerve tonic. It has a mild laxative effect, soothes mucous membranes and can dissolve LDL cholesterol buildup. Olive oil lowers blood pressure by thinning the blood to prevent harmful blood clots. Olive oil may inhibit breast cancer. A June 1995 issue of Cancer Causes by the Harvard School of Public Health noted that women who eat olive oil more than once a day have a much lower rate of breast cancer than women who use it less frequently.

—**Perilla oil** is rich in linolenic acid. Recent studies show that small amounts of perilla oil can suppress the development of aberrant *crypt foci* thus acting as a possible preventative agent in the early stage of colon carcinogenesis.

—**Safflower oil,** from safflower plant seeds, has the highest percentage of unsaturated fats and linoleic acid of any oil. It has the ability to neutralize uric acid better than water. (Water tends to bind with toxins and harden, causing emergemce of fatty tissue and cellulite.) Safflower oil has a soothing effect on the intestines and is reputed as a digestive aid. It has a tendency to go rancid quickly. Keep safflower oil refrigerated.

—**Sesame oil,** created from pressed seeds of the sesame plant, is rich in monounsaturated (40%) and polyunsaturated (42%) fatty acids. It contains sesamol, a natural preservative highly resistant to rancidity. Sesame oil is ideal in macrobiotic cooking. Also rich in lecithin, sesame oil can build the central nervous system, circulation and brain health, thus improving depression and stress symptoms. Massaging sesame oil on sunburn or minor skin eruptions will provide relief. I find it's a perfect skin-softening make-up remover.

—**Sunflower oil,** a 20% protein oil, is high in beneficial oils like lecithin, linoleic acid and vitamin E. Sunflower oil helps the endocrine and nervous systems form new tissue, resist disease and reduce cholesterol levels. Just one tablespoon daily may reverse polyneuritis paralysis, and substantially reduce symptoms of multiple sclerosis.

—**Walnut oil,** a good source of oleic and linoleic acid, can lower your chance of developing heart disease by increasing HDL - good cholesterol.

—**Wheat germ oil, from the embryo of the wheat berry,** is a premier antioxidant with measurable amounts of vitamin E and octacosonal. One tablespoon provides the antioxidant equivalent of an oxygen tent for 30 minutes. It's rich in inositol, a chemical that enhances fat metabolism, and contains a full range of B-vitamins to promote digestion, absorption of nutrients and bowel function. Wheat germ oil goes rancid within one week of opening; buy nitrogen-flushed packaging and keep refrigerated.

The hardest thing in life is learning which bridge to cross and which bridge to burn.

Dairy Foods in a Healing Diet

I believe you should avoid dairy foods during a cleansing diet, especially during a mucous cleansing diet. Dairy products interfere with the cleansing-healing process because their density and high saturated fats challenge both digestion and metabolism. Dairy foods are tremendous mucous producers that burden the respiratory, digestive and immune systems. Cow's milk in particular has clogging properties for many people. Pasteurized milk is a relatively dead food as far as nutrition is concerned. Even raw milk can be difficult to assimilate for someone with respiratory problems.

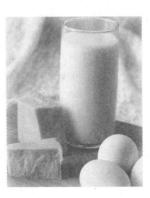

One-quarter of Americans have an intolerance to dairy foods. They experience allergy reactions, poor digestion and mucous build-up from dairy intake. Besides a lactose sensitivity, many people process some proteins in cow's milk poorly, throwing off excess from cheeses, cream, ice cream and milk. For humans, milk-digesting lactase levels are at their highest immediately after birth, decreasing after weaning. So dairy foods become harder to digest as we age, accumulating strain and mucous clogs on eliminative organs. Even people without great sensitivity to dairy foods report an energy rise when they reduce their dairy intake.

Children can be especially susceptible to dairy reactions. Besides childhood allergies, cow's milk can cause loss of iron and hemoglobin in infants by triggering blood loss from the intestinal tract. Heavy consumption of milk, especially by small children, may result in vitamin D toxicity. Some research shows that iron absorption is blocked by as much as 60% after dairy products are eaten in a meal. Studies in the New England Journal of Medicine show that children who are not given cow's milk products during infancy have a dramatically lower risk of diabetes later in life. The culprit appears to be a cow's milk protein — *bovine serum albumin,* which differs just enough from human proteins to cause an anti-body reaction. The antibodies attack and destroy insulin-producing beta cells in the pancreas, increasing the chance of diabetes.

When dairy foods are removed from the diet of mucous clogged children, enlarged tonsils and adenoids shrink, a clear sign of immune relief. Doctors who put children on dairy-free diets often report a marked reduction in colds, flu, sinus and ear infections.

Women do not handle dense dairy products as well as men. Their systems back up more easily, so less dairy (especially cheese) usually means easier bowel movements for women. Female problems, like fibroids, bladder and kidney ailments can also be improved by avoiding dairy. A sugar in dairy products, galactose, may even be fatal to a woman's eggs, impacting her fertility. When a women is having trouble getting pregnant, I usually recommend that she reduce her dairy consumption first.

Isn't calcium from dairy foods good for us? Contrary to advertising, dairy products are not a very good source of calcium for people. We don't absorb dairy calcium well because of an unbalanced ratio with phosphorus, high fat content, and pasteurizing and processing. Even in cattle tests, calves given their own mother's milk that had first been pasteurized, didn't live six weeks!

Hormone residues, pesticides and additives used in modern cattle-raising inhibit absorption of calcium and other minerals. In contrast, calcium from green leafy vegetables is easily absorbed. One study compared the absorption of calcium from a leafy green, kale, with the absorption from cow's milk. The absorbed amount of calcium from kale was 41%, compared to 32% from milk.

Besides leafy greens, other vegetables, nuts, seeds, fish and soy foods have measurable amounts of absorbable calcium, along with minerals like magnesium, potassium and zinc that are easy for us to assimilate. Herbs, like sea plants, borage seed, pau d'arco, valerian, wild lettuce, nettles, burdock and yellow dock offer healing concentrations of calcium.

Dairy foods aren't even a very usable source of protein for humans. Cow's milk has proteins that are harmful to our immune systems, (see previous page). Repeated exposure to these proteins disrupts normal immune response. Fish and poultry proteins are much less damaging; plant proteins pose the least hazard.

I advise soy milk, soy cheese, tofu, and nut milks in place of dairy products. At the least, use low-fat or non-fat products, and goat's milk, raw milk and raw cheeses instead of pasteurized. Kefir and yogurt, although made from milk, don't have the absorption problems of dairy foods. Unless lactose intolerance is severe, cultured foods don't cause a lactose reaction, and they help you heal through friendly cultures without the downside of dairy.

For long range diets, consider most dairy products as good for taste, but questionable for nutrition. **A little is fine - a lot is not.** Small changes in your cooking habits and point of view are all it takes - mostly a matter of not having dairy products around the house, and substituting dairy-free alternatives in your recipes. (See Food Exchanges section pg. 136.) Reducing your dairy intake usually means some weight loss, too, as well as lower blood pressure and cholesterol levels. Soon, you won't feel deprived at all, just delighted.

How specific dairy foods can affect your healing diet:

• <u>**What about butter?**</u> Surprise! Butter is okay in moderation. Although a saturated fat, butter is relatively stable, and like raw cream, is a whole, balanced food, used by the body better than its separate components. When butter is needed, use raw, unsalted butter, not margarine or shortening that are full of trans fats. Don't let it get hot enough to smoke. If you want less saturated fat, use clarified butter. Simply melt the butter and skim off the top foam. Let it rest a few minutes and spoon off the clear butter for use. Discard whey solids that settle to the bottom, and the foam.

• <u>**There's good news about eggs**</u>! "Eggsperts" are realizing what many of us in the whole foods world have long known. Although high in cholesterol, eggs are <u>also high in balancing lecithins and phosphatides</u>, so they don't increase the risk of atherosclerosis. Nutrition-rich fertile eggs from free-run chickens are a perfect food. The difference in fertile eggs compared to eggs from commercial egg factories is remarkable; the yolk color is brighter, the flavor fresher, the workability in recipes better. The distinction is most noticeable in poached and baked eggs, where the yolks rise higher. Eggs should be lightly cooked for the best nutrition, poached, soft-boiled, hard boiled or baked, never fried. Eggs are concentrated protein; use them with discretion.

• <u>**The saturated fats in cheese make it hard for a healing diet to succeed.**</u> Commercial cheeses, even when labeled "natural," contain bleaches, coagulants, emulsifiers, moisture absorbants, mold inhibitors and rind dyes that visibly leak into the cheese itself. Many restaurant and pizza cheeses are loaded with synthetic flavors, colors and preservatives. Processed cheese foods (like Velveeta) get their texture from hydrogenated fats rather than natural fermentation. Even if you're not on a healing diet, limit your cheese consumption to small amounts 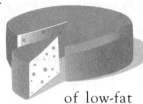 of low-fat or raw cheeses that provide usable proteins with good mineral ratios. Low sodium, low fat cheeses are a better choice for a healing program. Raw cheeses are superior in taste and health value to pasteurized cheeses, which have higher salts and additives.

<u>Options to make your cheese choice healthier:</u>

—**Rennet-free cheese** uses a bacteria culture, instead of calves' enzymes to separate curds and whey. Rennet, the dried extract of the enzyme rennin, is derived from the stomach of a suckling calf or a lamb. It speeds up the separation process of cheese making.

—**Goat cheese (chevre) and sheep's milk cheese (feta)** are both lower in fat than cow's milk cheeses, and more easily digested. There is a world of difference in taste.

—**Real mozzarella cheese** is from buffalo or sheep's milk - low fat, and delicious!

—**Raw cream cheese** is light years ahead of commercial brands with gums, fillers, thickeners.

—**Lowfat cottage cheese**, a cultured dairy product, is a good substitute for ricotta, cream cheese, and processed cottage cheese foods that are full of chemicals. Usually okay for those with a slight lactose intolerance, cottage cheese mixes well with non-fat or low-fat plain yogurt to add the richness of cream or sour cream to recipes without the fat.

—**Yogurt cheese** is easy to make, lighter in fat and calories than sour cream or cream cheese, but has all the richness and texture. See "Cultured Foods," page 56 for how to make fresh yogurt cheese.

—**Kefir cheese** is an excellent replacement for dairy products in dips and other recipes. (I like it better.) Widely available in health food stores, kefir cheese is low in fat and calories, and has a slightly tangy, rich flavor that really enhances snack foods. Use it cup for cup in place of sour cream, cottage cheese, cream cheese, ricotta or pot cheese.

—**Tofu**, a white digestible cheese-y curd made from fermented soybeans, is one of the best replacements for cheese, in texture, taste and nutritional content. It is high in protein, low in fat, versatile and easy to use in place of sour cream, cheese, milk and cottage cheese in cooking. Try tofu in place of eggs in quick breads, cakes, custard-based dishes, quiches and frittatas.

—**Rice cheese** is low in fat and sodium, and fairly high in calcium, and vitamins E and A. It is delicious, tastes amazingly like dairy cheese and comes in a variety of flavors (swiss, jalapeño jack, mozarrella and cheddar). Like rice milk from which it's made, rice cheese is easy to digest; its smooth texture makes it perfect for melting on snacks, veggie burgers or casseroles.

—**Soy cheese**, made from soy milk, is a non-dairy cheese free of lactose and cholesterol. A minute amount of calcium caseinate (milk protein) is added for melting. Mozarrella, cheddar, jack and cream cheese are available. Use it cup for cup in place of cheese.

Apart from how dairy foods affect healing ability, there are debatable issues surrounding the manufacture of dairy foods that influence your health. There is a whirlwind of controversy about rBST *(recombinant bovine somatotrophin)* and rBGH *(recombinant bovine growth hormone)*. The hormones increase milk production, but since America always has a surplus milk supply, and long-standing dairy subsidies, it's hard to see why an American dairy farmer would use a potentially harmful hormone in order to produce even more surplus milk. We know little about long-term effects of these hormones. We do know they increase mastitis infections in treated cows, leading to more use of antibiotics to treat the mastitis. This, of course, leads to higher levels of antibiotics in the milk, widely questioned by scientists and concerned consumers alike.

All over the world, modern medicine is losing the battle against the onslaught of new drug-resistant pathogens. <u>**Some researchers believe that even moderate use of antibiotics in an animal's feed can result in antibiotic resistance in the animal's bacteria, and a transfer of that resistance to human bacteria.**</u> A 1997 peer-reviewed study, in the *International Journal of Health Services*, says that genetically engineered rBGH may promote breast and colon cancer, acromegaly, hypertension, diabetes and breast growth in men. Even the milk itself from hormone-treated cows is not as wholesome. It has less protein and higher levels of saturated fat.

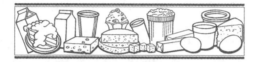

—<u>**Pesticides seem to concentrate in the milk of both farm animals and humans.**</u> A study by the Environmental Defense Fund found widespread pesticide contamination of human breast milk among 1,400 women in forty-six states (1997). The levels of contamination were twice as high among meat-and-dairy-eating women as among vegetarians.

—<u>**Ovarian cancer rates parallel dairy-consumption patterns around the world.**</u> The culprit is galactose, a milk sugar from lactose. Women with ovarian cancer often have trouble breaking down galactose. Test animals fed galactose develop ovarian cancer. There are no clear signs of digestive upset, but a new series of enzyme tests can tell you whether you lack the proper enzymes.

—<u>**Cow's milk is associated with insulin-dependent diabetes.**</u> The milk protein *bovine serum albumin* (BSA) leads to an autoimmune reaction in the pancreas impairing its ability to produce insulin. Exposure to large amounts of cow's milk in a child's diet may lead to juvenile diabetes.

—<u>**Dairy proteins may play a major role in onset of non-Hodgkin's lymphoma,**</u> an immune system cancer. A 1989 study and a growing consensus among scientists shows that high levels of the cow's milk protein beta-lactoglobulin are found in the blood of lung cancer patients as well.

—<u>**Bovine leukemia virus is found in 3 out of 5 dairy cows in the United States!**</u> In about 80% of U.S. dairy herds, a large percentage is contaminated when the milk is pooled for distribution. Pasteurization, if done correctly, kills the virus, but the issue continues to haunt, because the percentage of cattle with the virus is so large.

<u>Are you lactose intolerant?</u> Do you have gas, bloating, cramps, nausea or diarrhea from 30 minutes to 2 hours after eating dairy foods?

Good dairy substitutes. *(See also* FOOD EXCHANGES *section on pg. 136.)*
—**<u>Kefir</u>** is a cultured food made by adding kefir grains (natural milk proteins available at health food stores), to milk and letting the mixture incubate overnight at room temperature to milkshake consistency. Kefir has 350mg of calcium per cup. Use the plain flavor cup for cup as a replacement for whole milk, buttermilk or half and half; use fruit flavors in sweet baked dishes.

—**<u>Soy milk</u>** is nutritious, versatile, smooth, delicious, lactose and cholesterol-free, (substituting soy milk for dairy milk in your diet can help reduce serum cholesterol). Soy milk contains less calcium and calories than milk, but more protein and iron. It adds a slight rise to baked goods. Use it cup for cup for milk in cooking — plain flavor for savory dishes, vanilla for sweet dishes or on cereal. (Soy ice cream, frozen desserts, soy yogurt and soy mayonnaise are also available.)

—**<u>Rice milk</u>** is rich and creamy, but much lower in fat and calories than regular cow's milk. Rice milk contains vitamin E and calcium, and is an especially good choice for people with digestive problems or who have food allergies. Extremely popular, ice milk comes in a variety of flavors.

—**<u>Almond milk</u>** is a rich, non-dairy liquid. Use it 1 to 1 in place of milk in baking, sauces, gravies, cream soups and drinks. <u>For 1 cup almond milk</u>: place 1 cup blanched almonds in a blender; add 2 to 4 cups water, depending on consistency. Add 1 tsp. honey; whirl until smooth.

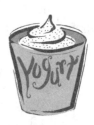

—**<u>Sesame tahini</u>** is rich, creamy, ground sesame seed butter. Use tahini as a dairy replacement in soups, dressings or sauces.... no cholesterol yet all the protein. Substitute tahini mixed with water to milk consistency as a milk substitute in baking. Use it in healthy candies and cookies, and on toast in place of peanut butter. Mix tahini with oil and seasonings for an excellent salad topping to greens and salad ingredients.

—**<u>Yogurt</u>** helps balance and replace friendly flora in the G.I. tract. It's culturing process makes it a living food. Yogurt contains more bioavailable protein and easily absorbed calcium than milk, a good thing for people at risk for osteoporosis.
Most yogurts contain the friendly bacteria *Lactobacillus bulgaricus, Streptococcus thermophilus* and *Lactobacillus acidophilus.* Even if you have a lactase enzyme deficiency, bacterial fermentation cultures in yogurt actually substitute for the missing enzyme to help you digest lactose. Yogurt also kills bacteria which causes most ulcers and gastritis. Yogurt boosts blood levels of gamma interferon, a component of the immune system that rallies killer cells to fight infections. The lactic acid bacteria in yogurt lowers levels of enzymes responsible for the development of colon cancer. Yogurt is also a good food treatment for children with diarrhea, especially if the diarrhea is aggravated by antibiotics.

<u>What's really low-fat?</u> Here's the strange low-down on low-fat milk.
—Two percent (reduced fat) milk is actually 35% fat.
—One percent (low-fat) milk is actually 25% fat by calories.
—Skim milk is called "fat free" or "non-fat."

Sugar and Sweeteners: Are They all Bad?

Is the bad health rap on sugar too extreme?

Sugar in America is synonymous with fun, good times and snacking. Our culture instills the powerful urge for sweetness from an early age. Sugar qualifies as America's favorite but most poorly understood drug, the food we eat to "cope" in times of stress and tension. Easily our most addictive food, it affects almost every body system with its highly concentrated power. (It takes 16 feet of 1-inch diameter sugar cane to produce 1 teaspoon of refined sugar.)

For the average American, almost 20% of daily calories come from refined white sugar. That works out to about 150 pounds of sugar per year - a substantial amount when you realize that sugar often replaces more nutritious foods in our diets.

Refined sugar actually first appeared as a "military drug" in The War of 1812 - as an energy source for Napoleon's army. (Interestingly, he lost his first battle.) Sugar existed this way, as a medicinal, all through the last century, only entering the food supply at the beginning of the 1900's.

There's some good news about sugar. It offers quick energy, helps metabolism, and brings closure to digestion, the reason we traditionally eat sweet things at the end of a meal. New research shows that some warnings about sugar have been overstated. For example, in regard to weight gain, a little sugar can actually suppress appetite, reducing the likelihood of overeating. The sugar in most snacks and desserts is less fattening than fat. Fat not only contributes more calories, but the calories are metabolized differently in the body, causing more weight gain than sugar. Sugar can also improve the taste of complex carbohydrate foods which are better for you than fatty foods.

But sugar can cause major interference in a healing program.

Refined sugar is sucrose, the ultimate naked carbohydrate - stripped of all nutritional benefits. Sugars include white, raw, brown and turbinado, yellow D and sucanat. All sugars can be addictive; most add nothing but calories to your body. Like a drug or alcohol, sugar affects the brain first, offering a false energy lift that eventually lets you down lower than when you started.

Large amounts of sugar-filled foods raise your insulin production resulting in problems like diabetes, hypoglycemia, high triglycerides and high blood pressure.

Raised insulin is also your body's signal to store fat. Sugar needs insulin for metabolism. Eating a lot of sugar means some of those calories become fat instead of energy. Excess sugar is metabolized into fat globules and distributed over storage areas like your stomach, hips and chin.

Too much sugar upsets mineral balances like magnesium and zinc. Sugar especially drains calcium, which accelerates aging and overloads your body with acid-ash residues responsible for much of arthritic stiffening. Sugar ties up and dissolves B vitamins, producing over-acid conditions that become gout, nerve, gum and digestive problems. A high sugar diet puts you more at risk for infection because it provides a breeding ground for staph and yeast infections. Funguses and parasites thrive on sugary foods.

91

Excess sugar depresses immune response. It's linked to high cholesterol, heart disease and coronary thrombosis. Studies implicate sugar in nearsightedness and skin problems like eczema and psoriasis. A study at the University of Alabama shows that people suffering from depression have less symptoms when they eat less sugar. Other research shows that when women switch from a diet high in sugar to a sugar-free, high nutrient diet, their food addictive behavior stops.

Personality-changing, mental and emotional signs of too much sugar:
—irritability, irrational mood swings
—chronic or frequent bouts of depression with manic-depressive tendencies
—difficulty concentrating, forgetfulness or absent-mindedness
—lack of motivation, loss of enthusiasm for plans and projects
—increasing undependability, inconsistent thoughts and actions
—moody personality changes with emotional outbursts

Physical effects of eating too much sugar:
—anxiety episodes and panic attacks
—bulimia eating disorder
—candidiasis and chronic fatigue syndrome
—diabetes and-or hypoglycemia
—food addiction with loss of B-vitamins and minerals
—menopausal mood swings and unusual low energy periods
—obesity
—high cholesterol and triglycerides leading to risk of atherosclerosis
—excessive emotional swings and food cravings, especially before menstruation
—tooth decay and gum disease

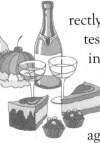

The inability to use glucose correctly affects millions of Americans. At least twenty million of us suffer from diabetes (high blood sugar) or hypoglycemia (low blood sugar). Glucose is the main sugar in the blood and brain. Under ideal conditions, glucose is released into the bloodstream slowly to maintain balanced blood sugar levels. Small blood sugar fluctuations disturb a normal feeling of well being. Large blood sugar fluctuations cause feelings of depression, anxiety, mood swings, fatigue, even aggressive behavior.

Foods that affect your sugar balance have a major impact on your healing program.

Hypoglycemia, often called a "sugar epidemic," in America is widespread in every industrialized country today. It's a direct effect of too much sugar and refined carbohydrates, coupled with low fiber foods. The pancreas reacts to too much sugar by producing too much insulin. The excess insulin lowers blood sugar too much as the body strives to achieve normal glucose-insulin balance. Hypoglycemia results.

Hypoglycemia is marked by dozens of unpleasant symptoms, especially in the way the brain functions. The brain requires glucose as an energy source to think clearly, and is the most sensitive organ to blood sugar levels. Worst case scenario reactions of hypoglycemia can even range to unconsciousness or death.

Diabetes, another "civilization" disease, also results from too much sugar, refined carbohydrates and caffeine. Chronic hypoglycemia often precedes diabetes. When your body doesn't use carbohydrates correctly, it may produce too little insulin, so blood sugar levels stay too high. The pancreas can't work properly, glucose can't enter the cells to provide energy. Instead, it accumulates in the blood, resulting in serious symptoms from mental confusion to uncontrollable obesity, to blindness, even to coma.

While seeming to be opposite problems, diabetes and hypoglycemia really stem from the same cause - an imbalance between glucose and oxygen in the body. Poor nutrition, the common cause of both disorders, can be improved with a high mineral, high fiber diet, adequate protein, small frequent meals, and regular mild exercise. Either condition requires diet and lifestyle change for there to be a real or permanent cure. Alcohol, caffeine, refined sugars and tobacco must be avoided.

Note: Even though poor sugar metabolism causes both diabetes and hypoglycemia, the different effects of each problem call for specific therapies. Get better body response by addressing low blood sugar and high blood sugar separately. See *Diabetes and Hypoglycemia Diets*, pg. 404 and 408.

There are many healthy alternatives to refined sugar.

Just because you follow a sugar-free diet doesn't mean you have to give up good taste or sweetness. Food sweeteners like honey, molasses, maple syrup, fruit juice or barley malt can satisfy your sweet tooth. Your body metabolizes them much more easily. These natural sweeteners are heroes in the effort to control sugar balance and sugar cravings. Clinical tests on crystalline fructose, and the herbs *stevia rebaudiana* and *gymnema sylvestre*, show good results even for people with sugar disorders. But they do not eliminate hypoglycemia or diabetes. Only a better diet and regular exercise make a permanent difference.

Note: When looking for a natural sugar, always look for the least processed product. Most commercial sweeteners bear no resemblance to their natural counterpart. For example, before sugar cane (the worst culprit), is refined and bleached, it is rich in vitamins and minerals.

Some sweet choices to consider for your healing diet:

• **Crystalline fructose** is a commercially produced sugar with the same molecular structure as that in fruit. It is called fruit sugar, but it's usually refined from corn starch today. It has a low glycemic index, meaning that it releases glucose into the bloodstream slowly. Fructose produces liver glycogen rapidly making it a more efficient energy source than other sweeteners. It is almost twice as sweet as sugar, so less is needed for the same sweetening power.

Fructose may be the sweetener of choice in a weight loss diet. In clinical tests before meals, subjects who drank liquids sweetened with fructose ate 20 to 40% fewer calories than normal, more than compensating for the 200 calories in the fructose. Those who drank liquids sweetened with table sugar ate 10 to 15% fewer calories; those who drank liquids sweetened with NutraSweet, Equal (aspartame commercial sweeteners) ate the same amount of calories as normal. Fructose also helps reduce cravings for fatty foods. In dental studies, dentists report less plaque and tartar with fructose than with sugar.

Fructose is as common in prepared foods as sucrose. Does it have drawbacks? Data on fructose's chemical structure shows that its highly reactive molecules bind to protein molecules. The protein-fructose interaction sometimes alters the structure of enzymes and their proteins, which results in tissue or organ damage and may be involved in diabetics. Fructose also inhibits copper absorption, essential to the production of hemoglobin and for maintaining a healthy cardiovascular system. New information indicates it may also stimulate high cholesterol levels levels.

Lack of critical information is another problem. Products labeled fructose can be pure fructose, 90% fructose or high fructose corn syrup (55% fructose which contains a high percentage of glucose needing insulin for metabolism).

Bottom line? It seems there are advantages to fructose, but if you are hypoglycemic or diabetic, fructose is still sugar and should be avoided.

• **Stevia rebaudiana,** (sweet herb), is a South American sweetening leaf. It is totally non-caloric, and about 25 times sweeter than sugar when made as an infusion with 1 tsp. leaves to 1 cup of water. Two drops of the infusion equal 1 teaspoon of sugar in sweetness. In baking, 1 teaspoon of finely ground stevia powder is equal to 1 cup of sugar.

Research shows that stevia can actually regulate blood sugar. (In South America, stevia is sold <u>as an aid</u> to people with diabetes and hypoglycemia.) Stevia helps lower high blood pressure but does not affect normal blood pressure. Frequent stevia users claim it inhibits tooth decay, aids mental alertness, counteracts fatigue and improves their digestion.

Stevia has been used as a natural sweetener in South America for over 1500 years; clinical studies indicate it is safe even in cases of severe sugar imbalance. In the 1970's, the Japanese refined the sweet glycosides from stevia to make a product called Stevioside, 300 times sweeter than sugar. Stevioside is currently used as a non-calorie sweetener in South America and the Orient where it enjoys a 42% share of the food sweetener market. While Stevioside does not affect blood glucose levels and is a good sweetener for both diabetics and hypoglycemics, it does not retain the extraordinary healing benefits of whole stevia leaves and extract.

Unlike other sweeteners, stevia is effective for weight loss and control because it contains no calories, yet significantly increases glucose tolerance. New research indicates that stevia may block fat absorption, too. People whose weight loss problems stem from sugar cravings benefit most from stevia, reporting that they experience reduced desire for sugary foods. Most stevia users also say they have less desire for tobacco and alcohol.

A facial mask of water-based stevia extract has gentle BHA activity, smoothing out skin wrinkles while healing skin blemishes. I have seen a single drop of stevia extract, applied directly on a blemish, work to reduce it.

Today, stevia has returned to the marketplace after a long FDA import ban, heavily influenced by Nutrasweet™ competition politics. Experts say that stevia may soon be regarded as one of the most good-for-you sweeteners on earth.

• **Gymnema sylvestre** is an herb that reduces blood sugar levels after sugar consumption. Gymnema's molecular structure, similar to that of sugar, can block up to 50% absorption of sugar calories. Both sugar and gymnema are digested in the small intestine, but the larger molecule of gymnema cannot be fully absorbed. Therefore, taken before sugar, the gymnema molecule blocks the passages through which sugar is normally absorbed, and fewer sugar calories are assimilated.

A person who eats a 400 calorie, high sugar dessert only absorbs 200 of the sugar calories when they use *gymnema*. The remaining sugar is eliminated as waste. *Gymnema* also helps curb cravings for sweet foods. Take with GTF Chromium for best results.

Gymnema has obvious uses for diabetes. Experimental studies show that gymnema may enhance endogenous insulin production in both Type I and Type II diabetics, actually regenerating pancreatic cells destroyed in the course of diabetes.

Take the gymnema taste test. Taste something sweet, then swish a sip of *gymnema sylvestre* tea in your mouth. Now taste something sweet again. You will not be able to taste the sugar, because gymnemic acid prevents your taste buds from being activated by sugar molecules in the food. *Gymnema* blocks the taste of the sugar in your mouth in the same way it blocks sugar in digestion.

• **Agave Nectar** is a new, high fructose sweetener. It's 90% solids, a percentage much greater than traditional high fructose corn syrup. (This amount of fructose may aggravate a copper deficiency linked to serious coronary problems.) Agave may cause disintegration of red blood cells, irritate the skin and the lining of the gastrointestinal tract, depress the central nervous system and immune response, and may cause miscarriage. More testing must be done, but agave nectar is a likely sweetener to look for soon.

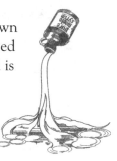

• **Amazake** is a pudding-like, whole-grain sweetener made from organic brown rice. The rice is cooked, then injected with koji, the Aspergillus enzyme culture used in miso and shoyu. Amazake is about 21% sugar, mainly glucose and maltose, and is high in nutrients, including available B complex and iron.

• **Barley malt and brown rice syrups** are mild, natural sweeteners made from barley sprouts, or cultured rice and water cooked to a syrup. Only 40% as sweet as sugar, barley malt's blood sugar activity is a slow, complex carbohydrate release that does not upset insulin levels.

• **Blackstrap molasses** is the liquid sludge left after sucrose is extracted from cane sugar refining. Rich in minerals and vitamins, molasses has more calcium, ounce for ounce, than milk, more iron than eggs, and more potassium than any other food. High amounts of B vitamins, pantothenic acid, iron, inositol and vitamin E make it an effective treatment for restoring thin and fading hair.

—**Sorghum molasses** is concentrated sorghum juice, a grain related to millet. It is similar to molasses but with lighter, milder flavor. Sorghum is made into a sweetener by crushing the plant stalks then boiling the extracted juice into a syrup.

• **Corn syrup** is commercial glucose made from chemically purified cornstarch with everything removed except the starch. Most corn syrup has sugar syrup added to it because glucose is only half as sweet as white sugar. It is highly refined and absorbed into the bloodstream very quickly.

• **Date sugar** is ground, dried dates. It is the least refined, most natural sweetener, with a high sucrose concentration. It has the same nutrient values as dried dates, and is about half as sweet as white sugar. Mix with water before adding to the recipe to prevent burning, or add as a sweet topping after removing your dish from the oven.

• **Fructo-oligo-saccharides** (FOS) are only half as sweet as sugar, and are found naturally in foods like bananas, onions, garlic, artichokes, barley, tomatoes, rye, honey and asparagus. FOS are not digested in the stomach; they pass untouched into the large intestine where beneficial bacteria consume them as nourishment. Even better, the by-products of FOS consumption are healthy EFA's, which are absorbed by the walls of the large intestine and used for energy. Studies show no harmful links for FOS. They do not affect DNA or promote cancer. FOS are available in health food stores.

Note: **FOS** can be used as a partial replacement for sugar in recipes. Too much (more than 40 grams) can cause loose stools, since FOS are not digested. I suggest FOS as a nutritional enhancement rather than a complete replacement.

<u>**Advantages of FOS**</u>:
—FOS feeds beneficial bacteria, while starving harmful bacteria.
—FOS relieves constipation.
—FOS stops antibiotic-induced yeast.
—FOS lowers cholesterol and triglyceride levels.
—FOS inhibits formation of cavities.
—FOS lowers blood sugar levels in diabetics.

• **Fruit juice concentrate** is a highly refined product with about 68% soluble sugar. It contains measurable levels of fiber, vitamins and minerals, and promotes slower digestion. Refined sugars raise serotonin levels in the brain, which can make you feel drowsy. Unrefined fruit sweeteners have less impact on brain chemistry because fruit sugars do not affect serotonin levels.

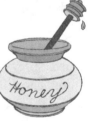

• **Honey** is a mixture of sugars formed from nectar in the bodies of bees by the enzyme invertase. It's a natural sweetener with bioactive, antibiotic and antiseptic properties. Honey contains all the vitamins, minerals and enzymes necessary for proper metabolism and digestion of glucose and other sugars. Still, honey is almost twice as sweet as sugar. Avoid it if you have candidiasis or diabetes; use it with great care if you are hypoglycemic.

• **Maple syrup** is concentrated from the sap of sugar maple trees. It takes 30 to 40 gallons of sap to make one gallon of syrup. Unless labeled pure maple syrup, it may be mixed with corn syrup and other additives to cut its cost.
—**Maple sugar** is concentrated, crystallized maple syrup.

• **Sucanat,** (an acronym from <u>su</u>gar <u>ca</u>ne <u>nat</u>ural) is the trade name for a sweetener made from dried granulated cane juice, available in health food stores. Its average sugar content is 85%, with complex sugars, vitamins, minerals, amino acids and molasses retained.

Use 1 to 1 in place of sugar. It is still a concentrated sweetener; use it carefully if you have sugar balance problems.

• **Turbinado sugar** is raw sugar refined by washing in a centrifuge so that surface molasses is removed. It goes through the same refining process as white sugar, just short of the final extraction of molasses, and is essentially the same as white sugar.

The following chart helps you convert your favorite recipes from sugar to natural sweeteners. If you have serious blood sugar problems, like diabetes or hypoglycemia, consult the appropriate diet pages in this book or your healing professional, about the kind and amount of sweets your body can handle.

Sweetener substitution amounts are for each cup of sugar:

Substitute Sweetener	Amount	Reduce Liquid in Recipe
• Fructose	$1/_3$ to $2/_3$ cup	....
• Maple Syrup	$1/_3$ to $2/_3$ cup	$1/_4$ cup
• Honey	$1/_2$ cup	$1/_4$ cup
• Molasses	$1/_2$ cup	$1/_4$ cup
• Barley or Rice Syrup	1 to $1^1/_4$ cups	$1/_4$ cup
• Date Sugar	1 cup	....
• Sucanat	1 cup	....
• Apple/Pear Juice	1 cup	$1/_4$ cup

What about aspartame, and its brand names, Nutrasweet and Equal?

The FDA has received more complaints about adverse reactions to aspartame than any other food ingredient in the agency's history! Yet we get an incredible amount of these chemical sweeteners in our food today. At least 30% of the U.S. population is sensitive to even moderate doses of aspartame and may suffer several symptoms.

Health problems related to synthetic sweeteners are nothing new. They've been a market-submerged health risk for decades. Saccharin has been used for 100 years, even though its undeniable link to bladder cancer was well known from the 50's. NutraSweet and Equal have taken the place of saccharin today and we're consuming more pre-prepared foods with these sweeteners than ever. Dangerous side effects are worse when aspartame sweeteners are used hot or in cooking (as it is in prepared foods). Adverse effects are reversible when aspartame sweetener consumption is stopped.

Aspartame, 200 times sweeter than sugar, is a combination of two amino acids with neurotransmitter activity - phenylalanine and aspartic acid. PKU seizures (phenylketonuria) result when the body can't effectively metabolize phenylalanine. High levels of the amino acid phenylalanine in body fluids can cause brain damage in anyone. All aspartame products include a warning that the sweetener contains phenylalanine.

Aspartame is clearly linked to sugar use problems — high blood pressure, insomnia, hypoglycemia, diabetes, ovarian cancer and brain tumors. A recent study shows that the more NutraSweet consumed, the more likely tumors are to develop. Aspartame is also associated with brain damage in fetuses. There are immediate, serious reactions to aspartame... severe headaches, dizziness, throat swelling, allergic effects, and retina deterioration attributed to methyl-alcohol, a substance released when aspartame breaks down.

Note: Avoid aspartame sweeteners if you have sugar sensitivities, if you have genetic PKU, advanced liver disease, are allergy-prone (especially children) or are pregnant.

How will the next generation of sweeteners affect you? Despite a huge health outcry, synthetic sweeteners aren't going away. They're just changing.

—**Acesulfame K,** *acesulfame potassium,* an organic salt in the U.S. market since 1988, (brand names Sunette, Sweet One and Swiss Sweet), is 200 times sweeter than sugar and boosts the sweetening effect of other sweeteners. It passes through the human digestive system unchanged, and is noncaloric. The FDA has ninety studies on its safety.

—**Sucralose,** *chlorinated sucrose,* is 400 to 800 times sweeter than sugar. Approved in Canada in 1991 for baking, its approval is pending in the U.S. I feel it would be treacherous to try and convert this concentrated sweetener to sugar amounts in baking.

Sucralose is seen as a chemical by your body, not as a carbohydrate, so it has no effect on insulin secretion or carbohydrate metabolism. Absorption of sucralose is limited; most of it passes through the body unchanged. The small amount that is absorbed is not metabolized for energy, which makes sucralose noncaloric.

Over 100 studies submitted to the FDA showed that sucralose is not carcinogenic and does not cause genetic change, birth defects, brain or nerve damage, or other health risks. Forty studies indicate it is biodegradable, safe for plant and aquatic life. Yet, new information has surfaced showing that these studies were possibly flawed and do not have clear results showing that sucralose is safe long term. Sucralose may cause thymus shrinkage, and enlargement of liver and kidneys. In addition, sucralose is a <u>chlorinated</u> sucrose derivative. Consuming it regularly means adding small amounts of potentially cancer-causing chlorine by-products into your body.

• **Alitame,** brand name ACLAME, is formed from the amino acids l-aspartic acid and L-alanine, chemically similar to aspartame. It is 2,000 times sweeter than sucrose with a clean, sweet taste. Alitame is hydrolyzed to release aspartic acid, which is metabolized normally in the body, then excreted in urine and feces as unchanged alitame. Fifteen studies indicate that alitame is safe at a dose of 100 mg/kg per day. However, the FDA, bowing to the negative publicity from aspartame (alitame is even more concentrated), is delaying approval in the U.S. pending further tests.

<u>Beware of these chemical sweeteners found on today's food labels.</u>
—**Dextrose,** a plant monosaccharide, often synthetically derived from cornstarch.
—**Lactose,** milk sugar, a di-saccharide sweetener mainly in infant foods and baked goods. Lactose intolerant people get gastrointestinal disturbances from consuming lactose.
—**Maltose,** malt sugar, is a disaccharide often synthetically derived from corn syrup. It does not normally stimulate insulin production.
—**Sorbitol,** derived from corn, is absorbed slowly. It is used in diabetic safe foods because it needs little insulin. It does not promote tooth decay, but can cause diarrhea and cramping.
—**Saccharin,** a solvent made from petroleum and toluene, used to prevent knocking in gas engines, is 300 times sweeter than sugar, calorie free, does not metabolize, is excreted quickly and does not build up in the body; but is linked to bladder cancer. The FDA tried to ban saccharin in 1977, but relented under pressure from the industry. It is now sold with a warning label.
—**Raw sugar,** a granulated, evaporated sugar cane juice product. It is 98% sucrose.
—**Xylitol,** from birchwood chips, may reduce cavities by neutralizing mouth acids.

Is it possible to eat a healthy diet that won't stimulate too much insulin but will allow normal blood sugar activity? Can we keep hunger under control all day, and manage our weight without starving? A low glycemic diet is a good answer.

A low glycemic diet is a diet that keeps insulin levels low so that fewer calories turn into fat and more are burned for energy, resulting in weight loss. A low-glycemic diet is low in fats and total calories, largely vegetarian, with most proteins from vegetable sources.

Whole grains and fresh vegetables have a low glycemic index. They don't elevate blood sugar after a meal like sugary, high-glycemic index foods that put blood sugar on a roller coaster and elevate it too rapidly. Insulin responds immediately to stimulate fat production. Too much insulin also causes extra sugar storage, which then results in low blood sugar. Low blood sugar causes stress-hormone release, fatigue and ultimately ravenous hunger, so the cycle begins all over again.

Plant fiber also regulates digestion for more balanced blood sugar levels. Plant fiber binds with most fats to prevent their absorption. In addition, plant fiber foods speed up bowel transit time to take stress off your liver so it can metabolize fats efficiently. When you add more plant fiber to your diet, you'll have less cravings for sugar.

Nutrients that help reduce sugar cravings and withdrawal are B vitamins, vitamin C, zinc, trace minerals, the amino acid L-glutamine and chromium. Chromium helps insulin work more efficiently at removing sugar from the blood. Glutamine is used directly by the brain and is helpful in reducing sugar craving. Some spices like cinnamon, clove and bay leaf also help control both blood sugar levels and sugar cravings.

A low glycemic diet can help you optimize brain biochemistry. You'll feel more comfortable while dieting and can diet without binging.

In sum: A low glycemic diet is based on whole grains, fresh fruits and vegetables, seafood, sea greens, soy foods and brown rice, largely high fiber foods that help stabilize blood sugar swings. It includes mono-unsaturated oils like olive or canola oil and plenty of cultured foods, like yogurt and kefir for optimum intestinal bacteria.

For longer life and better health, use sugar sparingly, on special occasions.

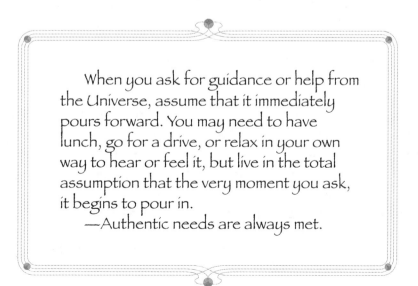

When you ask for guidance or help from the Universe, assume that it immediately pours forward. You may need to have lunch, go for a drive, or relax in your own way to hear or feel it, but live in the total assumption that the very moment you ask, it begins to pour in.
—Authentic needs are always met.

A Low Salt Diet and Healing

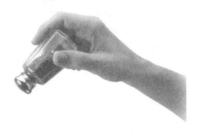

In the past generation, Americans have consumed more salt than ever in our history; too much restaurant food, too many refined foods and too many animal foods. Heart disease, hypertension and high blood pressure have increased correspondingly, so most people are aware that excessive salt is a diet problem. Too much salt constricts circulation, kidneys retain fluid, and migraines occur frequently. Like too much sugar, salt's a cause of hyperactivity and aggressive behavior. The average American adult consumes between 4,000 and 6,000mg of sodium a day.

Nutrition and medical studies are replete with the negative effects of salt. Yet, salt is necessary for good health; indeed it is essential to human existence. In ancient times, salt was so valuable that men traded it for its weight in gold. Today's sound-byte media medicine teaches us that salt is dangerous and that the public should avoid it. While some people must curb their intake during healing, most Americans do not suffer ill effects when they use salt sensibly in their diets.

Sodium occurs naturally in foods. Accompanied by its partner mineral, potassium, sodium regulates blood pressure, transmits nerve impulses and maintains muscle activity. Together, sodium and potassium pump nutrients into the cells to nourish, and drain waste products out of the cells to clean them. The sodium-potassium relationship also helps maintain fluid balance, so you don't retain excess fluid or get dehydrated.

Salinity is needed for good body tone because sodium helps muscles to contract. It is needed for strong blood, because without sodium, the body cannot use calcium. Sodium helps keep the body pH balanced as it transports nutrients and nerve impulses. It keeps glands and organs healthy, and produces hydrochloric acid so we can digest our food. Too little sodium leads to low vitality, stagnate blood and loss of clear thinking, because the brain depends on good fluid circulation.

When we change the natural salt balance in our bodies we get health problems. What makes our bodies lose necessary salts? Diuretics, excessive sweating, heat, even exercise can cause severe sodium imbalance, which results in poor kidney function. The high fever, vomiting or diarrhea you experience during an infection robs your body of fluids and salt.

Signs that you have too little salt? Signs of sodium deficiency include flatulence, diarrhea, and unexplained nausea. Tissue dehydration causes wrinkles and sunken eyes. Poor fluid circulation in the brain causes confusion, irritability, heightened allergies and low blood pressure.

Signs that you have too much salt? PMS symptoms like breast tenderness and bloating, constipation, headaches, dizziness, asthma, fatigue, ringing in the ears and body weakness.

What makes our bodies retain too much salt? Beyond eating extra salty food, excessive use of cortisone drugs or anabolic steroids cause us to build up salt. Congestive heart failure, kidney diseases (healthy kidneys control sodium levels), gastrointestinal disease and diabetes also affect salt balance.

What about salt and high blood pressure? Table salt is 40 percent sodium and 60 percent chloride; it's the sodium that affects blood pressure. A sodium-restricted diet for hypertension ranges from 1,000 to 3,000mg a day. Our bodies need about 500 milligrams ($^1/_4$ teaspoon) of sodium to help regulate distribution of body fluids. Sodium restriction has no effect on the blood pressure of people who have normal blood pressure.

It is a common myth that table salt is the major source of sodium in the average American diet. Ten percent of the sodium in the average diet occurs naturally in food, 15 percent comes from salt you add to your food, (one teaspoon of salt = about 2,000mg of sodium). But a whopping 75 percent is added to food during processing - up to 4,000 milligrams of sodium a day. A . Sodium-containing ingredients that you may not recognize on a label include *sodium caseinate, monosodium glutamate, trisodium phosphate, sodium bicarbonate* and *sodium sterol lactate.*

Junk and fast foods are the worst offenders for high blood pressure and it's an explosive health situation. Read labels carefully on medicines, too. Over-the-counter drugs like antacids, laxatives, and sleeping aids contain generous amounts of sodium. Effervescent antacid tablets, for example, contain 276mg sodium per tablet; Instant Metamucil has 250mg sodium per package.

Good ways to get the good salts that your body needs:
—Sea greens' salty taste is really a balanced mineral chelate.
—Herb salts and seasonings provide plant enzymes to make salts absorbable.
—Sea salt is a rich source of iodine, potassium and many minerals besides sodium.
—Tamari is a wheat-free soy sauce, lower in sodium and richer in flavor than soy sauce.
—Umeboshi plums are highly alkalizing, excellent for a macrobiotic diet.
—Naturally fermented foods like pickles, relishes, olives are also healthy cultured foods.
—Bragg's LIQUID AMINOS is an energizing protein broth, with valuable amino acids.
—Miso is a salty-tasting soy paste made from cooked, aged soybeans.
—Gomashio blends sesame seeds and sea salt, a delicious staple in oriental cooking.

A salt-free diet may be desirable for someone who eats too much salt. However, once the body's salinity normalizes, some salt should be brought back into the diet quickly.
Low salt, not no salt, is best for a permanent way of eating. Don't worry about sodium deficiency; even a low sodium diet has 2,400mg.

> The beauty of self-healing is reconnecting with nature and letting your body take care of the rest.
> —Ann Wigmore

Sea Greens Are Amazing Healers

Sea greens have superior nutritional content. They transmit the energies of the sea to your body as a rich source of nutrients. Ounce for ounce, along with herbs, they are higher in vitamins and minerals than any other food. Sea greens are one of nature's richest sources of vegetable protein, and they provide full-spectrum concentrations of beta carotene, chlorophyll, enzymes, amino acids and fiber. The distinctive salty taste is not just "salt," but a balanced, chelated combination of sodium, potassium, calcium, magnesium, phosphorus, iron and trace minerals.

Sea greens help re-mineralize us. They convert inorganic ocean minerals into organic mineral salts that combine with amino acids. Our bodies use this combination as an ideal way to get usable nutrients for structural building blocks. In fact, sea greens contain all the necessary trace elements for life, many of which are depleted in the earth's soil.

Sea plants can rebalance our body chemistry. Our body fluids have the same chemical composition as sea water. The same 56 elements course through our veins that circulate in the ocean. Sea greens are the ocean's purifiers. Their rich antioxidant qualities neutralize toxins for detoxification, and they perform many of the same functions for our bodies, also largely made up of salt water. Sea plant chemical composition is so close to human plasma, that perhaps the greatest benefit from sea greens is that they can normalize our bodies from the effects of a modern diet. They strengthen us against disease, and reduce excess stores of fluid and fat.

Sea greens are natural superfoods, some of our most powerful healers. They have anti-inflammatory, antiviral, antimicrobial, antifungal, and anticancer activity. Modern science validates many traditional benefits of sea plants, especially their algin, the component thought to be responsible for the success of seaweeds in the treatment of obesity, asthma, atherosclerosis and blood purification. Algin absorbs toxins from the digestive tract in much the same way that a water softener removes the hardness from tap water. Algin means less toxins enter the circulatory system

Sea greens are the most nutrition dense plants on the planet. They have access to all the nutrients in the ocean, acquiring their nourishment across its entire surface through wave action and underwater currents. Sea greens are rich in fiber and packed with vitamins, with measureable amounts of vitamins K, A, D, B, E and C, and a broad range of carotenes. Sea greens are almost the only non-animal source of Vitamin B-12 necessary for cell development and nerve function. They are full of amino acids, contain up to 20% protein, and have enzymes and essential fatty acids to rejuvenate us. They contain 10 to 20 times the minerals of land plants, and beyond their mineral quantities, their mineral balance is a natural stabilizer for building sound nerve structure and good metabolism.

Nutrition studies show that sea plants effectively lower blood pressure and cholesterol, help deter arteriosclerosis and reduce tumors. Immune-compromised diseases like chronic fatigue, HIV infection, arthritis and allergies respond to sea plant treatment. Sea plant iodine is a key to controlling and preventing gland disorders like breast and uterine fibroids, prostate inflammation, adrenal exhaustion, and toxic liver and kidney states.

More things sea greens can do for you:

1: <u>Sea greens protect us in a destructive environment</u>: Sea plants can protect us from a wide range of toxic elements in the environment, including heavy metals (most dental fillings still contain them) and radiation by-products, converting them into harmless salts that we can eliminate. The natural iodine in sea greens can reduce by almost 80% the radioactive iodine-131 absorbed by the thyroid. Still, although seaweeds contain the compounds that directly counteract carcinogens, most researchers believe that their success is in boosting the body's immune system so it can combat the carcinogens itself.

Sea greens contain powerful antioxidant and anti-cancer properties, working to stop the proliferation of cancer cells. Some experts consider them more potent than drugs used to treat breast and prostate cancer, especially as interceptive measures. Japanese studies show that a diet with as little as 5% sea greens inhibits cancer growth, even causing remission of active tumors.

2: <u>Sea greens protect against breast cancer</u>: Iodine deficiency and hypothyroidism are clearly involved with a higher incidence of breast cancer. Japanese women have less than one-sixth the breast cancer rate of American women of similar age. Japanese women who live in rural areas have a much lower breast cancer rate than Japanese women in urban areas. The determining factor seems to be diet. The rural Japanese women routinely eat sea plants - a food uncommon in the diets of American and urban Japanese women who eat many processed foods. In animal studies, rats exposed to chemicals known to cause breast cancer were fed sea greens and were protected against getting cancer.

Women with low iodine levels often have cervical dysplasia and breast fibroids, too. In clinical trials, dysplasia lesions have been corrected by sea plant supplements. My own experience with sea plant iodine shows that it reduces both breast and uterine fibroids, with significant anti-inflammatory and anti-scarring effects.

3: <u>Sea greens and bone health</u>: Sea greens have high magnesium, essential for the absorption of calcium. Magnesium stimulates production of calcitonin, the hormone which increases calcium in the bones. Sea greens are a good source of natural vitamin D, also essential for calcium absorption, bone health and muscle function. Many people don't store vitamin D very well; our indoor lives don't let us get into the sun as much as in times past. Forty percent of Americans (especially women) are deficient in this nutrient. Even many who take vitamin D supplements show a deficiency.

4: <u>Sea greens and your thyroid</u>: In our era of processed foods and iodine-poor soils, sea greens and sea foods stand alone as potent sources of natural, balanced iodine. Iodine is essential to life; the thyroid gland cannot make thyrozin, the enzyme that regulates metabolism, without it. Iodine is important for alertness and rapid brain activity, and a prime deterrent to arterial plaque.

Thyroid hormones are made from iodine and the amino acid tyrosine. Thyroglobulin, the mixture of tyrosine and iodine stored in the thyroid gland, is transformed into hormones that regulate our protein, carbohydrate and carotene use, and cholesterol distribution (sea greens help lower cholesterol). The amount of thyroid hormone released into the bloodstream determines our basic energy level and along with the adrenal glands, the rate at which sex hormones are made. Sea plants nourish an underactive thyroid and normalize adrenal functions to trigger increased libido.

Goiter, a thyroid disorder, develops when the pituitary gland stimulates the thyroid to make more hormones but the thyroid can't do it because it doesn't have enough iodine. It enlarges in the attempt and goiter develops. The rate of goiter in the U.S. is still relatively high - 6% of the population in some areas. It's a strange situation, because few people in the U. S. are iodine deficient (the average American intake of iodine is estimated at over 600 micrograms daily from iodized salt). Since the recommended adult allowance for iodine is quite small, 150 micrograms, experts believe that at least some of the high rates of goiter are really connected to too much sugar, alcohol, fats and caffeine, or to eating a lot of goitrogen foods, which block iodine absorption.

Goitrogens are cruciferous vegetables like broccoli, cauliflower or cabbage, legumes like beans, and peas, beets, and nuts like almonds and peanuts, which may cause a mild hypothyroid state when eaten raw. Cooking neutralizes the thyroid-blocking components. If you have a tendency to goiter or hypothyroidism, cook these healthy foods lightly.

5: <u>**Sea greens guard against birth defects:**</u> Low iodine has a profound effect on the health of a fetus early in conception. I recommend that a woman who wants to become pregnant consider adding sea greens to her diet while she is trying to conceive, rather than waiting until she realizes she is pregnant. Most American women get enough iodine, but in landlocked countries where iodine is not plentiful in food, infants are often born with cretinism which results in stunted growth, mental defects, puffy facial features and poor muscle coordination, all signs of low iodine.

<u>**Sea greens in a pregnant woman's diet help the health of the mother, too.**</u>
—Hemoglobin counts rise from 65% to 83%.
—Colds decrease in number and severity. Arthritic conditions improve.
—Hair color and quality improve; fingernails grow stronger.
—Skin texture improves; capillary strength increases, so there is less bruising.
—Eye conditions improve, especially if there is eye redness or inflammation.
—Constipation lessens and a sense of well-being increases.
—Stretch marks are less during pregnancy and skin heals better afterwards.

6: <u>**Sea greens are a valuable treatment for candida albicans yeast infections.**</u> Their high mineral, especially selenium content, builds up immunity against candida. Enzymes use the rich iodine in seaweeds to produce iodine-charged free radicals, which deactivate yeasts.

7: <u>**Sea greens help stop vaginal infections:**</u> Iodine-rich sea plants are effective against a wide range of organisms like trichomonas, candida and chlamydia. A douche solution with 1 tablespoon dried sea plants to 1 quart of water, used twice daily for 7 to 14 days, is effective against most of these pathogens.

8: <u>**Sea greens boost weight loss and deter cellulite build-up.**</u> Very low calorie and virtually fat-free (but with plenty of skin-nourishing EFA's), sea plants normalize thyroid metabolism, especially as you age. The detoxifying quality of sea plant algin stimulates lymphatic drainage to discourage cellulite, and reduces bowel transit time to aid weight loss. Rich antioxidant nutrients in sea plants increase your body's stamina and fat-burning ability during exercise.

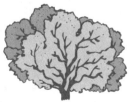

Both eating sea greens and bathing in them helps reduce the look of cellulite. Seaweed encourages absorption of minerals into skin tissue and fat cells. The minerals act like electrolytes to break the chemical bond that seals the fat cells. So seaweed temporarily opens the cells to allow trapped wastes to escape, releasing toxins into the lymph system and eliminating them through the kidneys and bladder. The best spas apply a sea plant solution as part of a body wrap or bath to do this very thing. It's called thalassotherapy, and it's been used for centuries to speed up metabolism and increase circulation to cellulitic areas.

9: Sea greens are a beauty treatment: Seaweeds add amazing luster to the skin. The sea-loving ancient Greeks said that Aphrodite, the goddess of love who rose out of the foaming sea, owed her supple skin, shiny hair, and sparkling eyes to the plants of the sea. A seaweed face mask increases circulation, stimulates lymphatic drainage and dilates capillaries to tone your skin. Seaweed returns mineral salts to your skin that stress and pollution deplete. Skin cells hold moisture better when they absorb the mineral salts, making the skin more supple and elastic. By retaining moisture, the skin plumps, removing the look of dry skin, lines and wrinkles. Many women report smoother skin texture after a seaweed treatment. Amino acid, mineral and vitamin content help nourish the skin, too. Certain types of seaweeds possess molecules similar to collagen.

A seaweed bath is a great way to get the benefits of sea plants all over your body.

Seaweed baths are Nature's perfect body-psyche balancer, and they're an excellent way to get your natural iodine. Remember how good you feel after a walk in the ocean? Seaweeds purify and balance the ocean; they can do the same for your body.

Noticeable rejuvenating effects occur when toxins are released from our tissues. A hot seaweed bath is like a wet-steam sauna, only better, because the sea greens balance body chemistry instead of dehydrating it. The electrolytic magnetic action of the sea plants releases excess body fluids from congested cells and dissolves fatty wastes through the skin, replacing them with depleted minerals - particularly potassium and iodine. As the natural iodine boosts thyroid activity, food fuels are used before they can turn into fat deposits. Vitamin K, a fat-soluble vitamin in seaweeds, aids adrenal regulation, so a seaweed bath also helps maintain hormone balance for a more youthful body. I find bathing in sea greens is great way to reduce cellulite and prevent it from recurring.

If an ocean near you has unpolluted waters, collect your own sea greens. Gather them from the water, (not the shoreline), in buckets or clean trash cans, and carry them home to your tub. If you don't live near the ocean, dried sea greens are available in health food stores. Whichever form you choose, run very hot water over the seaweed in tub, filling it to the point that you will be covered when you recline. The leaves will turn a beautiful bright green. The water will turn rich brown as the plants release their minerals. As you soak, the gel from the seaweed transfers onto your skin. This coating increases perspiration to release toxins from your system, and replaces them by osmosis with minerals. Rub your skin, especially cellulite areas with the sea leaves during the bath to stimulate circulation, smooth and tone the body, and remove wastes coming out on the skin surface. When the sea greens have done their work, the gel coating dissolves and floats off the skin, and the leaves shrivel - a sign that your seaweed bath is over.

105

Each bath varies with the individual, the seaweeds used, and water temperature, but the gel coating release is a natural timekeeper for the bath's benefits. Forty-five minutes is usually about right to balance the body's acid-alkaline system, encourage liver activity, cellulite release and fat metabolism. Skin tone, color, and better circulation are almost immediately noticeable. To get the most from a seaweed treatment, dry brush cellulitic skin before your seaweed bath or wrap to exfoliate dead skin, and open up pores for waste elimination and blood flow to the affected area.

Note: A hot seaweed bath is one of the most effective treatments in natural healing. It should be used with care. If you are under a doctor's care for heart disease or high blood pressure, check with your physician to see if a seaweed bath is okay for you.

Sea plants are green, brown, red and blue-green. A quick profile:

—**Kelp** (*laminaria*) contains vitamins A, B, E, D and K, is a main source of vitamin C, and is rich in minerals. Kelp proteins are comparable to animal protein quality. A brown marine plant, kelp contains sodium alginate (algin), an element that helps remove radioactive particles and heavy metals from the body. Algin, carrageenan and ager are kelp gels that aid digestion and rejuvenate gastrointestinal health. Kelp works as a blood purifier, relieves arthritis pain, and promotes adrenal, pituitary and thyroid health. Kelp is best known for its therapeutic iodine that can normalize thyroid-related disorders like overweight and lymph system congestion. It is a demulcent that helps eliminate herpes outbreaks. Kelp is rich — a little goes a long way; use it mostly as a seasoning.

—**Kombu** (*laminaria digitata, setchelli, horsetail kelp*), has a long tradition as a royal Japanese delicacy with great nutritional healing value. It is a decongestant for excess mucous, and helps lower blood pressure. Kombu has abundant iodine, carotenes, B, C, D and E vitamins, important minerals like calcium, magnesium, potassium, silica, iron and zinc, and the powerful skin healing nutrient germanium. Kombu is a meaty, high-protein seaweed, often used in soups and to flavor stocks for sauces. It is higher in natural mineral salts than most other seaweeds. Add a strip of kombu to your bean pot to reduce gas.

—**Hijiki** is a mineral-rich, high-fiber seaweed, with 20% protein, vitamin A, carotenes and calcium. Its crisp black strands are delicious sauteed with seafood or veggies, in soup or on rice. Hijiki has the most calcium of any sea green, 1400mg / 100gr of dry weight.

—**Nori** (*porphyra, laver*) is a red sea plant with a sweet, meaty taste when dried. It contains nearly 50% balanced, assimilable protein, higher than any other sea plant. Nori's fiber makes it a perfect sushi wrapper. Nori is rich in all the carotenes, iodine, iron, and phosphorus. Nori's high calcium content makes it a good choice for weight loss and bone density for menopausal women.

—**Arame** (*eisenia bycyclis*), is one of the ocean's richest sources of iodine. Herbalists use arame to help reduce breast and uterine fibroids, and through its fat soluble vitamins and phytohormones, to normalize menopausal symptoms. Arame promotes soft, wrinkle-free skin, enhances the growth of glossy hair and prevents its loss.

—**Sea Palm** (*postelsia palmaeformis*) the American species of arame, grows only on the Pacific Coast of North America. One of my favorites, it has a sweet, salty taste that goes especially well as a vegetable, rice or salad topping.

—**Bladderwrack** is packed with vitamin K - an excellent adrenal stimulant. It is still used today by native Americans in steam baths for arthritis, gout and illness recovery.

—**Wakame** (*alaria, undaria*) is a high-protein, high calcium seaweed, with carotenes, iron and vitamin C. Widely used in the Orient for hair growth and luster, and for skin tone.

—**Dulse** (*palmaria palmata*), a red sea plant, is rich in iron, protein, and vitamin A. It is a supremely balanced nutrient, with 300 times more iodine and 50 times more iron than wheat. New tests on dulse show activity against the herpes virus. It has purifying and tonic effects on the body, yet its "salt" nourishes as a mineral, without inducing thirst.

—**Irish moss** (*Chondrus Crispus, carrageen*) is full of electrolyte minerals — calcium, magnesium, sodium and potassium. Its mucilaginous compounds help you detoxify, boost metabolism and strengthen hair, skin and nails. Irish moss was traditionally used for a low sex drive.

Preventive measures may be taken against iodine deficiency problems or disease risk by adding just 2 tablespoons of chopped, dried sea greens to your daily diet.

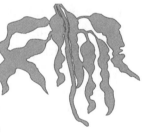

Sea greens are tasty. Crush, chop, veggies you like into soups and and salads. Roast them into any-etables, no other salt is needed, an Sundried, they are convenient to them in a moisture proof container variety of sea greens is available today. snip or crumble any mix of dry sea sauces, pizzas or focaccias, casseroles thing you cook. If you add sea veg-advantage for a low salt diet. buy, store, and use as needed. Store and they keep indefinitely. A wide

To be a winner,
all you need to give
is all you have.

Healing Powerhouses of the Desert

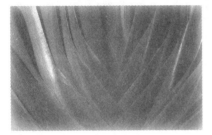

Aloe vera, the lily of the desert, is a unique, potent healing superfood with a wealth of new research. Over seventy-five healing compounds have been identified in aloe, including steroids, antibiotic and anti-carcinogenic agents, amino acids, minerals and enzymes (one enzyme has been isolated to treat burns). It has excellent trans-dermal properties, allowing it to penetrate deep skin levels.

Aloe gel has been used since Egyptian times as a skin lubricant and healer for cuts, sunburn, bruises, insect bites, sores, acne, eczema and burns. New research shows healing results for skin cancers, hemorrhoids and varicose veins.

Aloe juice is widely popular today because it boosts the body's self-cleansing action - balancing the system rather than using harsh irritant effects. Aloe has at least three anti-inflammatory EFA's that help the stomach, small intestine and colon. Even in the medical world, aloe is recommended for post-op healing, because it is a natural antiseptic and astringent. Aloe also stimulates lymphatic circulation, boosting antibody formation against infections.

Aloe juice is a core element in the alternative healing arsenal with unique nutritional and body balancing properties. It helps normalize fat metabolism, which helps reduce cholesterol and triglycerides. New research shows it's effective for immune disorders like candida, parasite invasions, fatigue syndromes like fibromyalgia, allergies, arthritis, eczema and psoriasis. Aloe juice alkalizes digestive processes to prevent overacidity - a common cause of indigestion, acid reflux, digestive tract irritations like IBS, colitis, Crohn's disease and ulcers. Ulcer patients taking aloe juice show up to 80% reduction in the number of ulcers being formed. Even after the formation of ulcers, healing is three times faster.

I call aloe vera an intelligent plant, because it can differentiate between normal cells, mutated cells (cancer) or diseased cells (HIV). It stimulates normal cell growth, while inhibiting cancer cell division (even lymphocytic leukemia) and virus spread. Aged aloe vera juice is widely used in AIDS treatment to block the HIV virus movement from cell to cell. *Acemannan,* an aloe derivative with powerful anti-viral effects, shows promise against herpes viruses.

Aloe vera is loaded with mucopolysaccharides, phytochemicals with profound healing qualities. Mucopolysaccharides are credited with aloe's immune enhancement qualities, antiviral-antibacterial activity, and its ability to eliminate toxic wastes. Rich in organic silicon, MPS's are a vital component of cell and artery walls, mucous membranes, and the connective tissues of bones, teeth and cartilage. They link with collagen and elastin to maintain tissues and organs, alleviate joint problems and rebuild degenerating cartilage. Essentially mucopolysaccharides and collagen hold our tissues together. MPS's also reduce inflammation and blood clotting time, lessening the risk for cardiovascular disease.

Nature's most energizing superfoods come from high desert beehives.

—Royal jelly is a nutritional powerhouse containing every nutrient necessary to support life. No other food source compares nutritionally to royal jelly, and it can't be duplicated in a lab. The exclusive food of the queen bee, royal jelly transforms a "cinderella" worker bee into a queen bee. Her life expectancy rises to an astounding 6 years, compared to a worker bee's 6 week life span - an amazing result of her royal jelly diet!

Royal jelly's rejuvenative powers have been used for centuries as a "fountain of youth" for humans, too. Modern herbalists say royal jelly is a fabulous nutrient for healthy skin and hair, nourishing the skin to ease wrinkles, dryness, even adult acne. Chinese herbalists advocate royal jelly for liver disease, arthritis, anemia, phlebitis, and stomach ulcers.

Royal jelly has extraordinary powers to strengthen and protect our immune systems. It is a rich source of B vitamins (one of the world's best natural sources of B-5, pantothenic acid), important minerals, sex hormones, enzyme precursors, and all eight essential amino acids. Royal jelly is effective against fatigue, depression, even premature senility. It is a natural antibiotic, supplies key nutrients for energy and mental alertness, combats stress, fatigue and insomnia. It is effective for gland and hormone imbalances that reflect in menstrual, menopause and prostate problems.

Royal Jelly is quite difficult to harvest and commands high prices because of its scarcity and consumer demand. The highest quality royal jelly products are preserved in their whole, raw, "alive" state for the best body absorption. As little as one drop of pure, extracted fresh royal jelly can deliver a daily supply.

Take panax ginseng and royal jelly in a dynamo drink for your healing diet. The attributes of ginseng and royal jelly are synergistic together.

—Propolis is a powerful natural antibiotic. Bee hives have been called "the most antiseptic places in nature," because propolis neutralizes all harmful organisms that enter the hive. Bees are prone to bacterial and viral infections; propolis protects the bees from these infections. The powerful antibiotic properties of propolis can also protect humans — specifically against *staphylococcus aureus*, a bacteria that causes serious infections, blood poisoning and a type of pneumonia. (Interestingly, *staph. a.* has become resistant to all but one pharmaceutical antibiotic.) New studies show that propolis inhibits the streptococcal bacteria that causes strep throat and dental cavities. Propolis even works well with two anti-staph drugs, streptomycin and cloxacillin, because it performs much like a prescription antibiotic — preventing bacteria cell division and breaking down bacteria cell structure. Even better, propolis works against viruses, something that antibiotics cannot do.

Bees collect the elements for propolis from the leaf buds on the bark of trees, then convert it with bee enzymes to a sticky material of 50-55% resin and balsam, 30% wax and 10% pollen. Rich in immune defense vitamins, minerals and amino-acids (all 22 of them), bees paste a propolis shield on the inner hive walls to guard against harmful microorganisms and to patch holes or cracks in the hive. Nature is incredibly efficient.

Propolis creates the same natural antibiotic shield for humans. Research shows that taking propolis during high risk "cold and flu" seasons reduces colds, coughing, and inflammation of mouth, tonsils and throat membranes. Look for a supplement that contains propolis, vitamin C and zinc for the best results. Further, propolis is rich in flavonoids and B-vitamins that work both internally and externally to heal scars, bruises and blemishes.

—Bee pollen is called nature's perfect food because it's nutritionally complete.
It has all 22 amino acids, 27 minerals, the full span of vitamins, complex carbohydrates, essential fatty acids, enzymes and co-enzymes. Bee pollen has 5 to 7 times more protein than beef! Bee pollen is so nutrient rich, it's been used worldwide for centuries to rejuvenate and rebuild the body after illness. I've experienced this healing ability myself. Pollen is a valuable aid to weight control. It can normalize body metabolism and stoke metabolic fires to keep calories burning and weight stable. Bee pollen also acts as a natural appetite suppressant through its amino acid phenylalanine (for people who need to gain weight, phenylalanine produces the opposite effect).

Bee pollen also:
—Increases energy levels and strength for athletes.
—Helps the body normalize diarrhea and constipation.
—Tranquilizes without side effects.
—Increases blood hemoglobin.
—Rids the body of toxins from drugs, alcohol, smoking, and chemicalized food.
—Chelates and flushes out artery-clogging biochemical deposits.
—Reduces the negative effects associated with radiation.
—Protects against skin dehydration and stimulates growth of new skin tissue.

Note: *Bee pollen has shown great effectiveness for the relief of allergy symptoms. However, a small percentage of the population may be allergic to bee products.*

—Jojoba benefits are attracting Americans.
Desert plants are full of natural, long-lasting moisturizers. For us, this means they are wonderful cosmetics as well as soothing healers. The jojoba plant is no exception. Jojoba nut oil has been used by Native Americans for hundreds of years to treat sores, cuts, bruises and burns.

Jojoba oil is actually like a liquid wax with rich antioxidant properties to keep it from turning rancid. This means that jojoba oil is a natural mimic of sebum oil secreted by the human skin. So it is an effective lubricant and protector in protecting human skin from aging and wrinkling.

Jojoba oil is rapid, penetrating, hypo-allergenic skin therapy. Besides moisturizing and soothing skin, jojoba gives your skin a healthy glow because it restores natural pH balance. In just one hour after application, jojoba oil increases skin softness by as much as 37 percent, and reduces superficial lines and wrinkles, especially around the eyes, by as much as 25 percent! Because of its purity and antioxidant freshness, herbal healers use jojoba to treat skin problems like adult acne, psoriasis, and neurodermatitis which are not responsive to chemical medicines.

Jojoba oil is the most effective natural scalp cleaning substance discovered so far. As it did in Native American medicine, jojoba helps restore non-hereditary hair loss that is linked to dandruff and clogged scalp follicles. Each single hair is lubricated by sebum, manufactured by sebaceous glands that lie next to the hair follicles. When too much sebum collects, hair follicles clog, resulting in unhealthy hair, poor hair growth, and shortened hair life. Jojoba dissolves excess sebum deposits, opens up hair follicles and encourages healthy hair growth.

Jojoba's versatile natural appetite suppressing activity comes from a constituent called *Simmondsia*. It's a delicious weight control aid, now made into tasty candy bars and chocolate-y beverages.

Foods are Some of Nature's Aromatherapy

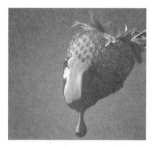

Sometimes we get so caught up in the constituents and nutritional values of our foods (amount of fat and calories, concentration of proteins, healing factors, etc.), that we lose the enjoyment of eating, and the one-ness we share with the living things that nourish us. Food affects the way we feel more than just through digestion. Eating creates health. It is an end as well as a means - something we do and react to every day.... a source of relaxation and pleasure.

It starts with aromatherapy. Aroma molecules enter the body first. We can smell something long before we can see it, touch it, hear it or taste it. How many times have you smelled a scent and had the "taste" almost instantly in your mouth? How often has a cooking food on the stove smelled so good you could literally "taste it?" Aroma starts the digestive process when your "mouth waters." As your diet becomes fresher and your appetite for whole foods increases, this sense sharpens, and even familiar scents become enhanced. Can the smell of a fresh lemon drive you wild?

For ancient man, smell was his first line of defense, his alarm bell. Today, we can use aroma as a first line of health care, especially for releasing stress and as a relaxation technique during healing. It can change our mind, mood and attitude almost instantly.

The aromatherapy of food affects every sense. Knowing this fact can make planning your healing diet meals much more interesting. Food colors for instance, generate many subtle feelings. Fresh foods are "solar grown and cooked." The solar vibrations from their growing are visible to us as their colors. Light, brightly colored foods, like fruits, make us feel lighter, and expansive. Darker colored root vegetables and grains make us feel more solid and earthbound. Traditionally, red-toned foods increase vigor and elimination, blue and violet foods relax, green foods promote strength and body balance, yellow and orange foods increase circulation and brain activity.

The shape and feel of fresh foods communicates to us even before we eat them, providing a certain anticipation about texture and temperature in the mouth.

Food sounds can be pure enjoyment; the crunch of a tart apple, the snap of a carrot or celery, the tender crisp sizzle of a fresh stir-fry, the slow bubble of a soup pot. Sound can tell you when just the right amount of cooking has been done.

But the taste is the test. In ancient times, our taste buds told us what was good and what was harmful for our bodies. For many of us today, years of eating over-processed, chemical-laced, or non-food foods have dulled this sensibility. Taste buds can be fooled by tobacco, chemicals and drugs. The recipes in this book can greatly improve your sense of taste. People are always amazed at how really good food tastes when their bodies begin to rebuild and rebalance from a better diet.

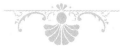

Cook with Herbs That Heal You

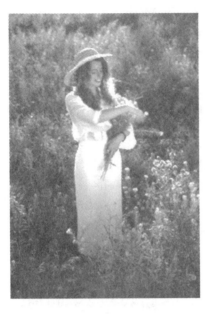

America is rediscovering herbal medicines with enthusiasm. Culinary herbs are the quintessential medicinal food. They enhance taste while enhancing healing activity in the body. A delight to cook with, every herb I know has medicinal properties, too. A little goes a long way.... both for healing and for seasoning.

Both dried and fresh herbs work medicinally. With the information in this section, you can use the herbs and spices in your recipes to enhance your everyday health! If naturally dried and stored airtight, herbs keep both their flavor and their healing potency for several years. I have worked with some herbs stored in a "time capsule" working pharmacy in one of California's State Parks. The pharmacy had been in operation from the early eighteen-sixties to the nineteen-forties. Some of the herbs I saw had been in storage for over hundred years, and when I touched and smelled them, they were still pungent and potent.

I use both fresh and dried herbs, but I think one of the nicest things you can do for your kitchen is to plant a fresh herb garden. It can be any size, from raised beds to a window box. Whatever you can manage is worth it for taste and health. Pick fresh only the amount you need each time. Dry the rest on screens or bunch them upside down on an herb drying rack when the season for an herb is over.

To substitute fresh herbs for dried in recipes, use three times as much as is called for.

Herbs can play a big part in your natural food pharmacy. The essence of human health is body balance, establishing and maintaining body chemistry that resists disease, and assures you energy and well-being. Herbs are at their best as body balancers.

Herbs pave the way for your body to do its own work, breaking up toxic accumulations, cleansing, lubricating, toning, supporting. Herbs are not instant panaceas, but they illustrate well how natural healing works- slowly, cumulatively, at the cause of the problem for system strength. Herbal formulas can be broad-based for over-all vitality, or specific to a special problem.

Herbs work like precision instruments in the body, not like sledge hammers. Herbal medicines work as natural, gentle activators to help the body heal itself.

—As nourishment, herbs can offer the body nutrients it does not always receive, either from poor diet, or deficiencies in the soil and air.

—As medicines, herbs work with your own body processes, so that it can heal and regulate itself. Herbs have the ability to address both the symptoms and causes of a problem.

Use herbs safely and effectively as medicines in your daily diet.

In ancient times, every household had an herb garden. Our forefathers did not distinguish between cooking herbs and healing herbs. Even up to just 150 years ago, a kitchen garden had a wide variety of herbs for family health. Herbal wisdom was passed from generation to generation.

We got away from this lifestyle for awhile, but herb gardens are coming back strong today — and these gardens don't just contain culinary herbs for cooking. They are healing gardens full of medicinal herbs. Healing herbs can help us get through many of the little health problems of life — and having them on hand for healing brings us back to one of the basics of the Earth and our life here.

Until the turn of the century, herbs were an integral part of American medicine, too. Herb use was taught in American medical schools until the discovery of penicillin. As pharmaceutical companies began to take over the medicine supply in the early 1900's, herbal remedies fell out of favor. The "flower children" of the 1960's and 70's brought back America's love of herbs. Today, there is a crescendo of herbal enthusiasm as the costs and difficulties of modern medical care rise. People, once again want the personal touch and convenience of having their medicines close at hand.

<u>Are herbs safe for you to use every day</u>? Most herbs, certainly culinary herbs, are as safe to take as foods. They go into your body as foods do, with your own enzyme activity. And they have almost no side effects as natural medicines. Herbs are not addictive or habit-forming, but they are powerful nutritional activators that should be used with care. The key to avoiding a negative reaction is moderation. Anything taken to excess can cause unwanted side effects. Occasionally, a mild allergy reaction may occur in a small number of people, the same as might occur to a food. This could happen because herb quality is poor, because it has been adulterated with chemicals in the growing - storing process, or in rare cases, because incompatible herbs were used together. Or it may be just an individual adverse response to a certain plant. Use normal common sense, reasonable care and intelligence when using herbs for either food or medicine.

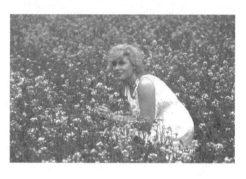

Balance is the key to using herbs for healing. Every person is different, with different nutritional needs. It takes a little more attention and personal responsibility than mindlessly taking a prescription drug... but the extra care is worth far more in the results you achieve for your health.

Herbs may be used as a primary part of your remedy system. I consider herbs a first line of defense in a lifestyle therapy program. They are a good starting choice for anyone who wants to take a measure of control over their own health care.

What about herb quality?

How can you tell if the herbs you buy have the potency and healing properties you're paying for? Thousands of herbs are available today at all quality levels. Communications and improved storage allow us to simultaneously obtain and use herbs from different climates, harvests and seasons, an advantage ages past did not enjoy. However, the natural variety of soils, seeds, and weather means that every crop of botanicals is unique. Every batch of a natural whole herb compound will also be slightly different, offering its own unique benefits and experience.

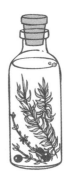

The way to insure high quality in the herb world is a firm commitment to excellence, because herb quality is never an accident. There is a world of difference between fairly good herbs and the best. If you are going to use culinary herbs as medicines, you must insist on superior stock. Superior plants cost far more than standard stock, but sell for proportionally far less - a true value for the alternative health consumer.

For therapeutic success, herbs must be **BIO-ACTIVE** and **BIO-AVAILABLE**. A good herbalist works with the naturally occurring bio-chemical properties, so high quality is not only a desired attribute, it is a mandatory element.

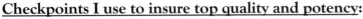

Checkpoints I use to insure top quality and potency:

• Use organically grown or wildcrafted herbs whenever available. They're easy to find today. Over 85% of the herbs I used in my Crystal Star Herbal Nutrition formulas were organically grown or wildcrafted. Botanical farms are springing up all over the U.S. Herb quality is historically prized in Asia; I find herbs from there are high quality.

• In general, herbs from small domestic suppliers are fresher and more potent. They buy small amounts of herbs frequently, rather than large amounts that may lose potency before they are used. Small suppliers are also more likely to buy fresh-dried, locally grown herbs immediately upon harvest, assuring short transportation time and fresher plants.

• Buy the best. In the herbal medicine world, price is generally a fair gauge of quality. Top quality plants may cost far more than standard herb stock, and more than vitamin supplements. But even herbs that seem outrageously priced are usually worth it in terms of their healing value. Herbal product results must be able to speak for themselves, and a little goes a long way.

• Store herbs in dark, sealed containers, cool and closed away from light and heat.

Common questions about how to use herbs:

Every person has a unique, wonderful body, and each body has the ability to bring itself to its own balanced and healthy state. Once people get started on the concept of taking responsibility for their own well-being, they discover that they know their own bodies better than anyone else. They also find that they can make wise health choices for themselves.

—**How do you incorporate herbal medicines into your daily diet?** Natural healing, including the use of herbs, is lifestyle therapy...... it's about incorporating elements that are available to you every day into a healing program. Staying healthy year-round is really a matter of staying in tune with the seasons. Herbs can help your body defenses target seasonal health risks all during the year. A good lifestyle healing program should also include diet, exercise, stress reduction techniques and mindset to achieve permanent health. Without these, you just get a quick fix.....a bandaid that doesn't last.

Herbs work like a cellular phone call, at the deepest levels of the body, at the cause, rather than the effect. They pave the way for the body to do its own work.

Herbs work better with a natural foods diet and a healthy lifestyle. Results increase dramatically when fresh foods and whole grains form the basis of your diet. The subtle healing activity of herbs is more effective when it doesn't have to labor through excess mucous, non-food material, or junk food accumulation. Studies show that many congested people carry around 10 to 15 pounds of excess density.

Herbs can help you overcome the problems of today's chemicalized foods, because they are rich in minerals and trace minerals, the basic elements missing or diminished in today's "quick-grow," over-sprayed, over-fertilized farming.

Minerals are a basic element in nutrient absorption. Mineral-rich herbs not only provide the healing activity to support your body in overcoming disease, but also the foundation minerals that allow your body to take them in! Mother Nature thinks of everything.

—When can I expect results from using herbs in my daily diet?
You'll often notice improvement from an herbal formula in 3 to 6 days. Some effects, like energy, relaxation or soothing may be felt in as little as half an hour. Effects for chronic and long-standing problems will, of course, take longer. **A good rule of thumb is one month of healing for every year you have had the problem.**

—How do you take herbal remedies for the best results?
Herbs are natural remedies.....products for problems. They work best when taken for a specific problem. They work best when used as needed. Take the best herb or herb combination for your goal at the right time - rather than all the time - for optimum results.

Herbs work better in combination than singly. Like the notes of a symphony, herbs work better in harmony than standing alone. Even in cooking, using several herbs in a dish offers a wider range of healing values while it adds more complexity to your recipe.

Herbs have broad, diverse benefits within an herbal compound..... even within a single herb itself. A good example of the wide range of activity from a single herb might be chamomile, which is good for the skin, for helping to dissolve gallstones, and as an aid to sleep. Another might be garlic, which has natural antibiotic properties, is an anti-fungal agent, and helps lower blood pressure.

Take only one or two herbal combinations at the same time. Rotating and alternating herbal combinations according to your changing health needs allows your body to remain most responsive to their effects. Reduce dosage as the problem improves. Allow your body to pick up its own work and bring its own vital forces into action. If you are taking an herbal remedy for more than a month, discontinue for one or two weeks between months to let your body adjust and maintain your personal balance. The idea is to stimulate your own vital healing force.... your immune system, to do its work.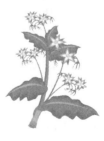

Take the herb or herbal formula that addresses your worst problem first. Alternate on and off weeks to allow your body to thoroughly use the herbal properties. One of the bonuses of an herbal healing program is the frequent discovery that other conditions were really complications of the first problem, and may take care of themselves as your body comes into balance.

How do herbs differ from vitamins and other supplements? Vitamins are not whole or naturally-occurring elements. Except for some food-grown vitamins, vitamins are partitioned substances, laboratory made. They do not combine with you systemically in the same way as foods or herbs do. What the body does not use is commonly flushed through and released. Vitamins, especially multiple vitamins, work best when strengthening a deficient or weak system, not as a substitute for a good diet.

Herbs are not like vitamins. Herbs are concentrated foods, not partitioned or isolated substances. Their value is in their wholeness and complexity, not their concentration. Herbs combine and work with the body's enzyme activity. They have restorative, body-energizing and tonic qualities. Herbs accumulate their nutrients instead of flushing excesses through.

Taking the same herbs all the time for maintenance and nutrient replacement would be like eating large quantities of a certain food all the time. The body would tend to have imbalanced nourishment from nutrients that were not in that food.

Don't take herbs like vitamins. Vitamins help shore up nutritional deficiencies, but with this benefit comes a problem. A vitamin that you take as a long term supplement is not very effective as a healing remedy. Vitamin C is a good example of this phenomenon. Herbs are remedies for problems. Use them when you need them, not all the time.

Most vitamins work best when taken with food for digestion. It is not necessary to take herbs or herbal formulas with food. Herbs are foods with their own enzymes for digestion.

How do herbs differ from drugs? Herbs go beyond vitamins because they can deal directly with a health problem. Two-thirds of the drugs in America today are still based on medicinal plants.

But modern herb-based drugs are not herbs — they are chemicals. Even when a drug has been derived from an herb, it is so refined, isolated and purified that only a chemical formula remains. Chemicals work on the body much differently than herbs do. As drugs, they cause many effects - only some of which are positive. Eli Lilly, a pharmaceutical manufacturer, once said "a drug isn't a drug unless it has side effects."

Drugs work pharmacologically; herbs work biologically. Drugs are highly focused medicines; generally one drug is used for one set of symptoms. Drugs are composed to treat the symptoms of a problem. America's science and big business orientation to health care means that we overlay this type of left brain thinking onto herbs, and try to make an herb fit the one-thing-for-one-thing mold.

Drugs work outside the body processes. Drugs aren't appropriate for many degenerative diseases, because they don't stimulate immune response, or help build the body up so it can take care of the problem. Viruses and pathogenic organisms often overcome, or develop immunity to drugs.

Herbal medicines are never just one thing for one thing. That's the wonderful thing about them. Herbs are living medicines - they may be our best hope for long lasting, healing results. Working at the body's deepest levels of the body, they become part of us through our own digestive activity.

Herbs in their whole form are not drugs, not even natural drugs. Do not expect the activity or response of a drug, which normally treats only the symptoms of a problem. In general, you have to take more and more of a drug to get continuing therapeutic effect.

Herbal medicines work differently.... just the opposite from drugs - much more than drugs in many ways. I find that, after starting with a good dose to "jump start" your body's healing processes, you need to take less and less of an herbal remedy, because your body picks up more of the healing work. Herbs are foundation nutrients. They work with the body, at the cause of the problem, improving body chemistry, reversing disease at its foundation, with more permanent effect. Results seem to take much longer, but the therapeutic effects also last much longer.

Even so, some improvement from herbal treatment can usually be felt in three to six days. Long standing problems take longer, but herbal remedies tend to work more quickly with each infection, and new infections grow fewer and further between.
A traditional rule of thumb is one month of healing for every year of the problem.

Herbs are not addictive, but they are natural medicines that should be used with care. As with other natural therapies, there is sometimes a "healing crisis" in an herbal healing program. This is known as the "Law of Cure," and simply means that you seem to get worse before you get better. Your body may eliminate toxic wastes heavily during the first stages of therapy. This is especially true in a traditional three to four day cleanse that many people use to begin a serious healing program. Temporary exacerbation of symptoms can range from mild to fairly severe, but usually precedes good results. Herbal therapy without a cleanse works more slowly and gently. Still, there is usually some weakness as disease poisons are released into the bloodstream to be flushed away. Strength shortly returns when this process is over. Watching this phenomenon allows you to observe your body at work healing itself.....an interesting experience indeed.

Herbs are amazingly effective in strengthening human immune response. But the immune system is fragile. It can be overwhelmed instead of stimulated. A virulent virus can mutate and be nourished by a supplement, instead of arrested by it. Sometimes taking an herb for too long can create an allergy to it, especially when taken in large amounts over a long period of time. Even when a good healing program is working and obvious improvement is being made, adding more of the medicinal agents in an effort to speed healing may aggravate symptoms and bring about worse results.

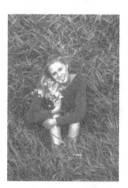

Don't overdo it. It takes time to rebuild health. Moderate amounts are much better than mega doses, even for serious health conditions. You'll get better results by giving yourself more time and gentler treatment.

Medical Science is changing fast. How does herbal healing fit in?

In many ways in America, and indeed around the world, we are in a paradigm shift.... especially in the global approach to healing. Clearly, American health care consumers are increasing their use of herbs as natural complements to drugs and drugstore medicines.

As the world grows undeniably smaller, people are interacting more, changing long-held beliefs. We see the earth as an intelligent being, evolving as we evolve and grow. Pathogenic organisms that cause diseases are also growing, replicating at an enormous rate, becoming more virulent.

Unfortunately, our immune defenses are weaker and the latest drugs aren't the answer. In fact, drugs are becoming less effective against organisms like powerful viruses, instead of more effective. New antibiotics now hardly last a year before the pathogenic organism they were designed to arrest develops immunity, mutates and grows stronger.

<u>It's a good example of a non-living agent like a drug trying to control a living thing</u>.

I call today's allopathic medicine "heroic medicine" because it was developed largely in wartime for the emergency requirements of triage, arresting death and infections until the body's healing powers could take over. But this type of medicine essentially hits the body with a hammer in this effort, so it isn't good at all against progressive and chronic diseases. In the end it overwhelms, instead of enhancing your own healing ability.

Drug therapy can't nourish and support, and drugs don't help your body by stimulating its immune response. In fact, most drugs and all surgery procedures create more body trauma along with their corrective benefits.

This is where complementary medicines, like herbs and homeopathic compounds are becoming so important. Natural remedies involve the work and cooperation of your own body in its healing. Our healing supports need to be able to work with us in our own way, for the best health.

I believe this is really the only way to permanent health because each of us is so individual. While we must be respectful of all ways of healing, most of us don't realize we have a choice. The only answer is something that is part of the larger picture, something worldwide that is living, that is big enough and intelligent enough to grow along with us.

<u>How can we use herbal medicines in today's health care</u>?

Herbs are one of the most important parts of alternative medicine, because they stimulate the body's own self-healing ability. When correctly used, herbs promote the elimination of waste matter and toxins from the system by simple natural means. They support nature in its fight against disease. I believe that in most cases, drugs are for emergencies and herbs are for lifestyle care.

Herbs can reach out to us with their marvelous complexity and abilities to help us address the problems of today just as they addressed ancient ones. We can count on the safety and efficacy of herbs in ways that the latest drug can never achieve. They may be our only hope to bring the balance back between the healing forces and diseases.

Watchword: Ask your pharmacist or health practitioner first if there is a known interaction between a prescription drug and the herb you wish to take. There have been a few studies checking botanicals for interaction with prescription drugs or over the counter medications.

<u>Are herbal remedies safe for children</u>?

Most herbs are very safe for children to take. Unless unusually or chronically ill, children have strong immune defenses. A child often needs only the subtle body-strengthening forces that nutritious foods, herbs or homeopathic remedies provide. The highly focused medications of orthodox medicines can have drastic side effects on a small body.

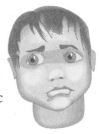

Sadly, the undeniable ecological, sociological and diet deterioration in America during the last fifty years has had a marked effect on children's health. Declining educational performance, learning disabilities, mental disorders, drug and alcohol abuse, hypoglycemia, allergies, chronic illness, delinquency and violent behavior are all evidence of reduced immunity and general health.

I find that you can get a lot of help from the kids themselves in an herbal healing program. Kids don't want to be sick; they aren't stupid; and they don't like going to the doctor any more than you do. We as adults tend to think that kids will reject herbal medicines, but they invariably recognize therapies that are good for them.

Children often don't need the heavy hammer of a drug. Children are naturally immune to disease. A nutritious diet and natural supplements can help keep them that way.

Here's how to use herbal remedies for children. Herb teas are the gentlest, easiest way for children to take herbal medications. If there is any taste rejection, simply give the herbs in juice or soup or other food.

Herb use normally goes by body weight. Base dose decisions on weight for children.
$^1/_2$ **dose for children 10-14 years**
$^1/_3$ **dose for children 6-10 years**
$^1/_4$ **dose for children 2-6 years**
Just drops for babies (I don't recommend giving herbs to tiny infants less than 6 months.)

Note: Herbs are good choices for many childhood diseases. My HEALTHY HEALING book offers a complete section on healing herbs for children.

Are herbal remedies a good choice for senior adults over 75?
Can they take herbal medicines safely? Even if their digestive processes are reduced? Senior citizens are America's fastest growing population. In many cases, drugs and drug interactions can be very harmful to them. I find that herbal combinations are a good choice for senior adults. They are gentle and mineral-rich to help a body with reduced stomach acid (HCl) take them in.

Most seniors have a wealth of long experience and common sense in their lives. They know their own bodies well and generally make very good choices for themselves. In addition, most senior adults are, and wish to remain, self-reliant.
Herbal medicines allow seniors to make many of their own healing choices, especially for disease protection or chronic ailments.

—Can you use herbal medicines if you currently take prescription medications?
In general, whole herbs are foods, and safe to take without drug interactions if you are taking prescription medication. For example, garlic is a strong herb with potent antibiotic properties. But you would not stop eating garlic just because you were taking a drug antibiotic.

Check the label of your herbal medicine to make sure the herbs are in their whole, naturally occurring state, not isolates or chemically concentrated. If you are unsure about which form the herbs are in, a naturopath, holistic pharmacist, or knowledgeable health food store professional can help. And, always ask your health professional if you're unsure whether an herb will react to a drug medicine.

119

Do herbs work differently for men and women?

Men and women clearly have different problems and different needs. Hormone and glandular secretions, at the deepest level of the body processes, are the basic cause of the differences in the sexes. The health and vitality for both men and women are based in the health of the glands.

Herbs are excellent answers for the problems that women face. It often all comes down to hormones for women - those incredibly important, potent substances that seem to be at the root of so many women's problems. Some have almost immediate effects on the system; some have a delayed reaction. Even in the tiniest amounts hormones have, as any woman can tell you, dramatic effects. A minute imbalance in ratio or deficiency can cause dramatic body swings. Many hormones are protein based, and we now know that proteins from herb and green plant sources can be very effective for human gland and hormone health.

Many serious hormone-driven conditions such as breast and uterine fibroids, endometriosis, menopausal problems, even breast cancer, are involved with thyroid imbalance, usually a low thyroid condition. Scientists believe that this is because estrogen levels are controlled by thyroid hormones. If the thyroid does not receive enough iodine, not enough thyroxine (a thyroid hormone), is produced, and too much estrogen builds up causing severe excess estrogen problems.

Drugs, chemicals and synthetic medicines, working as they do outside nature's cycle, often do not bring positive results for women. Herbal therapy nourishes in a broad spectrum, like the female essence itself. A woman's body responds to herbs easily without side effects. Herbs as foods are identified and used by the body's own enzyme action. I find that most women know their bodies well, and can instinctively pinpoint even deep level areas of imbalance that need support. Relief, and response time are often quite gratifying.

It's a little known health fact, but an unusual number of people born after WW II have thyroid problems, especially women. American industry started using many new chemicals during the war years that were not well tested. Some of them ended up in our food supply after the war, in fertilizers, preservatives and pesticides. Iodine-containing foods and herbs help bring the thyroid back into balance and stop the production of too much circulating estrogen.

One of the best therapy sources for natural iodine are sea greens. Americans think of sea greens in connection with Asian foods, but some of the best ones come from pristine, unpolluted waters off the northern shores of our own coasts - from Maine and the western San Juan Islands. They are delicious, sweet, and they can make a big difference to your health.

Just 2 tablespoons a day provide a therapeutic-strength dose. Buy them in sun-dried packages in any health food store, and snip them over a soup, salad or rice; or grind them in a blender with your favorite dried spices and herbs for a delicious vegetable seasoning.

Herbs can be a valuable answer for men, too. Today's fast pace and changing lifestyles seem to demand that men be Supermen. A man must be strong physically during workouts and sports, supportive emotionally in relationships, balanced under stress, mentally creative and quick, and sexually keen and virile.

While diet and exercise have been the main pillars of health for men, the quality of both are woefully deficient in the modern American man's life. Poor farming methods and processed foods have made us one of the earth's most nutritionally deficient nations. Today's men lead a hectic, but sedentary lifestyle that doesn't seem to allow for exercise unless a conscious effort is made.

Herbs can expand energy to the reproductive system, a primary area of male strength, increasing the health of a man's whole body. Herbs help give the male body solid foundation nourishment it needs to reproduce new cells and to improve vitality. Herbs, like ginseng, spirulina and ginkgo biloba are strong enough to specifically benefit a man's body without the side effects of drugs. They have broad spectrum activity for long term results, act quickly, yet are cumulative in the system to build a strong nutritional base.

Are herbs safe to take if you are pregnant? Or nursing?

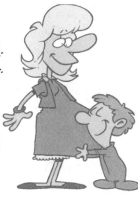

Herbs have been used successfully for centuries to ease hormone imbalances, stretching, bloating, nausea and other discomforts experienced during pregnancy, without impairing the development or health of the baby.

Herbs are mineral-rich foods, perfect for the extra growth requirements of pregnancy and childbirth. Herbs are accepted by the body's enzyme activity as food nutrients, lessening the risk of toxemia or overdose, while they provide gentle, quickly absorbed nutrition for both mother and baby.

Be extra careful taking herbs during pregnancy.

Even with gentle herbs, you need to know what you are doing. All regular maintenance supplements need to be re-examined during pregnancy, even if your program is holistically oriented. A mother's body is delicately tuned and sensitive at this time; imbalances can occur easily.

Mega-doses of anything are not good for the baby's system. Anything you take affects the tiny system of the baby. Fetuses and babies lack some of the ability to detoxify harmful chemicals in herbs. **Doses of all medication or supplements should almost universally be less than normal to allow for the infant's tiny capacity.** I recommend reducing dosage substantially during both pregnancy and nursing. Cutting dosage strength in half is usually about right. Ideal supplementation from food sources is best for absorbability.

Note: My HEALTHY HEALING book has a comprehensive list of herbs that you should avoid when you are pregnant, as well as those that are all right to take for problems you may face during pregnancy.

Watchwords for Using Herbs Safely:

1: **The vast majority of herbs would have to be ingested in almost impossible amounts to cause harm.** We are exposed to potentially toxic substances every day, yet in small amounts our bodies can normally metabolize them safely. According to U.S. mortality statistics, adverse effects of herbal medicines are among the least likely causes of poisoning or death in the U.S. Dosage is important - most negative reactions occur to the dose, or to overuse, not the herb itself. The herbs available for sale in natural food stores in America are legal and safe for normal use.

2: **Find out what the herb does, how to use it and the proper dosage.** If you get symptoms from taking a medicinal herb, stop taking it and contact a naturopath or herbalist, professionals trained to know the side effects or adverse effects of medicinal herbs. Though herbs are natural substances, they are strong medicines and should be used carefully. Each herb is a chemical factory on it's own. Taking too much or for too long means you run the risk, over long-term use, of creating a proving, meaning that symptoms an herb can cure in a sick person may manifest in you.

3: **Beware what a "scientific" study says about herbal safety.** There are very few good, honest evaluations of individual herbs, though there is research in the works to address that deficiency. Unfortunately, most herbal studies are done in labs as drugs; in other words, the isolated plant components, not the whole plant, are studied. Side effects to <u>chemicals</u> in herbs have been noted, but this method usually gives an incomplete picture of the safety of herbs. Whole plants, not isolated components of plants, contain hundreds of constituents, all with synergistic relationships. Nature, in its wisdom, builds in protective benefits that neutralize the harm that an isolated component might do.

4: **Be careful of the limited information you hear in the press.** As herbs re-emerge in our medical culture, they are subjected to increased scrutiny from the press. But a "sound bite" can rarely give the whole story..... and that's important with something as complex as herbs. News accounts usually focus on an isolated adverse reaction instead of looking at the long beneficial history of the plant. Some of our best natural medicines are lost to public use through this type of reporting.

5: **Learn as much as you can about the herbs you wish to take.** A helpful source of this information is my book, *How To Be Your Own Herbal Pharmacist.*

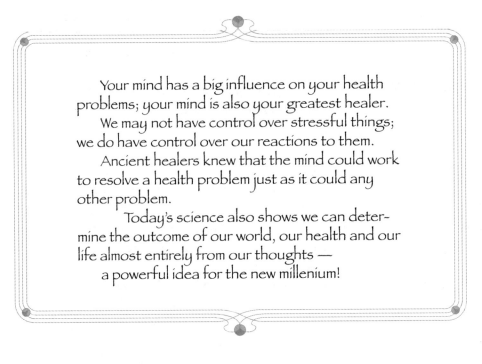

Your mind has a big influence on your health problems; your mind is also your greatest healer.

We may not have control over stressful things; we do have control over our reactions to them.

Ancient healers knew that the mind could work to resolve a health problem just as it could any other problem.

Today's science also shows we can determine the outcome of our world, our health and our life almost entirely from our thoughts —
a powerful idea for the new millenium!

You need Whole Foods for Healing

Whole Foods for Healing

<u>Promise yourself whole foods for your healing diet. They're the key</u>.
Before our "modern age," food was pretty wholesome. People were close to their gardens and farms, and animals and natural resources. Today, we live in a man-made jungle of food substances instead of foods - many of them highly processed, devoid of nutrients, chemical-laced, sugar-drenched and full of hidden fat.

<u>How does the food pharmacy keep you healthy</u>?
First and foremost - whole foods keep you whole. Your body isn't a lot of separate parts. It's all connected. The essence of human health is body balance, establishing and maintaining whole body chemistry that resists disease and assures you energy and well-being.

Left-brain oriented Science, western science, can only break things down, take them apart and look at the pieces to understand, so orthodox medicine today expresses diseases and health conditions in terms of different body elements. But, don't be fooled.... you are all one. Anything you do to any one part of your mind, body or spirit, affects every other part of you, too.

We are also learning this painful lesson about our planet. We have to keep all of Mother Earth healthy, so she can take care of all of us. It's a truth that Native Americans knew well. We are all one. The very material of our bodies comes from the Earth. Anything we do to the planet, we do to ourselves.

Whole foods are those that come to us as Nature intended, not broken down into separate "nutrients," or altered with chemicals or additives. Our bodies work best when we have whole foods to work with. Processed, refined, man-made foods make our bodies struggle to use them... and then the job is only a partial one.

<u>Organically grown foods are popular and easily available today. Seek them out. Eat with the seasons you live in</u>.
Flow with the season's changes for harmony. (Does your body really need strawberries in December?) If we look closely, Nature provides what is needed for each part of the Earth in tune with the time of year, like fruits in the summer for cooling, and root vegetables in the winter for building. It helps keep the balance around us right, reminding us that we are all part of the natural chain.

I find that a working kitchen garden can do wonders for harmony of mind and body. If you can't have a garden, eating fruits and vegetables from your own region is a wonderful way to keep a closer touch with where you are and who you are.

The Case for Eating Whole Foods

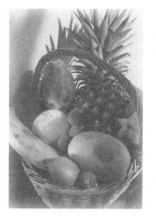

You're probably using this book because you're concerned about the health problems from eating refined, preserved, pasteurized, waxed, hydrogenated, canned, smoked, cured, irradiated, colored, additive-laden, chemically adulterated, even genetically altered foods. Modern processing removes many nutrients from foods. Chemically adding them back after processing doesn't make the altered food whole again. Not only are chemical additives incapable of supporting life themselves, when combined with foods, the food itself is chemically changed, its life-sustaining ability diminished. Many microorganisms develop resistance to ion radiation and other preservatives, too — your food may still appear edible when it is seriously contaminated.

Even when food values are labeled on a package, they are derived from test results of fresh, unsprayed, un-processed produce. Further, food value measurements are outdated. They were calculated in the 1950's or earlier before the enormous amounts of pesticides agri-business uses today.

Most of us have washed heads of lettuce and seen the water turn soapy, or peeled cucumbers, apples or eggplant to remove wax. Supermarkets brag that their produce is in the store the day after it is picked. Freshness-retaining chemicals are not needed for so short a time. Most processing is needed for economic, not nutritive, reasons - for longer shelf life, unnatural perfection of appearance, or import/export regulations.

A look at some wide ranging new studies reveals startling information on the health effects of adding chemicals to our food supply. Here's a small sampling about this trend:

—Up to 10,000 food additive chemicals may be used in pre-prepared foods before they reach our tables. The average American now consumes up to ten pounds of additives a year.

—More than 1000 of these chemicals have not been tested for their cancer causing potential or properties that may impact genetic damage or birth defects. Food processing methods compound the problem by removing many nutrients that might protect us from the harmful effects.

—More than 80% of all food purchased in supermarkets today is processed or refined. A typical fast food meal of a hamburger, shake and french fries, contains 22 chemical additives. Twelve of the twenty-two are considered toxic, even in fairly small amounts.

—Autopsies of American soldiers between the ages of 18 and 22 killed in World War II showed no signs of atherosclerosis. Almost every autopsy of an American soldier killed in Vietnam showed some stage of atherosclerosis or narrowing of the arteries.

—40% of Armed Forces volunteers in the last decade were rejected for physical or mental deficiencies.

—In the last decade, the number of patients admitted to hospitals for serious degenerative diseases increased 5 times faster than the growth of the population as a whole.

—In his book, *The Betrayal of Health: The Impact of Nutrition, Environment and Lifestyle on Illness in America,* Dr. Joseph Beasley says that "degenerative diseases afflict more than 100,000,000 Americans," a phenomenon he calls the Malnutrition-Poisoning Syndrome.

The Case for Eating Organically Grown Foods

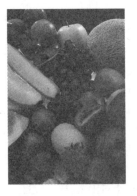

Over 77% of the 4.5 billion pounds of pesticides we dump yearly in the U.S. are used in agriculture to produce our food! Pesticide by-products are even used in our water! (See page 58.) In 1997 alone, pesticide costs totalled over 12 billion dollars. Although our government has recently taken steps to reduce pesticide use by "phase out" programs, it may be too little, too late, because so many of these chemicals have already contaminated our food and water supply. Pesticides can remain in the food chain for decades. DDT, chlordane and heptachlor are found in soils more than 20 years after their use.

More than 2 million synthetic substances are known, **25,000 are added each year** — over 30,000 are produced on a commercial scale, some so widespread we are unaware of them. But, they work their way into our bodies faster than they can be eliminated, and they're causing allergies and addictions in record numbers. Only a tiny fraction are ever tested for toxicity, and those that come to us from developing countries have few safeguards in place.

Recent World Health Organization studies show that chemical and environmental factors are responsible for 80 to 90% of all cancers. New studies also link pesticides and pollutants to hormone dysfunctions, psychological disorders and birth defects. The molecular structure of many chemical carcinogens interacts with human DNA, so long term exposure can result in metabolic and genetic alteration that affects immune response.

The chemical industry is quick to point out that the use of DDT and some other harmful pollutants containing environmental hormones is illegal in America. Yet, the U.S. is still the largest producer of DDT, selling it to the rest of the world. Many food-producing countries that supply America do not support pesticide bans, so imported foods from them still carry a toxic threat to us. Even if we ban the sprayed foods at our ports, the Earth's winds circle the globe, and all the Earth's waterways are connected, so chemical pollutants containing environmental hormones reach the entire world's food supply.

The newest statistics come from breast cancer research. The dramatic rise in breast cancer in the last decade is consistent with the increased accumulation of organo-chlorine (PCB) residues. In Long Island, for instance, women living in areas previously sprayed with DDT have one of the highest breast cancer rates in the U.S.

Israel's pesticide experience offers even more dramatic evidence of the pesticide-breast cancer connection. Until twenty years ago, breast cancer rates and contamination levels of organo-chlorine pesticides in Israel were among the highest in the world. An aggressive phase-out of these pesticides has led to a sharp reduction in contamination levels and breast cancer death rates.

Here's how the link between pesticides and breast cancer seems to work.

Pesticides, like other pollutants, are stored in fatty tissue areas like breast tissue. Some pesticides (including PCB's and DDT) compromise immune function, overwork the liver and disrupt the glands the way too much estrogen does.

A recent study showed up to 60% more dichloro-diphenyl-ethylene (DDE), DDT, and poly-chlorinated bi-phenols (PCB's) in the bodies of women who have breast cancer than in those who don't. Some researchers suggest that the reason today's older women experience a higher than normal rate of breast cancer may be that these women had greater exposure to DDT before it was banned.

What can we do to overcome these environmental health threats? More awareness of our food supply and more care for our own internal environment are a start.

Start with the foods you eat.

It's a quandary. The healthy fruits and vegetables we're all encouraged to eat are unfortunately very likely to contain unhealthy pesticides. (Grains have less because the milling process removes them.) Should you stop eating fresh produce? Of course not; fruits and vegetables clearly protect against cancer and heart disease.

Take steps to protect yourself from chemical residues in your food.

1: Buy organic produce whenever you can! Fix it yourself for the best results if you're on a healing diet. A rapidly growing group of Americans are seeking out farmer's markets and produce stands.... even growing some of their own foods.

2: Buy seasonal, local produce whenever you can. Avoid imported produce as much as possible. Foreign countries have different regulations for pesticide use, so produce from other countries typically contains higher levels of pesticides than locally grown. Developing countries have few regulations. Mexico, for instance, has only recently begun phasing out DDT and chlordane which have been banned in the U.S. for decades. Imported produce also carries the threat of dangerous microbes, like those found in Guatemalan and Mexican strawberries in 1997.

3: Eat more fruits and vegetables that have the lowest PCB residues - like avocados, onions, broccoli, bananas, cauliflower, sweet potatoes, corn and watermelon. Eat a wide variety of fresh foods to keep your exposure to any one pesticide low.

4: Always wash produce. Especially wash foods with the highest residues - strawberries, cherries, spinach, bell peppers, cucumbers and grapes.

5: Minimize your intake of high risk seafood. America's coasts are in crisis. The ecosystem of our planet has been drastically upset by overfishing and by incredible amounts of waste dumped into our waters. More than one-third of U.S. shellfish beds are closed due to contamination from industrial chemicals like PCB's and methyl mercury. Should you stop eating seafood? Of course not. Fish, seafoods and sea greens are some of the healthiest foods our planet offers. Fish like salmon and tuna, are loaded with Omega-3 fatty acids that clearly decrease risk of heart disease and cancer. Sea greens like nori, wakame and dulse are some of the few non-animal sources of B-12, needed for cell development and nerve function. They are rich in natural iodine to strengthen poor thyroid function, at the root of many energy and weight problems. Two tablespoons of dried sea greens into rice, soups and salads every day increase metabolism and energy.

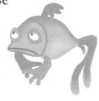

Unfortunately, some seafoods are not safe to eat. Fish like striped bass, rock cod, ocean perch, catfish, walleye, shark, caviar and lake trout, langoustinos and Maine lobster often contain high residues of DDT, chlordane, dioxin and PCB's. In addition, eating tuna, shark and swordfish from Connecticut is not safe for pregnant women or young children because of high mercury levels.

At this printing, the safest seafoods to include in your diet are farmed abalone, Dungeness crab, halibut, Pacific and farmed salmon, and shrimp. Wild abalone and swordfish are both so scarce they are on the endangered species list.

6: Be extra careful about your water supply. We've all heard scary things about our water supply lately. Experts estimate that 50% of the U.S. water supply is contaminated with giardia, which unlike bacteria, is not killed by chlorination. Giardia waterborne bacteria sickened 300,000 people and killed more than 100 in Milwaukee in 1993. Twenty-two American cities in 1996 were served by public water systems that violated minimum safety levels for contaminants.

Should you stop drinking water? Of course not. Water is critical to your very existence. But you can make sure your water is as clean as possible. —Drink quality water. Buy bottled water or invest in a purification system. Reverse osmosis systems are expensive (about $1,000), but they are the best at eliminating impurities. Carafes and pitchers are much cheaper (about $25). They remove some organic pollutants and lead. —Investigate the quality of your drinking water. Read the review on water safety on page 58. Ask your water utility for its latest contamination review. Call the Clean Water Hotline at 800-426-4791 for information on EPA standards for water safety.

7: Avoid foods that usually have environmental estrogens and androgens. How do environmental hormones affect you? Exogenous (literally outside the body) estrogens and androgens affect your endocrine system, a vital system of glands, hormones and cellular receptors that control your internal functions. Nearly 40% of pesticides used in commercial agriculture are suspected endocrine disrupters. They contain hormone-like substances, especially estrogens and androgens (the major male and female hormones), that spell disaster for our health.

Only in the last five years has anyone realized how common environmental estrogens are in our world. People who live in high pesticide agricultural areas, who eat a high fat diet, or hormone-injected meats are most at risk.

Science is just beginning to accept, even though naturopaths have known for some time, that man-made estrogens can stack the deck against women by increasing their estrogen levels hundreds of times over normal levels. Many scientists still believe that there is no significant difference between man-made and natural hormones, but it seems apparent from the evidence of thousands of women, that even if a lab test can't tell the difference, their bodies can.

Women's diseases linked to chronic exposure to synthetic estrogen mimics:
- breast and reproductive organ cancer.
- breast and uterine fibroids, and ovarian cysts.
- endometriosis, and pelvic inflammatory disease (PID).

Another indication of abnormally high estrogenic activity? American girls are reaching puberty at earlier and earlier ages. Nearly half of African American girls and fifteen percent of white girls start to develop sexually by age eight.

Women aren't the only ones endangered by the estrogen-imitating effects of these substances. There is substantial evidence that man-made estrogens threaten male health with reproductive disorders, too. The most alarming statistics relate to sperm count and hormone-driven cancers.

<u>**Environmental androgens**</u> (substances that mimic male sex hormones) in chemical pollutants are even more widespread and may reveal even more frightening results. Research on synthetic androgens is still too new to know all the hormonal health implications, but early indications show that these substances have widespread involvement in the development of some cancers. One in vitro study found that out of ten pollutants, five bound to human androgen receptors while only two bound to estrogen receptors.

Men's health problems linked exposure to environmental hormones.
- a 50% average decrease in male sperm counts over the past 50 years.
- a 32% rise in undescended testes, small penis size and male fertility problems.
- a dramatic rise in prostate disease, testicular cancer and male cancer deaths.

For the first time in history, large numbers of people worldwide are having trouble conceiving children. In America today, one in six married couples of child-bearing age has trouble conceiving and completing a successful pregnancy. Chemical pollutants seem to be a factor in the birth rise of female and intersex babies where males would normally be born. Both humans and animals are now being born with both male and female genitalia, a frightening sign that our hormonal health, and that of future generations, is in jeopardy. Other effects include birth defects, impaired immunity, diabetes, and liver damage.

Remind yourself that only whole foods are wholesome. A healthy detox twice a year may be a good way to rid yourself of the dangerous chemicals in your body.

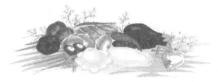

Unhappiness is
the hunger to get.
Happiness is the
hunger to give.

What About Genetically-Engineered Foods
Are they "superfoods" or a disaster in the making?

Food technology is expanding almost at the rate of the "big bang!" In the year 2000, up to 70 percent of the foods on American grocery shelves are genetically engineered to some extent (up 90% in less than a decade). GE foods are everywhere. Most of the soy, corn, potatoes, tomatoes, dairy foods and yellow squash at your local market is genetically engineered. More than one-third of U.S. farmland is planted with genetically-engineered seeds. All food is expected to be genetically engineered in the next five to ten years. By the end of the twentieth century there will be enough GE crops to cover Great Britain, Taiwan and New York's Central Park!

You may be shocked but should you be worried? Genetically engineered foods often contain DNA from widely different species. Plant, animal, insect, even bacterial or viral DNA are used to make the new "improved" foods.

Pros and Cons of the New Millennium Food Supply
Are GE foods really "Franken-foods?"

There are benefits from genetic engineering:
- Proponents of GE foods insist that genetic engineering can boost resistance to pests, decreasing the need for harsh pesticide sprays and incidence of plant disease.
- Genetic engineering improves shelf life by altering genes which lead to spoilage.
- GE companies hope to create "super crops" that will feed the Earth's exponentially growing population for generations to come. Genetic engineering is already here for some animal foods. "Super salmon" now grow to 10 lbs. in only 14 months.
- GE foods offer an easy delivery route for drugs and vaccinations. Genetically modified chickens now lay drug-enriched eggs to fight certain diseases. (For people who rely on natural therapies, drug delivery through foods is not desirable.)

There's also a downside risk to GE foods... a price to pay:
- Allergens are transferred at the molecular level. As we add genes into foods from substances that aren't normally in our food chain, new allergies could run rampant. We simply won't know what GE foods will cause reactions until it's too late. New reports show that soy allergies have gone up 50% since genetically engineered soy came into the food supply in 1997.
- Using genes in GE foods from known allergens (like peanuts) can trigger severe reactions in allergic people. Eating a GE food that contains an allergen could mean life or death for an allergic person! A 1996 study in the *New England Journal of Medicine* revealed that soybean spliced with a Brazil nut gene caused the same allergy reaction as eating the Brazil nut itself.
- Cross-pollination means pollen from GE crops will likely transfer into organic crops located nearby, so even organic foods may be exposed to genetically altered organisms.
- Crops that are genetically engineered to build resistance to pesticides may transfer into neighboring weeds creating "superweeds" which don't yield to herbicides.

• Research shows bioengineering may destroy healing properties and reduce nutrient content of foods! A 1999 study in the Journal of Medicinal Food shows that cancer-fighting phytoestrogens in genetically engineered soybeans are 14% lower than in natural soybeans.

• Genetic engineering means animal by-products make their way into vegetarian foods. Fish genes (which improve shelf life) are routinely added to GE tomatoes, outraging vegetarians who assumed that at least their fruits and vegetables were free of animal products.

• GE foods developed to create their own insecticides or herbicides are especially precarious. A GE food that can kill another living organism could be dangerous for consumption by both animals and people. Even the ability to kill a so-called harmful plant or insect is risky. Mother Nature has many pathways to the health and survival of the Earth's species; we know only a tiny portion of how nature really works. As our own Native Americans have long known.... we are all one.... unnaturally changing <u>ANY</u> species has far-reaching consequences for others.

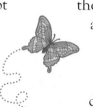

• Genetic engineering may prompt the development of "super" insects, that can resist normal methods of eradication and disturb the ecosystem. We already see disruptions in insect populations from GE technology. A European study shows ladybugs who eat aphids that dine on genetically engineered, insect-resistant potatoes live far shorter lives and produce one-third fewer eggs. California studies report monarch butterflies dying from eating GE corn pollen!

<u>Should we slow technology until we get a better handle on the health implications</u>?

We know some critical GE dangers already. For example, once you alter plant DNA you run the risk of risk of causing mutations that lead to cancer. Yet only 1% of the USDA's molecular biology budget is spent on exploring the risks of genetic engineering on our foods!

The "Flavr Savr" tomato introduced in 1994 is an example of GE food failure. Genes in the tomatoes conferred resistance to the antibiotics *kanamycin* and *neomycin* in the people who ate them. Antibiotic marker genes are used throughout the genetic engineering process today. Yet, more than 150 genetically engineered foods will be approved for sale this year (2000), virtually none of them tested for this type of risk. If we continue to rely on these techniques, genetic engineering may cause the rates of antibiotic-resistant bacteria coming from foods to skyrocket!

The massive genetic pollution of our population may be the ultimate price we pay for disrupting the natural balance within plant and animal species through genetic engineering. Once a living organism is genetically modified, it can reproduce, mutate and migrate at will. Even simple human mistakes could have disastrous consequences.

<u>Darwin may have been right</u>. Natural selection may be the key. Nature never does anything without good reason. Plants and animals change naturally with time to adapt to a changing environment. For instance, we know many plant species have lengthened their growing season to better use the effects of global warming. Over time, a plant may become more resistant to a disease or the effects of pollution. Some tomatoes growing in polluted areas actually become stronger, boosting their antioxidant nutrients to protect themselves from harsh conditions, in the process, becoming a more powerful medicinal food..... **without genetic engineering!**

Nature is the world's premier biochemist, making biological adjustments that keep humans <u>and</u> plants protected from changing conditions and diseases strains.

Today humans are breaking natural laws almost without thought to the consequences.... simply because we can do it. Never before in history have we so upset the boundaries between species set by Nature as we have now through genetic engineering. Europe has already rejected the new "frankenfoods." Other foreign markets threaten to stop buying U.S. exports until they are free of GMO's (genetically modified organisms). Americans are slowly waking up to dangers of genetic engineering. Gerber baby foods has announced they will be "GE-free."

For industry giant Monsanto, genetic engineering means new GE species to be patented, monopolized and sold at enormous profit. According to its own Director of Corporate Communications, Monsanto believes it is the FDA's responsibility to assure the safety of the foods they sell. Monsanto's interest is only to "sell as much of it as they can."

At this writing, no FDA labels are required on GE foods. There's no way to be sure whether the foods you buy are genetically altered. The FDA says GE foods don't need labelling because they are no different than hybrids created by cross breeding. Yet hybrids are vastly different than GE foods. Hybrids result from cross breeding two or more varieties of the same species. Genetically foods have no species boundaries. Genes from entirely different species can be used. Animal, viral and bacterial genes can all be inserted in a GE plant or animal. In reality, the FDA has no policy on how GE foods should be regulated because they are clearly not natural foods!

Surveys show that over 80% of Americans want GE foods to be labeled. Congress introduced a bill in December 1999 that may force manufacturers to label GE foods to allow consumers a choice. U.S. agricultural groups now warn member farmers about the consequences of genetic engineering in terms of consumer dissatisfaction and "massive lawsuit liability."

What can we do to protect ourselves? If you want GE foods to be labeled as I do, write to Jane Henney M.D., FDA Commissioner, at 5600 Fishers Lane, Rockville, MD 20857.

Protective measures you can take to avoid GE foods:

1. Stick with certified organic foods which are less likely to be affected by genetic tampering. Be aware however that the Organic Standards Board does allow processed organic food to contain 5% non-organic ingredients which could theoretically be genetically engineered although the vast majority of the industry opposes the practice.

2. Buy seasonal fruits and vegetables from organic local farmers whenever possible. Buying with the seasons in your local community helps strengthen small farmers and weaken gen-food corporations. Always ask if genetically engineered seeds are used.

3. Especially avoid non-organic foods containing soy, canola oil and corn ingredients- foods routinely genetically engineered.

4. Consider organic dairy. Most commercial dairy is injected with rBST, a GE hormone. *Note:* Research in the 1995 Cancer Letter shows cows treated with GE hormones have higher levels of insulin growth factor, a risk factor for breast and prostate cancer and child leukemia.

Perhaps Charles, Prince of Wales said it best: "The genetic engineering of foods "takes mankind into realms that belong to God and God alone."

Getting Junk Foods Out of Your Life

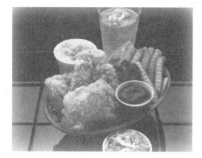

America is the world's richest nation, yet its population is one of the most poorly nourished. The American diet tends to make people sick instead of strong. Our cancer rate for hormone- driven cancers, like breast and uterine cancer is 500% greater than any other country. The American Institute For Cancer Research recognizes that 40 to 60 % of all cancers are related to poor diet choices.

You might think that after a decade of media attention and "food police" warnings, most Americans would have changed their diets and clamored for higher nutrient foods. This is simply not the case. Food products in supermarkets and most restaurants remain chemical-laced, highly-refined, enzyme impoverished and nutrient deficient. Junk food may be even more highly processed than when the warnings began; irradiation practices and virulent food-borne pathogens like *E. coli* show up regularly in fast foods.

Note: I've found that most restaurants are very responsive to the requests of their discriminating clientele. Many will even prepare a fresh or low fat dish exactly to your order at no extra cost.

New reasons to eliminate problem foods from your healing diet:

—Fried foods: Maybe you love them but your arteries and heart hate them! Frying temperature is from 400° F up to 700° F. At temperatures this high, CIS fatty acids are converted to trans-fatty acids; their molecules behave like saturated fats, raising cholesterol levels and increasing heart disease risk. Cancer studies document a high incidence of colon cancer in populations where saturated fat intake is high.

Even scarier..... when fat is reheated at high temperatures (as it is in deep fryers) the fat is likely to produce virulent carcinogens, like acrolein and benzopyrene. Burning or overcooking fats and oils contributes to the formation of free radicals, fragmented molecules that damage your cells.

Do you suffer from indigestion? Eliminate fried foods first. They cause bloating, gas and diarrhea in many people. A tasty alternative: mix bread crumbs with your favorite seasonings, coat the food, then bake for a crispy, "fried" taste without the health risks.

—Hydrogenated oils (trans fats): These fats are thought to be the culprits in the recent sharp rise in LDL cholesterol levels and obesity in America. They're widely used in today's snack foods of all kinds. Trans fats are present in most cooking oils (even some you thought were healthy, like safflower oil) because they undergo hydrogenation to extend their shelf life.

Hydrogenation or partial hydrogenation makes unsaturated fats into saturated fats. (See *Fats and Oils*, page 72.) Startling studies show that even butter, once thought to be the worst saturated fats, is better for health than hydrogenated margarine. A Univ. of Texas Southwestern study shows that cholesterol drops by more than 100 points when trans fats are dropped from the diet.

A study published in *Cancer Epidemiology, Biomarkers and Prevention* reveals that women with breast cancer have higher levels of trans fatty acids in their bodies than women without. Breast cancer risk increased an astounding 40% for women with high levels of trans fatty acid!

Trans fats double the risk of heart attacks and clogged arteries. They contribute to diabetes, obesity, rheumatoid arthritis and auto-immune diseases like fibromyalgia. Trans fats are difficult to release from the body. It may take up to 2 years to rid your blood and arteries of their deposits.

Consider reducing hydrogenated and partially hydrogenated foods right away. Avoid fast food restaurants. Use mechanically pressed oils like olive and canola oils in your recipes. Oleic acid, a mono-unsaturated fatty acid in mechanically extracted (rather than solvent extracted) olive oil, for example, retains most of its nutrients even after extraction and is less prone to oxidation.

—**White sugar:** White sugar is the most refined carbohydrate in our food supply. A little of this no-nutrition food goes a long way. Did you know it takes 16 feet of sugar cane to produce 1 teaspoon of sugar? Refined sugar first appeared as a "military drug" in the War of 1812 as a light-weight energy source. Interestingly, when Napoleon used it for his army, he lost his first battle.

Sugar began as a medicinal to help other medicine go down. It entered our food supply in a big way in the middle of the last century. Today, sugar qualifies as America's favorite but most poorly understood drug. The average American now consumes 150 pounds of white sugar per year. Some say we are a nation addicted to sugar.

Eating sugary foods regularly causes abnormal insulin production that results in problems like diabetes and hypoglycemia. Sugar robs your body of B-vitamins, critical minerals like magnesium and zinc, and trace minerals like chromium (effective for weight loss and blood sugar balance). Too much sugar is linked to circulatory diseases like thrombosis, chronic gum disease and severe depression. Each of these health conditions improves when sugar is eliminated from the diet. A University of Alabama study shows dramatically reduced symptoms when sugar is removed from the diet of hospitalized depression patients.

—**White flour:** White flour is the most common carbohydrate in the U.S. In the 19th century, when microscopes revealed bacteria on grain, white flour became the baker's standard. It didn't spoil quickly, so was thought safer than whole grains. But white flour's long shelf life is a result of stripped nutrients; at least 22 nutrients are lost in its milling. Only four are replaced when the flour is "enriched." White bread lacks copper, B vitamins and zinc, and has 75% less fiber than 100% whole wheat. Many of us remember our grammar school days when we mixed white flour with water to form paste. White flour sticks to everything, including your intestines!

—**Are all carbohydrates bad?** Carbohydrates are quick energy sources. Once metabolized, they supply your body with glucose for energy and brain function. Complex carbs from beans and grains, vegetables, fruit and nuts are generally considered to be healthful. But there is a dark side to eating too many carbohydrates of any kind.

<u>**Excess carbohydrates are stored in your body as fat.**</u> Excess carbohydrates cause blood sugar levels to rise triggering insulin release from the pancreas. The insulin removes excess glucose from the blood to be stored as glycogen, and then as fat, leading the way to obesity.

—**Additives and preservatives:** Most of us have no idea know what we're really eating when we buy foods with additives and preservatives. We certainly can't decode the long chemical chain names. But most of our foods have them to prevent spoilage and boost looks and flavor, even in foods we might think are fresh. Many of them are not innocent, inactive ingredients. In fact, they are often harmful, taxing our immune systems and triggering hyperactive responses in children.

I believe we could stop using many, if not most synthetic chemical additives. There are effective natural food preservers, which are harmless, and even enhance the nutritional value of foods. For example, vitamin C is a frequently added preservative in foods to prevent the "turning" of canned fruits or fruit juices. Vinegar, salt and wood smoke have a long history of safety when used in moderation. Vitamin E tocopherols, and rosemary extract are effective antioxidant preservers.

Beware of these food additives and preservatives.....
• **Monosodium glutamate (MSG)** used to enhance the flavor of Chinese food, chips, processed meats and packet soups, causes broad allergic responses in many people. Its powerful "excitotoxins" are implicated in destroying brain and nervous system tissue. Avoid it to reduce the risk of Alzheimer's or Parkinson's disease. I advise pregnant women to avoid MSG as well.

• **Yellow Tartrazine (E102),** a widely used food coloring is regularly linked to hyperactive misbehavior problems in children. If your child has ADD or ADHD, eliminate yellow tartrazine, other colorings, and all additives and preservatives from the child's diet. Most parents see improvement within a month if E102 is part of the behavior problem.

• **Nitrates and nitrites** are often added to processed meats (especially bacon, sausage and ham), and to dried fruits as color preservers. Both nitrates and nitrites convert to potentially carcinogenic nitrosamines linked to many types of cancer and thyroid problems. Choose organic meats and produce to stay clear of nitrates and nitrites.

• **Sulphur dioxide and sulfites** are used to kill sugar fermentation yeasts in food and alcoholic beverages. People with severe asthma or allergies should avoid wines, beer, soft drinks and restaurant foods that contain sulfites. Several anaphylactic shock cases and wide media attention on salad bars that use sulfites have resulted in less use of these chemicals.

• **Mineral hydrocarbons** were sprayed on dried fruit as non-stick additives until very recently when the U.S. Agriculture Dept. finally advised manufacturers of their health hazards. They are still used in non-stick sprays for baking. Mineral hydrocarbons accumulate in the lymphatic system, our body's chief detoxifier and blood waste cleanser, putting unneeded stress on your body's immune system. Check labels to make sure they don't become part of your food chain.

• **Artificial sweeteners** like sorbitol and xylitol replace sugar in sugar-free snacks, toothpaste, gum and diabetic products. But they can create even more health problems than refined sugar, and compound sugar-related diseases like diabetes and hypoglycemia. Sorbitol in particular, causes severe cramping and diarrhea symptoms. If you (or your child) are sugar sensitive, check labels for dextrose, lactose, maltose or saccharin. Synthetic sweeteners, like Nutrasweet and Equal, developed from powerful chemicals like aspartame, are everywhere. Aspartame, 200 times sweeter than sugar, has received more FDA complaints than any other food ingredient in the agency's history. Immediate, serious reactions to aspartame include severe headaches, extreme dizziness and throat swelling. Retina deterioration is attributed to methyl alcohol, a substance released when aspartame breaks down. Aspartame is also linked to high blood pressure, insomnia, ovarian cancer and brain tumors. (See *Sugar and Sweeteners,* page 97.)

Changing the Face of Your Diet

A healthy healing diet can change your way of cooking because it incorporates new, different ingredients. This may be a bit daunting to handle all at once - especially when you have a family, and want to keep everybody happy by fixing their favorite meals.

This section can help. Moving away from a meat-based, saturated fat, sugary foods diet doesn't mean you're depriving yourself. My staff and I have "done it all" over the last twenty-five years; changing over processed, pre-prepared foods to whole foods and ingredients, substituting new high protein foods for red meats, making recipes rich without dairy products, adding fiber to low residue dishes, lightening heavy recipes.... and lowering saturated fat in everything. The healing recipes in *Book Two: The Healing Recipes* are healthy versions of many popular dishes.

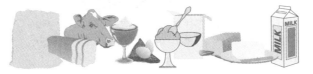

The Art of Food Exchanges for Healing

You can still enjoy your favorite dishes simply by making food exchanges. If you have food allergies or sensitivities, an increasing problem, food exchanges may be necessary so that you can enjoy eating while avoiding the foods that are causing the problems.

Protein exchanges for meats:
- **Tofu** (a cultured soy product) - use equally in exchange for ground meat in recipes. You can prepare tofu in almost every way you prepare meat. Tofu may be used fresh or frozen, thawed, squeezed out and sliced or crumbled. It may be baked or sautéed.
- **Tempeh** (a cultured soy product much like firm tofu, but with a nuttier taste and chewier texture) - use plain, or frozen and thawed, equally for red meats in recipes.
- **Dried beans and legumes,** soak and cook, then use as a one-for-one substitute for red meats. Note: Bean sprouts may also be used as a ground meat substitute in casserole recipes.
- **Falafel or grain burger mixes** - mix with liquid to use instead of ground meat.

Creamy exchanges for dairy foods: (See also *Dairy-Free Cooking* in *The Healing Recipes.*
—Milk and cream exchanges:
- **Soy milk, plain or vanilla** - use in equal amounts for milk or cream.
- **Yogurt** - blend with water to the consistency of milk as an equal exchange for milk.
- **Kefir** - an equal exchange for milk, buttermilk or half-and-half.
- **Fruit juice** - use to taste to replace milk in sweet recipes, or on dry cereals.
- **Almond milk** - use cup-for-cup in place of milk in gravies, soups, sauces.
- **Tahini milk** - make by adding 1 TB sesame tahini and 1 teasp. honey to 8-oz. water.
- **Rice milk,** substitute for milk in recipes. It's absolutely delicious.
- **Water** - it lends a dry, crunchy taste instead of smooth, moist texture.

- **Chickpea (light) miso** - mix with stock and seasonings, and substitute for milk.
- **Lecithin granules** - use to emulsify and thicken instead of milk or cream.

—**Ice cream exchanges:**
- **Rice Dream dessert** (in health food stores), or soy-based ice cream desserts.
- **Bananas** - chunk, peel and freeze, then blend with fruit or juice and refreeze.
- **Lecithin granules** - mix 1 - 2 TBS into frozen desserts; emulsifies without cream.

—**Cheese exchanges:**
- **Tofu** - sliced, marinated, steamed - use in cold or hot sandwiches.
- **Kefir cheese** - use 1 to 1 for sour cream, cream cheese or cottage cheese.
- **Soy cheese and almond cheese** - use equally as substitutes for cheese or cream cheese.
- **Cottage cheese** - one-for-one for cream cheese, ricotta and full fat cottage cheese.
- **Yogurt cheese (how to make, page 56) - use 1 to 1 for sour cream or cottage cheese.**
- **Mochi,** grate and substitute for cheese topping.... chewy, melted cheese texture.

—**Sour cream exchanges:**
- **Tofu** (use silken, soft texture) - substitute equally for sour cream.
- **Yogurt** - substitute equally for sour cream.
- **Yogurt and mayonnaise** - mix half and half and use instead of sour cream.

—**Butter exchanges:**
- **Vegetable oil** - use instead of butter in sauce, dressing, gravy, baking, sautees.
- **Vegetable broth** - exchange for butter in sautées, braising, sauces and gravies.
- **Clarified butter** - use in place of a saturated fat. Simply melt butter and skim off top foam. Use the clear butter in recipes in place of full fat butter, cooking oil or shortening.

—**Egg exchanges:**
- **Egg replacers** - useful for leavening and binding in recipes.
- **Dry yeast or sourdough starter** - use as a leavening agent in place of eggs.
- **Tofu,** fresh, crumbled, in place of scrambled or shirred eggs. Experiment.
- **Starchy vegetables** - like potatoes, sweet potatoes, cauliflower, applesauce or almond butter - use as binding agents instead of eggs.

Wheat, gluten and yeast exchanges: (Se*Wheat-Free Baking* in *The Healing Recipes.*)
- **Yeasted wheat bread substitutes** - rye bread, rice cakes, mochi, corn tortillas, chapatis, sprouted, flat or quick bread, pancakes made with baking powder.
- **Pasta** - corn or vegetable pasta, soba noodles and frozen/thawed tofu.
- **Cooked grains** like barley, millet, rice, buckwheat, amaranth.
- **Cereals** - rice, amaranth, corn, millet, buckwheat, oat cereal, or wheat-free granola.
- **Starchy vegetables** - puree and substitute in recipes for bread, grains or pasta.

Citrus exchanges:
- **Apple cider vinegar** - use one-for-one as a substitute in recipes for citrus.

Salt exchanges:
- **Mineral salt seasonings** like roasted sea greens-herb mixes - use to taste.
- **Herbal seasonings** (no or very low sodium) - use to taste.
- **Miso** - use to taste in casseroles, gravy, soups and sauces; a little goes a long way.
- **Shoyu or tamari** - use to taste in any savory dish needing more salt.
- **Spices and citrus zests** - use singly or mix for either sweet or savory recipes.

Sugar exchanges:
- **Honey** - use in a ratio of $^1/_2$ cup to 1 cup of sugar. Reduce recipe's liquid by $^1/_4$ cup.
- **Maple syrup** - use $^2/_3$ cup to 1 cup of sugar. Reduce recipe liquid by $^1/_4$ cup.
- **Molasses** - use $^1/_2$ cup to 1 cup of sugar. Reduce recipe's liquid by $^1/_4$ cup.
- **Malt syrup** - use 1 $^1/_4$ cup to 1 cup sugar. Reduce recipe liquid by $^1/_4$ cup.
- **Apple or fruit juice** - use 1 cup to 1 cup of sugar. Reduce recipe's liquid by $^1/_4$ cup.
- **Fructose** - use in a ratio of $^1/_3$ to $^2/_3$ cup to 1 cup of sugar.
- **Date sugar** - use in a ratio of one-for-one to 1 cup of sugar.
- **Stevia (sweet herb)** - make into a strong tea and use sparingly (stevia is 25 times sweeter than sugar) in drinks and as a liquid sweetener. Store in the fridge between uses.
- **Vanilla, cinnamon, cardamom** - use for sugar toppings and in dessert sauces.

Is Microwaving Your Food Safe?

Since their introduction microwave ovens have posed safety questions. Original owners were even told to stand at least four feet away during use, and not to watch the food while it was cooking. New research shows that microwave <u>packaging</u> is also questionable for health. Testing for migration of chemicals into food was only done up to 300°F. But microwave temperatures reach up to 500°F. Even microwave-approved materials show chemical instability at this high temperature. Packaging chemicals and adhesives at this temperature leach into food within 3 minutes of cooking. Many of them, such as *benzene, toluene* and *xylene* are suspected carcinogens.

Microwave "cookware" can leach chemicals into the food during heating. Many microwave packages contain a "heat susceptor," a piece of metallized plastic that gets hot and fries the surface of the food to crisp or brown it.

    —Put foods from microwave packages into covered glass or ceramic.
    —Make sure plastic wrap doesn't come in contact with food.
    —Use plastic containers to store foods only, not to heat them.

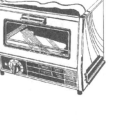

Japanese tests confirm that foods lose 10 percent or more of vitamins E and A after six minutes in a microwave; after twelve minutes they lose 40%.

<u>But the biggest problem with microwaving food is that it destroys enzymes</u>. Enzyme protection and our ability to use enzymes as therapy in a healing diet, are dramatically affected by a microwave. Enzymes are extremely sensitive to heat. Heat above 120°F. destroys them. Even low heat reduces digestion. Some experts say that if we microwaved all our food, we couldn't live. If you are on a healing diet, or sensitive to chemically altered foods, consider a conventional oven.

The Healing Diets

Chart Your Custom Healing Diet

It's so easy..... each diet program has all the information you need in order to use your diet to solve your health problem.

- Each diet reviews what you need to know about the health problem, and offers self-diagnosis signs and symptoms.
- Each diet has a complete step-by-step daily nutrition plan, and points you to the recipes that can heal your problem.
- Each diet offers herbs, supplements, bodywork and lifestyle choices.

140

Special Healing Diets

The healing diets are the heartbeat of this book. They are unique. <u>Your diet can be great medicine</u>… even for serious diseases. We tend to think that the healing powers of foods are subtle or mild, without the overwhelming potency of drugs. Yet healing doesn't always need to deal a hammer blow… even for serious problems.

All the advances made by modern medicine still don't address chronic diseases very well; they don't address disease prevention at all. Food science is advancing on two distinct tracks today. Genetically altered foods are increasing at an enormous rate (at this writing, over 70 percent of our foods are altered in some way). Yet a new, December 1999 poll shows that most Americans (81%) want these genetically altered foods labelled. On the other hand, new research is telling us much more about how food nutrients actually work in our bodies. Almost every day, another new study shows us that foods can heal, too. There's an enormous thirst for information about how to use this nutrition information for our health.

Most people are already actively trying to eat better. Everybody wants to build health and overcome disease with foods and herbs.

But most people don't know HOW to use foods as medicine. The healing diets in this book can help you navigate the healing path easily and effectively. It's all a matter of the way you direct what you eat.

<u>You'll have everything you need to do it yourself, day by day, and succeed.</u>

1: Detailed STEP-BY-STEP DIETS for a wide range of illnesses and health problems.
2: Detailed supplement and herb suggestions to enhance your healing progress.
3: Bodywork recommendations to enhance your healing program.
4: Recommended recipe sections that can help your diet the most.
   (Choose from a wide range of recipes in each section to keep your diet interesting.)

Remember: Medicines from foods and herbs work the opposite from drugs. They nourish the body and enhance the immune system. The food you eat changes your weight, your mood, the texture of your skin, the shape of your body, your outlook on life… and therefore your future.

A healing diet is the first step to the health and balance of your universe.

141

Detoxification Diets

Special Detoxification Diets

Body purification has been a part of mankind's rituals for health and well-being for thousands of years. Cleansing is a rich tradition that has helped humans through all ages and cultures. It is at the foundation of every great healing philosophy.

Today, we see how important detoxification is becoming once again — for everybody. No one is free from the enormous amount of environmental toxins assaulting us in the world today. No one is immune to every unhealthy lifestyle option. How do we remain healthy in a destructive environment?

The special detox diets in this section can offer your body the best start for your healing program. Each diet program includes the visible signs that your body needs a particular cleanse, step-by-step instructions for the initial diets, the supplements and herbs you'll need, along with tips that can give you the best results.

Detoxification programs are included for:

1: Colon and bowel cleansing
2: Bladder and kidney cleansing
3: Lung and mucous congestion cleansing
4: Liver and organ cleansing
5: Lymphatic cleansing
6: Skin cleansing
7: Blood cleansing for heavy metal toxicity, alcohol and drug addictions

For more information, see my new book, DETOXIFICATION ©1999, a comprehensive book on all aspects of cleansing for safe, effective personal detox programs. Over 250 pages, it includes delicious green cuisine cleansing recipes, detox plans for specific health problems, and extensive detox charts for easy use.

Do You Need to Detoxify?

What is detoxification? Our bodies naturally do it every day. Detoxification is a normal body process of eliminating or neutralizing toxins through the colon, liver, kidneys, lungs, lymph and skin. In fact, internal detoxification is one of our body's most basic automatic functions. Just as our hearts beat nonstop and our lungs breathe continuously, so our metabolic processes constantly dispose of accumulated toxic matter. It's a perfect natural set-up.... the catch is that today, body systems and organs that were once capable of cleaning out unwanted substances are now completely overloaded with toxic material from our environment.

We long for yesterday's pollution-free environment, whole foods and pure water. Today, we control our environment even less. But, since humans are born with a "self-cleaning system," this ideal probably never existed. Our bodies try to protect us from dangerous material by surrounding it with mucous or fat so it won't cause imbalance or trigger an immune reaction. **The body stores foreign substances in fatty deposits — a significant reason to keep your body fat low.** Some people carry around 15 extra pounds of mucous that harbors this waste! Keep pollutants to a minimum and periodically get rid of them through detoxification.

Detoxification through special cleansing diets may be the missing link to disease prevention, especially for immune-compromised diseases like cancer, arthritis, diabetes and fatigue syndromes like candida albicans. Our chemicalized, genetically altered foods radically alter our internal ecosystems, (that's not even counting too much animal protein, too much fat, too much caffeine and alcohol). Even if your diet is good, a body cleanse can restore your vitality against environmental toxins that pave the way for disease.

A detox program aims to remove the cause of disease before it makes us ill. It's a time-honored way to keep immune response high, elimination regular, circulation sound, and stress under control so your body can handle the toxicity it encounters. In the past, detoxification was used either clinically for recovering from addictions, or as a once-a-year "spring cleaning" for general well-being. Today, a regular detox program two or three times a year makes a big difference not only for health, but for the quality of our lives.

Should you detoxify? Today Americans are exposed to chemicals of all kinds on an unprecedented scale. Industrial chemicals and their pollutant run-offs in our water, pesticides, additives in our foods, heavy metals, anesthetics, residues from drugs, and environmental hormones are trapped within the human body in greater concentrations than at any other point in history.

Many chemicals are so widespread that we are unaware of them. But they have worked their way into our bodies faster than they can be eliminated, and are causing allergies and addictions in record numbers. **More than 2 million synthetic substances are known, 25,000 are added each year, and over 30,000 are produced on a commercial scale.** Only a tiny fraction are ever tested for toxicity. A lot of them come to us from developing countries that have few safeguards in place.

The molecular structure of some chemicals interacts with human DNA, so long term exposure may result in genetic alteration that affects cell functions. World Health Organization research implicates environmental chemicals in 60 to 80% of all cancers. Hormone-disrupting pesticides are linked to hormone problems, psychological disorders, birth defects, still births and now breast cancer.

As toxic matter saturates our tissues, antioxidants and minerals in vital body fluids are reduced, so immune defenses are thrown out of balance. Circumstances like this are the prime factor in today's immune compromised diseases like candidiasis, lupus, fibromyalgia, chronic fatigue syndrome, even arthritis (which now impairs over 50 million Americans).

Chemical oxidation is the other process that allows disease. The oxygen that "rusts" and ages us also triggers free radical activity, a destructive cascade of incomplete molecules that damages DNA and other cell components. If you didn't have a reason to reduce your animal fat intake before, here is a critical one: **oxygen combines with animal fat in body storage cells and speeds up the free radical process.**

Almost everyone can benefit from a cleanse. It's one of the best ways to remain healthy in dangerous surroundings. Not one of us is immune to environmental toxins, and most of us can't escape to a remote, unpolluted habitat. Technology is now seriously able to harm the health of our entire planet, even to the point of making it uninhabitable for life. We must develop our culture further and take larger steps of cooperation. Mankind and the Earth must work together – to save it all for us all.

What can we do?

We can start by keeping our own body systems in good working order so that toxins are eliminated quickly. We can take a closer look at our own air, water and food, and keep an ever watchful eye on the politics that control our environment. Legislation on health and the environment follows two pathways in America today.... the influence of business and profits, and the demands of the people for a healthy habitat and responsible stewardship of the Earth. (See "Fluoridation – An Unnecessary Poison in our Drinking Water," pg. 61.)

Is your body becoming toxic? Body signs can tell you that you need to detoxify.

We all have different "toxic tolerance" levels. Listen to your body when it starts giving you those "cellular phone calls." If you can keep the amount of toxins in your system below your toxic level, your body can usually adapt and rid itself of them.

Do you have:

—Frequent, unexplained headaches, back or joint pain, or arthritis?
—Chronic respiratory problems, sinus problems or asthma?
—Abnormal body odor, bad breath or coated tongue?
—Food allergies, poor digestion or chronic constipation with intestinal bloating or gas?
—Brittle nails and hair, psoriasis, adult acne, or unexplained weight gain over 10 pounds?
—Unusually poor memory, chronic insomnia, depression, irritability, chronic fatigue?
—Environmental sensitivities, especially to odors?

Laboratory tests like stool, urine, blood or liver tests, and hair analysis can also shed light on the need for a detox.

What benefits can you expect from a good detox?

A detox frees your body of clogging waste deposits, so you aren't running with a dirty engine or driving with the brakes on. Cleansing lets your body rebalance, so energy levels rise physically, psychologically and sexually, and creativity begins to expand. You start feeling like a different person — because you are. Your outlook and attitude change, because your actual cell make-up changes.

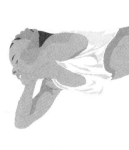

1: You'll clean your digestive tract of accumulated waste and fermenting bacteria.
2: You'll clear your body of excess mucous and congestion.
3: You'll purify your liver, kidney and blood, impossible under ordinary eating patterns.
4: You'll enhance mental clarity, impossible under chemical overload.
5: You'll be less dependent on sugar, caffeine, nicotine, alcohol or drugs.
6: You'll turn around bad eating habits... your stomach can reduce to normal size for weight control.
7: You'll release hormones that couple with essential fatty acids to stimulate your immune system.

You've decided your body needs a cleanse.

How long can you give out of your busy lifestyle to focus on a cleansing program so that all the processes can be completed? 24 hours, 2 or 3 days, or up to ten days? The time factor is important — you'll want to allocate your time ahead of time, to prepare both your mind and your body for the experience ahead.

A good detox program is in 3 steps — cleansing, rebuilding and maintaining.

Years of experience with detoxification have convinced me that if you have a serious health problem, a brief 3 to 7 day juice cleanse is the best way to release toxins from your body. Shorter cleanses can't get to the root of a chronic problem. Longer cleanses upset body equilibrium more than most people are ready to deal with except in a clinical environment. A 3 to 7 day cleanse can "clean your pipes" of systemic sludge — excess mucous, old fecal matter, trapped cellular and non-food wastes, or inorganic mineral deposits that are part of arthritis.

A few days without solid food can be an enlightening experience about your lifestyle. It's not absolutely necessary to take in only liquids, but a juice diet increases awareness and energy availability for elimination. Fresh juices literally pick up dead matter from the body and carry it away. Your body becomes easier to "hear," telling you via cravings what foods and diet it needs — for example, a desire for protein foods, or B vitamin foods like rices or minerals from greens. This is natural biofeedback.

A detox works by self-digestion. During a cleanse, the body decomposes and burns only the substances and tissues that are damaged, diseased or unneeded, such as abscesses, tumors, excess fat deposits, and congestive wastes. Even a relatively short fast accelerates elimination, often causing dramatic changes as masses of accumulated waste are expelled.

You will know your body is detoxing if you experience a short period of headaches, fatigue, body odor, bad breath, diarrhea or mouth sores that commonly accompany accelerated elimination. However, digestion usually improves right away as do many gland and nerve functions. Cleansing also helps release hormone secretions that stimulate immune response and encourages a disease-preventing environment.

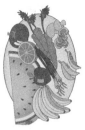

Is a water fast the fastest way to cleanse? I don't recommend it. Here's why:

Juice cleansing is a better evolution in detoxification methods. Detoxification experts agree that fresh vegetable and fruit juice cleansing is superior to water fasting. Fresh juices, broths and herb teas help deeply cleanse the body, rejuvenate the tissues and guide you to a faster recovery from health problems better than water fasting.

A traditional water fast is harsh and demanding on your body, even in times past before huge amounts of food and environmental toxins were part of the picture. Today, a water fast can be dangerous. Deeply buried pollutants and chemicals may be released into elimination channels too rapidly during a water fast. Your body is essentially "re-poisoned" as the chemicals move through the bloodstream all at once. Sometimes, the physical and emotional stress of a water fast even overrides the healing benefits.

Vegetable and fruit juices are alkalizing, so they neutralize uric acid and other inorganic acids better than water, and increase the healing effects. Juices support better metabolic activity, too. (Metabolic activity slows down during a water fast as the body attempts to conserve dwindling energy resources.) Juices are better for digestion — easily assimilated into the bloodstream. They don't disturb the detoxification process.

Step one: elimination. Clean out mucous and toxins from the intestinal tract and major organs. Everything functions more effectively when toxins, obstructions and wastes are removed.

Step two: rebuild healthy tissue and restore energy. With obstacles removed, activate your body's regulating powers to rebuild at optimum levels. Eat only fresh, simply prepared, vegetarian foods during the rebuilding step. Include supplements and herbal aids for your specific needs.

Step three: keep your body clean and toxin-free. Modify your lifestyle habits for a strong resistant body. Rely on fresh fruits and vegetables for fiber, cooked vegetables, grains and seeds for strength and alkalinity, lightly cooked sea foods, soy foods, eggs and low fat cheeses for protein, and a little dinner wine for circulatory health. Include supplements, herbs, exercise and relaxation techniques.

What Type of Cleanse Do You Need?

Cleanses come in all shapes and sizes. You can easily tailor a cleanse to your individual needs. Unless you require a specific detox for a serious illness, or recovery from a long course of drugs or chemical therapy, I recommend a short cleanse twice a year, especially in the spring, summer or early autumn when sunshine and natural vitamin D can help the process along.

The short detox program on the next two pages is a general cleanse that you can return to again and again, whenever your body needs a "wash and brush." Check out the rest of this detox chapter to access cleanses for specific body systems and problems.

3-Day Body Stress Cleanse

Do you need an overall body stress cleanse?

You change the oil in your car to make it run smoother and last longer. You plunge into spring cleaning to rid your home of health hazards. You buy air and water filters to clean out environmental toxins. You sink into a hot bath to cleanse your skin. If you stop there, you've left out an important part of the cleansing job. Cleansing on the inside improves everything on the outside. A stress cleanse revitalizes your whole body. It clears the junk out of body pathways so that wholesome nutrients can get in to rebuild energy and strength. I believe that much of the "food" in America's supermarkets doesn't really have much that your body can translate into nutrition. Some "foods" like designer fake fats or hormone-treated animal foods may even contribute to illness.

Is your body showing signs that it needs a stress cleanse?

—Is your immune response low? Are you catching every bug that comes down the pike?
—Are you unusually tired? Do you feel mentally dull? Do you feel like you need a pick-me-up?
—Have you had unusual body odor or bad breath lately? Have you gained weight even though your diet hasn't changed?

Stress Cleanse Detox Diet

Start with a 3 day juice-liquid diet like this one and follow with 4 days of fresh foods. Eat plenty of fresh veggies and fruits, and fiber foods like whole grains and beans. Avoid trans fats (page 74), but get plenty of essential fatty acids from sea greens, and herbs like ginger, ginseng or evening primrose oil. Drink plenty of water.

—**On rising:** take a glass of 2 fresh squeezed lemons, and 1 TB maple syrup in 8-oz. of water.
—**Breakfast:** have a nutrient-dense Kick-Off Cleansing Cocktail: juice 1 handful fresh wheat grass or parsley — extremely rich in chlorophyll and antioxidants, 4 carrots, 1 apple, 2 celery stalks with leaves, $\frac{1}{2}$ beet with top.
—**Mid-morning:** have a glass of fresh carrot or fresh apple juice. Add 1 TB. of a green superfood like Crystal Star ENERGY GREEN™ drink mix; Green Kamut GREEN KAMUT; Vibrant Health GREEN VIBRANCE.
—**Lunch:** have a Salad-In-A-Glass: juice 4 parsley sprigs, 3 tomatoes, $\frac{1}{2}$ bell pepper, $\frac{1}{2}$ cucumber, 1 scallion, 1 lemon wedge.
—**Mid-afternoon:** have a cup of Crystal Star CLEANSING & PURIFYING™ tea, green tea or mint tea.
—**Dinner:** have a warm Potassium drink for mineral electrolytes (page 568). Or Super Antioxidant Soup: 1 cup broccoli florets, 1 sliced leek, 2 cups peas, $\frac{1}{2}$ cup sliced scallions, 4 cups chard leaves, $\frac{1}{2}$ cup diced fennel bulb, $\frac{1}{2}$ cup fresh parsley, 6 garlic minced cloves, 2 tsp. astragalus extract (or $\frac{1}{4}$ cup broken astragalus bark), 6 cups vegetable stock, pinch cayenne, 1 cup diced green cabbage, $\frac{1}{4}$ cup dry, snipped sea greens. Bring ingredients to a boil. Simmer 10 min. Let sit 20 minutes. Strain and use broth only.

In the Recipe Book: See Detoxifocation and Cleansing Foods, and Healing Drinks for more info.

Herb and Supplement Choices

Choose 2 or 3 stress cleansing enhancers.

• **Cleansing boosters:** Crystal Star DETOX™ caps with goldenseal stimulates the body to eliminate wastes rapidly; or Crystal Star CLEANSING & PURIFYING™ tea.

• **Cleansing support formulas:** New Chapter LIFE SHIELD; or Futurebiotics OXY-SHIELD. When solid food is re-introduced, use Nature's Secret ULTIMATE CLEANSE.

• **Enzyme support:** Prevail DETOX ENZYME FORMULA; Transformation EXCELLZYME.

• **Antioxidants help remove toxins:** Biotec CELL GUARD; Rainbow Light MULTI CAROTENE COMPLEX.

• **Probiotics restore a friendly intestinal environment:** Jarrow Formulas JARRO-DOPHILUS+FOS; Wakunaga KYO-DOPHILUS; Prevail INNER ECOLOGY.

• **Electrolytes dramatically boost energy levels:** Nature's Path TRACE-LYTE LIQUID MINERALS.

• **Green superfoods:** Crystal Star ENERGY GREEN™ drink; Vibrant Health GREEN VIBRANCE.

• **Detoxing flower remedies:** Natural Labs STRESS/TENSION; Nelson Bach RESCUE REMEDY.

Bodywork and Lifestyle Techniques

Bodywork techniques accelerate your cleanse:

• **Enemas:** Flushing your colon on the first and the last day of your stress detox quickly releases toxins.

• **Especially helpful:** Guided imagery, biofeedback and aromatherapy techniques.

• **Stretch:** Body stretch daily during your cleanse. Repeat 5 times: Stand tall; raise your hands above your head. Stretch your arms and fingers to reach for the sky; move your hands and fingers as if you are climbing up into the sky. Rise on your toes as you reach; inhale deeply through your nostrils. Exhale slowly; gradually return to your starting position, arms loose at your sides. Follow your stretch with a brisk walk.

• **Deep Breathing:** Deep, relaxed breathing removes stress, composes the mind, improves mood and increases energy. 1. Take a full breath. Exhale, slowly. Slowly. 2. Take another deep, full breath. Release slowly. 3. And again. 4. Maintain a quiet rhythm, exhaling more slowly than you inhale.

• **Massage:** A massage therapy treatment further removes toxins and stimulates cleansing circulation.

Benefits that you may notice as your body responds to a body stress cleanse:

• Your digestion noticeably improves as your digestive tract is cleansed of accumulated waste.
• You'll feel lighter (most people lose about 5 pounds on this cleanse) and more energized.
• You'll feel less dependent on substances like sugar, caffeine, nicotine, alcohol and drugs as your bloodstream purifies.
• You'll feel healthier. Most people have noticeably better resistance to common colds and flu.
• You'll feel more mentally alert, less spacey, more emotionally balanced. Creativity begins to expand.
• You'll feel energized as your body rebalances. Energy levels rise physically, psychologically and sexually.

Can't find a recommended product? Call the 800 number listed in Product Resources for the store nearest you and for more info.

149

Body System Cleanses

You can target your detox to focus on a specific body system. Directing your detox to a particular body system often goes to the heart of a health problem right away, and frequently clears up other related conditions as well. Each body system shows tell-tale signs when it becomes overloaded with pollutants or congestion. Knowing what they are can help you deal with a problem quickly and correctly.

This chapter analyzes toxicity signals, detoxification techniques and cleansing diets for seven body systems that make a noticeable difference in your health after a cleanse.

Colon-Bowel Elimination Cleanse

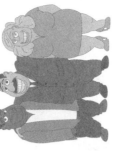

Most of us need a colon elimination cleanse. New estimates show that over 90% of disease in America is attributable in some way to an unhealthy colon. Over 100,000 Americans have a colostomy every year! An incredible fact. Hardly any healing program will work without a colon cleanse as part of it. It's understandable.... the solid waste management organ for the entire body, your colon is also the easiest breeding ground for putrefactive bacteria, viruses and parasites. (A nationwide survey reveals that 1 in every 6 people have parasites living somewhere in their bodies.)

Health problems like headaches, skin blemishes, bad breath, fatigue, arthritis and heart disease are linked to a congested colon. Colon and bowel malfunctions are a big factor in accelerated aging.... mental dullness is a sign of colon congestion. When colon waste backs up it becomes toxic, releasing the toxins from the bowel into the bloodstream. Real healing takes place at the cellular levels of your body, which are fed by your blood. The nutrients get to your blood by way of your colon. So a clogged, dirty colon means toxins throughout your body.

Is your colon toxic? Ask yourself these questions:

1: Is your elimination slow? Bowel transit time should be about twelve hours. Slow bowel transit time means wastes become rancid. Blood capillaries lining the colon absorb the rancid wastes into the bloodstream, exposing the rest of your body to the toxins.

2: Do you eat a lot of highly processed, chemicalized food, fast foods or synthetic foods? A clean, strong system can metabolize or eliminate many pollutants, but if you are constipated, they are stored in your tissues. As more and different chemicals enter your body they tend to interact with those already there, forming second generation chemicals more harmful than the originals. Colon cancer, now the second leading cause of cancer in the United States (only slightly behind lung cancer in men and breast cancer in women), is a direct result of accumulated toxic waste. Colitis, irritable bowel syndrome, diverticulosis, ileitis and Crohn's disease, all signs of waste congestion, are on the rise, too.

3: Is your digestion poor? The most common sign of toxic bowel overload is poor digestion. If you eat a lot of rich, red meats and cheeses, refined-flour bread, sugary, salty foods or fried foods, they're robbing your body of critical electrolytes and they have almost no fiber for digestion. High fiber moves food through your digestive system quickly and easily. A low fiber diet causes a gluey state — your intestinal contractions can't work efficiently. You can picture this if you remember the hard paste formed by white flour and water when you were a kid. A lot of the food we eat today is simply crammed into the colon, never fully excreted.

4: Do you eat enough fiber? America has focused so much media attention on high fiber foods, you'd think we would all have changed our diets to a more colon-health oriented pattern. This is simply not the case. But a gentle, gradual change from low fiber, low residue foods helps almost immediately. In fact, a gradual change is better than a sudden, drastic about-face change, especially when the colon is inflamed.

The protective level of fiber in your diet is easily measured: 1. The stool should be light enough to float. **2.** Bowel movements should be regular, daily and effortless. **3.** The stool should be almost odorless, signalling decreased bowel transit time. **4.** There should be little or no gas or flatulence.

Is your body showing signs that it needs a colon cleanse?

—Are you constipated most of the time? (a colon cleanse softens and removes cloging colon congestion)

—Do you feel heavy and logy? (a colon cleanse helps you lose colon congestive weight)

—Do you have gas or bloating after you eat? (a colon cleanse removes gluey materials impairing digestion)

—Do you catch a cold, or flu every few weeks? (a colon cleanse releases excess mucous that harbors viruses)

—Are you tired for no real reason? (a colon cleanse boosts immune and liver response for more energy)

—Do you have a coated tongue, bad breath or body odor? (a colon cleanse clears rancidity that causes smells)

—Do you feel mentally slow and tired? (a colon cleanse lets more blood circulation get to your brain)

—Is your skin unusually sallow and dull? (a colon cleanse removes toxin that come out through your skin)

—Do you have a degenerative disease like cancer, arthritis or lupus? (a colon cleanse removes toxic elements)

—Are your cholesterol numbers too high? (a colon cleanse increases absorption of cholesterol-lowering foods)

Use your stool as a tool to tell your body state:

Few of us are comfortable talking about what goes on (or doesn't go on) in our private moments in the bathroom — even with our own physician. That's too bad because your stool can be surprisingly revealing about your health status.

• Bloody or mucous-covered stools can be a sign of Crohn's disease, ulcerative colitis or even colon cancer. Or they may be a sign of hemorrhoid inflammation. Report symptoms like these to your physician right away.

• Thin, ribbonlike or flattened stools usually signal an obstruction like a polyp that narrows the elimination pathway. They may also be a sign of Irritable Bowel Syndrome or spastic colon.

• Stools that are large, messy and leave a film in toilet water can be a sign of malabsorption. If the problem is chronic, consult with a qualified health professional who understands malabsorption problems and nutritional deficiencies.

• Abnormally fatty stools may be a sign of pancreatitis, inflammation of the pancreas that can lead to diabetes.

• Extremely foul-smelling stools may mean you lack enough "friendly bacteria" in your intestines, and you eat a diet too high in red meat protein. Foul stools often signal Candida yeast overgrowth.

• Greenish stools may mean you need more whole grains in your diet and you should cut down on sugar.

• Pale, greyish stools can be a sign of liver or gallbladder problems.

• Black, tar-like stools may mean you have bleeding in your upper digestive tract. Report these symptoms to your physician.

• Reddish stools are usually the result of eating a lot red red foods. Beets are the frequent cause here.

• Dark brown stools can be the result of too much salt in the diet.

Colon Elimination Detox Plan

Start with a 3 to 5-day nutrition plan: The 4 keys: 1) high chlorophyll plants for enzymes; 2) fruits and vegetables for fiber; 3) cultured foods for probiotics; 4) eight glasses of water a day. *Bowel elimination problems are often chronic, and may require several rounds of cleansing. Space out more than one colon cleanse by alternating it with periods of eating a healthful diet.*

The night before your colon cleanse...

—Take your choice of gentle herbal laxatives, such as Herbaltone or Crystal Star FIBER &HERBS CLEANSE™.

—Soak dried figs, prunes and raisins in water to cover; add 1 TB. molasses, cover, leave over night.

The next day...

—**On rising:** take 1 heaping teaspoon of a fiber cleansing booster such as Crystal Star CHO-LO-FIBER TONE™ drink mix in apple juice. Add 1000mg vitamin C with bioflavonoids to raise body glutathione levels.

—**Breakfast:** discard dried fruits from soaking water and take a small glass of the liquid (eat several prunes to scrub wastes).

—**Mid-morning:** take 2 TBS. aloe juice concentrate in a glass of juice or water and another 1000mg vitamin C; or have a fresh apple or carrot juice with chlorella powder added.

—**Lunch:** take a small glass of potassium broth (page 568); or a glass of fresh carrot juice with Bragg's LIQUID AMINOS added.

—**Mid-afternoon:** take a large glass of fresh apple juice; or an herbal colon cleansing tea like Crystal Star LAXA-TEA™.

—**About 5 o' clock:** take a small glass of potassium broth, or fresh carrot juice, or a vegetable drink (page 569).

—**Supper:** take a glass of apple or papaya juice and 1000mg vitamin C with bioflavonoids.

(Note: On the last night, finish your cleanse with a small fresh salad. Sprinkle on lemon juice and nutritional yeast flakes.)

—**Before bed:** take a small glass of potassium broth, (potassium opens up tight intestinal organs); or a fresh carrot juice; or Crystal Star CHO-LO FIBER TONE™ drink mix in apple juice, or a cup of mint tea.

Watchwords: *If you're in the habit of taking drugstore laxatives...I've found that they aren't really body cleansers. They offer only temporary relief, are usually habit-forming and destructive to intestinal membranes, and don't even get to the cause of the problem. The bowels tend to expel debris simply because the colon becomes so irritated by the laxative that it expels whatever loose material is around.*

For best results from your colon cleanse....

1: A colonic irrigation is a good way to start a colon/bowel cleanse. (See how to take a colonic enema, page 572.)

2: Take a brisk walk for an hour every day to help keep your colon elimination channels moving.

3: Take several long warm baths during your cleanse. A lower back and pelvis massage, and dry skin brushing helps release toxins coming out through your skin.

◆ In the Recipe Book: See Detoxification and Cleansing Foods, and Healing Drinks for more info.

Herb and Supplement Choices

Choose 2 or 3 colon cleansing boosters.

•**Gentle herbal laxatives:** HERBALTONE tablets, Crystal Star LAXA TEA, M. D. Labs DAILY DETOX TEA. Note: If you have irritable bowel disease (IBS), avoid products with senna or psyllium. Use a gentle herbal cleanser with peppermint oil, like Crystal Star BWL TONE I.B.S.™ to lessen inflammation which makes the bowel more permeable to toxins.

•**Cleansing - flushing boosters:** Nature's Secret SUPERCLEANSE tabs; Crystal Star FIBER & HERBS COLON CLEANSE™; Herbal Magic COL-LIV HERBAL clears mucus from the intestinal walls; una da gato extract drops in water.

•**Chlorophyll sources:** Sun Wellness SUN CHLORELLA; Futurebiotics COLON GREEN; Crystal Star ENERGY GREEN™.

•**Enzymes:** Transformation DIGESTZYME; Biotec FIBERZYME.

•**Electrolyte boosters speed up the cleanse:** Nature's Path TRACE-LYTE MINERALS; Arise and Shine ALKALIZER.

•**Probiotics replenish healthy bacteria:** UAS Labs DDS-PLUS with FOS; Nature's Path FLORA-LYTE; Rejuvenative Foods VEGI-DELITE.

•**Antioxidants defeat pollutants:** Country Life SUPER 10 ANTIOXIDANT; NutriCology ANTIOX FORMULA.

•**Fiber support:** All One FIBER COMPLEX; Crystal Star CHO-LO FIBER TONE™ drink; AloeLife FIBERMATE.

Bodywork and Lifestyle Techniques

Bodywork techniques accelerate your cleanse:

—**Irrigate:** a colonic irrigation is a good way to start a colon/bowel cleanse. (See how to take a colonic enema, page 572.) Grapefruit seed extract (15 to 20 drops in a gallon of water) is effective, especially if there is colon toxicity along with constipation; or diluted liquid chlorophyll enema every other night during the cleanse. Catnip enemas may be given to children. Use smaller amounts for size and age. Allow water to enter very slowly; let them expel when they wish.

•**Exercise:** take a brisk walk for an hour every day to help keep your elimination channels moving, abdominal muscles toned and muscle action optimal.

•**Bathe:** take several long warm baths during your cleanse. A lower back and pelvis massage and dry skin brushing will help release toxins coming out through your skin.

Lemon Detox Bath: add into warm bath – 5 drops lemon and 2 drops geranium essential oil.

•**Massage therapy:** get one good lower back and pelvis massage during your cleanse.

•**Visualize your detox:** Close your eyes and inhale and exhale long and slowly. As you exhale, visualize toxins dislodging and leaving your colon. As you inhale, visualize pure, nourishing nutrients rebuilding your vibrancy.

Note: The second part of a colon health program, rebuilding healthy tissue and body energy, takes 1 to 2 months for best results. Focus on fiber rich foods from fresh vegetables and fruits to keep colon congestion loosened. Emphasize cultured foods to replenish healthy intestinal flora, green foods for enzyme production, and alkalizing foods to prevent irritation while healing. Avoid refined foods, saturated fats, fried foods, red meats, caffeine and pasteurized dairy foods.

Can't find a recommended product? Call the 800 number listed in Product Resources for the store nearest you and for more info.

Lung-Mucous Cleanse

Lung and respiratory diseases of all kinds have increased dramatically in just the last decade. Air, water and environmental pollutants may have finally reached an overload point on the general population where having a congestive "cold" is more common than breathing free. During high risk seasons, almost a third of Americans have a cold every two or three weeks. Cold symptoms are frequently your body's attempt to cleanse itself of wastes and toxins that have built up to the point where natural immunity cannot handle or overcome them. Your glands are always affected, (since the endocrine system is on a 6 day cycle, a cold usually runs for about a week) as the body works through all its detoxification processes.

Your lungs are on the front line of toxic intake from viruses, allergies, pollutants, and mucous-forming congestants. An occasional lung cleanse supports your respiratory system in releasing pollutant-caused infections. But your body works together. Extra pressure of disease or heavy elimination on one part of the body puts extra stress on another. Cleansing your kidneys, for example, takes part of the waste elimination load off your lungs so they can recover faster. Similarly, promoting respiratory health through a lung cleanse also helps digestive and skin problems.

Note: Consciously steer clear of air pollution. Environmental and heavy metal pollutants, like chlorofluorocarbons and tobacco smoke (even secondary smoke), contribute greatly to respiratory problems and can undo all your hard cleansing work.

Is your body showing signs that it needs a lung-mucous cleanse?

—Do you have a chronic phlegmy cough? or post nasal drip?

—Do you have a wheeze in your lungs when you inhale?

—Is your head stuffy with congestive allergies?

—Do you have bronchitis, severe sinusitis, or asthma?

—Do you have a runny nose in any weather?

—Are you a cigarette smoker?

—Are you highly sensitive to chemicals and pollutants?

Pointers for best results from your lung-mucous cleanse:

• Drink non-dairy fluids, like water, juices, herb teas or broth, to hydrate and flush the body. Milk congests and constipates.

• Stimulate your immune response - a primary way to support lung and respiratory health.

• Alkalize your body during a lung cleanse. Acid-forming foods aggravate or prolong colds, flus and other respiratory problems. Eat alkalizing foods like fresh fruits, green vegetables, sea greens and non-gluten grains like brown rice or millet in a ratio of about 4:1 over acid-forming foods like red meats or lunch meats, dairy foods, caffeine or fried foods during a lung and mucous cleanse.

• Chlorophyll-rich green foods like chlorella, spirulina and barley grass speed up lung cleansing, and increase oxygen in the body.

• Get plenty of quality sleep, fresh air and sunshine. Steer as clear as you can away from smoke and air pollution.

Lung-Mucous Detox Plan

A program to overcome chronic respiratory problems is usually more successful when begun with a short mucous elimination, lung cleansing diet. This allows the body to first rid itself of toxic accumulations that cause congestion before an attempt is made to change eating habits that support better health. Your body works together. Extra pressure of disease or heavy elimination on one part of the body puts extra stress on another. Cleansing your kidneys, for example, takes part of the waste elimination load off your lungs so they can recover faster. Similarly, promoting respiratory health through a lung cleanse also helps digestive and skin problems.

Begin with 3 days of fresh enzyme rich juices, and follow with 1 to 4 days of a diet of 100% fresh foods.

The night before your lung cleanse....

–Take your choice of gentle herbal laxatives.

The next day....

—**On rising:** take 2 squeezed lemons in water with 1 TBS. maple syrup; or take a glass of apple, grapefruit or cranberry juice; or a glass of apple cider vinegar (1-2 TB) with hot water and honey.

—**Breakfast:** have a water-diluted grapefruit juice or pineapple juice as natural expectorants with 1 TB green superfood, such as Crystal Star SYSTEMS STRENGTH™, Transitions EASY GREENS or Nature's Secret ULTIMATE GREEN; take 2 or 3 garlic capsules and $^1/_4$ teasp. ascorbate vitamin C or Ester C powder in water.

—**Mid-morning:** take a carrot juice or mixed fresh vegetable juice such as Personal Best V-8 (page 569); or a cup of comfrey-fenugreek tea, or Crystal Star RESPR-TEA™ or ASTH-AID TEA™.

—**Lunch:** have a Potassium Juice (page 568) to cleanse, neutralize acids and rebuild the body; or a hot vegetable, miso or onion broth; and take 2 or 3 garlic capsules and $^1/_4$ teasp. ascorbate vitamin C or Ester C powder in water.

—**Mid-afternoon:** have a mucous cleansing tea like Crystal Star X-PECT™ TEA; or a green drink with Monas CHLORELLA; add $^1/_4$ teasp. ascorbate vitamin C or Ester C powder in water.

—**Dinner:** Try this soup, soothing to gastric mucosa, rich in zinc, vitamin A, C, potassium and magnesium electrolytes: In 2 cups water, cook 1 cup fresh mixed vegetables (carrots, broccoli, dark leafy greens, celery and parsley) with 1 TB miso. Let cool slightly and blender blend (add 4 TBS sunflower seeds for a hearty soup). Or, have a Potassium Essence broth (page 568) for energy and mineral electrolytes.

—**Before Bed:** have fresh apple-cranberry, or apple-carrot juice.

Benefits you'll notice as your body responds to a lung-mucous cleanse:

Chest congestion and discomfort begin to clear almost immediately. Lung and respiratory system irritation and infection abates as the immune system strengthens. Long term resistance increases so you can better handle today's impure biosphere.

◆ **In the Recipe Book:** See <u>Detoxification and Cleansing Foods, and Healing Drinks</u> for more info.

Herb and Supplement Choices

Choose 2 or 3 supplements.

• **Lung cleansers:** Herbs Etc. LUNG TONIC; Nature's Secret ULTIMATE RESPIRATORY CLEANSE; Creation's Garden LNG-1 (assists respiratory ailments settling in the lungs) and LNG-3 (clears lung congestion, bronchial inflammation).

• **Lung anti-infectives:** Etherium Technology COLLOIDAL SILVER, SILICA, & GOLD; East Park OLIVE LEAF EXTRACT or NutriCology PROLIVE (olive leaf extract); Oregano oil thins mucous, stops excess mucous secretion, has antiviral and antibacterial properties that help eradicate lung infection conditions. Tea Tree has decongestant, antiviral and antibacterial properties; Crystal Star X-PECT-TEA™ aids mucous release.

• **Lung superfoods:** Country Life SHIITAKE/REISHI COM-PLEX; Chlorophyll-rich superfoods: like chlorella, spirulina and barley grass or Body Ecology VITALITY SUPERGREEN, speed up lung cleansing, increase oxygen in the body.

• **Enzymes:** Transformation Enzyme GASTROZYME clears mucous; PUREZYME strengthens immune system.

• **Electrolytes increase oxygen uptake:** Nature's Path TRACE-LYTE LIQUID MINERALS; Arise & Shine ALKALIZER.

• **Probiotics inhibit harmful organisms:** Source Naturals LIFE FLORA; Nature's Path FLORA-LYTE.

• **Antioxidants:** vitamin C 1,000mg 3x day raises body's glutathione levels to protect the lungs; Futurebiotics OXY-SHIELD; Source Naturals PROANTHODYN.

Bodywork and Lifestyle Techniques

Bodywork techniques accelerate your cleanse:

• **Enema:** Take an enema the first and last day of your lung cleansing program to thoroughly clean out excess mucous.

• **Deep Breathing Exercise:** Do this deep breathing exercise often during your cleanse to remove stress, compose your mind, improve your mood and increase your energy: Take a deep, full breath - engage the diaphragm so that the lungs are filled to capacity. Exhale it slowly.... slowly. Take another deep, full breath. Release slowly. And again. Maintain a quiet rhythm, exhaling more slowly than you inhale.

• **Exercise:** Take a brisk, daily walk on each day of your cleanse. Breathe deep to help the lungs eliminate mucous and help bring in cleansing oxygen.

• <u>**Compress:**</u> Apply wet ginger-cayenne compresses to chest to increase circulation and loosen mucous.

• **Essential oil support:** Assist your lung cleanse with oregano, tea tree and eucalyptus oils (singly or in combination). Put a total of 15 drops essential oils in 1-oz of a carrier oil (such as jojoba) and rub on the chest. As an inhalant: add 6 drops of the essential oils to one quart hot water – inhale the steam. Eucalyptus especially has antiviral action to loosen mucous, and treat asthma, bronchitis and sinusitis.

• **Bath or Sauna:** Take a hot 20 minute bath or sauna at the onset of a cold, flu or beginning of a respiratory cleanse to stimulate body defenses and increase toxin elimination.

Note: After your juice cleanse, a diet for lung health should be high in vegetable proteins and whole grains, low in sugars and starches. Include cultured foods like raw sauerkraut, yogurt and kefir for probiotics. Include lung-specific pitted fruits like apricots, peaches and plums. Include nutritional yeast 2 tsp. daily. Take a green superfood drink at least three mornings a week for a month after your cleanse to "set" the cleanse benefits.

Can't find a recommended product? Call the 800 number listed in Product Resources for the store nearest you and for more info.

Bladder-Kidney Cleanse

Do you need a bladder-kidney cleanse?

Kidney function is vital to health. The kidneys are largely responsible for the elimination of waste products from protein breakdown (such as urea and ammonia). If the movement of salts, proteins or other bio-chemicals goes awry, a whole range of health problems arises, from mild water retention, to major kidney failure, and mineral loss. Concentrated protein wastes can cause chronic inflammation of the kidney filtering tissues (nephritis), and can overload the bloodstream with toxins, causing uremia.

But your bladder and kidneys do more than just remove water wastes. They are primary removal sites for toxic and potentially toxic chemicals in the bloodstream, channeling pollutants and chemicals out before they build up in the tissues and contaminate cells. The urinary system is also part of a complex process that maintains your body's fluid stability. Urinary controls are involved with the brain, hormones, and receptors all over the body. They are smart controls that register what your body needs for fluids. Sometimes, they remove very little salt or water; at other times, they remove a lot. By the way.... dehydration is the most common stress on the kidneys. Natural medicine emphasizes the importance of ample, high-quality water for kidney health.

Check these signs to see if you need a bladder-kidney cleanse:

—Do you have chronic lower back pain?
—Does it hurt when you urinate?
—Do you have frequent unexplained chills or fever?
—Do you have nausea or unusual fluid retention?
—Do you have dark circles under your eyes?
—Do you have dark orange or even dark yellow urine, a sign that the urine is too concentrated?

Pointers for best results from your bladder-kidney cleanse.

• Drink 8-10 glasses of bottled water each day of your cleanse. Body purification systems can operate efficiently only if the volume of water flowing through them is sufficient to carry away wastes.

• Avoid dietary irritants on the kidneys, such as coffee, alcohol, and excessive protein.

Benefits you'll notice as your body responds to a bladder-kidney cleanse:

• The flow of urine increases; dark urine lightens to pale yellow.
• Infection and irritation abate, so pain is curtailed.
• As the kidneys normalize their filtering duties, your skin will return to a healthy color... more than likely, dark under-eye circles will disappear.

Bladder-Kidney Detox Plan

Start with a 3-day nutrition plan: Water is the key. Drink 8 to 10 glasses of water each day. Bladder and kidneys operate efficiently only if there is sufficient water volume flowing through them to carry away wastes. Avoid dietary irritants on the kidneys, such as coffee, alcohol, and excessive protein.

Note: Avoid commercial antacids during healing. Some NSAIDS drugs have been implicated in kidney failure cases.

The night before your bladder cleanse....

—Take a cup of bladder cleansing herb tea, like Crystal Star BLDR-K TEA™. Add ¹/₄ tsp. non-acidic C crystals.

The next day....

—**On rising:** take 1 lemon squeezed in a glass of water, with 1 teasp. acidophilus liquid and add ¹/₄ teasp. non-acidic vit. C crystals; or 3 tsp. cranberry concentrate in a small glass of water. (Cranberry juice reduces ionized calcium in the urine by over 50% to create an unfavorable environment for urinary tract infections.)

—**Breakfast:** have a glass of watermelon juice or cranberry juice with ¹/₄ tsp. non-acidic vitamin C crystals or a glass of organic apple juice with ¹/₄ tsp. acidophilus powder.

—**Mid-morning:** take 1 cup watermelon seed tea (grind seeds, steep in hot water 30 minutes, add honey); or a potassium broth (page 568) with 2 tsp. Bragg's LIQUID AMINOS; or an herbal bladder cleansing tea such as Crystal Star GREEN TEA CLEANSER™, or a kidney healing tea such as parsley/oatstraw, plantain tea, or cornsilk tea.

—**Lunch:** have a carrot-beet-cucumber juice, or a chlorophyll-rich drink like Monas CHLORELLA, Crystal Star ENERGY GREEN™ drink mix, Body Ecology VITALITY SUPERGREEN, or Ethical Nutrients FUNCTIONAL GREENS; or a glass of carrot juice.

—**Mid-afternoon:** a cup of bladder healing herb tea, like parsley/oatstraw, plantain, watermelon seed tea or cornsilk; or a cleansing herb tea like uva ursi, juniper, watercress, cleavers or couch grass.

—**Dinner:** have a carrot juice, add 1 tsp. spirulina powder; or another cranberry juice, add ¹/₄ teasp. ascorbate vitamin C crystals. A cleansing diet option: have a mixed greens salad with cucumbers, spinach, watercress and celery with lemon, a little olive oil and Bragg's LIQUID AMINOS.

—**Before Bed:** take a glass of papaya or apple juice with ¹/₄ tsp. acidophilus powder.

—**One week kidney flush option:** During watermelon season, try this excellent kidney flush. Drink three 8-oz glasses of watermelon juice per day (or 3 cups of watermelon cubes). Eat only fresh vegetable salads and fruit you need the highest natural water content available in your foods for this cleanse.

◆ In the Recipe Book: See <u>Detoxification and Cleansing Foods</u>, and <u>Healing Drinks</u> for more info.

Bodywork and Lifestyle Techniques

Bodywork techniques accelerate your cleanse:

• **Exercise:** Take a daily brisk walk to keep kidneys flowing.

• **Irrigation:** Take a spirulina or catnip enema at least one day of your kidney cleanse to help release toxins. See enema instructions (page 571) in this book.

• **Heat therapy:** Hot saunas release toxins and excess fluids, and flush acids out through the skin. Or, take alternating hot and cold sitz baths.

• **Compresses:** Apply wet and hot to lower back to speed cleansing. Combine your choice: ginger - oatstraw, or cayenne - ginger, or mullein - lobelia.

• **Massage therapy:** Have at least one massage during your cleanse to stimulate circulation.

• **Bladder-Kidney Baths:** Add 8-10 drops of essential oils to your bath (or use 15 drops essential oil in 4-oz of jojoba oil and rub on kidney area before your bath). Combine 2 to 3 of these oils: juniper, cedarwood, sandalwood, lemon, chamomile, eucalyptus or geranium. Stir bath water to disperse.

Herb and Supplement Choices

Choose 2 or 3 liquid supplements for this cleanse.

• **Take a liquid green drink each day of your cleanse:** Green Foods VEGGIE MAGMA; Monas CHLORELLA; Crystal Star ENERGY GREEN™ drink; spirulina powder in juice.

• **Bladder-kidney cleansers:** Crystal Star BLDR-K™ tea or extract; cornsilk tea; Nature's Apothecary DETOX FORMULA.

• **Antibiotic, anti-infective, anti-inflammatory:** Crystal Star ANTI-BIO™ extract in water; marshmallow tea; vitamin C-1,000mg 3x a day in juice; Nature's Answer BLADDEX or Nature's Plus AQUA-ACTIN.

• **Enzymes:** Transformation Enzyme EXCELL-ZYME (kidney antioxidant), and PUREZYME (protease breaks apart protein-based viscid matter that cements salts into stones).

• **Bladder-kidney healers:** Crystal Star GREEN TEA CLEANSER™, Herbs Etc. KIDNEY TONIC; Nature's Apothecary KIDNEY SUPPORT; dandelion tea; parsley tea.

• **Electrolyte minerals:** Nature's Path TRACE-LYTE LIQUID MINERALS; Arise & Shine ALKALIZER.

• **Probiotics:** Nutricology SYMBIOTICS + FOS; Wakunaga KYODOPHILUS.

• **Fiber supplements reduce risk of stones:** All One FIBER COMPLEX; Nature's Secret ULTIMATE FIBER.

Note: After your cleanse, eat plenty of fresh vegetables and fruits, drink plenty of water and other healthy liquids, add seafoods and sea greens, whole grains and vegetable proteins. Continue with a morning green drink, like Crystal Star GREEN TEA CLEANSER™ for the rest of the month along with kidney healing foods like garlic and onions, papayas, bananas, watermelon, sprouts, leafy greens and cucumbers. Avoid foods that inhibit kidney filtering - heavy starches, red or prepared meats, dairy foods (except yogurt or kefir), salty, fatty and fast foods. Kidney stones are linked to low fiber, large amounts of animal protein, refined sugar, alcohol, high fat, and high salt.

Can't find a recommended product? Call the 800 number listed in Product Resources for the store nearest you and for more info.

Liver-Gallbladder Cleanse

Your liver is your most important organ of detoxification. Your life depends on your liver. To a large extent, the health of your liver determines the health of your entire body. The liver is really a wonderful chemical plant that converts everything we eat, breathe and absorb through the skin into life-sustaining substances. The liver is a major blood reservoir, forming and storing red blood cells, and filtering toxins at a rate of a quart of blood per minute. It manufactures natural antihistamines to keep immune response high.

More than any other organ, the liver enables us to benefit from the food we eat. It is the primary metabolic organ for proteins, fats and carbohydrates. It synthesizes and secretes bile, a substance that not only insures good food assimilation but also is critical to the excretion of toxic material from the gastrointestinal tract. Blood flows directly from the gastrointestinal tract to the liver, where it deals with toxic substances from our food before they are distributed through our blood.

Unfortunately, the usual American diet is high in calories, fats, sugars and alcohol, with unknown amounts of toxins from preservatives, pesticides and nitrates, so almost everybody has liver damage to some extent. Health problems occur after years of abuse, when the liver is so exhausted it loses the ability to detoxify itself. Still, your liver has amazing rejuvenative powers, continuing to function when as many as 80% of its cells are damaged. More remarkable, the liver can regenerate its own damaged tissue, so that even in life-threatening situations, such as cirrhosis, hepatitis, acute gallstone attacks, mononucleosis or pernicious anemia, the liver can be rejuvenated, to avert major surgery, even death. You can help your liver take a "deep cleansing breath" ... something I've found you can almost feel as its miraculous powers of recovery begin to flow.

A liver detox is often the first vital step for the body to begin to heal itself. Gland function and digestion often improve right away. You'll have fewer instances of swollen glands during cold and flu season, and less lower back fatigue. Weight and cellulite control difficulties may be solved, especially if you've had unusual stomach distension, a clear sign of a swollen liver. Drug and alcohol cravings reduce. Women notice that PMS and other menstrual difficulties like endometriosis are far less severe. Seemingly unrelated problems like breast or uterine fibroids, infertility, and even osteoporosis may be corrected. Male impotence is normally improved. Inflammatory conditions like shingles flare-ups, neuritis pain, and herpes outbreaks abate. Brown skin spots and spots before the eyes (signs of liver congestion and poor elimination) begin to fade.

Is your body showing signs that it needs a liver cleanse?

—Unexplained fatigue, listlessness, depression or lethargy, numerous allergy reactions
—Unexplained weight gain and the appearance of cellulite (women), or a distended stomach (men) even if you are thin
—Mental confusion, spaciness; food and chemical sensitivities; unusually poor digestion, even unexplained nausea
—Sluggish elimination, general constipation alternating to diarrhea
—PMS, headaches and other menstrual difficulties; bags under the eyes
—A yellowish tint to the skin and/or liver spots on the skin; poor hair texture and slow hair growth; skin itching and irritation
—Anemia and large bruise patches indicate severe liver exhaustion

Liver-Gallbladder Detox Plan

I recommend a short liver detox twice a year in the spring and fall, using the extra vitamin D from the sun to help. Your liver is probably the most stressed in the spring and early summer (one of the reasons that people with skin problems get more flare-ups in the spring). As upward energy movement in the spring is mirrored in the human body, our bodies can more readily rid us of wastes accumulated during the winter.

Start with this 3-day nutrition plan:

Drink 8 glasses of water each day. Add $1/4$ tsp. vitamin C crystals (a natural chelator of heavy metal toxins that deteriorate liver function) to each drink you take. Follow with a diet of 100% fresh foods the rest of the week. Have a dark green leafy salad every day.

The night before your liver cleanse...

—Take a cup of miso soup with sea greens snipped on top.

—Make a liver tonic tea: 4-oz hawthorn berries, 2-oz. red sage, and 1-oz. cardamom seeds. Steep 24 hours in 2 qts. water. Add honey. Take 2 cups daily.

The next day....

—**On rising:** take 1 lemon squeezed in a glass of water; or 2 TBS. cider vinegar in water with 1 teasp. honey.

—**Breakfast:** take a potassium broth, (page 568) or carrot-beet-cucumber juice; or Crystal Star SYSTEMS STRENGTH drink™. Add 1 teasp. Monas CHLORELLA to any drink. Chlorella cleanses and protects against toxic injury to body organs.

—**Mid-morning:** take a green veggie drink (page 569); or a green superfood powder mixed in water or vegetable juice (superfood choices: Green Foods GREEN MAGMA, Crystal Star ENERGY GREEN or NutriCology PRO-GREENS).

—**Lunch:** have a glass of organic apple juice (helps soften gallbladder stones) or a glass of fresh carrot juice. Add 1 teasp. lecithin to your juice; or a cup of liver tonic tea (above).

—**Mid-afternoon:** have a cup of peppermint tea, green tea, or Crystal Star LIV-ALIVE TEA™.

—**Dinner:** have another carrot juice or a mixed vegetable juice; or have a hot vegetable broth (page 569).

—**Before Bed:** take another glass of lemon juice or cider vinegar in water. Add 1 tsp. honey or royal jelly; or a pineapple/papaya juice with 1 tsp. royal jelly.

Improvement signs show that your body is responding to the cleanse.

—Many skin conditions trace back to liver problems, so skin conditions show signs of clearing and skin becomes more radiant.

—Stiff, aching muscles experience relief.

—Warmth may return to cold hands and feet.

—Recurring headaches or migraines may disappear.

◆ In the Recipe Book: See Detoxification and Cleansing Foods, and Healing Drinks for more info.

Herb and Supplement Choices

Choose 2 or 3 liver cleansing supplements.

• **Bitters herbs stimulate liver and bile flow:** Crystal Star BIT-TERS & LEMON CLEANSER™; Floradix HERBAL BITTERS; Solaray turmeric caps; dandelion tea.

• **Liver cleansers:** Crystal Star LIV-ALIVE™ tea or caps, or GREEN TEA CLEANSER™; Nature's Apothecary LIVER SUP-PORT; Gaia Herbs SUPREME CLEANSE.

• **Liver tonics:** Milk thistle seed extract (speeds liver healing by a factor of four); Enzymatic Therapy SUPER MILK THISTLE COMPLEX / ARTICHOKE; Herbs Etc. LIVER TONIC.

• **Enzymes:** Transformation Enzyme LYPOZYME contains the highest amount of lipase (digests fats) found in any product. It aids in the breakdown of gallstones.

• **Lipotropics prevent fatty accumulation:** Phos. Choline or choline 600mg, or Solaray LIPOTROPIC PLUS; sea greens (any kind) daily; dandelion tea; gotu kola or fennel seed tea.

• **Liver antioxidants:** ALPHA-LIPOIC ACID by NOW. Lipoic acid is one of the most powerful liver detoxifiers ever discovered); CoQ$_{10}$ 60mg 3x daily; Solaray ALFA-JUICE caps.

• **Herbal sediment-stone dissolvers:** Crystal Star STN-EX caps (with dandelion, gravel root, milk thistle and hydrangea) and Planetary Formulas STONE FREE have a long successful history of helping to dissolve gallstone accretions.

Bodywork and Lifestyle Techniques

Bodywork techniques accelerate your cleanse:

• **Rest:** the liver does some of its most important work while you sleep! A complete liver renewal program can take from 3 to 6 months.

• **Enema:** take a coffee enema (1 cup coffee to 1 qt. water) the first and last day of your liver cleanse.

• **Massage therapy:** Massage the liver and gallbladder area to help remove congestion.

• **Exercise:** Take a brisk walk on each day of your cleanse. Breathe deep to help the liver eliminate toxins. The liver is dependent on the amount and quality of oxygen coming into the lungs. Exercise, an air filter, or time spent walking in the forest and at the ocean can be of great benefit.

• **Sunbathe:** Take an early morning sunbath or get out in early morning sunshine for 15 to 30 minutes when possible.

• **Undo liver stress:** Avoid eating late in the evening.

• **Essential oils:** To assist liver and gallbladder cleansing, use essential oils of lemon and rosemary. Put a total of 14 drops essential oil in 1-oz of a carrier oil and rub on skin. Or add the oils to your bath.

• **Flower Essence Remedies:** Bach Flower RESCUE REMEDY or Natural Labs Deva Flowers STRESS/TENSION oil.

Note: Keeping fat low is crucial to liver regeneration and vitality. Casein in dairy products increases formation of gallstones. Vegetable proteins from foods like soy, oat bran and sea vegetables help prevent gallstone formation. Beets, artichokes, radishes, and dandelion herb and greens promote the flow of bile, the major pathway for chemical release from the liver. A permanent diet for liver health should be lacto-vegetarian, low in fats, rich in vegetable proteins, with plenty of vitamin C foods for good iron absorption. Special foods and herbs for the liver and gallbladder include: cabbage, artichokes (organic only), dandelion greens, garlic, burdock root (cut up and use in soups), tumeric and rosemary (in soups and on salads), licorice tea (as a flavoring).

Can't find a recommended product? Call the 800 number listed in Product Resources for the store nearest you and for more info.

Blood Cleanse

Your blood is your river of life. Blood must supply oxygen to your body's sixty trillion cells, transport nutrients, hormones and wastes, warm and cool your body, ward off invading microorganisms, seal off wounds and much more. It is your body's chief neutralizing agent for bacteria and toxic wastes. Toxins ingested in sublethal amounts can eventually add up to disease-causing amounts. For example, slow viruses like those that lead to MS, a nerve disease, can enter the cells and remain dormant for years, feeding on toxic wastes, then reappear in a more dangerous form. Your body has a self-purifying complex for maintaining healthy blood, but to protect yourself from disease you need to keep those cleansing systems in good working order. Use a blood purifying diet for 1 to 2 months, or longer if needed. You can return to a blood cleansing regimen as needed.

Is your body showing signs that it needs a blood cleanse?

A simple blood-color test monitors blood improvement. Make a small, quick, sterilized razor cut on your finger. If the blood is a dark, bluish-purplish color, it is not healthy. A bright red color indicates healthy blood.

In addition: Do you have:
—A chronic, deep, choking cough?
—Unexplained depression, memory loss or unusual insomnia, schizophrenic behavior, seizures, or periodic black-outs?
—Sexual difficulties, such as impotence or lack of normal libido?
—Black spots on the gums, bad breath/body odor, unusual, severe reactions to foods and odors?
—Loss of hand/eye coordination, especially in driving?

Pointers for best results from your blood cleanse:

1: A key to changing unhealthy blood is to put a nourishing diet into place. Eliminate meats, dairy foods, any foods with saturated fats, concentrated sugars, canned foods, prepackaged foods, foods with preservatives and additives, and all refined foods. Drink at least 8 glasses during each day. Include mild herb teas and bottled mineral water. Inadaquate water causes the blood to get sticky, thick and clogging, hampering all the duties of the bloodstream.

2: Adaquate water is also at the core of blood health. Drink at least 8 glasses during each day. Include mild herb teas and bottled mineral water. Inadaquate water causes the blood to get sticky, thick and clogging, hampering all the duties of the bloodstream.

3: I have seen excellent results from special blood cleansing agents like plant based enzyme protease and olive leaf extract. See Herbs and Supplements on the page 167.

Benefits you may notice as your body responds to the blood cleanse:

—Overall energy levels improve. Chronic conditions such as headaches, allergies, arthritis, chronic fatigue, depression, chemical poisoning, and immune system deficiency ailments regularly improve.
—Skin disorders, such as rashes, psoriasis, eczema, acne, etc. clear or greatly improve.

164

Blood Detox Plan

Vegetable and fruit juices stimulate rapid, heavy waste elimination, a process that can generate mild symptoms of a "healing crisis." A slight headache, nausea, bad breath, body odor and dark urine occur as the body accelerates release of accumulated toxins. If you are detoxifying from alcohol or drug overload, take 5,000 to 10,000mg. of ascorbate vitamin C daily to help keep your system alkaline and encourage oxygen uptake. Sprinkle $1/2$ tsp. lactobacillus powder over any food to normalize body chemistry.

__Caution for people who suffer from severe blood toxicity:__ Most immune deficient diseases are the result of blood toxins and can benefit from a blood purifying diet. However, in serious degenerative conditions like AIDS, lupus, chronic fatigue syndrome or fibromyalgia, large amounts of toxins and pollutants may exist in the blood. __When this is the case, an all-liquid fast is not recommended.__ It is often too harsh for an already weakened system, and in fact may dump more toxins into the bloodstream than the body can handle. The initial diet in these severe cases, should be as pure as possible to be as cleansing as possible – totally vegetarian – free of meats, dairy foods, fried, preserved and refined foods, and saturated fats.

__Begin with a 3-day liquid diet:__ follow with 4 days of 100% fresh foods.

The night before your blood cleanse....

–Take your choice of gentle herbal laxatives, or Gaia Herbs SUPREME CLEANSE.

The next day....

–**On rising:** a glass of fresh carrot juice, green tea, or a green tea blood cleansing formula, like Crystal Star GREEN TEA CLEANSER™; or blender blend a half lemon with skin and 8-oz. aloe vera juice, 1 tsp. honey, 1 cup distilled water; and $1/2$ tsp. lactobacillus powder.

–**Breakfast:** have a blood cleanser-builder: juice 5 carrots, 1 beet, 2 celery stalks and add 1-oz. wheatgrass juice powder, 1 handful fresh parsley; or an 8-oz. aloe vera juice with $1/2$ teasp. powdered or a capsulated probiotic (see next column).

–**Mid-morning:** take a potassium broth (page 568) and $1/2$ teasp. ascorbate vitamin C crystals, and $1/2$ teasp. lactobacillus powder; and another fresh carrot juice with these supplements, or pau d'arco tea.

–**Lunch:** have a glass of fresh PERSONAL BEST V-8 juice (page 569) and add 1 teasp. of Pines BEET JUICE POWDER (beet detoxifies and also builds the blood) or a carrot or apple juice. Mix in 1 TB. of a green superfood such as Crystal Star ENERGY GREEN™; Pines MIGHTY GREENS SUPERFOOD, or NutriCology PRO-GREENS.

–**Mid-afternoon:** have a Blood Regenerator Juice: handful spinach, 4 romaine leaves, 4 sprigs parsley, 6 carrots, $1/4$ turnip.

–**Dinner:** have a cup of miso soup with 2 TBS dried sea greens (dulse, nori, wakame, kombu or sea palm) snipped over the top.

–**Before bed:** take 8-oz. of aloe vera juice with $1/2$ teasp. ascorbate vitamin C with bioflavs and $1/2$ teasp. lactobacillus powder.

◆ In the Recipe Book: See Detoxification and Cleansing Foods, and Healing Drinks for more info.

Keep your blood balanced after your cleanse:

This is the perfect time to put an optimum diet, rich in vegetables and fruits (organically grown if possible) into effect. The following food spectrum can give some easy checkpoints to make this transition. It works from the most cleansing foods (alkaline-forming) to the more building foods (acid-forming). If you are not a vegetarian, you may wish to add animal products back into your diet after cleansing. However, I believe animal foods should be used in moderation. Focus on vegetables, fruits, whole grains, legumes, seeds, seafoods and sea greens, and booster foods like bee products and nutritional yeast.

The Food Spectrum: Moving from Cleansing to Building Foods

Liquids: • Pure water • Cleansing and purifying herb teas • Fruit juices • Vegetable juices • Green drinks (fresh greens with wheat grass, barley grass, chlorella, spirulina, sea greens, etc.) • Vegetable broths, especially miso soup

Fresh foods: • Fruit, especially apples and enzyme-rich fruits like pineapple, mango and papaya • Sprouts • Vegetables • Cultured vegetables (raw sauerkraut, Japanese Tsunomono or Korean Kim Chee) • Sea greens (can be prepared by simply soaking and rinsing in water) • Superfoods like green grasses and micro-algae, manufactured at temperatures under 100° F.

Cooked foods: • Steamed leafy and root vegetables • Grains like brown rice, buckwheat (full of rutin) and millet • Legumes like mung beans, black beans and lentils

Healthy (in moderation) but not for cleansing: • Nuts and oily seeds • Healthy fats like flax oil, olive and canola oil, or grapeseed oil • Cultured dairy foods like kefir and yogurt • Low fat cheeses and eggs • Fish and hormone-free poultry.

When the blood is too acid, it weakens the respiratory system — less oxygen is brought into the lungs and therefore less oxygen is brought into the cells. A long term acidic condition provides an environment where auto-immune diseases like cancer and AIDS can flourish. An inadequate supply of oxygen leads to fatigue. Chronic exhaustion is a common symptom of candidiasis, chronic fatigue, cancer and AIDS. Eating a good amount of alkaline foods, deep breathing and exercise all contribute to getting more oxygen. A lack of mental clarity (forgetfullness, feeling disorganized, etc.) can be caused by an acidic blood condition. Clear thinking and precise action is supported by an alkaline body. Cells living for an extended time in an acidic body environment can mutate and become malignant.

For blood health, about 80% of your diet should be alkaline. Alkaline-forming foods include: • All vegetables, most fruits, sprouts • Cultured vegetables, like raw sauerkraut • Sea greens (dulse, nori, kombu, hijiki, wakame) • Grains like brown rice, millet, quinoa, amaranth, buckwheat • Seeds, except sesame seeds • Herbs and herb teas • Olive oil

Eat about 20% acid-forming foods. Acid-forming foods include: • Poultry, ostrich meat, eggs and seafood • Sunflower, safflower, canola oils • Wheat breads, oats, white rice • Acid fruits like pomegranates, cranberries, strawberries • the herb stevia

Acid-forming foods to avoid: • Sugar, candy, soft drinks, all processed foods with preservatives and chemicals, red meats, white flour products, beans, nuts (except almonds) and nut butters, alcoholic beverages, and commercially refined vinegar containing foods. Avoid sweeteners like Nutrasweet - use instead the healthful sweetener, the herb stevia.

Herb and Supplement Choices

Choose 2 or 3 blood cleansing supplements.

• **Enzyme support:** Transformation PUREZYME, a potent blood purifier, breaks down protein invaders in the blood so they can be destroyed by the immune system. Use: 20 to 30 caps per day, in-between meals, divided in 3 doses.

• **Herbal blood cleansers:** Olive leaf extract conquers most microbes. Take 4 caps per day, between meals. Crystal Star GREEN TEA CLEANSER™ or DETOX™ capsule blend. (One of the most potent blood cleansing formulas available, used successfully for over two decades to rebalance blood chemistry. DETOX is strong and fast-acting. Should you decide to use it, take it alone.... not with other herbs, or vitamins other than vitamin C).; M.D. Labs DAILY DETOX II tea; Planetary Formulas COMPLETE PAU D'ARCO PROGRAM; Herbal Magic PURIFY HERBAL with red clover and burdock.

• **Blood purifiers with immune stimulants:** Nature's Answer BLOOD SUPPORT; Planetary RIVER OF LIFE.

• **Electrolytes establish healthy blood:** Arise & Shine ALKALIZER; Nature's Path TRACE-LYTE LIQUID MINERALS.

• Chlorophyll enhances blood cleansing: Sun Wellness SUN CHLORELLA; Pines WHEAT GRASS or BARLEY GRASS.

• **Antioxidants strengthen white blood and T-cells:** MICROHYDRIN, available at Healthy House, is one of the fastest ways to alkalize your body. It reduces the acidity of the urine and saliva, discouraging the growth of unfriendly organisms; germanium 150mg; Vitamin E 1000IU - selenium 200mcg; CoQ$_{10}$ 180mg; Enzymatic Therapy GRAPE SEED PHYTOSOME 100; Bromelain 500mg 3x daily; shark cartilage 1400mg daily for interferon, interleukin, lymphocytes.

Bodywork and Lifestyle Techniques

Bodywork techniques accelerate your cleanse:

• **Live Blood Cell Analysis:** by a skilled live cell technician can give you a great deal of insight on the state of your blood. It shows your personal profile (enzyme deficiencies, vitamin and mineral deficiencies, free radical stress, digestion and metabolic absorption, toxic conditions, and chronic health conditions). It offers useful information to help you fine tune your unique dietary and supplement needs). Live Blood Cell Analysis contact: Hannah Ineson 207-563-7460. Also call NuLife Sciences 707-781-9557 for more information.

• **Irrigate:** Take an enema the first and last day of your blood cleanse to help release toxins; a colonic irrigation or Nature's Secret SUPERCLEANSE to remove infected feces.

• **Exercise:** Exercise daily in the morning, if possible.

• **Massage therapy:** stimulates blood circulation.

• **Essential oils for blood cleansing:** use rosemary, cypress and vetiver, or a combination of all three. Put a total of 15 drops essential oil in 1-oz carrier oil and rub on the skin.

• **Bath and Sauna:** Take several saunas or long hot baths during a blood cleanse for faster, easier detoxification. Add a total of 10 drops of essential oils (see above) to your bath. Stir the water briskly to disperse evenly.

Can't find a recommended product? Call the 800 number listed in Product Resources for the store nearest you and for more info.

Lymph System Cleanse

The lymph system is a key to your body's immune defenses and a major player in your health. Cleansing the lymph system and re-establishing its unblocked circulation throughout the body is a vital part of any healing process. The lymphatic system includes lymphatic vessels and nodes, thymus gland, tonsils and spleen. The spleen is the largest mass of lymphatic tissue. It destroys worn-out red blood cells, and serves as a reservoir for fresh red blood. During times of demand, such as hemorrhage, the spleen can release its stored blood and prevent shock from occurring. The bone marrow, also part of this system, is where the white blood cells originate (marrow also produces red blood cells and platelets). Lymph nodes are clustered around the neck, armpit and groin.

The lymphatic system is actually a network of tubing that drains waste products from tissues, produces disease-fighting white blood cells (lymphocytes) and antibodies, and carries the bulk of your body's waste from the cells to the final elimination organs. Experts call the lymphatic system a second circulatory system, because it manages body fluids, assisting the bloodstream with millions of tiny vessels and ducts throughout the body to collect tissue fluid not needed by the capillaries or skin and return it to the heart for recirculation. Special filtering lymph nodes in groups along the lymph ducts remove infective organisms.

But your lymph system is even deeper and more autonomic than your heart. The valves of the lymph system have no pump (like the heart). Lymph circulation depends solely upon breathing and muscle movement. So physical exercise and diaphragmatic deep breathing are critical to lymph health. Without the ability to flow, lymph becomes waste-burdened, sluggish, and even toxic from harmful bacteria, chemicals, drugs, allergens or viruses. These pathogens often multiply and drain strength from the immune system.

If your lymph pH is acid, it creates an environment favorable to the growth of viruses. You can get an idea of your lymph pH by checking the pH of your saliva. Healthy "resting" saliva has a pH of 6.4 (after eating it will rise to 7.2 but will return to the resting pH). You can buy test strips to measure saliva pH at drug stores and some health food stores. A neutral pH is 7. Lower than 7 is the acid range and higher than 7 is alkaline.

Your liver and lymph systems are symbiotic. The liver produces the majority of lymph in your body. In turn, the lymph system, rich in fat-soluble proteins, is a major route for nutrients from the liver. The integrity of the lymph system is dependent on special immune cells in the liver that filter out harmful bacteria and destructive yeasts. Liver health is a key to lymphatic health. Dr. Philip Princetta of Atlanta, GA says "swollen lymph nodes are a sign of liver congestion and the lymph nodes reduce in size when the liver is purified."

Is your body showing signs that it needs a lymph cleanse?

—Do you have low immune response with frequent colds or flus?
—Are you under chronic stress, and constantly tired (indicating liver exhaustion)?
—Is your skin is very pale? Are you are extremely thin? Is your memory is noticeably failing?
—Does your body look soft and pudgy? Do you have newly noticeable cellulite (too many saturated fats and sugary foods)?

Lymph System Detox Plan

Begin with a 3 day juice-liquid diet and follow with 1 to 4 days of a diet of 100% fresh foods. Vital foods are elemental. Nutrient deficiency is the most frequent cause of a sluggish lymph system. Immune-boosting vegetables for juicing: cabbage, kale, carrot, bell pepper, collards and garlic. Lymph-enhancing fruits for juicing: apple, pineapple, blueberry and grape.

—**On rising:** take a glass of lemon juice and water in the morning for lymph revitalization.

—**Breakfast:** have a fresh vegetable lymph juice builder: handful parsley, 1 garlic clove, 5 carrots, and 3 celery stalks. Add 2 TBS of a green superfood like Nutricology PRO-GREENS, Crystal Star ENERGY GREEN™ or Wakunaga of America KYO-GREEN.

—**Mid-morning:** have two cups of Crystal Star LIV-ALIVE™ tea for liver and lymph cleansing, or a lymph tonic tea blend of white sage, astragalus, echinacea root, Oregon grape root and dandelion root.

—**Lunch:** have a vitamin A/ mixed carotene/vitamin C rich drink: 3 broccoli flowerets, 5 carrots, 1 garlic clove, 2 celery stalks and $1/2$ green pepper. Add 2 TBS. of a green superfood like Vibrant Health GREEN VIBRANCE or Green Foods VEGGIE MAGMA.

—**Mid-afternoon:** a glass of apple or grape juice.

—**Dinner:** have a Potassium Essence Broth (page 568), for mineral electrolytes. Or a zinc-rich broth, with vitamin A and C, potassium and magnesium electrolytes: In 2 cups water, cook 1 cup fresh veggies (carrots, broccoli, dark leafy greens, celery and parsley) and 1 tsp. miso. Strain. Hearty version: blend warm broth and vegetables. Add 4 TBS sunflower seeds.

—**Before Bed:** have a glass of papaya juice.

Pointers for best results from your lymph cleanse:

• A lymph detox both cleanses the lymph system of harmful microorganisms or toxic substances and enhances its ability to boost immune response, through cellular repair and increasing cellular metabolism.
• Water is the best over-all body cleanser - drink 8 glasses of bottled water each day of your cleanse.
• Spicy foods like salsas, cayenne, horseradish and ginger boost sluggish lymph and cut mucous congestion.
• Include potassium-rich foods regularly — sea greens, broccoli, bananas and seafood.
• Omega-3 fatty acids from flax or fish oils boost the lymphocytes and accelerate the power of antibodies.
• Avoid caffeine, sugar, dairy foods and alcoholic drinks during your cleanse. They contribute to lymph stagnation.

Benefits you may notice as your body responds to the lymph cleanse:

—Most people notice a daily energy increase with far fewer stress reactions like headaches.
—Most people avoid seasonal colds that come their way, and the illnesses they do get don't last as long.
—Most people notice better weight control and less cellulite formation as congestion lessens.

◆ In the Recipe Book: See <u>Detoxification and Cleansing Foods</u>, and <u>Healing Drinks</u> for more info.

Herb and Supplement Choices

Choose 2 or 3 lymph cleansing supplements.

• **Deep lymph cleanser:** Gaia Herbs SUPREME CLEANSE; Echinacea and Astragalus extracts, effective deep lymph cleansers.

• **Lymphatic cleansers:** Crystal Star ANTI-BIO™ caps for white blood cell formation, a lymph purifier with immune-stimulant properties. Creation's Garden LYM-1 cleanses the lymphatic system of bacteria, viruses and toxins, also helps restore ear, sinus, throat and skin from infection and irritations. Herbs Etc. LYMPHATONIC with echinacea (reduces lymphatic swelling and congestion), red root (powerful lymphatic cleanser, synergistic with echinacea), and ocotillo (flushes lymph congestion); Nature's Apothecary LYMPH CLEANSE; Herbalist and Alchemist BURDOCK-RED ROOT COMPOUND; Gaia Herbs ECHINACEA-RED ROOT SUPREME.

• **Immune support:** Silica decisively affects lymphatic system activity, increasing phagocytes to strengthen the immune response. Eidon SILICA MINERAL SUPPLEMENT; Flora VEGE-SIL.

• **Supporting lymph nutrients:** vegetable protein and B-12; vitamins A, C, E, B-complex, carotenes, iron, zinc and selenium.

• **Lymph immune support:** Crystal Star REISHI-GINSENG™ extract; maitake mushroom; Grifron MAITAKE D-FRACTION.

• **Enzyme support:** Protease is a powerful lymph immune booster, Transformation Enzyme PUREZYME.

• **Electrolyte boosters:** Mineral electrolytes help remove acid crystals. Nature's Path TRACE-LYTE LIQUID MINERALS.

Bodywork and Lifestyle Techniques

Bodywork techniques accelerate your cleanse:

• **Colonic irrigation:** take a colonic irrigation or a Sonné BEN-TONITE CLAY CLEANSE once a week to remove lymph congestion and infected feces from the intestinal tract.

• **Exercise:** exercise is critical to lymphatic flow. To stimulate: activate muscles with regular exercise and stretching. Start every exercise period with deep, diaphragmatic breathing. Mini-trampoline exercise clears clogged lymph nodes.

• **Massage therapy:** elevate feet and legs for 5 minutes every day, massaging lymph node areas. Acupuncture and acupressure are both effective.

• **Shower:** an alternating hot and cold hydrotherapy treatment at the end of your daily shower stimulates lymph circulation.

• **Essential oils:** to assist your lymph cleanse use geranium, juniper and black pepper. Use one or a combination of all three oils. Put a total of 15 drops essential oil in 1-oz of a carrier oil (such as jojoba) and rub on the skin.

• **Bathe:** a relaxing mineral bath: Add 1 cup Dead Sea salts, 1 cup Epsom salts, $1/2$ cup regular sea salt and $1/4$ cup baking soda to a tub; swish in 3 drops lavender oil, 2 drops chamomile oil, 2 drops marjoram oil and 1 drop ylang ylang oil. Stir the water briskly to disperse evenly.

• **Eliminate aluminum:** cookware, food additives, and aluminum containing foods and deodorants.

Note: Poor nutrition profoundly impairs the immune system. Excessive dietary sugars and alcohol over consumption especially inhibit white blood cell activity. Be sure to eliminate or limit their use. Adequate protein intake is critical to immune health and the ability to heal. The best sources for immune response are those with plenty of EFAs: salmon and fresh tuna, sea vegetables, green superfoods like spirulina and barley grass, and sprouts.

Can't find a recommended product? Call the 800 number listed in Product Resources for the store nearest you and for more info.

Skin Cleanse

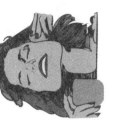

Do you need a skin cleanse? Your skin is the surest mirror of your lifestyle. Almost everything that's going on inside you shows on your skin. Your skin is your body's largest organ of elimination and detoxification. It acts as a backup for every other elimination organ. When your colon is overloaded with toxins, or your liver can't filter out impurities, your skin tries to compensate by releasing toxins from your body. It sweats them out, or throws them off through rashes or boils. Your skin is the essence of renewable nature.... it sloughs off old, dying cells every day, and gives your body a clean, new start.

Your skin is also your body's largest organ of absorption — both for nutrients and toxins. Good dietary habits show quickly. By the same token, food toxins and nutritional deficiencies from a poor diet show up first on your skin. For example, toxins eliminated through oil glands in the skin show up as acne. The skin mirrors our emotional state and our hormone balance, too. So, stress and hormone disruption show up as poor skin texture, or spots and blemishes.

Is your body showing signs that it needs a skin cleanse?

—Do you have sallow skin? Poor skin coloring may indicate build-up from liver wastes or drug residues.
—Do you have age spots? Brown mottled spots on the hands or face may reflect liver waste accumulation.
—Do you have adult acne, or uneven skin texture? Waste build-up from environmental pollutants, poor diet, liver exhaustion and stress allow increased free radical formation which attacks skin cell membranes.
—Do you have wrinkles, or sagging skin contours? Free radical activity also affects skin collagen and elastin proteins, resulting in wrinkling and dry skin. Poor skin tone is a sign of antioxidant deficiency.
—Do you have puffy, swollen eyes, dark circles under your eyes, or crusty, mucous formations in your eyes?
—Is your breath bad? Do you have body odor? They're pretty solid signs your body is overloaded with wastes.
—Do you have a skin disorder? Psoriasis, dermatitis and seborrhea all indicate it's time for a skin cleanse.
—Do you have skin sores or rashes that aren't healing? or hard skin bumps? You may not be eliminating wastes properly.
—Do you have unusually oily skin? or scaly, itchy skin? or chronically chapped and red skin?
—Is your circulation poor with cold hands and feet, and swollen ankles? Your body lacks tissue oxygen uptake.

Benefits you may notice as your body responds to skin cleansing:

—Most people see an appearance improvement in about 3 weeks. Skin texture appears smoother; fine lines less noticeable.
—Skin blemishes, blotches and spots diminish or disappear. Your face will look rested, rejuvenated and revitalized.
—Your skin's natural glow will return as capillary circulation and lymphatic drainage improve.
—The whites of your eyes will become whiter; dark circles will disappear.

171

Skin Detox Plan

1: Your diet is the quickest way to change your looks. Soft, smooth skin depends on a diet rich in fresh fruits and vegetables. Skin tissues need a rich, oxygen blood supply, and plenty of mineral building blocks. Silica, sulphur, calcium and magnesium are specific minerals for your skin. Plants are the most absorbable way for your body to get them.

2: Beautiful skin tone needs vitamin A, vitamin C, minerals and vegetable protein foods for collagen and interstitial tissue health. Eliminate or limit sugary foods, fried foods and trans-fats, like those in milk and dairy foods, margarine, shortening and hydrogenated oils. Avoid red meats and refined foods of all kinds.

3: Drink at least 8 glasses of bottled water each day of your cleanse — herbal "skin" teas are fine, too. Water keeps your body flushed so wastes and toxins won't be dumped out through the skin as blemishes or rashes. Fluoridated water may leach vitamin E out of your body.

Begin your skin cleanse with a 3-day liquid diet and follow with 4 days of a fresh foods diet.

—**On rising:** take a glass of lemon juice and water; add New Chapter GINGER WONDER syrup if desired.

—**Breakfast:** make a Complexion Booster: juice 2 slices of pineapple and 2 apples. Add 1 TB Crystal Star BIOFLAV, FIBER & C SUPPORT™, 1 teasp. nutritional Red Star yeast and 1 teasp. wheat germ oil.

—**Mid-morning:** have watermelon juice when available (rich in natural silica), or a skin tonic drink: juice 1 cucumber, 1 handful fresh parsley, one 4-oz. tub fresh sprouts and sprigs of fresh mint. Or, have a superfood green drink, like Crystal Star ENERGY GREEN™ or Transformation EASY GREENS.

—**Lunch:** have a fresh carrot juice; or a skin drink: juice 5 carrots, 2 apples, add 15 drops GINGER EXTRACT.

—**Mid-afternoon:** have a carrot/beet/cucumber juice once a week for the next month for a clean liver.

—**Dinner:** have a warm Potassium Essence Broth (page 568) for mineral electrolytes. Or, make a high luster skin broth: In 2 ¹/₂ cups water cook 2 cups chopped fresh mixed vegetables, add 1 teasp. miso and 2 TBS chopped dried sea greens. Vegetable protein aids faster healing for damaged skin because it's easier absorbed.

—**Before Bed:** have Crystal Star BEAUTIFUL SKIN™ TEA or green tea for skin support; or a pineapple-papaya, papaya or apple juice; or Red Star nutritional yeast broth for high B-complex vitamins.

Improvement signs show that your body is responding to the cleanse.

—Many skin conditions trace back to liver problems, so skin surface begins to clear and skin becomes more radiant.

—Stiff, aching muscles experience relief; warmth usually returns to cold hands and feet.

—Recurring headaches or migraines may disappear.

◆ In the Recipe Book: See Detoxification and Cleansing Foods, and Healing Drinks for more info.

Herb and Supplement Choices

Choose 2 or 3 skin cleansing supplements.

•**Deep skin cleansing:** Creations Garden TOTAL BODY CLEANSE, Crystal Star SKIN THERAPY #1™ and #2™ caps; sage or burdock root tea. Include a green superfood daily.

•**Smoothing-hydrating herbs for skin:** Crystal Star BEAU-TIFUL SKIN™ caps for blemishes and complexion beauty; Nature's Apothecary HEALTHY SKIN; Herbs Etc. DERMATONIC; burdock root normalizes production of the skin's beneficial oils; chamomile tea or CamoCare FACIAL THERAPY; lavender aromatherapy oil to reduce puffiness.

•**Skin vitamins and minerals:** Diamond HERPANACINE for superior skin support; Futurebiotics HAIR, SKIN & NAILS - results in just 2 weeks; Crystal Star MINERAL SPECTRUM™ caps.

•**Antioxidants are critical for skin health:** Beta carotene protects against the sun's free radicals; vitamin E protects against the lipid peroxidation caused by UV rays; Bioflavonoids improve vascularization of the skin.

•**EFA's in dry skin and wrinkling:** Evening primrose oil 2000mg daily; Spectrum ESSENTIAL MAX EFA OIL.

•**Enzymes:** Protease heals skin disorders; Transformation Enzyme PUREZYME or Enzymedica PURIFY.

•**Silica reduces dry, wrinkled skin:** Eidon SILICA MINERAL; Flora VEGESIL; Crystal Star SILICA SOURCE™.

•**MSM enhances skin pliability** and helps repair damaged, scarred skin: Nature's Path MSM-LYTE.

Bodywork and Lifestyle Techniques

Bodywork techniques accelerate your cleanse:

•**Sunlight:** Early morning sunlight on the body for natural vitamin D is a key.

•**Exercise** to get skin circulation flowing.

•**Dry brushing:** Use a natural bristle brush. Start with the soles of your feet - brush vigorously making rotary motions and massage every part of your body – work up to the neck.

•**Facial massage:** Improves skin circulation for better tone.

•**Healing, beautifying skin treatments:** Crystal Star BEAU-TIFUL SKIN™ gel, a restorative phytotherapy gel. Beautiful Face tea: steep chamomile, calendula, rosehips, juice of 1 lemon and 2 teasp. rose water. Strain; apply with cotton balls to face. Nature's Path SKIN-LYTE, a liquid electrolyte spray.

•**Aloe vera:** Herbal Answers HERBAL ALOE FORCE -THE SKIN GEL boosts circulation and stimulates new cell growth.

•**Fruit acid treatment:** Rub face with the insides of papaya or cucumber skins (natural AHA's) to neutralize wastes that come out on the skin and smooth skin.

•**Essential oils:** Use a combo of lavender, geranium, sandalwood and neroli. Use one or a combination of all three oils. Put 15 drops oil in 2-oz of a carrier oil, rub on the skin.

•**Skin mineral bath:** Add 1 cup Dead Sea salts, 1 cup Epsom salts, ¹/₂ cup regular sea salt and 4 TBS. baking soda to a tub; swish in 3 drops lavender, 2 drops geranium, 2 drops sandalwood and 1 drop neroli oil.

Continuing Diet Notes: Follow a whole foods diet. Eat mineral-rich foods such as leafy greens, bell peppers, broccoli, sesame and sunflower seeds, fish and sea vegetables. Include 4 to 5 servings of vegetables day–if possible eat half raw–as salads. Eat fruits once a day. Increase fiber to help keep your colon clean. Besides the fiber of vegetables and fruits include: flax seed meal, whole grains (like oats and rice), and beans (pinto and black beans).

Can't find a recommended product? Call the 800 number listed in Product Resources for the store nearest you and for more info.

Allergy Management Diets

Allergies are an epidemic at the turn of the millenium. Over 60 million Americans suffer from allergies - that's 20% of the population! Environmental toxins, acid rain, a depleted ozone layer, chemically treated and genetically altered foods, radiation levels, air and soil pollutants, and stress in our lives, result in lowered immunity and more allergens than our bodies can cope with or neutralize. Irresponsible use of antibiotics and steroid drugs taken over a long period of time for allergy symptoms greatly reduces immune response, and the ability to overcome allergens permanently. Allergy reactions are frequently an unrecognized cause of illness.

Substances that cause allergy reactions are called allergens. Most allergens produce congestion as the body tries to seal them off or work around them. The body forms a thick mucous shield and we get the allergy symptoms of sinus clog, stuffiness, hayfever, headaches and red, puffy eyes. Or our bodies try to throw the excess acids out through the skin causing rashes or boils, fever blisters, or a scratchy throat. There is growing evidence that some allergies alter personality, emotions, and one's sense of well-being.

Allergy origins fall into three main areas:

1: Allergies to Chemicals and Contaminants: Multiple chemical sensitivities are multiplying. We're exposed to more chemicals every day than any generation in history; 30% of Americans have sensitivities to chemicals! Over $2\,^{1}/_{2}$ billion pounds of pesticides are used in America every year! (300 million pounds are used in the home.) Benzene, formaldehyde, and carcinogens from carpeting and dry cleaning affect our brains. Repeated chemical exposures set off rampant free radical reactions and allergic responses. Those making the news today, environmental illness, sick buildings, Gulf War syndrome, breast cancer, nerve damage, attention deficit disorder in children, latex and insecticide allergies, are just the latest. Worse, our bodies use up enormous amounts of nutrients trying to detoxify us from these chemicals, nutrients that could have been used to keep us happy and healthy.

2: Allergies to Seasonal Environmental Conditions: Environmental pollutants, like asbestos and smoke fumes, and seasonal conditions, like dust, pollen or spores, affect the respiratory health of 35 million Americans. A seasonal allergic reaction is more likely to occur if the body has an excess accumulation of mucous which harbors environmental irritants. Common drugstore medications generally only mask symptoms and also have a rebound effect - the more you use them, the more you need them. The newest ones are strong medicine.... and have strong side effects like rapid heartbeat, even possible tumors. Steroid drugs for hayfever allergies, if taken for long periods, do not cure and often make the situation worse by depressing immune response, and impeding allergen elimination.

3: Allergies to foods and food additives: Food sensitivities are the fastest growing allergies as people become more exposed to chemically altered, enzyme-depleted, processed foods. A food allergy is an immune system antibody response to a food. A food intolerance is a non-immune reaction, usually an enzyme deficiency to digest a food. Celiac disease is a food sensitivity to gluten, a wheat protein (celiac disease affects up to 20% of Americans). Without enzyme action, your food is not all assimilated during digestion. Large amounts of undigested fats and proteins may be left that the immune system treats as toxic, releasing prostaglandins, leukotrienes, and histamines into the bloodstream that cause an allergy reaction. (See DIET FOR FOOD ALLERGIES, page 392.)

Is your body showing signs that it needs an allergy control diet?

Allergies to environmental allergens like air pollutants, asbestos or heavy metals, and seasonal allergens to dust, pollen, spores and mold, are called Type 1 allergies. This type of allergy develops more easily if your body has excess mucous accumulation to harbor the allergen irritants. Environmental allergens frequently interact in the bodies of allergy sufferers, both activating and aggravating other offending irritants. When this is the case, even the most powerful drugs do not relieve symptoms.

Signs that you may have a Type 1 environmental or seasonal allergy:

—Do you have chronic sinus congestion with itchy, watery nose and eyes? Do you have frequent bronchitis?
—Do you get headaches with sneezing, coughing and scratchy throat?
—Does your face swell up, with itchy, rashy skin? Do you have a skin rash on your arms or torso?
—Do you have trouble sleeping at night? Are you unusually tired during the day?
—Do you have unusual menstrual pain and congestion?
—Do you have hypoglycemia?

Allergies to chemicals and contaminant allergens are called Type 2 allergies. Chemical irritants occur from a wide range of petrochemicals like dry cleaning chemicals, estrogenic chemicals like pesticides, combustion residues from household appliances and products like chlorine bleach and insect repellents, and exhaust fumes. An allergic reaction to chemicals only occurs after the second exposure to the irritant when your body's histamine response is alerted. Repeated exposures set off massive free radical reactions as the body's contaminant toleration levels are reached; toxic overload results and a severe allergic reaction sets in. Worse, chemical sensitivities initiate other allergy reactions, so that the sufferer becomes allergic to nearly everything else.

Signs that you may have a Type 2 allergy to chemicals and contaminants:

—Unexplained migraine headaches? Usually with nausea or diarrhea?
—Frequent unexplained skin rashes?
—Low energy? Feel "under the weather" regardless of how much sleep you get?
—Hear your ears ringing, especially at night?
—Frequent colds and flu, or chronic respiratory infections?
—Frequently moody and depressed for no reason?
—Gained or lost weight recently for no reason? (Chemical allergies may cause poor metabolism.)
—Do friends and family tell you that your personality changes?
—Are often spacey? Is your memory is getting unusually bad?
—Do you have a child that's chronically hyperactive or who has difficulty learning?

Getting allergies out of your life will lift an unpleasant burden you have probably been putting up with for years. **How does the food pharmacy work to keep you healthy?** Making diet changes and taking therapeutic herbs are the most beneficial and quickest means of controlling allergies. A short 3 or 4 day mucous elimination diet can rid the body of excess mucous build-up, and pave the way for nutritional changes to have optimal effect. Herbal combinations help neutralize allergens, increase oxygen uptake, encourage critical adrenal activity and allow better sleep while therapy on the underlying allergy cause goes on. Aerobic exercise is pivotal to increase oxygen use in the lungs and tissues. Relaxation techniques overcome the stress reactions that aggravate allergies.

In addition to allergy reactions themselves, the allergy control diets in this chapter improve the following allergy-caused or associated problems: *Adrenal Exhaustion, Asthma, Hayfever, Chronic Sinusitis, Cyclical Headaches, Epilepsy Seizures, Digestive Disorders, Hypoglycemia, Candida Albicans Infections, Emotional Over-reactions.*

Mucous Elimination Diet for Allergies and Asthma

A mucous cleansing diet is a good way to start relieving allergy and asthma reactions. Toxin build up in the body is the most common trigger for allergy-asthma symptoms. Releasing toxic accumulations makes a big difference in relieving them.

Is your body overloaded with mucous congestion?

Your body needs some mucous. We're taught that mucous is a bad thing because it obstructs our breathing during a sinus infection, asthma or a cold. But mucous is also a needed lubricant and an important body safeguard. We take about 22,000 breaths a day. Mucous gathers up irritants like dirt, pollen, smoke and pollutants we take in along with our oxygen to protect mucous membranes in the respiratory system. Foods that putrefy quickly inside your body are the ones most likely to produce excess mucous like meat, fish, eggs and dairy products. These foods also slow down transit time through your gastrointestinal tract. Some of us carry around as much as 10 to 15 pounds of excess mucous!

Is your body showing signs that it needs a mucous cleanse?

    –Your breathing is labored. You have a chronic wheeze or cough. You have difficulty exhaling.

    –You have chronic bronchitis or sinus congestion, with a runny nose and sneezing.

    –You frequently use over-the-counter drugs for allergy or asthma (which often drives congestion deeper into lungs).

    –Allergies and asthma usually mean excess mucous in the colon, too, so you may experience constipation.

    –You catch every infection that goes around, (excess mucous is a breeding ground for infectious microbes).

Recipes that can help your mucous elimination diet: •DETOXIFICATION and CLEANSING FOODS; •HEALING DRINKS; •SOUPS - LIQUID SALADS.

Mucous Elimination Diet Plan

A 3 to 4 day nutrition plan

A program to overcome any chronic respiratory problem is more successful when begun with a short mucous elimination diet. This allows the body to rid itself of accumulations that cause congestion before attempting to change eating habits.

Benefits of a mucous elimination cleanse: 1: chest congestion clears as the non-mucous forming diet begins to work. 2: Bronchial inflammation and a chronic cough are relieved as the cleanse progresses. 3: Chronic lung and throat mucous are broken up and released. 4: Mucous from the colon is often expelled in a series of ropy, slimy stools. 5: Discomfort from colds or flu, allergies or asthma clears faster.

The night before your mucous elimination diet....

—Mash 4 garlic cloves and a large slice of onion in a bowl. Stir in 3 TBS. honey. Cover, let macerate for 24 hours; remove garlic and onion and take only the honey/syrup infusion - 1 teasp. 3x daily.

The next day....

—**On rising:** take 2 squeezed lemons in water with 1 TB maple syrup.

—**Breakfast:** take a glass of grapefruit, pineapple, or cranberry-apple juice.

—**Mid-morning:** have a glass of fresh carrot juice with 1 teasp. Bragg's LIQUID AMINOS added; or a cup of congestion clearing tea, like Crystal Star X-PECT™ TEA, an expectorant to aid mucous release, or Crystal Star RESPR TEA™, to help in oxygen uptake.

—**Lunch:** have a vegetable juice like V-8, or a potassium drink (page 568); or make a MUCOUS CLEANSING TONIC by juicing: 4 carrots, 2 celery stalks, 2-3 sprigs parsley, 1 radish and 1 garlic clove.

—**Mid-afternoon:** have a green veggie drink (page 569), or a teasp. of MONAS CHLORELLA powder or Sun Wellness SUN CHLORELLA granules in water; or a sea greens drink like Crystal Star ENERGY GREEN™.

—**Dinner:** take a hot vegetable broth (page 569), add 1 TB nutritional yeast. Add a small fresh salad the last night of the cleanse.

—**Before Bed:** apple or papaya/pineapple juice.

—**The next day....** Have toasted muesli or whole grain granola for breakfast, with a little yogurt or apple juice; a small fresh salad for lunch with lemon/oil dressing; a fresh fruit smoothie during the day; a baked potato drizzled with flax or olive oil and a light soup or salad for dinner.

Pointers for best results from your mucous cleanse:

1: Herbal teas are a good choice. They act as premier broncho-dilators and anti-spasmodics to open congested airspaces and break up mucous. They soothe bronchial inflammation and coughs. They are expectorants to remove mucous from the lungs and throat.

2: Drink 8 glasses of water each day of your cleanse to thin mucous and aid elimination.

3: Eliminate junk foods, fried foods, pasteurized dairy foods, and refined foods; they are a breeding ground for continued congestion.

4: Eat plenty of fresh enzyme-rich foods. They form little mucous and they are the easiest to digest.

Herb and Supplement Choices

•**Deep body cleanser for intestinal tract and lungs:** Use Nature's Way 5 SYSTEM CLEANSE caps after juice cleansing to help pull and clear intestinal mucous and mucous congestion from the respiratory system.

•**Mucous cleansers:** Crystal Star X-PECT-TEA™ aids mucous release; Herbs Etc. LUNG TONIC loosens and removes mucous; Herbs Etc. RESPIRATONIC loosens mucous and clears lung congestion.

•**Herbs to relieve mucous:** Mullein loosens and expels mucous; slippery elm removes excess mucous; nettles caps for allergic rhinitis; sage helps mucous discharge; white pine, an antioxidant expectorant, reduces mucous.

•**Maximize oxygen uptake:** Take 10,000mg ascorbate vitamin C crystals with bioflavonoids daily the first three days; just dissolve $\frac{1}{4}$ teasp. in water or juice throughout the day, until the stool turns soupy, and tissues are flushed. Take 5,000mg daily for the next four days. MICROHYDRIN available at Healthy House increases the body's oxygen uptake.

•**Antioxidants:** Crystal Star RESPR™ TEA and NutriCology GERMANIUM 150mg are good lung antioxidants that make a real difference.

•**Enzyme support:** Transformation DIGESTZYME; Herbal Products and Development POWER-PLUS ENZYMES; Transformation GASTROZYME relieves bouts of mucous congestion.

•**Electrolytes boost digestive efficiency up to 80%:** Nature's Path TRACE-LYTE LIQUID MINERALS.

•**Probiotics maintain proper mucous levels:** Nature's Path FLORA-LYTE; Ethical Nutrients INTESTINAL CARE; UAS Labs DDS-PLUS with FOS.

Bodywork and Lifestyle Techniques

•**Release mucous fast:** Take 1 teasp. fresh grated horseradish in a spoon with lemon juice. Hang over a sink to release great quantities of excess mucous fast.

•**Enema:** Take an enema the first and last day of your fasting diet to thoroughly clean out excess mucous.

•**Irrigate:** A colonic offers a more thorough colon cleanse.

•**Exercise:** Take a brisk daily walk each day of your cleanse, breathing deeply to help the lungs eliminate mucous.

•**Massage therapy with percussion:** a percussion massage loosens mucous. Most people have several congestion-releasing bowel movements and expectoration incidences within 24 hours after a massage therapy treatment.

•**Compress:** Apply wet ginger-cayenne compresses to the chest to increase circulation and loosen mucous.

•**Bathe and Sauna:** Take a hot sauna or a long warm bath with a rubdown to stimulate circulation and help loosen mucous congestion. Add to your bath 5 drops of eucalyptus, tea tree oil or oregano oil.

•**Essential oils:** aromatherapy oils help clear mucous.
—Eucalyptus (inhale) - antiviral action works on respiratory tract to loosen mucous - treats asthma, bronchitis and sinusitis.

—Tea tree oil (inhale) - antiviral, antibacterial decongestant.
—Oregano oil (inhale) - antiviral and antibacterial properties help eradicate lung infection.

•**Visualize your cleansing process:** Close your eyes. Inhale and exhale long and slowly. As you exhale, visualize mucous dislodging, and leaving your lungs and your colon. As you inhale, visualize oxygen and nutrients renewing all your cells.

Can't find a recommended product? Call the 800 number listed in Product Resources for the store nearest you and for more info.

Diet Plan to Control Seasonal-Environmental Allergies

Diet change is a powerful force for overcoming and neutralizing allergens of all kinds. In fact, diet improvement is the single most beneficial thing you can do to control allergic rhinitis reactions. • Cut fats, especially fatty animal products. Your body stores more saturated animal fats (and allergens along with them). • Drink more water. Good water intake reduces histamine production in histamine-generating cells. • Make sure your diet stays nutrient-rich. Eat plenty of plant foods — fresh vegetables, fruits, sea greens, whole grains, nuts, seeds and beans. Include fresh vegetable and fruit juices, cultured foods for friendly digestive flora, and flax and canola oils for EFA's. Eat a fresh salad every day. • Strengthen your adrenals with low fat, fresh foods. The better your adrenals work, the less sensitivity you'll have to allergens. Low adrenal function leads to more severe allergies and to multiple allergies. • Boost your immune response with superfoods. Concentrated nutrients from foods like green and blue-green algae (chlorella and spirulina), green grasses (barley, wheat grass and alfalfa) and bee pollen decrease your body's sensitivity to allergens.

Start with this 3-day light cleansing plan to address underlying allergy causes.

The night before your allergy cleanse....

—Have a green leafy salad for dinner to give your bowels a good sweeping.

The next day....

—**On rising:** take 2 squeezed lemons in water with 1 TB maple syrup; or take a glass of cranberry, apple, pineapple or grapefruit juice; or a cup of green tea each morning.

—**Breakfast:** have a vitamin E-rich drink (vitamin E has antihistamine activity): one handful spinach, 5 carrots, 4 asparagus spears; or mix Crystal Star SYSTEMS STRENGTH™ drink into hot water and add 1 tsp. nutritional yeast and a pinch of cayenne pepper.

—**Mid-morning:** have a glass of fresh carrot juice with 1 tsp. Bragg's LIQUID AMINOS added; or a cup of a congestion clearing tea, like Crystal Star X-PECT™ TEA, to aid mucous release, or Crystal Star RESPR-TEA™, to aid oxygen uptake.

—**Lunch:** have a fresh mixed vegetable juice, or a potassium broth (page 568); or make this Mucous Cleansing Tonic by juicing: 4 carrots, 2 celery stalks, 2-3 sprigs watercress or parsley, 1 radish and 1 garlic clove. Take hot miso or chicken soup to release mucous. For solid food, have a fresh vegetable salad. Add a little olive oil, squeeze of lemon and Bragg's LIQUID AMINOS to taste.

—**Mid-afternoon:** have a veggie drink (page 569), add in 1 TBS. of Monas CHLORELLA; or a greens and sea greens mix, such as Crystal Star ENERGY GREEN™ DRINK (add to water or juice).

—**Dinner:** have a hot vegetable broth (page 569) with 1 TB nutritional yeast; or miso soup with sea greens snipped on top; or a mixed fresh vegetable juice or fresh carrot juice with 1 TB of a green superfood mixed in.

—**Before Bed:** have a glass of apple juice or papaya/pineapple juice.

Recipes that can help your seasonal allergy diet: •LOW FAT and VERY LOW FAT RECIPES; •ENZYME-RICH RECIPES; •SALADS ; •DAIRY FREE COOKING; •SOUPS -LIQUID SALADS; •CULTURED HEALING FOODS

Herb and Supplement Choices

• **Natural antihistamines:** Crystal Star ALRG™ (address cause) or ANTI-HST™ caps (address symptoms); Trimedica MSM 1000mg daily to counter IgE anti-body response; Ester C up to 5000mg daily with bioflavonoids, and CoQ$_{10}$ 30mg 3x daily to help the liver produce antihistamines; Grapeseed PCO's 100mg; Herbs, Etc. ALLER-TONIC with nettles and eyebright; Pure Essence Labs ALLER-FREE (especially good for chronic runny nose).

• **Green superfoods are potent immune builders:** Crystal Star ENERGY GREEN™ drink; NutriCology PRO-GREENS with EFA's; Country Life SHIITAKE/REISHI with CHLORELLA.

• **Bee foods noticeably strengthen your system against pollen allergies:** CC Pollen ALLER BEE-GONE; Beehive Botanicals ROYAL JELLY caps, or ROYAL JELLY-GINSENG caps for pantothenic acid; CC Pollen PROPOLIS caps.

• **Antioxidants are a key:** Crystal Star BIOFLAV, FIBER and C SUPPORT™, MICROHYDRIN available at Healthy House; Nutricology GERMANIUM 150mg; Vitamin E 400IU with selenium 200mcg; CoQ-10 60mg 3x daily.

• **Flush mucous congestion:** Crystal Star ANTI-BIO™ caps 6 daily; Zand DECONGEST HERBAL; AloeLife FIBER-MATE.

• **Feed your adrenals:** B-complex 150mg; Crystal Star ADRN-ACTIVE™ extract or caps; Planetary SCHIZANDRA ADRENAL; Herbs, Etc. ADRENO-TONIC.

• **Stabilize reaction to hayfever allergens:** Crystal Star GINSENG-REISHI drops in RESPR-TEA™; Quercetin 2000mg daily with bromelain 1500m; Zand ALLERGY SEASON.

• **Homeopathics remedy attacks without side effects:** Euphrasia drops; BioForce POLLINOSAN; Nova HAYFEVER; Bio-Allers POLLEN-HAYFEVER; Boericke & Tafel ALLERAIDE.

Bodywork and Lifestyle Techniques

• **Identify your allergens:** Use Coca's Pulse Test or muscle testing to identify allergens. (See page 570.)

• **Avoid allergens:**
  –Stay indoors, especially in the morning.
  –Exercise indoors on dry, windy days. Invest in an air filter.
  –Stop smoking; avoid secondary smoke. It magnifies allergy reactions.

• **Topical applications:**
  –MSM gel topically to skin rashes.
  –BREATHE RIGHT post nasal strips.
  –Cayenne-ginger chest compresses.

• **Exercise:** Exercise increases oxygen uptake. Take a daily walk with deep breathing exercises.

• **Use relaxation techniques:** Stress depresses immunity and aggravates allergies. –Acupuncture and chiropractic have both proven effective for allergies.

  –**Try the following calming technique:** when your mind races and you feel anxious, shift your focus. Turn your attention to your breathing. The connection between breathing and your state of mind is a basic principle of yoga relaxation. It's the simplest form of concentrative meditation.
  1: Consciously take slow, deep regular breaths, for at least one minute. 2: Recall a pleasant past experience. Recount the good things and people you have in your life. It works.

• **Effective acupressure points:**
  1–During an attack, press tip of nose hard for relief.
  2–Press hollow above the center of upper lip as needed.
  3–Press underneath cheekbones beside nose, angling pressure upwards.

Can't find a recommended product? Call the 800 number listed in Product Resources for the store nearest you and for more info.

180

Diet Plan To Control Chemical-Contaminant Allergies

Chemical and heavy metal poisoning is a major problem of modern life. There seems to be no way to avoid toxic exposure. Toxic effects are serious.... we have moved from fetid air to undrinkable water to severe allergy reactions, birth defects, even cancer caused by pollution. The main impact of chemical toxins is on immune response, because our filtering organs, the liver and kidneys, are overwhelmed. Periodic detoxification needs to be a part of life to keep our bodies able to defend us.... against yet more pollutants. (An astounding twenty-five thousand NEW chemicals enter our society every year.) A hair analysis can help you determine nutrient deficiencies caused by chemical toxins and which heavy metals are lodged in your body.

Is your body showing signs that it needs a pollution/heavy metal cleanse?

–Are you far more sensitive to odors like perfumes and strong cleansers than most people?

–Do you have an unusually small tolerance for alcohol?

–Are there medications you can't take? some vitamins or other supplements that make you feel worse?

–Do you have small black spots along your gum line? Unusually bad breath or body odor?

–Is your reaction time when driving noticeably poorer in city traffic?

–Do you have unexplained seizures, memory failure or psychotic behavior?

–Have you become infertile or impotent?

Watchwords for your chemical-contaminant allergen cleanse:

1— I don't recommend an all-liquid diet if you're trying to release heavy metals or chemicals. They may enter the bloodstream too fast and heavily for your body to handle and can poison you even more. Eat solid cleansing foods instead, like brown rice and steamed vegetables to release the toxins more slowly and safely.

2—Chemical exposure sets off rampant free radicals. Green drinks are key detoxifiers and blood builders, (see page 569 for recipes), or consider •Crystal Star ENERGY GREEN™ drink, •Green Foods GREEN MAGMA, •Herbal Answers ALOE FORCE juice, •Futurebiotics VITAL K, •Sun Wellness CHLORELLA, especially against radiation, •Green Foods CARROT ESSENCE, •Pines MIGHTY GREENS.

3—Eat organically grown foods as much as possible. Avoid canned foods, and foods sprayed with colorants, waxes or ripening agents. Drink only bottled or distilled water.

4—For quickest toxin release, eat sea greens every day. 2 TBS is a therapeutic dose. Just snip dry greens over soup, a salad, rice, even a pizza.... delicious. Or eat 6 pieces of sushi a day.

5—Reduce saturated fats and trans fat intake; add good omega-3 oils with essential fatty acids: sea greens, flax, canola and olive oils for resistance.

6—Avoid fried foods, red meats, pasteurized dairy products, fatty and sugary foods. Avoid caffeine - it inhibits liver filtering.

7—Eat legumes and sea greens to excrete lead. Have an apple a day. Apple pectin removes metal toxins.

Start with a short 3 to 7 day purifying cleanse to begin toxin release.

Note 1: A heavy metal, pollutant detox is one of the most likely cleanses for a "healing crisis" to occur. You may feel headachey, with a slight upset stomach as toxins are released. The feelings should pass quickly, usually within 24 hours.

Note 2: Avoid commercial antacids - they interfere with enzyme production, and the ability of the body to carry off heavy metals. Use plant enzymes for digestive help instead.

—**On rising:** 2 TBS. cranberry concentrate in water with $^1/_2$ tsp. vitamin C crystals; or Crystal Star GREEN TEA CLEANSER™; or blend 2 tsp. lemon, 1 tsp. honey, 1 cup water and 1 tsp. acidophilus in 8-oz. aloe vera juice.

—**Breakfast:** have a glass of fresh carrot juice with 1 TB. green superfood like Crystal Star ENERGY GREEN™ or Green Foods GREEN MAGMA, and whole grain muffins or rice cakes with kefir cheese; or a cup of soy milk or plain yogurt blended with a cup of fresh fruit, walnuts, and $^1/_2$ teasp. acidophilus in 8-oz. aloe vera juice; or a bowl of high fiber cereal to bind / eliminate toxins in the G.I. tract. Sprinkle on nutritional yeast, toasted wheat germ and lecithin granules.

—**Mid-morning:** take a cup of green tea, with $^1/_2$ teasp. ascorbate vitamin C crystals; or a fresh vegetable juice with 1 TB green superfood such as Nutricology PRO-GREENS with beneficial EFA's, or Wakunaga KYO-GREEN. Mix of $^1/_4$ cup each: wheat germ, molasses, lecithin granules and nutritional yeast (or Biostrath LIQUID YEAST). Take 2 TBS daily in juice or a green drink.

—**Lunch:** have a leafy salad with lemon-flax oil dressing; or a cup of miso soup with brown rice; or steamed veggies with brown rice; and green tea with $^1/_2$ teasp. vitamin C and $^1/_2$ teasp. acidophilus powder.

—**Mid-afternoon:** have a carrot juice with 1 TB. green superfood like Crystal Star ENERGY GREEN™; or a cup of miso soup with sea greens snipped on top.

—**Dinner:** have a baked potato with Bragg's LIQUID AMINOS and a fresh salad with lemon-flax dressing; or a black bean or lentil soup; or a Chinese steam/stir fry with vegetables, shiitake mushrooms and brown rice.

—**Before Bed:** an 8-oz. glass of aloe vera juice with $^1/_2$ teasp. vitamin C and another carrot juice or another cup of miso soup.

—Follow with a diet that helps fight contaminant allergies:

Keep a large percent of your diet rich in enzymes by bringing in more fresh vegetables and fruit. Enzymes break down protein allergens and help prevent the process that causes an allergic reaction. Other wholesome foods that fight chemical and contaminant allergies are whole grains, legumes, seeds, seaweeds, superfoods, seafood, etc. Use foods like eggs, dairy (except yogurt) and poultry only occasionally. Eliminate foods which contribute to toxic accumulation, like sugar, animal fats, processed-refined foods, etc. Obviously avoid any foods which you know are causing an allergic response. Use organically grown produce and hormone-free meats whenever possible.

Recipes to help your chemical allergy diet: •LOW FAT and VERY LOW FAT RECIPES; •ENZYME-RICH RECIPES; •LIGHT MACROBIOTIC EATING; •HEALING DRINKS; •SOUPS-LIQUID SALADS; •CULTURED HEALING FOODS

Herb and Supplement Choices

•**Release contaminants from the body:** Transformation PUREZYME, a protease, binds to heavy metals, sparing metabolic enzyme destruction (high doses effective in lowering blood mercury toxins); Crystal Star HEAVY METAL CLEANSE™ or DETOX™ caps for 2-3 months. For lead poisoning in children: take vitamin C with CLEANSING & PURIFYING™ tea daily. For radiation poisoning: vitamin C powder with bioflavonoids $\frac{1}{2}$ teasp. every hour to bowel tolerance as a tissue flush.
•**Oral Chelation cleanses heavy metals:** Metabolic Response Modifiers CARDIO-CHELATE; Golden Pride FORMULA ONE.
•**Stimulate liver activity:** Lipoic Acid 600mg daily for 2 months.; Crystal Star LIV-ALIVE™ caps or tea with MILK THISTLE SEED extract; Dandelion extract; Enzymatic Therapy LIVA-TOX caps.
•**Build immune defenses with immune enhancers:** •Astragalus extract; •Propolis extract or lozenges; •Garlic 6-8 caps daily; •Siberian ginseng extract caps; •Spirulina 2 teasp daily, or •Spirulina MICROCLUSTERS, available at Healthy House (especially for radiation/chemotherapy toxins); •Monas CHLO-RELLA 2 teasp. daily for chemical toxins. Kelp 10 tabs daily, especially for suspected radiation poisoning.
•**Protect yourself with powerful antioxidants:** Carnitine 1000mg 3x daily for 1 month; NAC (N-acetyl-cysteine) 500mg 3x daily; CoQ-10, 60mg 4x daily; Nutricology GERMANIUM 150mg daily. Beta carotene 150,000IU with extra lycopene 5-10mg; Vitamin E 400IU with selenium 200mcg; Glutathione 100mg daily; MICROHYDRIN available at Healthy House; Source Naturals CHEM-DEFENSE; Enzymatic Therapy THYMUPLEX. Biotec CELL GUARD 8 daily.

Bodywork and Lifestyle Techniques

•**Lifestyle measures to avoid contaminants.**
—Seek out trees to live around. Trees produce oxygen and remove many air pollutants.
—Avoid antacids.... they interfere with enzymes, and your body's ability to carry off chemical residues.
—Invest in an air filter. Pay attention to unhealthy air alerts; stay indoors if you have chemical sensitivities.
—Avoid as much as possible: smoking and secondary smoke, pesticides (sprinkle pepper on anthills instead), fluorescent lights, aluminum cookware and deodorants.
—Protect against radiation syndromes: avoid foods labeled irradiated or electronically pasteurized.
—Use vinegar, baking soda and salt as cleansers.
—Protect yourself from EMF fields: avoid non-filtered computer screens, cell phones, electric blankets, microwave ovens. (Don't use plastic wrap in a microwave. Its heat can drive plastic molecules into the food.)
—Get plenty of oxygen. Take a walk every day, breathing deeply. Do deep breathing exercises on rising, and in the evening on retiring to clear the lungs. Spray Earth's Bounty O₂ SPRAY on soles of feet every 2 days for tissue oxygen.
—Take a hot seaweed bath, or a sweating bath, like Crystal Star POUNDS OFF BATH™. Use a dry skin brush before and after the bath to remove toxins coming out on the skin.
—Acupuncture, chiropractic, massage therapy are effective for chemical allergies. Spring Life POLARIZERS have notable success against environmental pollutants.
—Use Coca's Pulse Test or muscle testing to identify allergens. (See pg. 570)

Can't find a recommended product? Call the 800 number listed in Product Resources for the store nearest you and for more info.

Asthma Control Diet

Asthma is the most serious Type 1 allergy reaction. Twenty million people in the U.S. have asthma, up from 10.4 million reported by the National Institute of Health in 1990. Two million have needed emergency treatment. Asthma is a chronic, breathing disorder characterized by bronchial spasms which restrict the flow of air in and out of the lungs. A person with healthy lungs can empty air in about 2-3 seconds. An asthmatic's lungs take 6-7 seconds! During an asthma attack, a person has extreme difficulty breathing, especially great difficulty in exhaling because the lungs cannot breathe air out. The bronchioles, tubes which carry air through the lungs, become thick with mucous, causing muscle spasms and choking. Asthma attacks are serious, sometimes even fatal – about 5,000 people die of asthma every year. Asthma treatments cost Americans over $6 billion every year. $1 billion is lost from loss of school days alone.

Sadly, asthma is the leading serious illness among children under the age of ten, (a 2:1 ratio of boys to girls), and it's on the rise. The number of children hospitalized for asthma has increased fivefold over the past 20 years! Kids miss 10 million school days each year from asthma-related problems. Children have smaller lungs and bronchial tubes, and less breathing reserves during an asthma attack than adults. They also have more cold and flu infections that trigger asthma attacks. Heredity, diet and lifestyle are all involved with asthma's development and severity. A child whose mother has asthma is more likely to develop it than other children. Some studies show a greater risk of asthma with childhood vaccinations.

Why has asthma experienced almost a 50% rise in the last decade?

–Environmental toxins are becoming a clear cause for the rise in asthma attacks. We take in chemical contaminants as we breathe. Unless we're eating organic foods and pure water we take in more chemicals from pesticides and additives in our foods, and chemical toxins in our water. **The average American eats his or her own weight per year of these chemicals.**

–Asthma is an immune deficient illness. The huge increase in prescription drug use over the last decade means more immune suppression. Even simple medications like aspirin may provoke asthma; leukotrienes involved in allergic reactions. Inappropriate use of asthma drugs may be playing a role in the upswing of attacks. Prescription bronchodilators and inhalers for asthma work short-term, by relaxing constricted airways during an attack. When overused, these drugs can lose their effectiveness and cause side effects like tremors, dizziness, nausea, even strokes. Bronchodilators relieve symptoms temporarily, but they don't address underlying asthmatic inflammation. Corticosteroid drugs, also inhaled, can help prevent asthma attacks and mini- mize their severity. However, using steroid inhalers long term for asthma may increase risk for glaucoma, cataracts and interfere with normal growth in children. Most inhalers also contain chlo- rofluorocarbons (CFCs) linked to the depletion of the Earth's protective ozone layer.

and NSAIDS may aggravate asthma because they can elevate

–Be very cautious when switching from oral steroid drugs to the new inhaled steroid drugs (like FLOVENT) to treat asthma symptoms. The new inhaled steroids are less active than oral steroid drugs. A warning now appears in the 1999 PDR advising caution because deaths due to adrenal insufficiency have occurred in some patients who switched their medication abruptly.

Asthma Control Diet Plan

Pointers for best results: 1: Eat fish, like salmon, swordfish, halibut, etc; they contain Omega-3 fatty acids that help control asthma. 2: You must avoid all chemical food additives when trying to control asthma. Read labels on every packaged food you buy. 3: Drinking 8 -10 glasses of water daily makes a big difference. Water thins mucous secretions, and there is a link between dehydration and excess histamine production in the body. 4: Add green leafy veggies - their magnesium relaxes bronchial muscles. 5: Take daily vitamin C; low vitamin C is linked to asthma.

Start with this 2 to 3 day nutrition plan. *Note: During an attack - eat only fresh foods. Include fresh apple or carrot juice daily.*
The night before your asthma diet: Make a syrup of pressed garlic juice, cayenne, olive oil and honey. Take 1 teasp. each day of your diet as a liver cleansing, bile stimulant for fatty-acid metabolism.

—**On rising:** take a glass of fresh apple, grapefruit juice or cranberry juice; or lemon juice in hot water with 1 teasp. honey; or a glass of apple cider vinegar, hot water and honey.
—**Breakfast:** take a hot potassium broth (page 568); or Crystal Star SYSTEMS STRENGTH™ drink; or apple juice with 1 teasp. Monas CHLORELLA. Add 3 garlic caps and ¹/₄ teasp. ascorbate vitamin C or Ester C powder with bioflavonoids in water.
—**Mid-morning:** have a glass of fresh carrot juice; and/or a cup of comfrey/fenugreek tea, or Crystal Star ASTH-AID TEA™.
—**Lunch:** have a hot vegetable, miso or onion broth, or Crystal Star SYSTEMS STRENGTH™ drink. Add 3 garlic caps and ¹/₄ teasp. ascorbate vitamin C or Ester C powder with bioflavonoids in water.
—**Mid-afternoon:** have an herb tea, such as alfalfa/mint or Crystal Star GREEN TEA CLEANSER™; or add Monas CHLORELLA, or Crystal Star ENERGY GREEN™ to a fruit or vegetable juice.
—**Dinner:** have a hot veggie broth, or miso soup with sea greens snipped on top; or another glass of carrot juice with 1TB Ethical Nutrients FUNCTIONAL GREENS. Add 3 more garlic caps and ¹/₄ teasp. ascorbate vitamin C or Ester C powder with bioflavonoids.
—**Before Bed:** take another hot water, lemon and honey drink; apple or cranberry juice.

Recipes to help your seasonal allergy diet: • **LOW FAT and VERY LOW FAT RECIPES;** • **ENZYME-RICH RECIPES;** • **SALADS HOT and COLD;** • **DAIRY FREE COOKING;** • **SOUPS -LIQUID SALADS;** • **CULTURED HEALING FOODS**

—Food sensitivities play a major role in asthma attacks. The food allergy-asthma link has long been established, especially from triggers like foods with (MSG) and sulfating agents used widely in wine, beer and snacks. New food colorants and additives are on the rise. Avoid high gluten breads, oily and fried foods, soft drinks and sugary foods that contain a lot of these additives. Reduce salt. Asthma is common when salt intake is high. Avoid dairy products; they generate the most mucous. Limit animal foods in general. Leukotrienes that contribute to asthma reactions are derived from arachidonic acid found only in animal products.

Herb and Supplement Choices

• **Deep lung cleansers:** Creation's Garden LNG-3 (clears lung congestion, bronchial swelling, inflammation). Use Nature's Way 5 SYSTEM CLEANSE caps after juice cleansing to help pull and clear intestinal mucous and lung mucous congestion.

• **Mucous release:** Crystal Star X-PECT-TEA™; Herbs Etc. LUNG TONIC; Medicine Wheel CONGEST-EASE. Herbs to relieve mucous: *mullein, slippery elm, sage, white pine*.

• **Plant sterols help control asthma:** Natural Balance MODUCARE STERINOL, for high circulating IgE antibodies.

• **Increase oxygen uptake:** Nature's Path TRACE-LYTE and Arise & Shine ALKALIZER; Crystal Star RESPR™ CAPS and TEA; NutriCology GERMANIUM 150mg.

• **Antioxidants are a key:** MICROHYDRIN, available at Healthy House; NutriCology ESTEROL (Ester C with bioflavonoids, Vitamins A and E and selenium, important in breaking down allergic leukotrienes). Biotec Foods CELL GUARD, 8 daily; Country Life SUPER 10 ANTIOXIDANT; Source Naturals PROANTHODYN.

• **Reduce swelling and inflammation:** Transformation PUREZYME; Gaia Herbs GRINDELIA/CAMELLIA SUPREME; BD Herbs HYSSOP FORMULA.

• **Magnesium, effective for acute asthma attacks:** People who get extra magnesium in their diets have stronger lungs. Nature's Path CAL-LYTE is a 1 to 1 calcium and magnesium ratio. Magnesium has a reciprocal relationship with calcium and they work best when they are in the proper balance.

• **Boost immunity:** Rainforest Remedies STRONG RESISTANCE; Jarrow Corp. JARRO-DOPHILUS+FOS; Nature's Path FLORA-LYTE; Arise & Shine POWER UP.

Bodywork and Lifestyle Techniques

• **Enema:** Take an enema the first and last day of your mucous elimination diet to thoroughly clean out excess mucous. Or, have a colonic for a more thorough colon cleanse.

• **Vaporizer:** Use one of the aromatherapy oils below to help clear mucous congestion in the lungs (inhale from vaporizer or from steam when mixed into hot water), or food grade H_2O_2, 3% dilute solution in 8-oz. water in a vaporizer at night for relief and tissue oxygen.

–*Eucalyptus*: antiviral action works on respiratory tract to loosen mucous - treats asthma, bronchitis and sinusitis.

–*Tea tree oil*: antiviral and antibacterial decongestant.

–*Oregano oil*: antiviral and antibacterial properties help eradicate lung infection.

• **Chest compress:** Apply wet *ginger/cayenne* chest compresses to increase circulation and loosen mucous.

• **Flower remedies:** Natural Labs DEVA FLOWERS ALLERGIES/ASTHMA; Nelson Bach RESCUE REMEDY for stress.

• **Bath and Sauna:** long warm baths or saunas loosen mucous congestion. Add to your bath 5 drops of *eucalyptus* or *tea tree oil*. Food grade 35% H_2O_2 may be used to increase tissue oxygen via the skin. Use $1\frac{1}{2}$ cups to a tub of water.

• **Massage therapy with percussion:** a rubdown stimulates circulation and loosens mucous. Most people have several congestion-releasing bowel movements and expectoration incidences within 24 hours after massage therapy.

• **Visualize easier breathing:** Close your eyes; inhale and exhale long and slowly. As you exhale, visualize mucous dislodging and leaving your lungs. As you inhale, visualize oxygen and nutrients renewing all your cells.

Can't find a recommended product? Call the 800 number listed in Product Resources for the store nearest you and for more info.

Arthritis Healing Diets

Arthritis is already the country's number one crippling disease, affecting up to 80% of people over 50. When you add to that number, people suffering from arthritis-like diseases - gout, bursitis, tendonitis, rheumatism, ankylosing spondylitis (arthritic spine), and lupus, the figure becomes staggering. Up to 50 million Americans are afflicted by one or more of these crippling conditions. Arthritis isn't a simple disease in any form, affecting not only the bones and joints, but also the blood vessels (Reynaud's disease), kidneys, skin (psoriasis), eyes and brain. Its origins range from metabolic disorders brought on by stress and adrenal exhaustion, to faulty elimination, an over-acid system, long emotional resentments and pessimism about life, and overuse of prescription drugs.

Arthritis is unique in its close ties to emotional health. Emotional stress frequently brings onset of the disease. Negative emotional resentments and obsessive-compulsive actions aggravate arthritis. Most arthritis sufferers have a marked inability to relax (relaxation techniques are essential to arthritis healing). Many have a negative attitude toward life that locks up their body's healing ability.

Because its causes are rooted in immune response as well as wear-and-tear effects, conventional medicine has not been able to address arthritis successfully. Many patients show little improvement from arthritis drugs; some patients who receive drug therapy become progressively worse and suffer serious side effects. The array of new products for arthritis is rising at an almost exponential rate as the baby boomer generation creeps into the "age of arthritis." NSAIDS drugs, cortisone drugs, even biogenetic drugs for arthritis have side effects and unknowns in terms of immune response. Some steroid drugs may depress immune response so dramatically that even minor infections can be life-threatening. They cause calcium depletion and adrenal gland depression, a primary cause of arthritis (and osteoporosis) in the first place.

Natural therapies, based in lifestyle changes, work extremely well, addressing the causes of arthritis while reducing pain and discomfort. Natural treatment relies on improved diet and nutrition to create an environment for the body to support its own healing functions. Even in advanced inflammation and joint degeneration, major digestive problems, and depression and fatigue, diet change can affect improvement. I have personally seen notable reduction of swelling, and deformity in long-standing cases.

Even though the medical focus of diagnosis has been on organic mineral (especially calcium) depletion as a cause of arthritis, I find that hormone imbalance and adrenal exhaustion are the keys to repair therapy. Arthritic conditions are degenerative processes that take years to develop. Small or subtle changes are not successful in reversing them. **Vigorous diet therapy is the most beneficial thing you can do to control the causes and improve the symptoms of arthritis.** Additional actions you can take for noticeable benefits are seaweed baths (pg. 461), hot and cold hydrotherapy showers (pg. 463), an arthritis sweat bath (pg. 464), and morning sunbaths for Vitamin D and better calcium use.

In addition to arthritis itself, the diets in this chapter improve the following arthritis associated problems: *Rheumatism, Bursitis, Bone Spurs, Corns and Carbuncles, Chronic Constipation, Gout, Shingles, Lupus, Prostate Inflammation, Post-Menopausal Bone Loss, Gum Diseases.*

187

Do you have signs of arthritis?

—Do you notice marked stiffness and swelling in your fingers, shoulders or neck in damp weather?
—Are you unusually stiff when you get up in the morning, especially when the weather is damp?
—Have you noticed bony bumps on your index fingers? Or bony spurs on other joints? Do your joints crack and pop?
—Are you anemic? Is your skin unusually pale? Have you lost weight lately but weren't on a diet?
—Do you have food sensitivities? Are you more than 20 pounds overweight with extra weight in your knees and hips?
—Do you experience back or joint pain when you move? Does it get worse with prolonged activity?
—Do you have long-standing bronchial congestion? Are you usually constipated? Do you suffer from ulcerative colitis?
—Do you take more than 6 aspirin a day on a regular basis? Are you on a long-term prescription of corticosteroid drugs?

A Three-Day Arthritis Cleansing Diet

Does your body need an arthritis detox for better joints, connective tissue and immune response? An arthritis detox diet helps dissolve and flush out inorganic mineral deposits, replacing them with healing nutrients. For best results, use Vitamin C powder with bioflavonoids, $1/2$ teasp. at a time, in juice or water 4 to 6 times daily, and omega-3 flax oil, 3 teasp. daily in juice or water.

Lack of water is linked to arthritis pain and stiffness. Chondroitin sulfate, a specific nutrient for arthritis, is the molecule in cartilage that attracts and holds water. Healthy joints are 85 to 90% water, but since cartilage doesn't have its own blood supply, chondroitin sulfate aids the chondroitin "molecular sponge" in providing joint nourishment, waste removal and lubrication. Water often helps restore healthy cartilage as it relieves osteoarthritis symptoms. Include eight 8-oz. glasses of water daily in your arthritis healing diet. Limit your alcoholic beverages since they are especially dehydrating.

—**On rising:** take a glass of lemon juice and water; or a glass of fresh grapefruit juice (Acidic citrus fruits help enzymes alkalize the body); or Crystal Star GREEN TEA CLEANSER™.

—**Breakfast:** take a potassium broth or essence (pg. 568); or a glass of carrot/beet/cucumber juice.
—**Mid-morning:** have black cherry juice; or a green drink, like Green Foods GREEN MAGMA or Crystal Star ENERGY GREEN™.
—**Lunch:** have a cup of miso soup with sea greens snipped on top, and a glass of carrot juice with 1 tsp. Bragg's LIQUID AMINOS.
—**Mid-afternoon:** have another green drink, or alfalfa/mint tea, or Crystal Star CLEANSING & PURIFYING™ tea.
—**Dinner:** have a glass of cranberry/apple, or papaya juice, or another glass of black cherry juice.
—**Before Bed:** take a glass of celery juice, or a cup of miso soup with 1 TB of nutritional yeast.

Recipes to help your arthritis sediment cleanse: •DETOXIFICATION and CLEANSING FOODS; •HEALING DRINKS; •SOUPS - LIQUID SALADS.

188

Diet to Change Body Chemistry and Control Arthritis

This alkalizing, anti-inflammatory diet can change your body chemistry and the way your body uses the nutrients you give it. It is particularly useful for gland nourishment where extreme inflammation is evidence that the body is not producing enough natural cortisone from adrenal cortex. It is free of nightshade plants, like potatoes, tomatoes, chilies, peppers, eggplant, etc. that impair calcium absorption. (If you take MOTRIN, remember its origin is a nightshade plant.) It is rich in Vitamin C for connective tissue, full of fiber for regularity, and free of alcohol, caffeine and sugar that aggravate acidity. It is low in fat and meats to reduce pain, and high in whole grains and vegetables for better-formed bone and cartilage.

—**On rising:** take a glass of lemon juice and water, or grapefruit juice; or a glass of apple cider vinegar in water with honey.

—**Breakfast:** Bioflavonoids help connective tissue. Eat and drink cranberries, cherries (10 times stronger anti-inflammatory than aspirin!), papayas and citrus fruits, or Crystal Star BIOFLAV., FIBER and VIT. C SUPPORT™ drink. Mix 1 TB each: sunflower seeds, lecithin granules, Red Star yeast and toasted wheat germ. Add 2 teasp. into yogurt, or sprinkle on fresh fruit or greens, but have some every day.

—**Mid-morning:** take a potassium drink (pg. 568); or for osteoarthritis, have an Arthritis V-8 Special: add to a bottle of Knudsen's VERY VEGGIE JUICE, 4 TBS each: wheat germ, lecithin granules and brewer's yeast flakes. Take 8-oz. twice daily; for rheumatoid arthritis, have a green drink such as Sun Wellness CHLORELLA or Green Foods GREEN MAGMA with 1 teasp. Bragg's LIQUID AMINOS added.

—**Lunch:** have a green leafy salad with lemon/oil dressing; and a hot miso broth or onion soup. There is a link between a sulfur deficiency and arthritis. Eat sulfur-containing veggies like broccoli, onions, cabbage and garlic.

—**Mid-afternoon:** have a cup of miso soup with sea greens on top; or alfalfa/mint tea, or Crystal Star AR-EASE TEA.

—**Dinner:** have a Chinese greens salad with sesame dressing; or a large dinner salad with soy cheese, nuts, tamari dressing, and a cup of black bean soup; or steamed vegetables with nutritional yeast sprinkled on top and brown rice for absorbable B vitamins. Have cold water fish like salmon for high omega-3 oils twice a week.

—**Before bed:** have a cranberry or black cherry juice; or a cup of miso soup with sea greens snipped on top; and/or celery juice.

Pointers for best results from your arthritis control diet:

1: Avoid arthritis trigger foods: corn; wheat; rye breads; bacon and pork; beef; eggs; coffee; oranges; milk; nightshade foods like peppers, eggplant, tomatoes and potatoes; mustard; colas; chocolate.

2: Cut down on: alcohol, fried foods, dairy foods, salty foods.

3: Add balancing foods: green tea, artichokes, cherries, cabbages, brown rice, oats (not for rheumatoid arthritis), shiitake mushrooms, sea foods, sea greens, fresh fruits, vegetables, leafy greens, garlic, onions, olive oil, sweet potatoes. Add ginger and parsley daily.

4: Fiber keeps crystalline wastes flushed. Eat whole grains like brown rice.

5: Make sure to drink 6 to 8 glasses of bottled water daily to keep inorganic wastes releasing quickly from the body.

Recipes to help your arthritis control diet: •BLENDING EAST and WEST FOODS; •BREAKFAST and BRUNCH; •SOUPS - LIQUID SALADS; •ENZYME-RICH; •DAIRY-FREE; •MINERAL-RICH FOODS; •HIGH FIBER RECIPES.

189

Herb and Supplement Choices

• **Repair joints, reduce pain, protect cartilage:** GLU-COSAMINE-CHONDROITIN 4 daily; Shark cartilage has natural chondroitin sulfates. Use with CMO (cetyl-myristoleate), 500mg, like Jarrow TRUE CMO for EFA's. Omega-3 flax or fish oil 3x daily - expect pain diminishment in 2 to 4 months.

• **Effective anti-inflammatories for arthritis:** DLPA 1000mg; Crystal Star AR EASE™ caps; Quercetin 1000mg with Bromelain 1500mg daily; or Nature's Plus INFLAMACTIN; MSM with MICROHYDRIN, available at Healthy House. Herbal anti-inflammatories: nettles extract; cat's claw caps; Earth's Bounty NONI liquid. Green-lipped mussel and sea cucumber caps 2000mg for 2 months.

• **Antioxidants help regenerate cartilage:** SAMe protects cushioning synovial fluid and blocks enzymes that degrade cartilage. CoQ$_{10}$ 60mg 3x daily; Carnitine 1000mg 2x daily; Grapeseed PCO's 300mg daily; Vitamin E 800IU daily; Ester C 500mg with bioflavs for collagen.

• **Chlorophyll sources stimulate cortisone:** Solaray ALFA-JUICE caps; Crystal Star ENERGY GREEN™ drink NutriCology PRO-GREENS; Wakunaga KYO-GREEN; Body Ecology VITAL-ITY SUPERGREEN; Vibrant Health GREEN VIBRANCE.

• **Enzymes help normalize body chemistry:** Transformation PUREZYME (protease) carries protein-bound calcium; Crystal Star BITTERS & LEMON CLEANSE™ extract.

• **Stimulate natural cortisone production:** Alfalfa tabs 10 daily or Solaray ALFA-JUICE caps; Crystal Star ADR-ACTIVE™ caps daily with Evening Primrose Oil 3000mg daily; CHLORELLA 1 teasp. daily; YS royal jelly/ginseng 2 tsp. daily; Enzymatic Therapy ADRENAL CORTEX COMPLEX.

Bodywork and Lifestyle Techniques

• **An arthritis sweat helps right away.** See page 464.

• **To relieve pain:** Press the highest spot of the muscle between thumb and index finger. Press in the webbing between the two fingers, closer toward the bone that attaches to the index finger. Press for 10 seconds at a time into the web muscle, angling the pressure toward the bone of the index finger.

• **Exercise:** Lack of exercise weakens muscles putting more stress on joints. A daily stretching program and yoga are my favorites for keeping skeletal muscles strong.

• **Effective bodywork:** Massage therapy (relieves pain, improves the circulation and hastens elimination of harmful deposits), acupuncture, hot and cold hydrotherapy (page 463), epsom salts baths, chiropractic treatments and overheating therapy .

—Crystal Star ALKALIZING ENZYME™ HERBAL WRAP normalizes body pH almost immediately.

• **Healing applications:**
—Transitions PRO-GEST wild yam cream.
—Wakunaga GLUCOSAMINE SOOTHING CREAM.
—Biochemics PAIN RELIEF lotion.
—Nature's Way CAYENNE PAIN RELIEVING OINTMENT or other capsaicin creme.
—Emu oil (with omega-3, omega-6 EFA's.)
—Herbal Answers HERBAL ALOE FORCE.
—Ayurvedic Boswellin creme
—Crystal Star ANTI-BIO™ gel with una da gato.
—Cayenne/ginger compresses on affected areas.
—DMSO on clean skin as directed.
—B & T TRIFLORA gel.

Can't find a recommended product? Call the 800 number listed in Product Resources for the store nearest you and for more info.

190

Intervening Against Osteoporosis

Few things age a person as quickly as osteoporosis (porous bone), a disease that robs bones of their density and strength, making them thinner, and more prone to break. Eventually, bone mass decreases below the level required to support the body. Over 35 million Americans suffer from osteoporosis today. Long considered a woman's problem, because of its female hormone involvement, osteoporosis affects from 35 to 50% of women in the first 5 years after menopause. Most of these are vibrant women at the height of their careers with no outward signs of poor health. Most have no idea their bones are becoming weaker and more brittle until they actually break. For women, osteoporosis is greater than the combined risks of breast, uterine and ovarian cancers.

Osteoporosis also affects men, just at a later age and with less ferocity. Some bone loss normally occurs in both sexes around 45 years of age. But a greater testosterone supply and more bone tissue offer men some protection from osteoporosis. Yet today's men, in ever-increasing numbers are suffering from the disease. In America, by age 75, one-third of all men are affected.

Are you at risk for osteoporosis? Check the following risk factors:

1) post-menopausal, small-boned white or Asian women, with a family history of osteoporosis.
2) women and men over 75 years; women over 45 with a history of calcium and vitamin D deficiency.
3) women and men who have a consistently high consumption of tobacco, caffeine and animal proteins.
4) women and men who take long courses of cortico-steroid drugs. Research shows that over a long period of time these drugs tend to leach potassium from the system, weakening the bones.
5) women and men with long use of synthetic thyroid. The drug Synthroid increases risk for both osteoporosis and high cholesterol, and may also aggravate weight problems.
6) women who had their ovaries removed before menopause, who are childless, or who had an early menopause (before 45 years old), or those with a history of irregular or no menstrual periods. Hormone and calcium deficiencies appear regularly in women with irregular menstrual cycles, most notably in women who exercise excessively or who have eating disorders. Over 50% of American women suffer from calcium deficiency.

You can check for early warning signs of osteoporosis:

If you think you're at risk, ask your physician or local pharmacy about bone mineral density screening, and review this symptom list.

1: Bone loss is greatest in the spine, hips and ribs, so osteoporosis begins to show up as chronic back and leg pain. Bone pain may also occur in the spine, affecting the cranial nerves.

2: Look for loss of bone in the jaw and tooth sockets. Bone may draw away from the teeth, causing them to loosen, or fall out. Look for unusually frequent dental problems, too.

3: Vision defects or facial tics may also occur due to bone marrow obliteration.

Bone loss is greatest in the high weight-bearing bones - hips, spine and ribs. In America, almost one-third of all women and one-sixth of all men will fracture a hip during their lives. For a person over 65, a simple fall can cause a fatal hip fracture due to recovery complications. Each year, 1.5 million bone fractures occur as a direct result of osteoporosis (costing the economy up $13.8 billion).

Why is the rate of hip fractures in the United States so high?

Our bone-stealing diet and lack of exercise are at the heart of the problem. If you eat a lot of highly processed, additive-laden foods, you're setting the stage for bone loss. Experts list these bad-to-the-bone diet and lifestyle habits:

Is your diet putting you at risk for osteoporosis?

—**If your diet is low in minerals, you're endangering your bones and your digestion.** Minerals are critical for a strong skeleton, and they are the bonding agents between you and your food. Low minerals means low thyroid function and poor collagen protein development, also part of osteoporosis.

—**If your diet is low in fresh foods, your body is low in essential enzymes.** Osteoporosis is at least in part, a result of enzyme deficiency. I find this is especially true for older men who try to correct digestive problems with handfuls of antacids.

—**If your diet is excessively high in protein, your bones are probably low in calcium.** The American Dietetic Association says "when protein consumption is doubled, calcium loss increases 50%!" There is a clear relationship between high protein consumption and osteoporosis. Protein from animal sources is an even bigger danger for osteoporosis. The kidneys pull calcium from the bones trying to rid the body of the excess nitrogen found in animal protein. Studies of vegetarians and non-vegetarians from age 60 to 90, reveal that the mineral content in meat eater's bones decreased 35% over time, while mineral content of a vegetarian's bones decreased only 18%.

—**If your diet is high in red meats, sodas, caffeine foods and alcohol, you probably have over-acid blood which puts you at risk for bone loss.** Your body's pH is critical to healthy bone. It's a fairly new idea, but some experts feel that health (or disease) is directly related to the degree of alkalinity or acidity in body tissues and fluids. Just as the body works to maintain a normal temperature of 98.6, so your metabolism works to maintain normal blood pH at around 7.3 . The blood tries to balance body pH by withdrawing calcium from your bones. About 80% of your diet should be alkaline; about 20% acid-forming foods.

—Alkaline-forming foods: All vegetables, most fruits, sea greens, cultured vegetables, sprouted seeds and beans, seeds (except sesame), almonds, grains like millet, quinoa, amaranth and buckwheat, olive oil, herbs and herb teas.

—Acid-forming foods: Animal foods (meat, fish, poultry, eggs, cheeses, milk, butter),wheat, oats, white rice, breads, acid fruits like pomegranates, cranberries and strawberries, sunflower, safflower and canola oils, the herb stevia (a sugar replacement).

—Acid-forming foods to avoid: Sugar, sweeteners such as saccharin and Nutrasweet, candy, soft drinks, all processed and chemicalized foods, flour products, nuts (except almonds) and nut butters, alcoholic beverages, and commercial vinegar containing foods. USDA research finds that men who consume five cans of cola a day for three months absorb less calcium, increasing risk for bone deterioration and breaks! High levels of phosphorous in meat and highly processed foods also deprive the body of calcium.

—**If your diet is high in milk and dairy products you may be MORE at risk for osteoporosis!** Most of us have been told from childhood to drink milk for strong bones. Advertising tells us that dairy foods are the best source of dietary calcium for bone protection. The ads don't tell you that it's been a hotly debated myth in the natural foods industry for years. The truth about drinking milk for strong bones? A twelve year, Harvard Nurses Health study of over 78,000 women reveals that high intake of milk and dairy products does NOT reduce bone breaks. In fact, proteins in milk can actually CAUSE calcium loss through the urine. Beyond calcium loss, for up to 25% of all Americans, lactose intolerance means little of the calcium and minerals in dairy foods is even digested. Further, most commercial milk today is loaded with saturated fat, hormone-disrupting chemicals and antibiotics, no good for health!

—**Your weight loss diet may be weakening your bones.** A recent study shows that for each 10% drop in weight, there is a two-fold increase in the risk of hip fractures in older women. When blood calcium levels become low from a severe weight loss diet, your bones release their calcium to keep the rest of the body running smoothly. Even taking calcium supplements may not be enough to maintain bone mass during dieting. Women who crash diet regularly show up with estrogen deficiency, also involved in bone loss. Doubly discouraging is the fact that many studies show most women gain all of their weight back after strict dieting. After many years of developing natural weight loss programs, I find dieters get better results when they add minerals via green drinks and vegetable juices. Women who drink high mineral juices don't gain the lost weight back, either as quickly or as much. Since a majority of American women admit to being on a weight control diet most of the time, maintaining a low fat diet, and adding high mineral drinks from food or herb sources to avoid bone loss while dieting is a better choice..

Beyond diet, your lifestyle influences osteoporosis.

—Too little exercise stunts healthy bone development. Too little sunlight means less vitamin D is available for bone building.
—Smoking interferes with your body's calcium and estrogen production. Women smokers have 10% lower bone density and are more vulnerable to fractures than non smokers.
—Depression may cause bone loss. People with a history of severe depression have 15% less bone density in their lower spines than non-depressed people.
—Overusing steroids, antibiotics or tobacco, and too much alcohol severely reduces mineral absorption.
—Ovary removal puts you at greater risk for osteoporosis.
—Drinking fluoridated water is a risk factor! New studies link hip fractures to fluoridated water. Fluoridated water literally leeches calcium from the bones. Research from the *Journal of American Medical Association* reveals hip fracture rates are much higher in people residing in fluoridated communities. New studies are proving that fluoride's cumulative effect on bone is devastating. Evidence of increased hip fracture has been reported in at least nine studies from five countries even at relatively "low" water fluoride levels. The World Health Organization says "individuals consuming between 2.0 - 8.0 mg of fluoride/day (2-8 litres of fluoridated water), can develop the pre-clinical symptoms of skeletal fluorosis," (arthritis-like symptoms). If you drink the health recommended amount of water (6 to 8 glasses per day) you may be at risk. Fluoride comes from other sources than your water. Fruits and vegetables, juices, soft drinks, beverages, and dental products all increase your fluoride intake.

Can you beat osteoporosis without drugs? How do hormones fit into the bone health picture?

Clearly estrogen is involved in bone-building and bone loss. Estrogen has been the mainstay of orthodox medicine therapy for decades. Yet while some tests find estrogen does inhibit bone cell death, other tests find that as many as 15% of women on estrogen therapy continue to lose bone! **Most experts agree that declining estrogen levels after menopause do not by themselves cause osteoporosis.** I believe hormone balance (not merely replacement) is the key. We know progesterone is highly involved in laying down and strengthening bone, and may even help reverse osteoporosis in some women. Thyroid function and collagen development are critical as well for women. Low androgen hormone levels of DHEA and testosterone play a role in men's osteoporosis.

—Ipriflavone, synthesized from isoflavones (plant estrogens), is a new leader in natural osteoporosis treatment. Studies find ipriflavone inhibits bone cell death and may even increase new bone growth. Three different two year studies from Italy show that 200mg of ipriflavone 3 times daily is effective against bone loss.

—**What about progesterone creams derived from wild yam roots?** Can they really stave off osteoporosis? In a recent study on women with osteoporosis, a bone scan showed up to 5% new bone density in an eighteen month period after the women used a natural wild yam progesterone cream, along with a good nutritional program. A four-year study shows that plant-derived progesterone creams increased bone density anywhere up to 40% for women from 45 to 60 years of age. Results were even better when a germanium supplement was added orally. I respect the work of California physician John Lee M.D. who finds some women with severe osteoporosis experience an amazing 30% increase in bone density after using progesterone cream in combination with lifestyle therapy.

A man's testosterone supply protects against osteoporosis. Can extra testosterone help women arrest osteoporosis? Testosterone drugs are not a good option for women. Male characteristics such as voice deepening, facial and chest hair growth surface quickly. Herbal research centers on phyto-testosterone sources like Panax Ginseng, and hormone balancers like saw palmetto and sarsaparilla for bone loss.

What about calcium? It's a cornerstone of medical treatment for osteoporosis. Calcium is the most abundant mineral in the body, and 98 percent of all calcium is stored in our bones. But calcium isn't the only mineral involved in bone. Osteoporosis is the result of much more than a calcium deficiency and **preventing osteoporosis is not just about adding more calcium to your diet.**

—**How do you know if you have a calcium deficiency?** Calcium deficiencies show up pre-menstrually as back pain, cramping, or tooth pain. (A calcium supplement before your period helps these symptoms disappear if this is your problem.) Note: women who think they are helping themselves by taking calcium-containing antacids may be doing just the opposite. Antacids are linked to easy fracture because they block stomach acids, which some specialists say, causes reduced bone growth and poor nutrient absorption.

Boost all your minerals instead! Other minerals, like silica and magnesium are just as important to bone health. Bone strength is best enhanced when calcium is used with other nutrients, such as B vitamins, magnesium, silica, manganese and boron.

In addition to osteoporosis itself, the diets in this chapter improve the following bone-related health problems: *Osteomalacia, Ankylosing Spondylitis, Back, Nerve and Muscle Pain, Skin, Hair and Nails, Menstrual Disorders, Hyperactive Behavior and Attention Deficit Disorder, Low Energy Levels, Indigestion and Bad Breath, Emotional Instability, Hyperthyroidism, Easy Bruising, Tendency to Motion Sickness.*

A Healthy Healing Program for (Almost) Unbreakable Bones

Osteoporosis is far more complex than was thought even just 5 years ago. Bone and cartilage are living tissue, an ever-changing infrastructure. Osteoporosis involves both mineral and non-mineral elements, so your bones need a full range of supportive nutrients. Even though it is a life-threatening disease, osteoporosis is a lifestyle disease.... and that means we can do something about it. Bone loss can be arrested; remaining bone can be preserved; new bone mass can even be rebuilt with a vigorous osteoporosis intervention program. Once you know what contributes to bone weakening, and what contributes to bone building, you have the power to keep your bones strong. I find the most successful treatment involves not only balancing (normalizing) hormone levels, but also improving lifestyle and dietary habits that we know accelerate bone loss. It's not just a case of adding estrogen, progesterone or even testosterone.

Successfully intervention against osteoporosis isn't a pill.... it's a program.

Osteoporosis - Bone Building Diet

You don't have to let osteoporosis steal your health! Nutritional therapy offers a broad base of both treatment and protection. I've seen natural therapies literally transform people crippled by osteoporosis. Start with diet improvements.

1: Eat vitamin C bioflavonoid rich foods regularly: kiwis, oranges, grapefruit and potatoes to enhance collagen production.

2: Add sea greens to your diet. 2 TBS daily, snipped on salad, soup, rice, even pizza. Sea greens offer bone building minerals and vitamins, like D, E and K which boost adrenal production of steroidal hormones like estrogen, progesterone and DHEA – prime supports for bone health. Consider a supplement like Nature's Path TRACE-MIN-LYTE (contains 500mg sea plants and electrolytes).

3: Eat calcium, magnesium and potassium-rich foods: broccoli, seafoods, eggs, yogurt, kefir, carrots, dried fruits, sprouts, miso, green and black beans, leafy greens, tofu, bananas, apricots and molasses. Mineral-rich veggies and herbs like oatstraw, burdock, dandelion and borage seed come without heavy protein, and they offer high levels of vitamin K, which helps calcium attach to bone tissue. Avoid sugar, salty snack foods, caffeine, tobacco, and nightshade plants that interfere with calcium absorption.

4: Consider more deep green veggies for bones of steel. They provide all essential minerals for rebuilding bone. Use green superfoods too, if you're already at risk for osteoporosis. Green foods have a pH close to 7 which buffers uric acid and lactic acids, and helps the body change from catabolic (breaking down) to anabolic (building up) bone mass. Try Crystal Star ENERGY GREEN™ drink; Nutricology PRO GREENS with EFA's; Ethical Nutrients FUNCTIONAL GREENS; Green Kamut GREEN KAMUT or JUST BARLEY.

5: Reduce protein from red meat and dairy foods. They disrupt pH balance and lead to mineral loss. Get protein from fish, legumes, and sea greens instead. Drink juices like carrot and orange instead for extra calcium. One 8-oz. glass of fresh carrot juice has 400mg bioavailable calcium. (An 8-oz. glass of fortified milk has only 250mg with low assimilation.)

Recipes to help your osteoporosis diet: • FISH and SEAFOODS; • ENZYME-RICH RECIPES; • HIGH FIBER • HIGH PROTEIN without MEAT; • DAIRY FREE COOKING; • MINERAL- RICH RECIPES; •CULTURED HEALING FOODS

Herb and Supplement Choices

• **Balance your hormones** (don't just add estrogen): Ipriflavone 600mg daily, or Metabolic Response Modifiers OSTEO-MAX 200mg ipriflavone with 200mg MCHC; Crystal Star OSTEO DE-FENSE, 4 daily, with extra EFA's; Crystal Star PRO-EST OSTEO™ roll-on, or Transitions EMERITA PRO-GEST. Crystal Star MALE PERFORMANCE™ caps, 4 daily, for men.

• **Boost your minerals** (not just calcium): Calcium citrate 1500mg / magnesium 1000mg / boron 3mg (too much boron alone actually causes bone loss); Eidon SILICA for 6 mos., or Ethical Nutrients BONE BUILDER with silica. Crystal Star CALCIUM SOURCE™ and SILICA SOURCE™ extract (for collagen-calcium). Nature's Path TRACE-MIN-LYTE (500mg sea plants and electrolytes); • Nutricology BONE CALCIUM COMPLEX; Enzymatic Therapy OSTEOPRIME; Nature's Path CAL-LYTE.

• **Boost mineral absorption:** Vitamin D 1000IU; marine carotene 100,000IU, or PHYCOTENE MICROCLUSTERS available at Healthy House; zinc 30mg; vitamin K 100mcg; Alacer EMERGEN-C or Nature's Path TRACE-LYTE for electrolytes and pH balance; MICROHYDRIN available at Healthy House for alkaline pH & better calcium absorbtion.

• **Boost bone health with EFA's:** Crystal Star EVENING PRIM-ROSE oil w. E, 6 daily; Spectrum Naturals 1300mg EPO; Barlean's OMEGA TWIN flax-borage; Nature's Secret ULTIMATE OIL.

• **Add enzymes to boost nutrient absorption:** for men -Herbal Products Dvlpt. POWER PLUS ENZYMES or Nature's Secret REZYME; for women- Transformation DIGESTZYME.

• **Bioflavonoids boost collagen/ connective tissue:** Vitamin C or Ester C with bioflavs. up to 5000mg daily; or •HAWTHORN, •BILBERRY, or •GINKGO BILOBA extracts.

Bodywork and Lifestyle Techniques

• **Smoking leaches bone nutrients:** Smoking a pack a day results in a 10% loss in bone density. Smoking also appears to interfere with estrogen production.

• **Get early morning sunlight** on the body every day possible for vitamin D.

• **Avoid:** fluorescent lighting, electric blankets, aluminum cookware, non-filtered computer screens, etc. All tend to leach calcium from the body.

• **Exercise is as important as a good diet for bones:** Exercise is a nutrient in itself. Duration of exercise is more important than intensity. Note: if you already have low bone density, start on a weight bearing exercise program after improvements from diet changes are seen in your bone scans in order to avoid injury. The best exercises are often water workouts. The water limits overdoing it, and is very forgiving to fragile bones.

Numerous studies make it clear that physical exercise (at least one hour of moderate exercise 3 times a week) can prevent bone loss and actually increase bone mass. A lack of exercise doubles the rate of urinary and fecal calcium excretion, resulting in a significant negative calcium balance.

• **Pump a little iron for your bones:** People who do regular weight bearing exercises have denser bones than those who don't. Your bones can rebuild themselves, but only when they're used. A sedentary lifestyle increases osteoporosis risk. Power walking is good for bones, so are aerobic workouts, like Tae Bo, or weight bearing exercise 3-4 times a week (especially for men and women under 35 whose bone mass is still growing).

Can't find a recommended product? Call the 800 number listed in Product Resources for the store nearest you and for more info.

196

Building Strong Bones

Bone is living tissue that interweaves a mineral, inorganic matrix, and a non-mineral, organic matrix framework. A solid mineral base is of prime importance to bone health. Healthy bones are critical to your body's mineral needs because they act as your body's mineral reservoirs when it doesn't get enough minerals from your food.

Minerals and trace minerals are the building blocks of your cells, the basic elements your body needs for proper metabolism. Minerals are the bonding agents between the body and food. Without them, the body cannot absorb or utilize nutrients. Minerals regulate pH balance, transport body oxygen, and control electrolytic movement between cells, nerves and tissue. They play a key role in heart health, sugar and blood pressure regulation, and cancer prevention. Even small mineral deficiencies imbalance your body by mobilizing needed elements out of the various body 'reservoirs' to compensate. Immediate effects of this process are irritability, nervousness, or depression. A mineral-poor diet can mean osteoporosis, premature aging, hair loss, brittle nails, dry, cracked skin, forgetfulness, food allergies, back pain, P.M.S., poor motor coordination, joint deformity, difficult pregnancy, taste and smell loss, slow learning, poor attention span, and the inability to heal quickly. This is only a partial list.

MINERALS ARE IMPORTANT!

Our bodies don't make minerals. They must be taken in through food, drink or mineral baths. Unfortunately, today's fruits and vegetables lack good mineral quality. Years of pesticides, non-organic fertilizers, and chemical sprays have leached them out of the soil. High stress lifestyles and habits inhibit mineral absorption. Eating too much meat protein and too many preserved and over-refined foods, a lack of vitamin D from sunlight, and too little exercise, are involved in our lack of minerals. Excessive steroid and antibiotic use, tobacco, and too much alcohol, all contribute to mineral depletion and weakening of bone structure. Mineral needs increase as the body ages, and requires more digestive and enzyme help. Calcium is not even the main mineral for bone regeneration; silicon is. Over a third of our population, and more than 50% of American women, suffer from calcium deficiency alone.

You need a constant supply of mineral-rich foods and nutrients to replenish the organic matrix of bone. Organically grown foods, sea plants and herbs are becoming the best way to get them. Foods and herbs are used by the body's own enzyme action, as a whole, (not a partial substance), and this is a key to their effectiveness. Vegetarians traditionally have denser, better-formed bones, because the most usable minerals come from leafy greens, sprouts, whole grains, soy foods, eggs, and vegetable complex carbohydrates.

Do you have weak bones?

To find out more about the state of your bones, ask your physician or local pharmacy about bone mineral density screening, and ask yourself the following questions.

1: Do your bones break easily? And heal slowly?
2: Do you have lots of dental plaque? Do you have gum disease? Do your teeth shift? Are they loose?
3: Do you have prematurely gray hair (before 40)? Or unusually thin skin?
4: Do your nails break easily and often?
5: Are your muscles weak? Are your joints and tendons chronically sore? Do you have chronic lower back pain?

Critical nutrients for strong bones:

—**Calcium** is the most abundant mineral in the body. Green leafy vegetables, sea greens and seafoods are rich sources of calcium.

—**Silica** strengthens the bone's connective tissue matrix by crosslinking collagen strands. Silica is found in mother's milk, leafy greens, brown rice, and bell peppers. Good herbal sources: horsetail, boneset, oatstraw, dandelion, alfalfa and sea vegetables.

—**Magnesium** is involved in many biochemical reactions in bone. Chlorophyll-rich plants and superfoods are rich in magnesium.

—**Vitamins:** B-6, B-12, folic acid and K help convert inactive osteocalcin, the major noncollagen protein in bone to its active form. Green leafy vegetables are excellent sources of vitamin K. Vitamin D (especially from exzposure to sunlight) stimulates the absorption of calcium.

—**Enzymes** transport nutrients and remove waste products; enzymes increase absorption of calcium and other bone nutrients.

Strong Bones Diet

Get serious early about taking care of your bones. Deposit enough structure building nutrients in your bone banks so you don't end up with low bone strength. Teenagers build the majority of their skeleton bones during adolescence. Most women stop building bone mass between 21 and 35 years of age. Bone mass for everyone can decrease by about 1% a year. At menopause, and for men at andropause, bone loss can rise to a high 8% for years. The high mineral diet below is designed to correct deficiency problems.

—**On rising:** take a high "green protein" drink, such as Green Kamut Corp. GREEN KAMUT or JUST BARLEY in apple or orange juice.

—**Breakfast:** mix 2 TBS each: toasted wheat germ, sesame seeds, Red Star yeast and lecithin granules. Sprinkle 2 teasp. on your breakfast foods - yogurt with fresh or dried fruits, poached or baked eggs on whole grain toast, or whole grain cereal or pancakes with apple juice, soy milk, honey or yogurt.

—**Mid-morning:** a potassium drink (page 568), Crystal Star SYSTEMS STRENGTH™ drink; or a green drink (page 569); or fresh carrot juice and miso soup with sea greens snipped on top; and some crunchy veggie sticks with kefir cheese dip.

—**Lunch:** have a veggie omelet and a carrot/raisin salad or a three bean salad; or a green salad with spinach, green peppers, sprouts and lemon-oil dressing; or a veggie sandwich with avocado, soy cheese on whole grain bread.

—**Mid-afternoon:** have a hard boiled egg with a yogurt dip and an herb tea like rose hips, nettles, dandelion, or a green drink like Nutricology PRO GREENS; or have some low-fat cheeses with whole grain crackers, and a small bottle of mineral water.

—**Dinner:** have a mushroom, asparagus, or broccoli quiche; or a salmon souffle, or baked salmon with brown rice and peas; or a light Italian veggie pasta meal with tomatoes and onions; or an oriental stir-fry with veggies and brown rice, and miso soup. Have a glass of wine for extra boron BEFORE dinner - liquids with meals inhibit mineral absorption.

—**Before bed:** have a glass of apple, pear or papaya juice, or a cup of Red Star yeast broth.

Recipes to help your bone building diet: •SEAFOODS; •ENZYME-RICH RECIPES; •BREAKFAST FOODS •HIGH PROTEIN without MEAT; •DAIRY-FREE COOKING; •MINERAL RICH RECIPES; •CULTURED HEALING FOODS

Herb and Supplement Choices

•**Add more bone nutrients to build bones:** Herbs are one of the best ways to get bone-builders. Add silica: Crystal Star SILICA SOURCE™, Eidon SILICA; Body Essentials SILICA GEL for collagen formation. Add balanced calcium: Crystal Star CALCIUM SOURCE™ caps or extract; Ethical Nutrients BONE BUILDER; Calcium ascorbate C 3000mg.

•**Improve assimilation of bone nutrients:** Magnesium, 400mg daily; Vitamin D 400IU daily; B-complex 100mg daily with extra B-6 100mg and folic acid, 400mcg. Manganese, 5mg; Jarrow MINERALBALANCE; Transformation DIGESTZYME; MICROHYDRIN, available at Healthy House, facilitates the absorption and the transport of bone nutrients. Magnesium and vitamin D dramatically increase calcium absorption. Nature's Path TRACE-LYTE also helps increase calcium absorption.

•**Keep your glands healthy for good bones:** Effective estrogen-progesterone balancing herbs: Crystal Star PRO-EST BALANCE roll-on; Moon Maid PRO-MENO WILD YAM CREAM or •royal jelly-ginseng capsules; DHEA 25mg daily; Transitions PROGEST CREAM; •Enzymatic Therapy OSTEO PRIME.

•**Help your body remodel your bones:** Jarrow BONE UP caps; Vitamin A & D 25,000IU/1000IU daily; Nature's Path TRACE-MIN-LYTE; Vitamin E 400IU; CoQ₁₀ 60mg 2x daily; Bilberry extract (herbal bioflavonoids); Lane Labs ADVACAL.

•**Effective bone knitters and healers:** Country Life sublingual B-12, 2500mcg every 3 days; Nettles caps or Horsetail extract; Glucosamine-Chondroitin capsules 1000mg daily; or shark cartilage 1400mg daily.

•**For suspected bone cancer:** *yarrow* tea, or Natural Energy Plus CAISSE'S TEA.

Bodywork and Lifestyle Techniques

The British LANCET states:

•<u>**Some medicines put bone health at risk if you take them for a long period of time:**</u> L-thyroxine, a thyroid stimulant; cortico-steroid drugs like hydrocortisone, cortisone and prednisone; phenytoin and phenobarbital (anti-seizure drugs); heparin, a blood thinner; furosemide, a diuretic; and No-DOZ, a stimulant.

•<u>**Some drugs can hamper your body's ability to maintain and repair bone:**</u> Ibuprofen, NSAIDS drugs like Naproxen, Fenclofenac, Indomethacin, Sulindac, Keto-profen, Diclofenac, Aspirin, Piroxicam, Flurbiprofen, Asopro-pazone.

•**Exercise and Bodywork:**
—Aerobic exercise and light weight training are primary bones builders and strengtheners.

—Get some sunlight on the body every day possible for natural vitamin D.

—Don't smoke. It increases bone brittleness and inhibits bone growth.

—Swim or walk in the ocean when possible.

—Avoid aluminum pots and pans, deodorants and fluorescent lighting. Both leach calcium from the body.

•**Helpful bone healers:** Homeopathic Arnica Montana; apply Arnica gel for swelling; or apply a Comfrey poultice.

•<u>**Want to know your mineral status?**</u> Eidon's MINERAL BALANCING PROGRAM analyzes your mineral levels through hair analysis tests, and designs you a personalized mineral supplement program to get your body back in balance. Call 800-700-1169 to learn more.

Can't find a recommended product? Call the 800 number listed in Product Resources for the store nearest you and for more info.

Controlling Cancer - Restoring Health

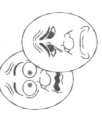

What do we know about cancer development today?

Cancer is the second most common cause of death today, led only by heart disease. 200 different diseases currently fall under the cancer label. Today, one in four deaths in the U.S. is from cancer. Cancer used to be extremely rare... the seventh cause of death at the turn of the last century in America. Right now, eleven million Americans are living with cancer. Over 1 million more will be diagnosed with cancer this year. In 1999, over 550,000 people died from cancer. Sadly, the latest statistics show conventional therapies fail 50% of the time. The numbers are even higher in cases of lung and advanced breast cancer, and cancers of the pancreas, liver, bone, ovary and colon.

In 1971, when the highly publicized National War on cancer was declared, the chances of falling victim to cancer were one in six. By 1983 those chances doubled to one in three. Today, 30 years after the National Cancer Act, the incidence of cancer is rising almost exponentially. Cancer treatment costs the economy $107 billion every year, making it the most expensive disease in the U.S. by far.

Obviously, cancer used to be an uncommon disease. The dramatic, late 20th century increase is only minimally due to new diagnostic tests, or to calling old diseases, like consumption, cancers. The devastating disease we know as cancer today appears to have emerged gradually and then started rising at extraordinary rates as industrial societies became more and more dependent on technology instead of nature. Is our lifestyle really that bad?

Is the cure worse than the disease? More than $30 billion has been invested in cancer research since America's "National War on Cancer," yet chemotherapy drugs, radiation and surgery are still the only "approved" cancer therapies, and they are treatments that can come at great cost. Cancer experts at Duke University estimate that 40% of cancer patients actually die from malnutrition, largely as a result of the severe nausea, vomiting, lack of appetite and poor nutrient intake that follows chemotherapy treatment. Analysis of 100 clinical studies published in the Surgical Forum showed no benefits, but did show significant damage when chemotherapy was the sole treatment for breast cancer patients! Chemo drugs don't distinguish between healthy cells and cancer cells, so many healthy cells are damaged during chemo treatments. Immunity is greatly compromised, leaving many patients wide open to the supergerm infections running rampant in today's hospitals. In fact, one of my research assistants lost a friend suffering from leukemia not to his cancer, but to a virulent lung fungus he caught in the hospital while in chemotherapy treatment. Chemo treated patients often look more like holocaust victims than people who have found a cure for their cancer. Still, chemotherapy is the treatment of choice for an astounding 75% of all cancer patients.

Radiation treatment, given to about 60% of cancer patients, has debilitating side effects, too. Painful swallowing, great fatigue and skin reactions are acute. Long-lasting ulcers, painful sores, reproductive malfunction and chronic diarrhea are frequently reported. Many patients actually develop other cancers because the risk for leukemia and internal scarring is so greatly increased.

Where do we go from here?

American science now has several decades of state-of-the-art research into cancer. There are a few bright spots, but still very few answers. Testicular cancer, Hodgkin's disease and childhood leukemia are now treatable, followed by radiation, instead of a radical mastectomy. Colon cancer techniques, a disease that almost always required a colostomy in times past, now allow most patients to keep significant amounts of colon structure. Overall, cancer survival rates have risen from 38% in 1971 to 50% today. Still, for ovarian cancer and cancers of the liver and pancreas, deaths can be as high as 1 in 20. Even the medical community recognizes the downsides and limitations of traditional chemotherapy and radiation treatments.

Today, new drugs and technologies in conventional cancer treatment are aimed at killing cancer, but not patients. For example, a new class of drugs, angiogenesis inhibitors, in early testing stages, starve the blood vessels that feed oxygen and nutrients to cancerous tumors. In animal tests, some of the angiogenesis inhibitors do arrest tumor growth. In some cases, tumors actually shrivel up and disappear. Human testing of two angiogenesis inhibitors, angiostatin and endostatin, is now underway.

Cancer vaccines are being designed to stop cancer recurrence for non-Hodgkin's lymphoma. The vaccines work by fusing tumor cells to antibody-producing cells, while boosting the immune system's ability to fight cancer growth. But we won't know if the vaccine works or not for another 6 to 8 years, too late for the 25,000 non-Hodgkin's lymphoma patients who die each year.

Other new drugs target cancer genes to stop tumor growth. Herceptin, a new breast cancer drug, pinpoints the gene HER2, which appears to fuel aggressive tumor growth. Unlike chemo drugs and radiation, Herceptin attacks only the tumor while leaving healthy cells intact. Studies show it can extend lifespan for women with the gene who have advanced breast cancer. But Herceptin is useless for the 70% of cases that don't involve this gene, and it may weaken the heart muscle, leading to congestive heart failure.

Some medical professionals are experimenting with "cryotherapy" to freeze tumors of the breast and prostate, and then surgically remove them, a process which experts say is less harmful to the body and more effective than other therapies.

Molecular biologists have spent the past 25 years trying to pry the lid off the "black-box" of the cancer cell. Molecular research convinces most scientists that cancer is a genetic disease in which mutations damage the genes that control cell division. Scientists are re-designing cells to contain cancer-killing properties that nature doesn't provide, such as an immune cell with a gene for TNF (tumor necrosis factor). Naturopaths know that harmful genetic mutations can also result from a diet with excess fat, because fat is involved in gland and hormone activity, or from environmental influences, like exposure to radiation or carcinogenic chemicals.

I believe that while being respectful of all ways of healing, we should also be quite careful about the long range consequences of genetic engineering. The drug world is already crowded with drugs that increase the risk of cancer, drugs that work at far less elemental body levels than our genes. Heroic medicine like this tends to hit the body over the head with a chemical hammer, does not address the cause of the problem, and in my opinion, can never fathom or take into account all of the complexities and ramifications of "playing God" through genetic construction. The "Jurassic Park syndrome" may only be the first terrifying forerunner of science trying hopelessly to control and predict Nature, which is fundamentally illogical, uncontrollable and unpredictable.

Do we know more today about what causes cancer to develop?

— **DIET:** The foods you're eating (or not eating) could be skyrocketing your cancer risk. 40 to 60% of cancer risk is determined by your diet choices! Studies show a lack of fruits, veggies and fiber is the biggest link to cancer. A high fat diet is another offender. Trans fatty acids from fried fast foods and commercial snack foods are especially dangerous; European studies show breast cancer risk is 40% higher in women who have high body levels of trans fatty acids! New studies reveal a diet high in protein (especially from animal sources, like the popular "Zone" and "Zone" clone diets) may increase cancer risk. Alcohol abuse, too much sugar and red meat (barbecue-charred meat is the most carcinogenic) can also be traced back to cancer development.

— **LIFESTYLE:** If you live on your couch, you're boosting your cancer risk. While one out of three Americans falls victim to cancer, only one out of seven <u>active</u> Americans does. Exercise acts as an antioxidant to enhance body oxygen use, alters body chemistry to control fat retention, and accelerates passage of cancer-causing waste out of the body.

We all know tobacco smoke is a carcinogen. The American Cancer Society directly attributes 173,000 cancer deaths in 1999 to tobacco use. Don't smoke! Protect yourself from second hand smoke by asking smokers to smoke away from you!

— **ENVIRONMENT:** Up to 90% of cancer risk is determined by environmental factors like overexposure to the sun's UV rays, air pollution, radiation, and chemicals like estrogen-containing pesticides. Clinical studies show that environmental toxins can damage cell DNA, which leads to cell mutation and tumor development. The chemical link to cancer is becoming undeniable. After World War II, America's use of synthetic chemicals exploded. Billions of tons of new chemicals were dumped into our water and onto our land. Only a meager 3% were ever tested for safety. Cancer rates begin rising at astronomical rates!

U.S. industries alone generate 88 billion pounds of toxic waste per year. The EPA estimates 90% is improperly disposed of. Environmental toxins can damage cell DNA, which leads to cell mutation and tumor development. Moreover, many chemicals have hormone mimicking effects – a primary reason they're implicated in hormone-driven breast and prostate cancers.

Women, in particular, have been hit hard. Human breast milk contains more dioxin, PCBs, DDT and other pesticides than any other food on the planet! A study in the International Journal of Epidemiology shows breast cancer mortality rates increase the closer women live to toxic waste dumps. Until about 20 years ago, both breast cancer rates and contamination levels of PCB pesticides in Israel were among the highest in the world. An aggressive phase-out of these pesticides has led to a sharp reduction in contamination levels, followed by a dramatic drop in breast cancer death rates for Israeli women. Here in the U.S., breast cancer rates have more than doubled since 1950. Today, one in eight American women will develop breast cancer in their lifetime.

Women aren't the only ones in danger. Men are getting a wake-up call of their own. Testicular cancer is on the rise in young men. The rate of prostate cancer has doubled since the WWII chemical era.

The chemical link to cancer has been vastly <u>understated</u> in medical literature. Hydrogen peroxide used in teeth whitening toothpastes and dental bleaches may accelerate mouth cancer. Research from University at Buffalo Dental Medicine shows hydrogen peroxide may cause precancerous cells to turn into full-blown cancer, promoting lesions already present to grow even larger!

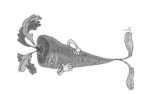

— **EMFs (electromagnetic fields):** Do electric fields cause cancer? It's still hotly debated, but today even the National Institute of Environment Health Sciences (NIEHS) says exposure to strong electromagnetic fields from power lines and electric appliances may be a cause of cancer. Most notable are studies which show high rates of leukemia in children living near high voltage power lines and increases in lymphoma among electric-utility workers exposed to EMFs on the job. Exposure to EMFs causes enzyme, and cell behavior changes. EMF's suppress the hormone melatonin, a cancer protector. To learn more about EMFs and cancer, visit the web site: www.niehs.nih.gov/emfrapid.

All electricity generates an electric field, but you can reduce exposure: 1: Call your electric company. Get a reading on EMFs in your home and recommendations to reduce emissions. 2: Avoid electric blankets; keep electric devices at least 5 feet from your bed. 3: Reduce TV and computer use. Make sure your computer has built-in protectors in the screen to lower emissions from the monitor.

Do you know the early detection signs of cancer? Bring on your risk reducers early if you see tell-tale signs.

1: **a change in bowel or bladder habits, especially blood in the stool.**
2: **chronic indigestion, bloating and heartburn, especially difficulty swallowing.**
3: **unusual bleeding or discharge from the vagina.**
4: **lumps or thickening of the breasts or testicles.**
5: **a chronic cough or constant voice hoarseness; bloody sputum.**
6: **changes in warts or moles, or scaly skin patches that never go away, especially if they become inflamed or ulcerate.**
7: **unexplained weight loss.**

Can you cut your risk? Most cancer is preventable.

It seems like we're assaulted from all sides by cancer activators that we can't control. It's easy to get the idea that anything and everything can cause cancer. Yet, ninety percent of all cancers relate to diet, lifestyle habits and chemicals (20,000 of the 70,000 chemicals people come in contact with regularly are toxic). Hereditary factors account for 5% of cancer cases, but even these are largely influenced by diet and environment. Lifestyle causes mean that we can positively affect most cancer sources ourselves - both to prevent cancer from occurring and helping ourselves when it has.

Diet is the first place to look no matter what kind of cancer you have. Improving your diet directly improves your defenses against cancer. The latest estimates list nutritional factors as accounting for 60% of women's cancers and 40% of men's. Extrapolating from that number means that good food choices could have helped prevent 395,000 to 750,000 new cancer cases, and between 180,000 to 350,000 cancer deaths in 1996 in the United States alone. Breast, uterine, kidney and colon cancers are closely related to the kind of protein and fat we eat, especially protein and fat from meats, and saturated fats from junky fried foods.

Fortunately, we know that certain foods also act as anti-carcinogens ...preventing and altering cancer occurrence and growth. In general, anti-carcinogenic foods can inhibit tumor development and growth, inhibit or prevent metastasis of cancerous growths, and help normalize cancer cells. Our bodies are built from, fueled by, and repaired by our food. Nutritional therapy for cancer relies on re-establishing metabolic balance.

Seven Ways to Cut Your Cancer Risk. Seven watchwords I recommend for cancer prevention:

—Improve your diet first.

1: Reduce your intake of fat. Environmental toxins become lodged in the fatty tissue of the animals in our food chain, and in tissue of humans who eat them. One of the best ways to protect yourself from chemical overload is to buy organic produce and meats whenever possible and incorporate a detoxification program in your life at least twice a year.

2: Reduce your intake of red meats. Cancer is closely related to the protein and fat, in red meats, fast foods and fried foods, and sometimes the added hormones injected into red meats.

3: Eat fruits and vegetables every day. People who eat plenty of fruits and vegetables have half the risk of people who eat few fruits and vegetables. Even small to moderate amounts of fruits and vegetables make a big difference. Two fruits and three vegetable servings a day show amazing anti-cancer results. Eating fruit twice a day, instead of twice a week, can cut the risk of lung cancer by 75%, even in smokers. Berries, citrus fruits and cruciferous veggies are among the most potent cancer fighters.

4: Use enzyme therapy. High enzymes are essential to cancer protection and in fighting cancer. Have a fresh green salad every day and use a supplemental proteolytic enzyme (like Transformation PUREZYME, protease) to stimulate immune response.

5: Use free radical-neutralizing antioxidants. Free radical damage to cellular DNA and RNA causes the loss of normal cell regulatory control, allowing cells to deviate and begin to multiply at a much faster rate contributing to cancer.

6: Detoxify and cleanse your body at least twice a year to defend against chemical overload. Superfoods like barley grass and chlorella, and vegetable juices accelerate natural body detox activity and prevent the genetic ruin of cells, a prelude to cancer. (See the special DETOX DIETS on pages 142-173 for details.)

7: Keep your immune system strong. Each of our 60 trillion body cells undergoes from 1,000 to 10,000 potential cancer-causing DNA breaks every day. Yet, our DNA repair mechanisms and immune defenses are able to keep genetic damage under control 99% of the time. Minerals set the baseline for your immune system. They're the foundation your body works with to build everything else. In addition, minerals increase body enzyme production and help establish normal pH levels, vital for immune maintenance and disease prevention. Electrolyte minerals are superior to colloidal products for maximum absorption. Try Nature's Path TRACE-LYTE.

Can diet and alternative therapies really help?

Cancer treatment is a place where conventional treatments and alternative therapies can come together for the good of the patient. More and more physicians and patients are embracing the complementary approach — using both today's technologies and natural healing therapies like biofeedback, imagery, acupuncture and nutrition in the battle against cancer. The use of supplements and herbs to beat cancer is exploding. Studies in the New York Academy of Sciences reveal 50% of cancer patients are using some type of unconventional cancer therapy!

(*See my book* **HEALTHY HEALING** *11th Edition for the latest information.*)

A diet to control cancer can also help the following conditions: *Systemic Cancers (Colon, Bowel, Stomach, Organ and Lung); Melanoma; Malignant Tumors; Leukemia; Pernicious Anemia; Multiple Sclerosis; Muscular Dystrophy; Cerebral Palsy.*

Your diet is the place to start

Your diet is your major weapon against cancer. Whole food nutrition allows the body to use its built-in restorative and repair abilities. A healthy diet can intervene in the cancer process at many stages, from its conception to its growth and spread. Even if your genetics and lifestyle are against you, your diet may still make a tremendous difference in your cancer odds. For example, certain body chemicals must be "activated" before they can initiate cancer. Food can block the activation process. Antioxidant foods can snuff out carcinogens, nip free radical cascades in the bud, and even repair some cellular damage.

Certain foods accelerate body detoxification, and prevent the genetic ruin of cells, a prelude to cancer (one of the reasons I emphasize a detoxification diet as part of cancer control). Healthy food chemicals in cells can determine whether a cancer-causing virus, or a cancer promoter like too much estrogen will turn tissue cancerous. Even after cells have massed into structures that may grow into tumors, food compounds can intervene to stop more growth. Some actually shrink the patches of precancerous cells.

Although far less powerful at later stages, diet can still influence the metastasis or spread of cancer. Wandering cancer cells need the right conditions in which to attach and grow. Food agents can foster a hostile or a favorable environment. So even after cancer is diagnosed, the right foods may help prolong your life. Massive new research is validating what naturopaths have known for decades. The more fruits and vegetables you eat, the less your cancer risk, from colon and stomach cancer, to breast and even lung cancer. People who eat plenty of fruits and vegetables have half the risk of people who eat few fruits and vegetables.

Most studies show that even small to moderate amounts of fruits and vegetables make a big difference. Two fruits and three vegetable servings a day have shown amazing anti-cancer results. Eating fruit twice a day, instead of twice a week, can cut the risk of lung cancer by 75% even in smokers. One National Cancer Institute spokesman said it is almost mind-boggling, that ordinary fruits and vegetables could be so effective against such a potent carcinogen as cigarette smoke. The evidence is so overwhelming that some researchers are beginning to view fruits and vegetables as powerful preventive drugs that could substantially wipe out the scourge of cancer. What an about-face this has been for cancer study!

The foods that provide prime cancer-fighting nutrition:

1) Fruits and vegetables rich in vitamin C, like citrus fruits, tomatoes, peppers and broccoli, offer anti-oxidant protection.

2) Active cultures in yogurt help neutralize carcinogens and de-activate enzymes that allow body substances to turn into cancer.

3) Antioxidant foods, such as wheat germ, soy products, yellow, orange and green vegetables, green tea, citrus fruits, and olive oil help normalize pre-cancerous cells, and neutralize cancer-causing free radicals.

4) Fiber-rich foods like whole grains, fruits and vegetables absorb excess bile and improve healthy intestinal bacteria.

5) Phyto-chemical foods, especially those in cruciferous vegetables, break down carcinogens and remove them from the body. These same vegetable compounds also break down excess estrogens that are responsible for some types of breast cancer.

6) Folic acid foods like whole wheat and wheat germ, leafy vegetables, beets, asparagus, fish, sunflower seeds, and citrus fruits are potent cancer fighters. Folic acid is critical to normal DNA synthesis so healthy cells do not mutate and turn cancerous.

Should you go on a macrobiotic diet for cancer control?

A macrobiotic diet is effective against cancer, helping to rebuild healthy blood and cells, and preventing diseased tissue from continued growth. This way of eating is non-mucous forming, low in fats that can alter body chemistry and enhance cancer potential in the cells, and it's high in vegetable fiber and protein. Asian foods like miso, bancha green tea, and shiitake mushrooms stimulate heart and circulatory systems. It is high in potassium, natural iodine and other minerals. Its greatest benefit is that it is cleansing and strengthening at the same time, and offers a balanced way of eating that is easily individualized for one's environment, the seasons, and the constitution of the person using it. The form recommended here for an intensive healing program should be followed for three to six months.

—**Before each meal, and before bed:** take 2 to 4 TBS aloe juice concentrate in water (detoxifies and eases nausea if you are undergoing chemotherapy or radiation).

—**On rising:** take a potassium drink (page 568); or carrot-beet-cucumber juice to clean liver and kidneys; or cranberry concentrate (2 tsp. in water) or red grape juice; or a ginseng restorative tea like Crystal Star GINSENG SIX™ tea; or Crystal Star SYSTEMS STRENGTH™ drink; or a vegetable superfood drink like Green Foods CARROT ESSENCE.

—**Breakfast:** make Pulsating Parsley Juice for vitamin A and carotenes: juice 6 carrots, 1 beet with top, a large handful of spinach leaves and $\frac{1}{4}$ cup fresh parsley; then, make a mix of: Red Star nutritional yeast, wheat germ, lecithin granules, CC Pollen HIGH DESERT BEE POLLEN granules. Sprinkle some daily on granola, or mix with yogurt and fruit, or on fresh fruit like strawberries or apples with kefir or kefir cheese; or have a breakfast pilaf like brown rice or Kashi, with apple juice or kefir cheese topping.

—**Mid-morning:** take a cup of Crystal Star CLEANSING & PURIFYING™ TEA; or a veggie drink (pg. 569); or Monas CHLORELLA, Green Foods GREEN MAGMA, Crystal Star ENERGY GREEN™ or fresh wheat grass juice. Or take an herb tea, like pau d'arco, Natural Energy Plus CAISSE'S TEA, Essiac tea, or Crystal Star CAN-SSIAC™ drops in water as a tea; or a glass of fresh carrot juice; or a cup of miso soup with fresh ginger and sea greens snipped on top. (Have 2 TBS dry sea greens daily.)

—**Lunch:** have Super V-7 veggie juice: juice 2 carrots, 2 tomatoes, a handful each spinach and parsley, 2 celery ribs, $\frac{1}{2}$ cucumber, $\frac{1}{2}$ green bell pepper. Add 1 TB green superfood: Crystal Star ENERGY GREEN™; NutriCology PRO-GREENS drinks with EFA's; Ethical Nutrients FUNCTIONAL GREENS; Vibrant Health VITALITY SUPERGREEN. Have steamed broccoli with brown rice, or an oriental stir fry with brown rice and miso sauce; or a green salad; or a black bean, onion or lentil soup, or a 3 bean salad.

—**Mid-afternoon:** a cup of green tea, or Crystal Star GREEN TEA CLEANSER™, and some whole grain crackers with kefir cheese.

—**Dinner:** have brown rice and steamed vegetables with shiitake mushrooms. Snip on dry sea greens, 1 TB flax or olive oil, and 1 TB Red Star nutritional yeast; or have a whole grain casserole with tofu, or tempeh and some steamed vegetables, or a dinner salad with sea greens, nuts and seeds, and whole grain bread or chapatis; or baked or broiled fish or seafood with rice and peas or other veggies, or stuffed cabbage rolls with rice, and baked carrots with tamari and a little honey.

—**Before bed:** have a cup of shiitake mushroom or ginger broth, or green tea - for chemoprotective effects; or organic apple juice; or a glass of papaya-pineapple juice to enhance enzyme activity; or 1 tsp. cranberry concentrate in chamomile tea.

Herb and Supplement Choices

•**Macrobiotic cleansing support:** DAILY DETOX by M.D.; Arise & Shine CLEANSE THYSELF PROGRAM - a specific for cancer patients, with many reports of success.

•**Enzyme support:** Transformation PUREZYME (proteolytic enzymes) dissolves the fibrin coating on cancer cells allowing immune defenses to work. Purifies the blood by breaking down protein invaders. Source Naturals COENZYME Q₁₀ ULTRA POTENCY; Herbal Answers HERBAL ALOE FORCE.

•**Immune supoport:** *Herbs:* panax ginseng, echinacea, ashwagandha, Siberian ginseng, goldenseal, licorice, astragalus, ligustrum, suma, dandelion and cayenne. Supplements: Allergy Research GLUTATHIONE with vitamin C; NutriCology LAKTOFERRIN with colostrum; Eidon SILICA MINERAL.

•**Green superfood support:** Crystal Star ENERGY GREEN™; NutriCology PRO-GREENS; Vibrant Health GREEN VIBRANCE; Country Life SHIITAKE/REISHI COMPLEX.

•**Antioxidants:** MICROHYDRIN & PHYCOTENE MICROCLUSTERS available at Healthy House. Biotec CELL GUARD; NutriCology ANTIOX FORMULA II.

•**Macrobiotics is all about balancing your body:** Avoid: — red meat and poultry; preserved, smoked or cured meats of all kinds; dairy products, coffee, and carbonated drinks; sugars, corn syrup and artificial sweeteners; and tropical and sweet fruits. — Avoid all refined and processed food, white vinegar and table salt. Limit hot spices, and nightshade plants like tomatoes, potatoes, peppers and eggplant if you also have rheumatoid arthritis.

Bodywork and Lifestyle Techniques

•**Sunlight:** Get some sunlight on the body every day possible (esp. for organ cancers).

•**Guided imagery:** effective in helping immune response, balancing hormones, and reducing production of abnormal cells.

•**Enemas:** Enemas are a specific for cancer detoxification: Take an enema the first, second and the last day of your cleansing program to help release toxins out of the body.

•**Irrigate:** a colonic once a week for thorough elimination.

•**Exercise:** Regular exercise is almost a "cancer defense" in itself. Exercise acts as an antioxidant to enhance body oxygen use and boost immune response; it accelerates waste passage out of the body. Exercise alters body chemistry to control fat retention, a key involvement with cancer.

•**Rest:** Immune power builds the most during sleep—essential to long-term recovery from cancer.

•**Overheating therapy:** highly effective against cancer.

•**Deep breathing exercise:** Deep, relaxed breathing removes stress, composes the mind, improves mood and increases energy levels. 1. Shift your focus away from your racing mind to focus attention on your breath. 2. Consciously take slow, deep, regular breaths, the mind will become calm. 3. Recall a pleasant experience. 4. Physically feel thankfulness or love about the good things and people you have in your life. 5. Sincerely question your inner intuition to help find a health solution, or a better response to the situation.

Recipes to help your cancer control diet: •**DETOXIFICATION and CLEANSING FOODS;** •**HEALING DRINKS;** •**SOUPS, LIQUID SALADS;** •**BLENDING EAST and WEST;** •**LIGHT MACROBIOTIC EATING.** •**ENZYME-RICH FOODS;**

Can't find a recommended product? Call the 800 number listed in Product Resources for the store nearest you and for more info.

Cancer Control and Prevention Diet

Research links good nutrition to the prevention of 70% of all cancers. One-third of all cancer deaths are related to poor nutrition. Dramatic diet changes can mean dramatic results. The nutritional therapy plan on this page can help you prevent cancer recurrence.

Watchwords: 1—Boost your intake of veggie juices, citrus juice and green tea. Add a glass of red wine a day. 2—Have miso, shiitake mushrooms, sea greens and nutritional yeast 3 times a week. 3—Reduce red meat, dairy proteins and fat. 4—Drink 8 glasses of water daily.

The best cancer-fighting foods: • carotene-rich foods: all red, orange and yellow fruits and veggies; tomatoes; green vegetables; • antioxidant foods soak up free radicals: garlic, onions, broccoli, wheat germ, sea greens, leafy veggies, chile peppers, grapes, berries, carrots; • steamed cruciferous vegetables: broccoli and broccoli sprouts, cabbage, cauliflower, kale; • protease inhibitors: beans (esp. soy), potatoes, corn, hibiscus tea, brown rice; • high fiber foods: whole grains, especially brown rice, apples, fruits and vegetables; • lignan foods: fish, flax oil, walnuts, berries.

—**On rising:** take 2 TBS Herbal Answers HERBAL ALOE FORCE, in orange juice; or Crystal Star BIOFLAV, FIBER & C SUPPORT.

—**Breakfast:** make a mix of 2 TBS each Red Star nutritional yeast, lecithin granules, toasted wheat germ, CC Pollen HIGH DESERT BEE POLLEN granules and flax seeds. Sprinkle some on your breakfast choice of fresh fruits, plain or with yogurt; or a whole grain granola with apple juice, yogurt, or soy milk topping; or whole grain toast or muffins with a little kefir cheese; or a baked or poached egg or omelet; and/or a Crystal Star SYSTEMS STRENGTH™ as a hot broth for optimum mineral/amino acid absorption.

—**Mid-morning:** a green drink (page 569) or Monas or Sun Wellness CHLORELLA, (chlorella's high beta carotene fights tumor formation); Green Foods GREEN ESSENCE, Green Kamut JUST BARLEY, or Crystal Star ENERGY GREEN™ drink in apple juice; or a tonifying herb tea, such as Siberian ginseng, red clover, Natural Energy Plus CAISSES'S TEA, or Crystal Star GINSENG 6™ TEA.

—**Lunch:** have a leafy green salad with a cup of miso or ramen noodle soup; or a cup of black bean, lentil, or other protein soup with baked potato and kefir cheese or yogurt sauce; or a fresh fruit salad with cottage cheese or yogurt cheese, and whole grain baked chips or crackers; or a light seafood or organic turkey salad; or a hot spinach pasta salad.

—**Mid-afternoon:** have whole grain crackers, rice cakes or crunchy raw veggies with a vegetable, soy or kefir spread, and a cup of light broth; or a cup of ginseng tea, or add Y.S. ROYAL JELLY-GINSENG blend to hot water, or mint tea, or Crystal Star FEEL GREAT™ TEA;

—**Dinner:** have a hearty high protein vegetable, nut and seed salad with soup and whole grain muffins or cornbread; or an oriental stir-fry with brown rice and miso soup with sea greens; or a baked veggie, tofu and whole grain casserole; or baked or broiled fish or seafood with a green salad and brown rice or steamed veggies. Have a glass of white wine for digestion and relaxation.

—**Before Bed:** have a cup of chamomile tea or apple or papaya juice, or a cup of Red Star nutritional yeast broth.

Recipes to help your cancer control diet: •BLENDING EAST AND WEST; •FISH and SEAFOOD; •ENZYME-RICH FOODS; •SALADS HOT and COLD; •LOW FAT RECIPES; •DAIRY-FREE; •MINERAL-RICH RECIPES.

Herb and Supplement Choices

• **Detoxification support:** Crystal Star DETOX™ capsules as directed, and GREEN TEA CLEANSER™ every morning. Give yourself a weekly vitamin C flush (also relieves pain) - up to 10g daily (or until stool turns soupy). Una da gato, especially if liver fluke parasites are involved (many cancers).

• **Discourage tumor growth:** Ginger extract; Ginkgo Biloba extract; European mistletoe helps repair damaged DNA; Nutricology MODIFIED CITRUS PECTIN as directed for metastasis; MICROHYDRIN available at Healthy House; Crystal Star SYSTEMS STRENGTH™ drink; probiotics, like UAS Labs DDS-PLUS with FOS; Jarrow IP-6; Crystal Star CAN-SSIAC caps™ 6 daily; Flora FLOR-ESSENCE.

• **Ginseng reinforces tumor immunity:** Imperial Elixir Siberian Ginseng-Royal Jelly, or Siberian ginseng extract.

• **Protect against free radical damage:** Glutathione 150mg daily; Lipoic acid, or Jarrow ALPHA LIPOIC ACID 600mg daily.

• **Enzyme therapy:** Protease enzymes have remarkable activity against cancer; Transformation PUREZYME. Bromelain 1500mg with Quercetin 1000mg daily; CoQ₁₀ 200mg 3x daily.

• **Boost anti-angiogenesis to block tumor nourishment:** Shark cartilage - Lane Labs BENE-FIN caps; Phoenix Biologics BO-VINE TRACHEAL CARTILAGE. Garlic 10 tabs daily; Pau d'arco tea, 4 cups daily.

• **Polyphenol compounds:** red wine, green tea, aloe vera juice, Maitake mushroom, Grifron PRO MAITAKE D-FRACTION.

• **Natural anti-neoplastic substances reduce tumors:** Green tea; folic acid 800mcg. EFA's and Omega-3 oils: Evening Primrose oil 3000mg daily; fish or flaxseed oil, 1-oz daily for cancer; selenium 400mg daily with vitamin E 800IU.

Bodywork and Lifestyle Techniques

• **Exercise regularly:** an antioxidant nutrient in itself, no healing program makes it without some exercise.

• **Sunlight:** get some on the body every day possible (esp. for organ cancers).

• **Guided imagery:** effective in helping the immune system work better, and the hormone system to stop producing abnormal cells.

• **Enemas can clean out putrefaction fast:** Take a coffee enema once a week for a month (1 cup strong brewed in a qt. of water) or chlorella implants, or a wheat grass retention enema.

• **Poultices to reduce external growths:**
  −Herbal Answer's HERBAL ALOE FORCE GEL.
  −Garlic/onion poultice.
  −Comfrey leaf poultice.
  −Green clay poultice.
  −Crystal Star GINSENG SKIN REPAIR™ GEL or ANTI-BIO™ gel with una da gato. PHYCOTENE CREME (contains a complex of 17 carotenoids) available from Healthy House.

• **Lifestyle measures:**
  −Avoid tobacco in all forms, synthetic hormones (particularly estrogen), X-Rays, excessive alcohol (especially beer) and caffeine.
  −Experts have finally linked alternating electromagnetic fields (not static as appear in nature) and some types of cancer.
  −Watch your barbecue - blackened meat has carcinogenic hydrocarbons.

Can't find a recommended product? Call the 800 number listed in Product Resources for the store nearest you and for more info.

Normalize your Body after Chemotherapy and Radiation

Chemotherapy and radiation treatments are widely used by orthodox medicine for most types, stages and degrees of cancer. While some partial successes have been proven, the effects of both treatments are often worse than the disease in terms of healthy cell damage, body imbalance, and reduced immunity. Medical therapists know the drawbacks to chemotherapy, but under current government and insurance restrictions, neither they nor their patients have alternatives.

Amazingly, even with so much new information on alternative methods, new procedure successes, and even new drugs, surgery, chemotherapy, radiation and a few extremely strong drugs are still the only protocols approved by the FDA in the U.S. for malignant disease. The cost for these treatments is beyond the financial range of most people, who, along with physicians and hospitals must rely on health insurance to pay the expense. Medical insurance will not reimburse doctors or hospitals if they use other healing methods. Thus, exorbitant medical costs and special interest regulations have bound medical professionals, hospitals, and insurance companies in a vicious circle where no alternative or new measures may be used to control cancer. Everyone, including the patient, is caught in a political web where it comes down to money instead of health. This is doubly unfortunate, since the advanced research and health care choices are easily available in Europe and other countries to which Americans are denied access.

Scientists admit that current treatments have been pushed to their limits. But new testing and research are extremely expensive. Even today, the vast majority of funds provided by the National Cancer Act support research to improve the effectiveness of existing therapies – radiation, surgery and chemotherapy. This practice is easier and cheaper, but it leaves patients with the same three therapies, just a more precise use of them. Even when a new treatment is substantiated, there is no reasonable investment certainty that government (and therefore health insurance) approval can be obtained through the maze of red tape and politics.

Some of this is changing as cancer patients refuse to become victims of their medical system as well as the disease. The American people are demanding access, funding and insurance approval for alternative health techniques and medicines. Slowly, state by state, legislators and regulators are listening, health care parameters are expanding, and insurance limitations are lessening

Conventional medicine rarely treats cancer as a systemic the way lab science and our left brains work, breaking things ing, identifying.... in consequence, hardly ever seeing the healers regard cancer as an unhealthy body whose defenses that a healthy body with strong immune response does not a whole rather than a disease in one part. Alternative therapy. highly toxic modalities like radiation and chemotherapy. treatments which rely on bio-chemistry, metabolic, nutri-

illness, defining it only by location and symptomatology. It's down into one-for-one causes and effects, assaying, isolating, whole person or the whole picture. By contrast, alternative can no longer destroy abnormal cells. Naturopaths believe develop cancer, and that cancer is a reflection of the body as pists seek to strengthen immune response, and generally shun They use a multifaceted, non-toxic approach, incorporating tional and herbal therapies, and immune enhancement.

A Healing Diet after Chemotherapy

You can help your body clean out drug residues and get over treatment side effects by following a healing diet. A healing diet can help minimize damage to healthy cells, and rebuild strength after chemotherapy and radiation. You can live with this diet for health on a lifetime basis, for cancer resistance to disease recurrence, and for good immune strength. It is high in absorbable vitamins and minerals, oxygenating foods, and immune and liver stimulating nutrients. It is generally seasonal eating, with a continued emphasis on the body building properties of whole grains and complex carbohydrates. Keep your diet about 60% fresh foods for the first month after chemotherapy.

—**On rising:** take ALL 1 VITAMIN/MINERAL drink or Nature's Plus SPIRUTEIN or Crystal Star BIOFLAV., FIBER & C SUPPORT™ drink in orange juice; or make your own fresh V- 8 juice (page 569) and add 1 TB. Bragg's LIQUID AMINOS.

—**Breakfast:** have a high fiber, whole grain cereal with yogurt, kefir or soy milk, and add your choice of nuts, seeds and dried fruit. Make a mix of 2 TBS each: Red Star nutritional yeast, lecithin granules, and toasted wheat germ, and sprinkle it every morning over whatever you eat for breakfast; such as some fresh fruit, or yogurt, or a baked or poached egg.

—**Mid-morning:** have some raw crunchy veggies with kefir or yogurt cheese or a veggie/soy spread; or a glass of carrot juice (at least once a week). Have a green supplement drink like Monas CHLORELLA (chlorella's high beta carotene content fights tumor formation) or Crystal Star ENERGY GREEN™ at least twice a week; take aloe vera juice as needed for nausea.

—**Lunch:** have a seafood salad, or a large green salad with cucumbers, kiwi, and peas, and yogurt or lemon-flax oil dressing; or a cabbage cole slaw salad with yogurt or lemon dressing; or a quiche with asparagus, broccoli, or artichokes and a whole grain crust; or aji tuna salad sandwich, or a tofu burger on a whole grain bun; or a baked potato with a little butter and a mushroom salad side dish.

—**Mid-afternoon:** a cup of green tea; or miso soup with sea greens snipped on top; or baked tofu chunks with low-fat dressing.

—**Dinner:** have a light Italian whole grain pasta meal, with fresh mozzarella cheese or soy mozarella; or a sweet potato pie, or baked yams and carrots with a little butter and brown rice; or a broccoli-Chinese cabbage stir-fry with miso soup; or steam-sautéed broccoli, cauliflower, green beans or zucchini with toasted walnuts and dressing; or a salmon souffle with rice and green beans; or fresh grilled or baked fish with peas and rice; or a zucchini and rice frittata; or a tofu or tempeh casserole with millet or rice.

—**Before bed:** have a cup of relaxing herb tea, or a glass of apple juice.

Recipes to help a chemo detox diet: •CULTURED HEALING FOODS; •HEALING DRINKS; •SOUPS, LIQUID SALADS; •ENZYME-RICH FOOD; •MINERAL-RICH; •FISH & SEAFOODS; •LIGHT MACROBIOTICS; HIGH FIBER.

Herb and Supplement Choices

• **For 3 months after chemo or radiation take daily:**
—Crystal Star **SYSTEMS STRENGTH™** broth daily.

—**Maitake mushroom** has a powerful anti-cancer punch to shrink tumors. In combination with the chemotherapy drug mitomycin-C (MMC), it produces an amazing 99% tumor reduction. Side effects from chemo like nausea, vomiting and hair loss are reduced by maitake. Grifron MAITAKE D-FRACTION.

—**CoQ₁₀** capsules, 360mg; in combination with germanium 150mg daily, and beta carotene 50,000IU daily, and Vitamin C crystals with bioflavonoids, ¹/₄ teasp. in liquid every hour, about 5 to 10,000 mg daily. An adjunct to chemotherapy treatment as a heart protector.

—**MGN-3,** "possibly the most powerful immune booster known to man," from Lane Labs.

—**800mcg folic acid** to normalize DNA synthesis, especially if methotrexate was used in your treatment.

—Floradix **HERBAL IRON,** 1 teasp. 3x daily, or Crystal Star ENERGY GREEN™ drink to counteract the anemia that causes such extreme fatigue after chemo treatments.

—**Healthy House PHYCOTENE MICROCLUSTERS,** 17 carotenoids that scavenge free radicals caused by chemo.

—**Protease enzymes** have remarkable activity against cancer; Transformation PUREZYME. Co-enzymate B complex sublingual, for hair regrowth.

—**Lactoferrin** blocks cancer angiogenesis and boosts strength against infection from chemotherapy. NutriCology LAKTOFERRIN. Caution: Lactoferrin is contraindicated during pregnancy as high of levels of lactoferrin may cause rejection of the fetus. Also contraindicated for leukemia.

Bodywork and Lifestyle Techniques

• **Regular exercise is a healing nutrient in itself.** Exercise can actually change body chemistry. Exercise with regular, moderate sunshine is the best choice of all.

• **Avoid tobacco in all forms.** Curtail caffeine intake. Avoid alcohol except for moderate wine.

• **Even small amounts of radiation are sometimes proving to engender cancer growth in delicate tissue.** Be extremely cautious of having X-rays, mammograms, etc. If you feel you are at risk for breast, uterine, ovarian, cervical or prostate cancer, avoid hormone replacement therapy, consciously avoid meats and dairy products that are regularly injected with hormones.

• **Reduce the effects of chemotherapy and radiation:** Reishi or Maitake mushroom extract; Astragalus extract; Nettles tea to dissolve adhesions. Apply kukui nut oil for chemotherapy or radiation burning.

Can't find a recommended product? Call the 800 number listed in Product Resources for the store nearest you and for more info.

212

Immunity: Building a Strong Defense System

Your immune response is critical. Your health throughout your life depends on it. Have you ever wondered why some people get sick more than others or why some seniors stay healthy in their later years while others get sick prematurely? Even though you may have inherited a strong immune system, good nutrition, lifestyle and exercise play a significant role in maintaining robust immunity.

Every single person's immune system is unique, individual and personal in every way. Science has found it impossible to develop an "immunity drug." It would have to produce over 6 billion drugs (the world's population today) to make one for everybody.

Integrate immune enhancing techniques into your life no matter how good you feel. Your immune system is challenged daily by at least 25,000 new chemicals that enter our environment every year - many of them from third world countries that don't have safeguards in place. These chemicals affect our air, our water, our food supply, and our basic hormone balance. We can't get away from them, their numbers are growing, and it means we live in an increasingly destructive world. A lot of us don't have very much to fight with. Today immune compromised fatigue diseases like candida albicans, chronic fatigue syndrome (CFS), fibromyalgia, Hashimoto's, lupus, sexually transmitted diseases, hepatitis and cancer are taking hold in almost epidemic proportions.

How can we stay well in a toxic environment? It isn't easy. There is no "magic bullet." But, there are tried and true "golden rules" that give you more control. Small but significant changes in your diet, and some simple natural therapies added to your daily life can add years to your health. Using natural therapies to build immunity is incredibly rewarding. You experience a feeling of empowerment, of control over the fate of your life, as well as a sense of well-being that comes from renewed health.

Your immune system is truly is amazing. Immune defense is automatic and subconscious. It works on its own to set up a healing environment for your body. It is this quality of being part of us, yet not under our conscious control, that is the great power of immunity. It is as if God shows us his face in this incredibly complex part of us, where we can just glimpse the ultimate mind-body connection. Our immune system shows us that there is so much more to healing than the latest wonder drug. We can see that we are the ultimate healer of ourselves.

The immune system is the most complex and delicately balanced infrastructure of your body, your personal defense team that comes charging to the rescue at the first sign of an alien force — like a harmful virus, fungus, pathogenic bacteria or parasite. The immune system is always vigilant, constantly searching for proteins, called antigens, that don't belong in our bodies. It can deal with a wide range of them, even recognizing potential antigens, like drugs, pollens, insect venoms, malignant cells and chemicals in foods. It can identify and react to foreign tissue, such as transplanted organs or transfused blood, rejecting the tissue it perceives as harmful. In an allergic reaction, the immune system may even overreact, and respond to substances that really aren't harmful.

The workings of other body systems are well known, but the dynamics of the immune system are still largely a mystery.

Part of the puzzle is its highly individual nature. Another puzzle is its incredibly complex character.

We know the main elements of the immune system itself: bone marrow, the thymus gland, the lymphatic system, the spleen, and a complex system of enzymatic proteins called the complement system. Mobilizing these elements can be a "big deal" for your body, requiring many of its resources. So Nature in her wisdom gives you "first line of defense" shields to repulse infectious organisms - like your skin's protective acid mantle, and mucous membranes that line your respiratory, digestive and urogenital tracts. Disease happens when harmful microorganisms slip by these barriers and your immune response can't come to the rescue.

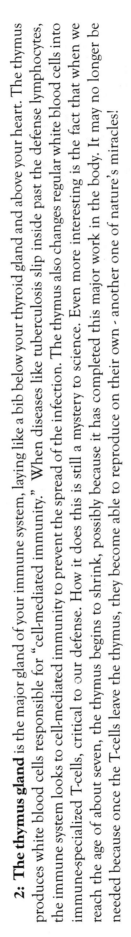

Here's how your immune system defends you. It's like a chain reaction.

1: Lymphocyte defense cells are divided into T-cells and B-cells, called eater cells or phagocytes. Lymphocytes form your body's overall defense system, attacking anything they perceive as foreign. But they don't identify microbes specifically, so some microorganisms can get past them. Pneumonia bacteria slip past for example, and so do viruses. B-cells, though, can turn into plasma cells that produce specific antibodies, like immunoglobulins, that can neutralize specific invading antigens, including viruses. Lymphocytes and phagocytes also release chemicals called cytokines which send signals to integrate the immune system's efforts. Two well known cytokines are interferon, active against viral infections, and tumor necrosis factor (TNF), which destroys cells that grow abnormally fast, like cancer cells. When infected cells become inflamed, lymphocytes attack them in order to confine the pathogen. This defensive backup is vital in resisting infections from mold-like bacteria, yeast, fungi, parasites and viruses.

2: The thymus gland is the major gland of your immune system, laying like a bib below your thyroid gland and above your heart. The thymus produces white blood cells responsible for "cell-mediated immunity." When diseases like tuberculosis slip inside past the defense lymphocytes, the immune system looks to cell-mediated immunity to prevent the spread of the infection. The thymus also changes regular white blood cells into immune-specialized T-cells, critical to our defense. How it does this is still a mystery to science. Even more interesting is the fact that when we reach the age of about seven, the thymus begins to shrink, possibly because it has completed this major work in the body. It may no longer be needed because once the T-cells leave the thymus, they become able to reproduce on their own - another one of nature's miracles!

3: The lymphatic system is like a secondary circulatory system, complementing the bloodstream. Lymph nodes filter and remove infective organisms, with large cells called macrophages that engulf foreign particles like bacteria and cellular debris. The lymph doesn't have a pump, like the heart, to move fluids around, so lymph circulation depends upon breathing and muscle movement. It's one of the reasons exercise is an important part of any immune enhancing program; among other things, exercise improves circulation in the lymphatic system so it can remove waste materials that block immune response. **The spleen** is the body's largest mass of lymphatic tissue. It destroys worn-out red blood cells and platelets, and serves as a reservoir for new ones. During a hemorrhage, the spleen comes to the rescue, by releasing stored blood and preventing shock.

4: The complement system is a complex series of 12 enzymatic proteins that circulate in the blood, reacting both to other immune substances and to antigens. The complement system promotes efficient T-cell function, by making lethal holes in harmful bacteria cells so they can be penetrated by the T-cells and B-cells, and by enhancing the immune inflammatory response.

5: Fever, mucous and the skin also form part of the body's immune defenses. Mucous in the GI and respiratory tract kills both bacteria and viruses to keep the body protected against invasion. The skin contains sweat and sebaceous glands which produce substances capable of killing bacteria and fungus on contact.

A fever is actually one of Mother Nature's defenses. A slight fever is your body's normal mechanism for clearing up an infection or toxic overload quickly. You might get better faster when you're sick if you let Nature take its course for a little while. Fever helps to destroy bacteria and improves the flow of interferon to fight off viral infections. Your immune system raises body temperature to literally "burn out" harmful poisons, throwing them off through heat and then through sweating. The heat from a fever can also deactivate virus replication. (Modern orthodox medicine is rediscovering heating therapy for diseases as serious as AIDS.) Unless a fever is exceptionally high (over 103° for kids and 102° for adults) or long lasting (more than two full days), it may be a wise choice to let it run its natural course, even with children.

6: Your liver is your body's personal chemical plant for immune strength. The liver lays down the raw materials for your lymphatic system. It produces most of lymph in the body, and the special types of macrophages in the liver give the lymphatic system its power to filter harmful bacteria, especially harmful yeasts like candida albicans, and toxic compounds in the gastrointestinal tract.

What depresses your immune response?

—**Long term courses of drugs:** antacids (reduce nutrient assimilation), antibiotics (destroy friendly bacteria vital to GI immunity), anti-inflammatory drugs like acetaminophen, aspirin and ibuprofen (inhibit white cells that fight infection).

—**Long term exposure to pollutants:** second hand smoke and chemicals put a strain on your body's detox mechanisms.

—**Repeated exposure to allergy-causing foods or chemicals.** Allergies cause immunity to take a dive because immune defenses are all channeled to deal with the allergen rather than to fight infection. (In turn, many allergies are the result of low immunity.)

—**A diet high in refined, chemicalized foods.** Low intake of protective, antioxidant, enzyme-rich fruits and vegetables. Fake fats like olestra that rob cancer-fighting carotenoids are especially disrupting.

—**A diet high in trans fats** (deep fried foods, fast foods, and almost all snack foods), saturated fats and refined sugars. Trans fatty acids increase LDL (bad) cholesterol and decrease HDL (good) cholesterol, and are found at high levels in women with breast cancer. Saturated fats interfere with prostaglandin E1 which regulates immune T-cell activity. Excessively sugary foods suppress white blood cell activity for hours! Eating these foods regularly may mean your immune system takes a nose dive all day long!

—**Excessive dieting** or low nutrient intake (depresses interferon activity). Overeating also depresses immune response.

—**Children born to parents who smoke, drink to excess or abuse drugs** have more predisposition to illness and infections.

—**A lifestyle low on rest.** Your body builds the most immune power during sleep. Sleep deprivation lowers the percentage of T-cells in your blood. In clinical tests performed at U. California at San Diego School of Medicine, killer cell activity is reduced by as much as 28% when sleep is cut by 4 hours!. Choose natural sleep aids rather than drugs for safe sleep with no side effects.

—**Not being breast-fed as a child.** Breast milk is rich in antibodies, essential fatty acids and interferon that strengthen a child's developing immune system.

—**A poor outlook on life or severe, long lasting depression.** Laughter lifts more than your spirits. It also boosts immune strength. Really! Laughter decreases cortisol, an immune suppressor, allowing the body's defense boosters to function better.

—**Stressed out people** who overextend themselves are unusually susceptible to immune system malfunction. Listen to soft music. Your pulse rate will actually follow the mellow beat to de-stress your body. Enjoy a long bath, take a sauna, or get a massage therapy treatment. These relaxation techniques last a whole week in terms of reducing stress and enhancing immune response.

—**Lonely, solitary people.** Build a strong support system of family and friends into your life. Research from the Carnegie Mellon University shows that having friends actually lowers your risk of catching a cold by 30%!

—**Couch potatoes.** Exercise 2 or 3 times a week. Exercise improves immunity by increasing lymphatic flow to keep your body toxin-free. Exercise keeps system oxygen high, too, and disease does not readily attack in a high oxygen, high potassium environment. Clinical tests on senior women show that those who exercise even moderately have marked improvement in immune response.

Is your immune response low?

I've worked for years to develop ways people can communicate with their bodies. It's hard to measure immune health. Every person is different and the character of immune response varies widely. Here's a quick personal quiz to monitor your immune status:

1: Do you suffer from chronic infections, colds, respiratory problems or allergies? Are you always tired?
2: Do you have, or have you had any immune-deficient diseases, like chronic fatigue syndrome, Hashimoto's or fibromyalgia?
3: Do you have a history of malabsorption problems, like irritable bowel syndrome (I.B.S.), or chronic diarrhea or constipation?
4: Do you have diabetes or liver disease? Have you ever been the recipient of an organ transplant?
5: Have you had long-term treatment with antibiotics or steroid drugs? Do you have candida yeast infections that don't go away?
6: Do you have a skin disorder like adult acne or Rosacea?
7: Have you recently undergone surgery, chemotherapy or radiation treatment?
8: Do you have periodontal disease? Do you have circulation problems or a history of claudication?
9: Do you drink 2 or more drinks of hard alcohol 4 to 5 times a week or take recreational drugs on a regular basis?
10: Are you a smoker or are you exposed to second-hand smoke on a regular basis?
11: Do you live in an area of heavy pesticide use? Are you regularly exposed to industrial heavy metals, like asbestos or mercury?
12: Do you drink untreated tap water? Do you eat meats, like pork or beef that are injected with antibiotics and hormones?
13: Do you suffer from chronic stress, anxiety, panic attacks or depression? Do you suffer from chronic insomnia?

Cleansing Diet Plan for Immune Strength

Do you need a pollutant or heavy metal cleanse?

Chemical pollutants and toxic by-products affect every facet of our lives, from our water and food supply to the workplace and our homes. Heavy metal poisoning and toxic pollutants are major health problems of the American culture. We have moved from fetid air to undrinkable water, to severe allergy reactions and serious diseases caused by pollution. The main effect of an unhealthy environment is reduced immune response, especially impacting our filtering organs, the liver and kidneys. Periodic detoxification needs to be a part of life to keep our bodies able to defend us against pollutants. (A hair analysis can help you determine nutrient deficiencies and which heavy metals are lodged in your body.)

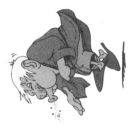

Is your body showing signs that it needs a pollution-heavy metal cleanse?

—**Are you far more sensitive to odors like perfumes and strong cleansers than most people?**
—**Do you have an unusually small tolerance for alcohol?**
—**Are there medications you can't take, or some vitamins or other supplements that make you feel worse?**
—**Do you have small black spots along your gum line? Unusual bad breath or body odor?**
—**Is your reaction time noticeably poorer when driving in city traffic?**
—**Do you have unexplained seizures, memory failure or psychotic behavior?**
—**Have you become infertile or impotent?**

7-Day Chemical Pollutant Detox Diet

A good way to begin fortifying the immune system, especially if you're feeling noticeably logy or tired, have had a series of exposures to chemical pollutants, or a history of frequent infections and virus invasions, is to go on a simple, detox diet for 7 days. A pollution cleansing detox re-establishes normal body chemistry, eases the energy your body has to expend on processing cooked or heavy foods, and releases hormone secretions that stimulate the immune complex and clear the way for its regeneration.

For best results from your pollutant-heavy metal cleanse:

(1) A heavy metal, pollutant detox is one of the most likely cleanses for a "healing crisis" to occur. You may feel head-achy, with a slight upset stomach as toxins are released. The feelings should pass quickly, usually within 24 hours. I don't recommend an all-liquid diet if you're trying to release heavy metals or chemicals. They may enter the bloodstream too fast and heavily for your body to handle safely. Eat solid cleansing foods instead to release the toxins more slowly and safely.

(2) Drink 8-10 glasses of bottled water each day to clear toxins more rapidly.

(3) Chlorophyll is the most powerful cleansing agent in nature. Green veggie drinks and green superfoods are key.

(4) Sea greens are powerful releasers of chemicals, heavy metals and radiation from the body. Sprinkle 2 TBS daily on any food or drink during your cleanse. Keep sea greens high on your immune list with at least 6 pieces of sushi a week.

(5) Fresh fruit and vegetable juices maximize your body's immune power. Try a carrot, beet, celery and parsley combo to rejuvenate the liver and gastro-intestinal health, and a banana, strawberry or blueberry combo for vitamin C and potassium. • Key juices for immunity: **garlic** - antibacterial and antifungal properties, especially combined with tomatoes, celery and carrots; **alfalfa sprouts** - an ideal source of protein that also helps keep your body clean. Sprouts are rich in vitamin A, B-complex, C, D and E, enzymes, essential fatty acids and antioxidant minerals which are natural immune strengtheners; **apples and celery** - improve lymphatic health by drawing toxins out of your tissues to be flushed away; **beets** - keep your liver functioning well. Combine them in a potassium juice with spinach, carrots and celery. In addition to juices, **eat cruciferous vegetables like broccoli, cabbage and cauliflower regularly** - they help flush out environmental estrogens in meats and pesticides.

(6) Have a tonic broth several times during your cleanse to boost immunity. Here's a delicious, proven favorite to prevent winter respiratory illness: mix miso, onions, garlic, shiitake mushrooms, and astragalus root, (an immune-boosting Chinese herb from the health food store). The miso represses carcinogens and neutralizes toxins. The onions and garlic fight off pathogens. The immune-boosting shiitake mushrooms (easy to find today in gourmet stores) produce a virus which stimulates interferon in the body.

(7) Add $^1/_4$ teasp. of a potent lactobacillus or acidophilus complex to each juice during the cleanse to stimulate friendly G.I. flora, and build enzyme strength, a key factor of strong immunity.

—**On rising:** have a drink of 2 TBS. cranberry concentrate in water with $^1/_2$ tsp. vitamin C crystals; or Crystal Star GREEN TEA CLEANSER™; or blend 2 tsp. lemon, 1 tsp. honey, 1 cup water and 1 tsp. acidophilus in 8-oz. aloe vera juice.

—**Breakfast:** have a glass of fresh carrot juice or veggie juice (see above) with 1 TB green superfood like Crystal Star ENERGY GREEN™ mix or Wakunaga KYO-GREEN, and whole grain muffins or rice cakes with kefir or yogurt cheese; or a cup of soy milk or plain yogurt blended with a cup of fresh fruit, walnuts, and $^1/_2$ teasp. acidophilus.

—**Mid-morning:** take a cup of green tea, with $^1/_2$ teasp. ascorbate vitamin C crystals; or a fresh vegetable juice with 1 TB green superfood such as Nutricology PRO-GREENS with EFA's, or FUNCTIONAL GREENS from Ethical Nutrients.

—**Lunch:** have a leafy salad with lemon-flax oil dressing; or a cup of miso soup with sea greens and brown rice; or steamed veggies with brown rice and sea greens; and green tea with $^1/_2$ teasp. vitamin C and $^1/_2$ teasp. acidophilus powder.

—**Mid-afternoon:** have carrot juice with 1 TB green superfood like Crystal Star ENERGY GREEN™ drink or a tonic broth (see above).

—**Dinner:** have a baked potato with Bragg's LIQUID AMINOS and a fresh salad with lemon-flax dressing; or a black bean or lentil soup; or a Chinese steam/stir fry with vegetables, shiitake mushrooms and brown rice.

—**Before Bed:** an 8-oz. glass of aloe vera juice with $^1/_2$ teasp. vitamin C and another carrot juice or green tea.

Recipes to help a chemical detox diet: •DETOXIFICATION FOODS; •HEALING DRINKS; •SOUPS, LIQUID SALADS; •ENZYME-RICH FOODS; •SALADS, HOT - COLD; •MINERAL-RICH FOODS •LIGHT MACROBIOTICS.

Herb and Supplement Choices

• **Pollutant-heavy metal cleansers:** Crystal Star HEAVY METAL CLEANZ™ caps or DETOX™ caps for 3 months. Oral chelation Metabolic Response Modifiers CARDIO-CHELATE; Golden Pride FORMULA ONE w/ EDTA. **For radiation poisoning:** vitamin C powder with bioflavonoids $\frac{1}{2}$ teasp. every hour to bowel tolerance.

• **Enzyme support:** Protease binds to heavy metals, sparing metabolic enzyme destruction. Transformation PUREZYME (high doses effective in lowering blood mercury toxins).

• **Liver enhancers:** Alpha Lipoic Acid 600mg daily for 2 months; Jarrow Formulas ALPHA LIPOIC ACID or GLUCOTIZE by MRI; Crystal Star LIV-ALIVE™ caps or tea or Enzymatic Therapy LIVA-TOX caps and *Milk thistle seed* extract; *Dandelion* extract; EVENING PRIMROSE oil caps 4 daily; Biostrath LIQUID YEAST.

• **Antioxidants defeat pollutants:** Carnitine 1000mg 3x daily for 1 month; NAC (N-acetyl-cysteine) 500mg 3x daily; CoQ-10, 60mg 4x daily; • Nutricology GERMANIUM 150mg daily. Beta carotene 150,000IU with extra lycopene 5-10mg; PCO's from grapeseed or white pine 100mg 3 daily; Vitamin E 400IU with selenium 200mcg; Glutathione 100mg daily; MICROHYDRIN available at Healthy House; Source Naturals OPTI-ZINC 30mg daily, and CHEM-DEFENSE; Enzymatic Therapy THYMUPLEX; Biotec CELL GUARD 8 daily.

• **Build strong immune defenses with herbal immune enhancers:** Astragalus extract; Propolis extract or lozenges; Garlic 6-8 caps daily; Echinacea extract; Cat's Claw caps; Siberian ginseng extract caps; Spirulina 2 tsp. daily, or Spirulina MICRO-CLUSTERS, available at Healthy House; Monas CHLORELLA 2 teasp. daily for chemical toxins.

Bodywork and Lifestyle Techniques

• **Protect against radiation syndromes:** avoid foods labeled irradiated or electronically pasteurized.

• **Use an air filter to remove toxins in the air.** Use vinegar, baking soda and salt as cleansers if you are very sensitive.

• **Protect yourself from EMF fields:** avoid non-filtered computer screens, cell phones, electric blankets, microwave ovens. (Don't use plastic wrap in the microwave, Its heat can drive the molecules into the food.)

• **Tobacco/nicotine in any form is an immune depressant.** The cadmium content causes zinc deficiency. It takes 3 months to rebuild immune response even after you quit.

• **Get plenty of tissue oxygen.** Take a walk every day, breathing deeply. Do deep breathing exercises on rising, and in the evening on retiring to clear the lungs and respiratory system.

—Use Earth's Bounty O_2 SPRAY on soles of feet every 2 days to keep tissue oxygen high.

• **Take a hot seaweed bath, or a sweating bath,** like Crystal Star POUNDS OFF BATH™. Use a dry skin brush before and after the bath to remove toxins coming out on the skin.

• **Spring Life POLARIZERS** have notable success against environmental pollutants.

• **Relaxation techniques are immune-enhancers.** A positive mental attitude makes a big difference in how the body fights disease. Creative visualization establishes belief and optimism. Biofeedback or massage therapy to reduce stress.

• **Stimulate immunity with a few minutes of early morning sunlight every day.** Avoid excessive sun. A sunburn depresses immunity.

• **Get quality rest:** immune power builds most during sleep.

Can't find a recommended product? Call the 800 number listed in Product Resources for the store nearest you and for more info.

Healing Diet to Restore Immune Strength

(1) Take a close look at the fruits and vegetables you're eating, especially during the winter months when your body needs more stability and a little more substance from your diet. Warm weather fruits and vegetables like cucumbers, head lettuce, kiwis, melons, summer squash or tomatoes, are too light for winter (high risk season) health. Switch to vegetables and legumes- like carrots, potatoes, lentils, black beans and squash. Good winter fruits are cranberries, pears and apples. Apples are a hydrating energy food, full of enzymes to help you use the other foods you eat. Apples are rich in pectin, an amazing food fiber that binds to and helps eliminate gut toxins to keep your GI tract healthy and digestion smooth. An apple a day may truly keep the doctor away. Cruciferous vegetables like broccoli, cabbage and cauliflower offer a megaload of nutrients for immune health, like vitamin C, beta carotene, calcium and fiber. They also have excess estrogen flushing activity against the environmental estrogens we get today from our meats and pesticides.

(2) Add more high fiber foods for high risk seasons. Whole grains and sprouts are full of fiber. Sprouted seeds and grains are living foods, some of the healthiest foods you can eat. My favorite whole grain all year round is brown rice. In the winter, a combination of wild rice and root vegetables provides mineral building blocks and complex carbohydrates for strength. I make up a big pot of rice every 2 or 3 days with 1 teaspoon of miso for every cup of rice. Miso helps to set up an immune-enhancing environment in the body.

(3) Eat cold water sea foods for essential fatty acids, vitamin E and Omega-3 oils for immune health. World Health Organization studies show that societies using fish and seafood as their primary source of fat and protein have much lower incidence of heart disease and cancer.

(4) Add to your healing enzyme supply during high risk seasons. Food enzymes are basic to immune response for natural enzyme therapy. Foods like alfalfa sprouts, garlic, pineapple and papaya provide more of their enzymes to work with yours.

(5) Drink enough quality water. Dehydration is at the root of a lot of disease, especially age-related conditions (like creaky joints, wrinkling skin, hemorrhoids, varicose veins and kidney stones).

(6) Eat cultured foods like yogurt, kefir, kefir cheese, cottage cheese and raw sauerkraut for friendly intestinal flora. Cultured foods help maintain the body's acid-alkaline balance, and strengthen the nerves and immune system. If you like wine, (a cultured food) have a little wine with dinner. More than an alcoholic drink, wine is a complex living food with absorbable B vitamins, and minerals like potassium, magnesium, organic sodium, iron, and calcium.

An immune enhancing program is also effective for: *Viral / Bacterial Infections, Staph / Strep Infections, Premature Aging, Mononucleosis, Meningitis and Rheumatic Fever, Respiratory Infections, Measles, Drug Overuse, Herpes, Environmental, Chemical and Heavy Metal Poisoning.*

7-Day Immune Stimulation Diet

Natural healing is not extravagant or heroic medicine; it is body normalization, rebuilding your body from the inside out. Your diet is the first place to start. Powerful immune-enhancing foods can be directed at "early warning" problems, like the ones you might have spotted in your quiz. Since immunity is the body system most sensitive to nutritional deficiency, good nourishment is the main key to keeping this system functioning at its peak. Incorporating some of these diet recommendations is well worth it. The inherited immunity and health of you, your children and your grandchildren is laid down by you and your choices.

Watchwords: The American diet of processed foods, 20% sugars and 37% fat, suppresses immunity. Saturated fat in pastries, fried foods, dairy foods and red meats is the worst culprit. Eat plenty of fresh foods, fiber foods, whole grains, sea foods, eggs and cultured dairy foods, like yogurt and kefir for friendly G.I. flora. Food enzymes are basic to immune response. Include a cup of green tea, fresh fruits and vegetables in your diet every day. Add enzyme-rich sprouts, garlic, papaya and sea greens. Environmental pollutants, particularly pesticides, lower immunity. Eat organically grown foods whenever possible. Green superfoods supply a "mini-transfusion" to detoxify your bloodstream. Take a green superfood drink twice a week.

—**On rising:** take 2-3 TBS. cranberry concentrate in 8-oz. water or 8-oz. aloe vera juice; or an immune stimulating drink like Crystal Star BIOFLAVONOID, FIBER & C drink or GREEN TEA CLEANSER™; or Unipro PERFECT PROTEIN.

—**Breakfast:** make an immune-stimulating mix of nutritional yeast flakes, lecithin granules, pumpkin seeds and flax seed. Sprinkle some on your choice of whole grain granola with almond, rice or soy milk, fresh fruit and yogurt, baked or poached eggss, or whole grain muffins or rice cakes with kefir cheese. Add a cup of green tea daily.

—**Mid-morning:** a green superfood like Crystal Star ENERGY GREEN™, GREEN KAMUT from Green Kamut Corp. or Green Foods GREEN MAGMA; or a fresh vegetable juice with 1 TB. green superfood like Nutricology PRO-GREENS with EFA's or Wakunaga KYO-GREEN.

—**Lunch:** have a leafy salad with lemon/flax oil dressing; or a whole grain sandwich with plenty of sprouts, nuts, seeds, veggies and yogurt or soy cheese; or a turkey or seafood salad or sandwich with a light yogurt dressing; or a cup of miso soup with brown rice and sea greens snipped in; or a stir fry or steamed vegetables with onions, brown rice and tofu.

—**Mid-afternoon:** have a carrot juice or a cup of immune stimulating herb tea like ginseng tea, or Crystal Star FEEL GREAT™ tea; and have some rice cakes with a soy spread or veggie dip.

—**Dinner:** have baked or broiled seafood or fish with brown rice and veggies; or a high protein soup or sandwich on whole grain bread; or a light Italian spinach pasta meal; or an Oriental stir-fry with veggies and seafood, a clear broth soup with sea greens snipped on top; or a tofu and veggie casserole with brown rice and a low-fat yogurt, cheese and wine sauce.

—**Before bed:** take a hot lemon and honey drink; or hot apple or cranberry juice; or green tea, or Red Star nutritional yeast broth, or miso soup with sea greens; or Crystal Star BIOFLAV., FIBER & C SUPPORT™ drink.

Recipes to help boost immune response: •DETOXIFICATION FOODS; •HEALING DRINKS; •SOUPS, LIQUID SALADS; •ENZYME-RICH FOODS; •SALADS, HOT and COLD; •MINERAL-RICH •LIGHT MACROBIOTIC EATING.

Bodywork and Lifestyle Techniques

• **Relaxation techniques are immune-enhancers.** A positive mental attitude makes a big difference in how the body fights disease. Creative visualization establishes belief and optimism. Biofeedback or massage therapy to reduce stress.

• **Exercise keeps system oxygen high, circulation flowing.** Disease does not readily overrun a body where oxygen and organic minerals are high in the vital fluids. Reduce prescription drugs if possible, especially antibiotics and steroid drugs that depress immunity over the long term.

• **Stop and smell the roses.** A conscious, free-flowing emotional life is fundamental for inner harmony. Have one good laugh every day.

• **Aromatherapy immune oils:** lavender or rosemary oil.

• **Eliminate recreational drugs.** Reduce prescription drugs, especially antibiotics and cortico-steroids that depress immunity.

• **Tobacco/nicotine in any form is an immune depressant.** The cadmium content causes zinc deficiency. It takes 3 to 6 months to rebuild immune response even after you quit.

• **Stimulate immunity by a few minutes of early morning sunlight every day.** Avoid excessive sun. A sunburn depresses immunity.

• **Get quality rest,** immune power builds the most during sleep.

Herb and Supplement Choices

• **Stimulate white blood cell activity with natural antibiotics:** Allergy Research Group LAKTOFERRIN caps with colostrum; Olive Leaf extract; NAC (N-acetyl-cysteine) 600mg.

• **Immune modulators act as response tonics:** Crystal Star HERBAL DEFENSE TEAM™ formulas, or Natural Balance MODUCARE caps for 2 months. Siberian ginseng, Panax ginseng or Suma root; Propolis caps 4 daily during high risk seasons; Earth's Bounty NONI liquid or Penny Saved Enterprises NONI caps; Zand HERBAL INSURE extract; Futurebiotics VITAL K.

• **Medicinal mushrooms enhance interferon production:** Reishi, shiitake and maitake mushrooms; Planetary Formulas REISHI SUPREME; Grifron MAITAKE; Metabolic Response Modifiers CORDYCEPS.

• **Enhance thymus gland activity:** Nutricology Organic Thymus; Nature's Path THY-LYTE; Enzymatic Therapy THY-MULUS; (Tap thymus with knuckles each morning to stimulate.)

• **Enzymes for immune response:** Biotec CELL GUARD w. SOD 6 daily for 6 weeks; Transformation PUREZYME; Milk Thistle Seed extract; Licorice root tea for a month.

• **Sea plants help your body remove toxins:** Sea greens of all kinds, 2 TBS daily, provide therapeutic iodine, potassium and sodium alginate to help purify your body; or take Crystal Star SYSTEMS STRENGTH™ caps, or POTASSIUM-IODINE sea plant complex; or Biotec PACIFIC SEA PLASMA tablets 6 daily; Nature's Path TRACE-MIN-LYTE (sea greens).

• **Antioxidants build immune strength:** PCO's, 100mg daily; vitamin E 400IU with selenium 200mcg; vitamin C or Ester C with bioflavonoids 3000mg, and zinc 50mg daily; CoQ$_{10}$ 200mg daily; MICROHYDRIN, available at Healthy House.

Can't find a recommended product? Call the 800 number listed in Product Resources for the store nearest you and for more info.

Immune Breakdown Diseases

There's a war going on today and your body is the prize. The human body is under tremendous assault from substances and lifestyles that make us vulnerable to disease. We have defenses, but no real early warning process. Our miraculous immune system is so automatic and so subconscious that we are able to function, even go on our merry way until our body uses up almost all its defenses and reserves. Sometimes the first signs of the state of our immune response are when an infection from an "opportunistic" micro-organism (usually a devastating, virulent virus) overwhelms our depressed immune system. This type of infection is serious and exceedingly difficult to overcome. Natural healing focuses on neutralizing the harmful organism, while vigorously nourishing and rebuilding a weakened defense system…. like a medieval castle under siege that holds the siege engines at bay, and tends to its wounded, while refortifying its walls and ramparts against attack.

Are you at risk? What causes immune response to sink to such drastically low levels?

—**Things that alter thymus gland activity, and its immune-controlling ability -** prolonged use of antibiotics or steroid drugs (or pleasure drugs); years of taking birth control pills without a break; unnecessary childhood vaccinations or travel immunizations.

—**Sexual contact with infected, contagious persons** who pass on opportunistic organisms.

—**Living a high stress lifestyle** that depletes basic body reserves.

—**Living with a fast food / chemical food diet,** that causes nutritional deficiencies on a wide scale, so your body can't replenish or refuel. A poor diet also imbalances your body chemistry so that disease elements are able to exist and grow.

—**Auto-toxemia** through poor waste elimination and constipation (essentially you're poisoning yourself).

—**Exhausted liver and adrenal glands,** your body's core defenses.

AIDS, autoimmune diseases like Lupus, M.S., sexually transmitted diseases, fatigue syndromes and parasite infections, are the result of a body unable to defend itself. Even though AIDS is officially caused by HIV (human immunodeficiency virus), a retro-virus that affects DNA and T-cells, there is a growing body of evidence that AIDS is influenced by nutritional factors. AIDS occurs in stages: an asymptomatic state (when the disease is most often passed), a mononucleosis-like stage with one or more AIDS-related complexes, and "full blown" AIDS. The proto- cols here are for those who are diagnosed with HIV, but are asymptomatic, for those who decide to reject orthodox AIDS treatment for alternative methods, and for those who have tried orthodox treatment, but showed no improvement and have decided to use alternative techniques (evidence shows that even new highly acclaimed drugs are failing, and may increase diabetes risk). If you decide to use a combination of orthodox and alternative treatments, seek out advice from a knowledgeable naturopath. Mixing natural products with the powerful drugs used for AIDS can be dangerous.

The goal for overcoming HIV infection is staying strong. System strength greatly reduces the chances of succumbing to full-blown AIDS or to another infection. In some cases, a strong person can develop resistance to the virus effects for many years.

Is there hope if you are HIV positive?

Testing "anti-body positive" does not mean that you have AIDS, only that you have been exposed to the HIV virus. Being HIV positive does not even mean that you will develop AIDS. It is a warning, not a sentence. Some research attests that only 60% of people diagnosed as HIV positive develop full-blown AIDS. HIV positive people are recognizing that the destructive lifestyle factors leading to their diagnosis can be changed to prevent further re-infection, and that they can greatly improve their health condition with lifestyle therapies that can help keep them symptom free. Protease inhibitor "cocktails" and genetic modifying drugs, coupled with a healthy diet, elimination of recreational drugs and responsible sexual behavior are showing promise in HIV status and are dramatically changing the face of AIDS in America. There are thousands of long term infected people in America who co-exist with HIV, lead a normal life and are even free of symptoms.

Holistic therapies show more promise than ever for AIDS, and its related immune syndromes. New drugs may offer new hope, but researchers find that even when 99% of the virus seems to be destroyed, resistant strains can appear within days. It is the alternative treatments that have made the difference in survival or inevitable fatality. Holistic programs are the key to abating symptoms, and they can even slow the advance of the virus itself while improving the quality of life. Alternative expertise is coming into the field via holistic physicians, homeopaths, naturopaths, chiropractors, therapists, nutritional counselors and others. The protocol in this book is a well-received holistic therapy program that has achieved measurable success with AIDS and its attendant conditions. Doses are generally quite high in the beginning. They may be reduced as improvement is observed. Treatments may be used together or separately as desired by each individual, along with the recommendations of a competent professional who has personal case knowledge.

Note: Address allergies and malabsorption before beginning alternative HIV treatment.

AIDS risks and symptoms you may not know.

—It is relatively easy to transfer HIV virus through anal intercourse, more difficult through vaginal or oral sex. Powerful proteins in tears, saliva and pregnant women's urine, friendly flora in the intestinal tract, and HCl in the stomach produce a hostile environment that destroys HIV. There is no such protection in the colon. Suppression of the immune system is believed to occur when the HIV virus slips through the intestinal wall and into the bloodstream. Your immune system normally attacks a virus with macrophages that then die and are removed by the lymphatic system. The toxic wastes are finally dumped into the colon on its last leg of clearance from the body, but in an unprotected colon without friendly bacteria or a good defensive environment, new HIV viruses hatch from the dead macrophages and multiply in the feces all over again, repeating the cycle. The immune system cannot detect the virus in the colon and does not marshal its forces until the infection is in the bloodstream.... often too late if immune defenses are exhausted.

—Symptoms can appear anywhere from 6 months to 3 years after infection. If you feel you are at risk, here are the early symptoms: swollen glands and lymph nodes in the neck area, armpits and groin; inability to heal even minor ailments like a small cut, bruise or cold; unusual fatigue; white patches in the mouth and trouble swallowing (thrush), nail ringworm fungus.

—You can continually re-infect yourself! The most destructive immune-suppressing lifestyle elements are continual exposure to HIV and other STD's through sexual excess and multiple sex partners, and excessive use of chemicals, drugs and alcohol.

—HIV never stands alone as the only culprit in the AIDS connection. Immuno-suppression comes before HIV. Syphilis is usually present in AIDS victims, along with parasites and other viruses that set the stage. Parasites are a co-factor in the development of AIDS. Amoebic parasites rupture immune defense cells that have engulfed the HIV virus in an effort to destroy it allowing the virus to spread. If you are frequently diagnosed with a bacterial infection and treated with antibiotics that don't help, have your stool tested for parasites. If your lifestyle is immuno-suppressing, parasites can easily take hold, and they are becoming an epidemic in the U.S.

—Hepatitis predisposes you to AIDS, because the liver is so weakened it cannot play its part in resisting infection. On the other hand, HIV also predisposes you to hepatitis by grinding down liver defenses.

—Environmental factors, such as water, air and soil, are now full of chemical pollutants that affect delicate immune balance. You must consciously make healthy choices for yourself in relation to these basics of life in order to rebuild your immune defenses.

—Symptoms that mean that AIDS is undeniable: purplish blotches that look like hard bruises occurring on or under the skin, inside the mouth, nose, eyelids or rectum that do not go away (Kaposi's Sarcoma); swollen glands that never go away; persistent dry, hacking cough (unrelated to smoking) that doesn't go away; fevers and night sweats that last for days or weeks; severe, unexplained fatigue; persistent diarrhea; rapid weight loss; visual disturbances; personality changes; memory loss, confusion and depression.

Malnutrition is the number one reason for low immune response.

HIV itself isn't deadly. It simply weakens the immune system to the point where it can't fight. A high resistance, immune-building diet is the key to success. Your intestinal environment must be changed to create a hostile site for the pathogenic bacteria. (Immune-depressing, pathogenic viruses thrive on dead and waste matter.) AIDS victims need about 4000 calories a day, double the usual amount, to sustain body weight. The liquid / fresh foods diet on the next page represents the first "crash course" stage of the change from cooked to living foods. It is an ultra pure diet to control the multiple allergies and sensitivities that occur in immune deficient diseases, yet still supplies the needs of a body that is suffering primary nutrient depletion. For most people, this way of eating is a radical change, with major limitations, but it has been extremely helpful in keeping an HIV positive person free of symptoms, and in symptom recession during full-blown AIDS. This program also helps prevent other attendant diseases, like hepatitis, fibromyalgia and M.S. associated with immune deficiency. The space in this book only allows for a "jump start" form of this diet.

Immune compromised diseases must be approached with vigorous energy, commitment and treatment. For several months at least, your diet should be vegetarian, low in dairy and gluten foods, and very low in saturated fat. This means eliminating all meats, dairy foods except yogurt, fried and fatty foods, with no yeasted breads, coffee, alcohol, salty, sugary or refined foods of any kind; and of course, no drugs, even prescription ones if possible. (See also BUILDING IMMUNE POWER page 213).

A diet protocol for immune compromised diseases works for: *AIDS and AIDS Related Syndromes, Lupus, M.S. Multiple Sclerosis, Candida Albicans, Muscular Dystrophy, Herpes, Rheumatic Fever, Mononucleosis, Chronic Fatigue Syndromes, Human Papilloma Virus (HPV), Lyme Disease, Parasite Infestations, Eczema and Psoriasis, Hepatitis, Toxic Shock Syndrome.*

Cleansing Diet Plan for HIV Infection

The extreme toxicity, fatigue and malabsorption of AIDS forestalls a liquid detox plan ~ it is too harsh for an already weakened system. The suggested step-by-step program below is a modified, enhanced macrobiotic diet, emphasizing more fresh than cooked foods, and mixing in acidophilus powder with foods that are cooked to convert them into living nourishment with friendly flora.

Watchwords:

1—Drink mild, cleansing herb teas and distilled water throughout the day for additional toxin cleansing and system alkalizing.
2—Add $^1/_2$ teasp. ascorbate vitamin C powder with bioflavonoids to any drink throughout the day until the stool turns soupy.
3—Get a good juicer. Three glasses of fresh carrot juice and a potassium drink (pg. 568) daily keep detoxification ongoing.
4—Eat organically grown produce. Eat plenty of foods with anti-parasitic enzymes: cranberries, pineapple, papaya.
5—No fried, fatty foods (they aggravate diarrhea). Avoid concentrated sweeteners, highly processed and chemicalized foods.
6—Rebalance body pH with micro-flora ~ an acidophilus complex with bifidus, and whey protein to inhibit HIV.

—**On rising:** 3 TBS cranberry concentrate in 8-oz. water with $^1/_2$ tsp. vitamin C crystals with bioflavs and $^1/_2$ tsp. Natren BIFIDO FACTORS.
—**Breakfast:** have a glass of fresh carrot juice with 1 teasp. Bragg's LIQUID AMINOS, and whole grain muffins or rice cakes with kefir cheese; or a cup of plain yogurt blended with a cup of fresh fruit, sesame seeds, walnuts, or oatmeal with yogurt and fresh fruit; and $^1/_2$ teasp. Nutricology SYMBIOTICS with FOS, or Transformation PUREZYME powder mixed in aloe vera juice.
—**Midmorning:** take potassium broth (page 568), with 1 teasp Bragg's LIQUID AMINOS and $^1/_2$ tsp. ascorbate vitamin C crystals with bioflavonoids; and have another fresh carrot juice, or pau d'arco tea, with $^1/_2$ teasp. Natren BIFIDO FACTORS added.
—**Lunch:** have a green salad with lemon-flax oil dressing, with avocado, nuts, seeds and alfalfa or broccoli sprouts; or a whole grain sandwich or a chapati with fresh veggies and kefir cheese; or a cup of miso soup with rice noodles, and some steamed veggies and tofu with brown rice; and a cup of pau d'arco tea with $^1/_2$ teasp. ascorbate vit. C, and $^1/_2$ teasp. Natren BIFIDO FACTORS added.
—**Midafternoon:** a carrot juice with Bragg's LIQUID AMINOS and $^1/_2$ tsp. Natren BIFIDO FACTORS added; and a green drink like VITALITY SUPERGREEN from Body Ecology, or Crystal Star ENERGY GREEN™, with $^1/_2$ tsp. vitamin C crystals and bioflavs.
—**Dinner:** a baked potato with Bragg's LIQUID AMINOS, low-fat cheese or kefir cheese and a green salad, and black bean or lentil soup with $^1/_2$ tsp. Jarrow Formulas JARRO-DOPHILUS + FOS added; or a fresh spinach or artichoke pasta with steamed veggies and lemon/flax oil dressing; or a Chinese steam stir-fry with shiitake mushrooms, brown rice and vegetables. Sprinkle $^1/_2$ teasp. Natren BIFIDO FACTORS over any cooked food, and add egg lipids from egg yolk lecithin like Jarrow Corp. LECITHIN: EGG.
—**Before Bed:** take papaya juice, or body chemistry balancing drink such as Crystal Star SYSTEMS STRENGTH™.

Recipes to help immune compromised disease: •DETOXIFICATION FOODS; •HEALING DRINKS; •SOUPS, LIQUID SALADS; •ENZYME-RICH FOODS; •SALADS; •MINERAL RICH FOODS; •LIGHT MACROBIOTICS.

Herb and Supplement Choices

• **Plant anti-virals are effective treatments against HIV:** Advanced Enzyme Formula PROTEASE 375K (only available through practitioners); Olive leaf extract, Licorice root, Nettles, Calophyllum lanegirum and Hyssop inhibit HIV replication; Milk thistle seed protects the liver; Turmeric (curcumin) inhibits TNF, a cytokine that increases HIV in T-cells; Garlic inhibits TNF, and is a leading selenium source; Una da gato and St. John's wort extracts, effective against retro-viruses; Siberian ginseng extract or Imperial Elixir SIBERIAN GINSENG, T-cell helpers; Evening primrose oil, 6000mg daily, cracks and kills infected cells with GLA.

• **TCM immunomodulators effective against HIV:** Lane Labs MGN-3; *Astragalus, Reishi, Shiitake* mushrooms; Grifron MAITAKE D-FRACTION extract; *Atractylodes, Schizandra, Ligustrum*; Chinese bitter melon and wheat grass juice are anti-tumor.

• **Detoxification / purifying supplements:** Egg yolk lecithin. Active lipids help make cell walls virally resistant; American Biologics DIOXYCHLOR or Crystal Star DETOX™ caps as directed; Enzymatic Therapy LIVA-TOX caps, or Jarrow LIPOIC ACID 150mg 3x daily or MRI GLUCOTIZE, Herbal Answers ALOE FORCE JUICE, 2 to 4 TBS daily to curb virus spread with *Echinacea* extract to stimulate interleukin; Nutricology GERMANIUM 150-200mg daily for interferon production.

• **Body normalizers:** Chlorella 20-60 tabs daily; Vitamin C powder with bioflavonoids, 10-30g daily, injection or orally; 300,000IU mixed carotenes to stimulate T-cell activity; Quercetin (blocks HIV the same way as AZT) with BROMELAIN 1500mg daily; CoQ_{10} 360mg daily, with GLUTATHIONE 200mg daily.

Bodywork and Lifestyle Techniques

• **It is absolutely necessary to detoxify the liver for holistic healing to be effective.** See the LIVER CLEANSING program in this book (page 161-163).

• **Remove infected feces from the intestinal tract.** Take a weekly colonic and a weekly enema implant with either supergreen foods like chlorella and spirulina; or micro-flora; or Enzymatic Therapy PHYTO-BIOTIC HERBAL FORMULA; or aloe vera or wheat grass until recovery is well underway.

• **Acupuncture, meditation, massage therapy and visualization** help in normalizing from AIDS symptoms.

• **Get fresh air and sunlight on the body every day.** Take a brisk walk for exercise and morning sunlight. Get plenty of rest. Do deep breathing exercises morning and evening.

• **Overheating therapy helps kill the virus.** Overheating therapy is effective for inhibiting growth of the invading virus. Hydrotherapy is effective in re-stimulating circulation. Take a sauna (pg. 462) or overheating bath (pg. 571).

• **Lifestyle practices to avoid HIV:**
 –Practice safe sex.
 –Avoid anal intercourse.
 –Avoid needle-injected pleasure drugs.
 –Make sure any blood transfusion plasma has been tested for HIV virus.

Can't find a recommended product? Call the 800 number listed in Product Resources for the store nearest you and for more info.

Healing Diet for Lupus and M.S.

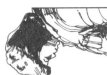

Lupus is a multi-system, auto-immune, inflammatory, viral disease affecting over half a million Americans, more than 80% of them black and Hispanic women. As in other immune breakdown diseases, immune response becomes disoriented and the body develops antibodies that attack its own nerve and connective tissue. Arthritis-like symptoms are severe. Kidneys and lymph nodes become inflamed; in severe cases there is heart, brain and central nervous system degeneration. Orthodox treatment has not been very successful for lupus. Natural therapies focus on rebuilding a stable immune system and relieving pain and stress. My experience shows that you feel worse for 1 or 2 months until toxins are neutralized. Then, suddenly, as a rule, you feel much better. A natural program works, but sometimes requires 2 to 3 years until blood tests clear.

Multiple sclerosis, for another half a million Americans, usually between age 30 and 45, is a progressive, central nervous system disease in which the myelin sheath that wraps the nerves is damaged. M.S. is also triggered by an auto-immune reaction to viruses where the immune system attacks itself. After recognizing the viruses, the immune system creates antibodies to the brain's myelin, which bears an uncanny resemblance to the viruses. M.S. must be treated vigorously. A little therapy does not work, but long lasting remission is possible. Natural therapies take 6 months to a year. Strong immune defense is essential.

Early symptoms for lupus and M.S. are similar. If you have these signs, see a health professional right away:

—Have you had recent seizures, amnesia or unexplained mental disturbance?
—Do you get periodic unpleasant numbness, or prickling sensations in your hands, feet and face?
—Do you have bouts of great fatigue where you are too tired to stand or walk? Are you depressed for no real reason?
—Do you have periods of bad eyesight, preceded by blurring, double-vision and eyeball pain? Are you photosensitive to light?
—Do you have bouts of difficult breathing and slurred speech not related to heart disease?
—Do you have nerve degeneration signs like poor motor coordination, a staggering gait, tremors or dizziness?
—Do you have unexplained rough, red skin patches or chronic nail fungus? Are your mouth, cheeks and nose inflamed?
—Have you had a persistent Candida yeast infection? Or long bouts of chronic fatigue syndrome? Or a chronic low-grade fever?
—Have you taken long courses of antibiotics or prescription drugs from Hydrazine derivatives?
—Are you allergic to certain chemicals? Do you have strong food allergy reactions?
—Do you have latent diabetic or hypoglycemia tendencies? Is your skin overly pale?
—Have you had chronic constipation for years? Do you have chronic bladder and kidney problems?
—Have you had long exposure to lead or heavy metals? Do you have mercury fillings?

An enhancement program for this type of immune breakdown is effective for: *Viral, Bacterial, Respiratory Infections, Staph / Strep Infections, Premature Aging, Mononucleosis, Meningitis, Rheumatic Fever, Measles, Drug Overuse, Herpes, Environmental, Chemical / Heavy Metal Poisoning.*

Immune Stimulating Diet for Lupus and M.S.

A poor diet and long standing stress usually precede M.S. and Lupus. Diet therapy, especially eliminating food allergens, is successful in reducing the symptoms of both diseases. A daily potassium drink (page 568) is critical for the first month of healing. Continue with the drink every other day for another month, then once a week for a third month for sometimes dramatic results. Take 2 glasses of aloe vera juice daily. Drink green tea each morning or Crystal Star GREEN TEA CLEANSER™ to restore homeostasis.

After you follow the immune stimulating diet on this page for at least a month, a low fat, vegetarian diet is strongly recommended.... about 75% fresh foods, with plenty of salads and green drinks and about 10% vegetable proteins from sprouts, legumes and seeds. Eat brown rice every day for B vitamins. Eat fish and sea greens with the rice at least three times a week for EFA's. Keep sugar levels low. Avoid all refined and fried foods, full-fat dairy foods, and caffeine foods. Eliminate meats except fish. Reduce high gluten foods. For lupus, avoid nightshade plants that aggravate arthritis symptoms (like eggplant, tomatoes, tobacco).

Superfood therapy is a significant part of the healing protocol. Here are some of the drinks I recommend: Wakunaga KYO-GREEN drink, Transitions For Health EASY GREENS, Crystal Star SYSTEMS STRENGTH with EFA's, All One GREEN PHYTOBASE for pain, YS Organic Bee Farm ROYAL JELLY with *ginseng*, or YS ROYAL JELLY 2 teasp. daily, Monas CHLORELLA or Sun Wellness CHLORELLA 20 tabs daily to stimulate B and T cells, Crystal Star BIOFLAV, FIBER & C SUPPORT™ drink to rebuild nerve tissue.

—**On rising:** take 2 TBS cranberry concentrate in 8-oz. water or 8-oz. aloe vera juice; or an immune stimulating drink like green tea or Crystal Star GREEN TEA CLEANSER™ or BIOFLAV. FIBER & C™ drink; or Unipro PERFECT PROTEIN.

—**Breakfast:** mix: Red Star nutritional yeast, lecithin granules, pumpkin and flax seeds. Sprinkle some on whole grain granola with almond or rice milk, or fresh fruit and yogurt, or baked or poached eggs, or whole grain muffins or rice cakes with kefir cheese.

—**Mid-morning:** take a green superfood like Crystal Star ENERGY GREEN™, Monas CHLORELLA or Green Foods GREEN MAGMA; or a fresh vegetable juice with 1 TB. green superfood such as Nutricology PRO-GREENS with EFA's or Wakunaga KYO-GREEN.

—**Lunch:** have a leafy salad with lemon-flax oil dressing; or a whole grain sandwich with plenty of sprouts, nuts, seeds, veggies and yogurt or soy cheese; or a turkey or seafood salad sandwich with a light yogurt dressing; or a cup of miso soup with brown rice and sea greens snipped in; or a stir fry or steamed vegetables with onions, brown rice and tofu.

—**Mid-afternoon:** carrot juice or an immune stimulating ginseng tea, or Crystal Star FEEL GREAT tea; rice cakes w. soy spread or veggie dip.

—**Dinner:** have baked or broiled seafood or fish with brown rice and veggies; or a vegetable protein soup or sandwich on whole grain bread; or a light spinach pasta meal; or an Oriental stir-fry with veggies and seafood, a clear broth soup and sea greens snipped on top; or a tofu and veggie casserole with brown rice and a low-fat yogurt, cheese and wine sauce.

—**Before bed:** take a hot apple or cranberry juice; or green tea, or Red Star nutritional yeast broth, or miso soup with sea greens.

Recipes to help lupus or M.S.: •DETOXIFICATION FOODS; •HEALING DRINKS; •SOUPS, LIQUID SALADS; •ENZYME-RICH FOODS; •SALADS, HOT and COLD; •MINERAL-RICH • LIGHT MACROBIOTIC EATING.

Herb and Supplement Choices

• **Reduce inflammation and manage pain:** Transformation PUREZYME, Allergy Research BIOGEN GH; MSM caps 800mg daily or MSM with MICROHYDRIN available at Healthy House; Solaray Centella Asiatica caps 6 daily to rebuild nerves; Quercetin 1000mg and bromelain 1500mg daily.

• **Relieve arthritis-like symptoms:** Acetyl-L-Carnitine 2000mg daily; Chondroitin 1200-Glucosamine 1500mg daily; Crystal Star AR-EASE™; Penny Saved Enterprises NONI, Nutricology or Premier GERMANIUM 150mg.

• **Magnesium, B-vitamins for muscle pain:** Magnesium 800mg daily, or Ethical Nutrients MALIC/MAGNESIUM; B-complex 150mg 3x daily, or Nature's Secret ULTIMATE B tabs.

• **Relieve stress:** SAMe (S-adenosyl methionine) 800mg daily; Reishi mushroom extract or Crystal Star GINSENG-REISHI extract 4x daily; Kava extract or Crystal Star RELAX™ caps with kava for muscle spasms; Crystal Star ADRN-ACTIVE™ caps; St. John's wort 300mg daily or Crystal Star DEPRESS-EX™ for depression.

• **Clean out trigger toxins:** Source Naturals LIPOIC ACID 300-600mg; Crystal Star LIV-ALIVE™ caps 6 daily and LIV-ALIVE™ tea; Vitamin C, $1/4$ teasp. every hour to bowel tolerance, daily for a month; reduce to 5000mg daily. Enzymedica PURIFY.

• **Essential fatty acids:** Evening primrose oil 4000mg daily; or Omega-3 rich flax oil 3x daily; Crystal Star PRO-EST BALANCE™ for DHEA boost; DHA 200mg daily, or New Chapter Supercritical DHA 100. Beta carotene 150,000IU and Jarrow EGG YOLK LECI-THIN for M.S.-related eye damage.

• **Rebuild strong nerve structure:** Crystal Star RELAX caps (highly successful); CoQ$_{10}$ 60mg 4x daily; Ginkgo biloba extract for tremor; Source Naturals MYELIN SHEATH (long-term support).

Bodywork and Lifestyle Techniques

• **Over-medication for lupus, especially by steroid drugs is dangerous;** they weaken the bones, cause excess weight gain and eventually suppress immune response.

—The risk of lupus is 40% more likely in users of oral contraceptives than in women who have not used them. Birth control pills, penicillin, allergenic cosmetics, and phototoxins from UV rays may result in a flare-up of lupus.

• **Sunlight and vitamin D influences remission of M.S.** There are far less incidences of the disease in sun-belt regions.

• **Get plenty of rest and quality sleep.**

• **To heal lupus rough skin patches:** apply Crystal Star ANTI-BIO™ gel with una da gato.

• **Overheating therapy is effective for M.S.** See pg. 571 for an at-home technique.

• **Exercise, guided imagery, massage therapy and mineral baths** are useful in controlling M.S.

• **Effective stress reduction techniques for lupus:** biofeedback, meditation, yoga and acupuncture.

• **Accumulations of aluminum may be a factor.** Avoid it in pots and pans, deodorants and commercial condiments.

• **Remove mercury amalgam fillings.**

• **Take a catnip enema or spirulina implant** once a week for several months.

• **Avoid emotional stress and excessive fatigue.** Keep your diet healthy to keep from triggering the onset of M.S. attacks.

• **Avoid smoking and secondary smoke.** You need all the oxygen you can retain.

Can't find a recommended product? Call the 800 number listed in Product Resources for the store nearest you and for more info.

Healing Diet for Herpes and STD's

Today, sexually transmitted diseases are a factor in every choice we make about our sexuality and our reproductive lives. No treatment for impotence, no questions about fertility or sterility, no decision about child conception can be made without considering the STD quotient. Sexually transmitted diseases are more prevalent, more insidious and more dangerous than ever. Experts say that one out of every five Americans has a sexually transmitted infection. Vaginosis, a little-known, but now common vaginal infection, puts women at risk for far more serious pelvic inflammatory disease (PID), even for contracting AIDS. Whether you believe our culture is paying for years of sexual freedom, (turning out not to be free, after all), or whether you believe that STD's are the result of irresponsible behavior and misinformation, they can't be ignored.

Herpes Simplex II Virus is the most widespread of all STD's, affecting 60 to 100 million Americans (up to 500,000 new cases per year). It is a lifelong infection that alternates between virulent and inactive stages. It may be transmitted even when there are no symptoms, by contact with infected fluids from saliva, skin discharges or sexual liquids. Babies pick up the virus in the birth canal, risking brain damage, blindness, even death. Recurring outbreaks may be triggered by emotional stress, poor diet, food allergies, menstruation, drugs and alcohol, sunburn, fever, or a minor infection. Men are more susceptible to recurrence than women. Outbreaks are opportunistic, taking over when immunity is low and stress is high. Optimizing immune response is of primary importance.

Cervical dysplasia (precancerous cervical lesions), is the newest sexually transmitted epidemic. The infected person often isn't aware of it. It's usually discovered through an abnormal PAP smear. Two sexually transmitted viruses, Human Papilloma Virus (Condyloma warts), and Herpes Simplex II are involved, (these viruses also play a role in cervical cancer). Both are extremely contagious diseases. Natural treatments deal with the causes of genital warts and require strong commitment and significant lifestyle changes.

Avoid the risks for an STD. 1: Early age of first intercourse; 2: multiple sexual partners; 3: nutrient-poor diet; 4: smoking since a teenager; 5: early and long use of oral contraceptives; 6: multiple drug use; 7: oral sex or intercourse with an infected person.

Do you think you have an STD? Early signs usually appear two to three weeks after sexual contact.

—**Cervical dysplasia:** heavy painful periods; usually bleeding between periods.

—**Herpes:** itching, painful blisters appears below the waist, over the groin, thighs and buttocks, accompanied by a fever and flu-like symptoms, and swelling of the groin lymph glands. Blisters swell and fester, rupture, then slowly heal in another 3 to 5 days.

—**Venereal Warts (HPV):** pain during intercourse; chronic yeast infection with heavy, pus-filled discharge; painful, infected sores in the genital area; high fever during infection.

—**Gonorrhea:** cloudy discharge for both sexes; frequent, painful urination, yeast infection symptoms; pelvic inflammation.

—**Chlamydia:** thick discharge in both men and women with pelvic pain. (Constant douching may put you more at risk.)

—**Trichomonas:** caused by a parasite; severe itchiness and thin, foamy, yellowish discharge with a foul odor.

—**Vaginosis:** vaginal discharge with highly unpleasant odor.

Cleansing Diet for Herpes and STD's

Body chemistry balance and strong immune response are essential to healing from STD's. Good nutrition is critical. The diet here should be used for 6 months to 1 year. It emphasizes changing the intestinal environment to strengthen immunity.

Watchwords:

1–Increase high fiber fresh fruits and vegetables, especially cruciferous veggies like cabbage and broccoli.

2–Add high folic acid foods like leafy greens, lima beans, soy foods, brown rice, whole wheat and nutritional yeast.

3–Have a potassium drink (pg. 568) each day. Add other vegetable juices and green drinks (pg. 569) for immune support.

4–Keep your diet alkaline with miso soup, brown rice and vegetables. Normalize intestinal flora with cultured foods.

5–Avoid dairy foods, especially hard cheeses. Avoid red meat and poultry foods. They are often treated with estrogens or other hormone treatments. Eliminate fried foods, nitrate-treated foods, and nightshade plants like tomatoes and eggplant.

6–Add 2 TBS chopped sea greens for protective ocean carotenes. Add fish like salmon and tuna for omega-3 oils and lysine.

7–Reduce caffeine and hard liquor. Particularly avoid foods that aggravate herpes-type infections like sugary and fried foods.

8–For herpes especially, a high lysine-low arginine diet has merit since arginine-containing foods aggravate herpes. Avoid until blisters disappear: chocolate, peanuts, almonds, cashews, walnuts, sunflower and sesame seeds, coconut. Eat wheat, soy, lentils, oats, corn, rice, barley, tomatoes, squash with discretion. Avoid citrus during healing. Increase your fresh fish (rich in lysine).

—On rising: take 2 TBS cranberry concentrate in 8-oz. water or 8-oz. aloe vera juice; or an immune stimulating drink like green tea or Crystal Star GREEN TEA CLEANSER™; or Unipro PERFECT PROTEIN, or Solgar WHEY TO GO protein drink.

—Breakfast: mix 2 TBS each: nutritional yeast, wheat germ and lecithin granules. Sprinkle on what you have for breakfast - a poached egg on a whole grain muffin with kefir cheese; or whole grain cereal or pancakes with apple juice; or yogurt and fresh fruit.

—Mid-morning: a cup of miso soup with sea greens; or more fresh fruit and an herb tea like peppermint (a specific for STD's); or a green drink like Body Ecology VITALITY SUPERGREEN, or Crystal Star ENERGY GREEN™ drink with raw crunchy veggies and kefir cheese.

—Lunch: a small omelet or baked eggs with a green salad; or a high protein sandwich on whole grain bread, with sprouts, nuts, seeds and tofu; or a baked potato with black bean or onion soup and a salad; or a vegetable soup with brown rice and sea greens.

—Mid-afternoon: have some whole grain crackers with raw veggies and kefir cheese; and an herb tea, such as red clover, or Crystal Star FEEL GREAT TEA™, or fresh carrot juice, or another green drink with 1 TB Bragg's LIQUID AMINOS if desired.

—Dinner: have whole grain or spinach pasta with a light sauce and a cup of onion soup; or have some marinated, baked tofu with brown rice and steamed veggies; or have a vegetable stew with a green salad and lemon/flax oil dressing; or have a broccoli stir-fry with brown rice and miso soup with sea greens on top; or have grilled fish or seafood with brown rice and peas or green beans.

—Before bed: have a cup of nutritional yeast broth, or miso soup; or a glass of apple, papaya, or aloe vera juice.

Recipes to help an STD infection: •DETOXIFICATION FOODS; •HEALING DRINKS; •SOUPS, LIQUID SALADS; •ENZYME-RICH FOODS; •SALADS; •MINERAL-RICH •LIGHT MACROBIOTIC EATING; •DAIRY-FREE RECIPES.

Herb and Supplement Choices

•**Control herpes infection:** Olive leaf extract or Nutricology PRO-LIVE olive leaf extract as directed; Lemon balm extract drops in water, and apply lemon balm extract or tea directly to sores (remarkable anti-herpes activity); or Enzymatic Therapy HERPILYN caps and ointment (with lemon balm). Take Crystal Star ANTI-VI™ with St. John's wort, (proven against HSV2); Vibrant Health GIGARTINA red algae (more potent against HSV than dumontiaceae), or Pure Planet RED MARINE ALGAE PLUS.

•**Reduce inflammatory outbreaks:** Crystal Star HRPS™ capsules 6 daily; Quercetin 1000mg with bromelain 1500mg instant relief; Ascorbate vitamin C, or Ester C powder $^1/_4$ teasp. every hour in water up to 10,000mg or to bowel tolerance, daily during an attack. Lysine 1000mg caps 4 daily until outbreaks clear. Peppermint tea is a specific against herpes.

•**For venereal warts:** Dilute oregano oil, 6 drops daily (1 part oregano oil to 4 parts olive oil); apply East Park OLIVE LEAF extract cream. Make up Goldenseal-Chaparral vaginal suppositories (mix powders with vitamin A oil), extremely helpful for venereal warts or dysplaysia, rendering many disease-free. Heal the sores: Crystal Star ANTI-BIO™ caps.

•**For cervical dysplaysia:** Take B-complex with extra 800mcg folic acid daily and sublingual B-12, 2500mcg daily; a vitamin C flush (see above); vitamin A up to 100,000IU for a month (not if pregnant), or beta-carotene 200,000IU; Crystal Star CALCIUM SOURCE™ caps or black cohosh extract to prevent pre-cancerous lesions from becoming cancerous.

•**Prevent future outbreaks:** Take selenium 600mcg daily for a month; Premier Labs LITHIUM .5mg arrests viral replication; MICROHYDRIN available at Healthy House.

Bodywork and Lifestyle Techniques

Note: Long courses of antibiotics and steroid drugs for STD's weaken both the immune system and bone density. Nonoxynol-9 contraceptive gel can put both men and women at more risk for STD's.

•**For herpes:** Apply ice packs to lesions for pain and inflammation relief. Ice may also be applied as a preventive measure when the sufferer feels a flare-up coming on.

–Get some early morning sunlight on the sores every day for healing Vitamin D.

–Take hot baths frequently for overheating therapy to arrest the virus (pg. 571).

–Stress reduction methods like biofeedback and imagery help prevent outbreaks. Acupuncture is effective for herpes.

–If you have an outbreak, don't touch the sores; especially don't touch your eyes if you have touched the sores.

•**For cervical dysplasia:** Nutribiotic GRAPEFRUIT SEED extract, Eidon SILICA MINERAL SUPPLEMENT, or chlorella powder paste, placed against the cervix draws out toxins and sloughs abnormal cells. (See page 572 to learn how to make a vag pack.)

–Alternating hot and cold hydrotherapy promotes healing activity to the pelvic area.

•**Venereal warts:** Earth's Bounty O$_2$ SPRAY daily for a month.

–Overheating therapy is effective in controlling virus replication. Even slight body temperature increases can lead to reduction of infection. See page 571 for effective technique.

–Smoking and a poor diet increase risk because they reduce immune defenses to create an environment for infection. Smokers are 3 times more at risk than non-smokers.

•**For crabs (pubic lice):** wash pubic hair well; tweeze out diehard lice; comb through with a vinegar-water solution.

Can't find a recommended product? Call the 800 number listed in Product Resources for the store nearest you and for more info.

Detox Diet for Parasite Infestation

Parasite invasions have become a major assault on the American population. Some experts estimate that one in six people have a parasite living somewhere in their bodies today. Since a common target for parasites is someone with low immune defenses, almost all victims of immune break-down diseases like candida, HIV and chronic fatigue syndrome, also have parasites in addition to their disease!

Worm and parasite infestations can range from mild and hardly noticeable to serious, even life-threatening in a child. Giardia and Cryptosporidium, caused by exposure to contaminated water, can be serious, acute, unremitting diarrhea, and are usually contracted from parasite infested water or food in third world or tropical countries. Amoebas cause dysentery, acute, unremitting diarrhea, and are usually body, including the brain, weakening the entire system. Pin-worms are the most common parasite in America, affecting 20-42 million people every year, mainly school age children. Nutritional therapy is a good choice for thread and pin worms, but is very slow in cases of heavy infestation. Short term con-ventional medical treatment is often more beneficial for masses of hook and tape worms, and blood flukes. Although a short course of antibiotics may help, a strong immune system and good nutrition are the best defenses against parasites, many of which have become antibiotic-resistant. Very little is being spent on parasite research. Today's drugs that fight parasites do very little to prevent reinfection, and can cause side effects ranging from rash and headache, to vomiting, abdominal pain, Candida yeast overgrowth and toxic psychosis.

Are parasites living in your body? Here are the warning signs:

—Do you have frequent stomach cramps? Is your abdomen distended? Do you have chronic constipation or diarrhea?
—Do you have chronic bad breath, flatulence and unusually foul smelling stools?
—Do you have food sensitivities and allergies? Have you had a fever, or nausea? Are you always tired and weak?
—Are you either excessively hungry or don't want to eat anything? Have you had sudden weight loss or weight gain?
—Do you have bouts of rectal itching? Do you have white thread-like objects or other unusual looking things in your feces?

If you think you may be suffering from a parasite infection, seek expert help right away. Long term parasitic infection can deplete essential nutrients, wreck immunity and destroy overall health.

—**Round worms:** fever, intestinal cramping
—**Hookworms:** anemia, abdominal pain, diarrhea, lethargy
—**Blood flukes:** lesions on the lungs, hemorrhages under the skin - typical in AIDS cases
—**Protozoa, (amoebas):** arthritis-like pain, leukemia-like symptoms, uncontrollable running of the bowels, pain, dehydration.
—**Tapeworms:** intestinal obstruction (even from a single worm); cancer-like symptoms
—**Giardia:** diarrhea, weakness, weight loss, cramping, bloating and fever.
—**Liver flukes:** may be a cause of, and have some of the same symptoms as cancer.

Cleansing Diet to Overcome Parasite Invasions

Emphasis must be on optimal nutrient foods for body regeneration and building a strong immune system. During acute stages, I recommend a short liquid cleanse with vegetable juices, green drinks and soup broths for three days. Complete the week using a cleansing fresh foods diet with plenty of fresh salads and greens to improve body chemistry. Avoid all sweets, pasteurized milk and refined foods. No fast foods or fried foods!

Parasite-cleansing soup broth for minerals and electrolytes: Cover with water in a soup pot - 1 onion, 6 cloves garlic, 4 carrots, 3 stalks celery, handful fresh parsley, 2 potatoes with skins, $^1/_2$ head cabbage, $^1/_2$ bunch broccoli. Simmer 30 minutes. Strain and discard solids. Add 2 TBS Red Star nutritional yeast, $^1/_2$ teasp. acidophilus powder and $^1/_2$ dropperful echinacea extract to broth.

—**On rising:** take 8-oz. organic apple juice or aloe vera juice with a dropperful of garlic extract, like Wakunaga KYOLIC, added; or a glass of lemon juice, 1 teasp maple syrup and water with $^1/_2$ teasp. acidophilus added.

—**Breakfast:** buy a fresh papaya - take papaya juice with 1 TB wormwood tea, and 1 TB molasses; mix 8 of the seeds with honey and chew them. Have an amaranth (only) cereal with apple juice (no milk); a cup of vanilla yogurt with 2 teasp. bee pollen granules.

—**Mid-morning:** take a glass of senna-peppermint tea with 1 TB castor oil, or senna/pumpkin seed tea, and eat a handful of raw pumpkin seeds. For tapeworms, take 4-oz. cucumber juice with honey and water. Drink down at once.

—**Lunch:** Eat a daily green salad with sea greens and shiitake mushrooms; have a cup of vanilla yogurt with 2 teasp. bee pollen granules added.

—**Mid-afternoon:** take a glass senna-peppermint tea with 1 TB castor oil, or senna/pumpkin seed tea with $^1/_2$ teasp. acidophilus added, and eat a handful of raw pumpkin seeds. For tapeworms, have another glass of cucumber juice (see above).

—**Dinner:** Have a bowl of miso soup with 1-oz. shiitake mushrooms and 1 TB. sea greens snipped on top; have another salad, with a bowl of amaranth grain seasoned with Bragg's LIQUID AMINOS.

—**Before bed:** take 8-oz. organic apple juice or aloe vera juice with a dropperful of garlic extract, like Wakunaga KYOLIC, added; take 1 dropperful milk thistle seed extract for liver support and detoxification each night.

Green superfoods really help build immune strength. I have used with success: Monas CHLORELLA; AloeLife ALOE GOLD juice; Crystal Star ENERGY GREEN™ Drink; Wakunaga KYO-GREEN with EFA's; Nutricology PRO-GREENS with EFA's; Vibrant Health GREEN VIBRANCE; Green Foods GREEN MAGMA, Transitions EASY GREENS; Body Ecology VITALITY SUPERGREEN.

Note: Some success has been achieved for amoebic dysentery: Take carrot/beet/cucumber juice once a day for a week to cleanse kidneys. Take a lemon juice/egg white drink each morning. Take 2 TBS epsom salts in a glass of water to purge bowels. Eat a high vegetable protein diet with cultured foods, like yogurt.

Recipes for a parasite infestation: •DETOXIFICATION FOODS; •HEALING DRINKS; •SOUPS, LIQUID SALADS; •ENZYME-RICH FOODS; •SALADS •MINERAL RICH •LIGHT MACROBIOTIC EATING; •DAIRY FREE.

Herb and Supplement Choices

• **Release and cleanse parasites:** Crystal Star VERMEX™, or Ayurvedic TRIKATU tablets; Arise & Shine WORM SQUIRM liquid, Herbal Magic PARASITE KIT, or Farmacopia IMMUN-NEEM capsules, 4 daily with 2 garlic oil caps after every meal for 2 weeks, and 4 cups fennel tea daily. Refrain from eating or drinking until bowels have moved. Repeat for 3 days.

—Then take Creation's Garden PARASINE and keep intestines cleansed and flushed with Crystal Star BITTERS & LEMON CLEANSE™ or Transformation PUREZYME caps each morning.

• **Anti-infectives:** Crystal Star ANTI-BIO™ caps 4 daily with Black walnut hull or Myrrh extract; Una da gato caps 6 daily; Basil tea; Cayenne-Garlic capsules 8 daily; Uni-Key PARA SYSTEM or East Park OLIVE LEAF EXTRACT, a potent parasiticide.

• **Relax bowels to release worms:** Valerian caps 4 daily; Slippery elm tea 2 cups daily; Magnesium 400-800mg daily.

• **Remove infected fecal matter and mucous build-up:** Solaray GARLIC-BLACK WALNUT caps; Enzymatic Therapy PUMPKIN SEED EXTRACT; Ayurvedic BITTER MELON caps; Homeopathic IPECAC as directed.

• **Probiotics restore intestinal health:** Jarrow JARRO-DOPHILUS + FOS; Natren TRINITY powder, $^1/_2$ teasp. 3x daily.

• **For giardia:** Nutribiotic GRAPEFRUIT SEED extract internally; BLACK WALNUT or MYRRH extract, 10 drops under the tongue every 4 hours, or tea tree oil, 4 drops in water 4x daily, or goldenseal extract in water for 10 days.

• **Immune enhancers for parasites:** Nature's Secret PARASTROY; Earth's Bounty OXY CAPS; Floradix HERBAL IRON; Beta carotene 50,000IU daily; B-complex.

Bodywork and Lifestyle Techniques

• **Take garlic enemas** daily during healing.
• **Take a high colonic irrigation** to clean the colon fast and thoroughly.
• **Drink extra water at least 8 to 10 glasses a day** to flush out dead parasites.
• **Apply zinc oxide to opening of anus.** Then take a warm sitz bath using $1^1/_2$ cups epsom salts per gallon of water. Repeat for 3 days. Worms will often expel into the sitz bath.
• **For crabs and lice apply one of the following around anus:**
   −Thyme oil (dilute with a carrier oil)
   −Sassafras oil
   −Tea tree oil
   −Myrrh extract and tea tree oil mixed.

236

Can't find a recommended product? Call the 800 number listed in Product Resources for the store nearest you and for more info.

Anti-Aging - Look and Feel Young Longer!

It's happening to everybody, most of the time faster than we'd like. But even though the hourglass tells us we're older, the passage of time isn't really what ages us. It's the process that reduces the number of healthy cells in our bodies. Whenever the gold and silver years begin for you, it's when the fun begins. Hectic family life quiets down, financial strains ease, business retirement is here or not far off, and you can do the things you've always wanted to do but never had time for - travel, art, music, a craft, gardening, writing, quiet walks, picnics, more social life..... doing what you want to do, not what you have to do.

We all look forward to the treasure years of life, and picture ourselves on that tennis court, bike path or cruise ship, healthy and enjoying ourselves. But, there's a catch - our freedom comes in the latter half of life, and many of us don't age gracefully in today's world. **Still, youth is not a chronological age. It's good health and an optimistic spirit.** Today, the concept of anti-aging is gaining momentum as more people realize they can positively affect their own aging process.

We can see anti-aging in today's elite athletes who perform at world class levels well into their thirties or even forties. And there are sparkling pockets throughout the world of people living healthy lifestyles past the century mark, proving that the downward spiral associated with aging need not happen.

Human lifespan can be increased. Scientists have gathered a wealth of clear data that shows living to 100 or even 120 in a disease-free state is entirely possible, indeed may be a natural state of human life.

This means that the human life span is at least 20 to 30 years longer than most of us actually live today. It's astonishing to realize that we are living only two-thirds of the years our bodies are capable of!

I believe the Fountain of Youth has been available all along. A balanced life is the key to longevity. Good food, pure water, energizing herbs and vitamins, exercise, proper rest, fresh air, sunshine, and a positive outlook on life, really work to keep you young.

Life expectancy lengthens as you age. It's an interesting paradox about aging: The average American child born in 1993 has a life expectancy of 75.4 years.

But average life expectancy at 85 years is six more years. The longer you live, the longer your total expected life span becomes! **Age is not the enemy.... illness is.**

Health is not just the absence of disease. Health is feeling alive, energetic, enthusiastic, with a zest for life. Our bodies are made to live in vibrant health for all but the last few days of our lifespan. Anti-aging is really a way of living our lives, as a fabulous adventure, consciously affirming vitality with our whole being - body, mind and spirit.

Here's what you can look forward to .....a better memory without senility, better skin with fewer wrinkles, a strong heart, healthy bones and immune response, flexible joints and muscles, a good metabolic rate and an active sex life, (good organ and endocrine activity keeps your whole body youthful), along with plenty of energy.

Our cells don't age; they're sloughed off as their efficiency diminishes, to be replaced by new ones. Given the right nutrients, cell restoration continues - well past current life expectancy. But in industrialized countries, pollutants, diets full of chemical-laced, refined foods, nutrient deficiencies, overuse of prescription drugs, all prevent our seniority dreams from becoming a reality.

Today, eighty percent of industrial country people over 65 years old are chronically ill. Yet, loss of vitality and the onset of disease are usually the result of diet, life-style or environment - things we can do something about. Youthfulness is restored from the inside, by strengthening lean body mass, boosting metabolism, increasing immune response with good nutrition and enzymes, getting regular exercise and fresh air, and having a positive outlook.

Are you aging faster than you want to? Don't be overly harsh, but an honest evaluation of the following widely accepted aging signs may identify areas where you can take action to slow down some of aging's effects.

Anti-Aging Check-Up:

• Is your energy level at an all-time low? Have your arms or legs become more flabby? Are your muscles noticeably weaker?

• Have you noticed brown spots around your eyes, nose and hands?

• Has your hairline receded? Is your hair showing a lot of gray?

• Has constipation or irregular bowel movements become a problem for you?

• Do you have some hearing loss or annoying ringing in the ears?

• Do you have joint crackling on one side? Do you have knobs on your index fingers? Are you stiff when you get up in the morning?

• Does it take longer for you to recover from colds and flu? Do colds frequently become pneumonia for you?

• Is your eyesight worsening? Are you afraid you have macular degeneration, glaucoma or cataracts?

• Is it more difficult for you to lose weight? Have you put on 10-15 pounds that you just can't get rid of?

• Are your eyes noticeably dry? Do you have trouble tearing? Are your mouth and nasal passages always dry? If you are a woman, do you have chronic vaginal dryness?

• Is the skin on your hands, arms and neck crepey, thinner, bruising easily or getting strawberry marks?

• Nothing makes you look older than poor teeth. Are your teeth discolored, brittle, or chipped? Have you lost teeth to gum disease?

• Do you experience heartburn, indigestion or gas regularly after eating (a sign of low hydrochloric acid)?

• Have you lost some height? Look in the mirror. Is your neck starting to hunch over at an angle?

• Have you had a recent bone fracture in a fall or accident that would never have meant a break in the past?

• Do you have poor circulation? Are your hands and feet cold even in mild weather?

• Do you have regular insomnia (a sign of adrenal deficiency)?

• Have you noticed a slight but constant trembling of your hands? Are you unsteady when you walk?

• Do you find yourself becoming seriously forgetful? Do you sometimes forget friends' names?

• Have you started to have heart palpitations? or small chest pains?

The biggest complaint I hear is the annoying drop in energy levels! People are always somewhat shocked when they don't have the energy to do something that used to come easily. We never thought it would happen to us, of course. The most worrisome part is that these signs of aging seem to be coming on sooner than we were led to believe.

Start restoring your looks and your energy by addressing the factors which affect aging the most:

—**Take a look at your prescription drugs:** Many drugs lead to serious body imbalances by impairing nutrient uptake, and they can spur a free radical assault that accelerates aging. They also tend to interact, especially hormonal drugs, like Viagra or Propecia.

—**Take a look at your habits:** If you're still a smoker (more than a pack a day), or live with one, nicotine saps your body's antioxidants, and is a sure link to skin wrinkling, let alone its links to degenerative diseases.

—**Take another look at your diet:** You've probably already cut down on fat and fried foods. But the chemicals and additives in foods like lunch meats, and most pre-prepared foods are the real culprits for early aging. They can create an over-acid condition that aggravates arthritis, are the triggers for many allergies, and like drugs, set up a free-radical cascade favorable to disease.

—**Take a look at your sugar intake:** If you eat a lot of sweets or drink hard alcohol regularly, your diet is probably high in sugar. Sugar is also a hidden ingredient in most processed foods. A high sugar diet wipes out immunity and reduces tissue elasticity. Artificial sweeteners with aspartame are linked to degenerative nerve disorders.

—**Take a look at your teeth and gums:** Almost nothing shows age faster than discolored teeth, lost teeth or red, receding gums. Take CoQ-10 right away for gum problems, about 200mg daily, for the first month. See a holistic dentist for discoloration problems.

—**Take a look in the mirror:** If you're starting to see that your neck is no longer straight, but is at a slight forward angle, or if your shoulders are looking hunched, you may be losing bone density: start a strengthening exercise program right away. Make sure it includes elongating, smooth muscle stretches and stick with it. This is one aging sign that exercise can rapidly reverse.

—**Take a look at your workplace:** Radical early aging used to show in coal miners. It happens today to people working around chemicals in the automotive, pesticide or household cleaning products industry; these chemicals overload your body's natural detox system.

—**As we age, many of us move to southern climates:** 90% of skin cancers and wrinkles are traced to sun exposure. Make sure you're using SPF 40 for your face, up to SPF 26 for your body and wear a hat, or face those fine lines in your mirror. Healthy House PHYCOTENE MICROCLUSTERS and MICROHYDRIN offer significant protection against sun exposure.

Your age is only a statement of time. Vibrant health doesn't have to end as you grow older. The idea is to have all the experiences, all the memories and all the wisdom your years give you. They contribute to the richness of your life, to the character of your looks, and to the hope for your future. As for sexuality, I think it only gets better. I personally wouldn't give up a single year of my life to recapture my so-called youth. Not even the hard ones. Natural therapies are ideal for antiaging because they support rejuvenation. With the right focus, you can look young longer and make the second era of your life the best ever.

A diet program for anti-aging is also effective for: *Immune Health, Healthy Sexuality, Poor Digestion, Heart and Circulatory Health.*

Longevity Begins with a Good Diet

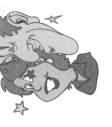

A nutrition rich diet is the centerpiece of a vibrant long life. Health experts agree that the food health pyramid needs to be modified as we age. Your diet must become even more nourishing, even higher in antioxidants as the years pass. A good diet improves health, provides a high energy level, maintains harmonious system balance, keeps memory and thinking sharp, staves off disease, and contributes to a youthful appearance. The aging process slows down if your internal environment is good.

Lower your daily calories to reduce the signs of aging. Your body needs fewer calories and burns calories slower as you age; optimum body weight should be 10 to 15 pounds less than in your 20's and 30's. A low calorie diet protects DNA from damage, and prevents tissue degeneration. An easy way to control a slow upward weight gain is to compose your diet of 50% fresh foods.

Focus on whole, fresh, organically grown foods to protect your skin from the signs of aging. Your skin is a window on your diet. The American diet was already saturated with chemicals from pesticides, preservatives and additives. Now over 70% of our foods are genetically altered. The brown age spots and rough texture we see on our skin are signs that our bodies are less able to process our foods correctly.

Keep your glands young! Trace minerals, essential fatty acids and protein are important for youthful gland function. Good gland foods: sea foods and sea greens, fresh figs and raisins, pumpkin and sesame seeds, broccoli, avocados, yams and dark fruits. Herbal digestive tonics with ginger, mineralizers from dark leafy greens like spinach, and herbal adaptogens like ginseng are gland boosters.

The Best Anti-Aging Foods:

—**Fresh fruits and vegetables!** Fresh produce gives you the most vitamins, minerals, fiber and enzymes. Plants have the widest array of nutrients and are the easiest for your body to use. Enzyme-rich fruits and vegetables are the essential link to stamina levels. Eat organically grown foods when possible to insure higher nutrient content and avoid toxic sprays. Have a green salad every day! European research reveals the immune cells of vegetarians are twice as effective as meat eaters in killing cancer cells!

Note: Fresh fruit and vegetable juices offer quick absorption of high-quality nutrients, especially antioxidants, which protect the body against aging, heart disease, cancer, and degenerative conditions.

—**Sea greens are the ocean's superfoods.** They contain all the necessary elements of life and transmit the energies of the ocean to us as proteins, complex carbohydrates, vitamins, minerals, trace minerals, chlorophyll, enzymes and fiber. Sea greens and sea foods stand almost alone as potent sources of natural iodine. By regulating thyroid function, they promote higher energy levels and increased metabolism for faster weight loss after 40.

—**Whole grains, nuts, seeds and beans for protein, fiber, minerals and essential fatty acids.** Sprouted seeds, grains, and legumes are some of the healthiest foods you can eat. They are living nutrients that can go directly to your cells.

—**Cultured foods for friendly digestive flora.** Yogurt tops the list, but kefir and kefir cheese, miso, tamari, tofu, tempeh, even a glass of wine at the evening meal also promote better nutrient assimilation. Raw sauerkraut is especially good for boosting friendly bacteria. (Avoid commercial sauerkraut processed with alum.)

—**Plenty of pure water every day** keeps your body hydrated and clean. Drink six to eight glasses of bottled water daily on a regular basis. See "Water" on pg. 58 for more info.

—**Keep your body chemistry balanced** for optimum health with green drinks, green foods, miso, and grains like rice.

—**Healthy, unsaturated fats and oils,** 2 to 3 tablespoons a day are enough to keep your body at its best.

—**Fish and fresh seafoods** two to three times a week enhance thyroid and metabolic balance for weight control and brain acuity.

—**Eat poultry, other meats, butter, eggs, and dairy in moderation.** Avoid fried foods, excess caffeine, red meats, highly seasoned foods, refined and chemically processed foods altogether.

—**On rising:** take a high nutrient drink, like Omega Nutrition VITALITY SUPERGREEN DRINK, or ALL 1 VITAMIN/MINERAL DRINK in orange or apple juice; or a glass of aloe vera juice. Add 2 teasp. CC Pollen HIGH-DESERT bee pollen granules.

—**Breakfast:** make a mix of 2 TBS each: nutritional yeast, lecithin granules, toasted wheat germ, bee pollen granules and flax seeds. Sprinkle some on your breakfast choice - fresh fruits, plain or with yogurt; or whole grain granola with apple juice, yogurt, rice milk or almond milk; or whole grain muffins with a little kefir cheese; or a baked or poached egg or omelet.

—**Mid-morning:** have a green drink (page 569) or Monas CHLORELLA, Green Foods GREEN MAGMA, or Crystal Star ENERGY GREEN™ drink in apple juice; or a tonifying herb tea, like Siberian ginseng tea, or Crystal Star GINSENG 6 SUPER™ tea; and some more fresh fruit with yogurt; or Crystal Star BIOFLAV, FIBER & C SUPPORT drink™.

—**Lunch:** have a leafy green salad with a cup of miso or ramen noodle soup; or a cup of black bean, lentil, or other protein soup with baked potato and kefir cheese or yogurt sauce; or a fresh fruit salad with cottage cheese or yogurt cheese, and veggie baked chips or crackers; or a light seafood or turkey salad; or a hot or cold vegetable pasta salad.

—**Mid-afternoon:** have fresh or dried fruits with yogurt; or crackers or rice cakes with a vegetable, soy or kefir spread, and miso broth; or a cup of ginseng tea, mint tea, or Crystal Star FEEL GREAT™ tea, and some crunchy veggies with a yogurt or soy cheese dip;

—**Dinner:** a hearty high protein vegetable, nut and seed salad with soup and whole grain muffins or cornbread; or an Asian stir-fry with brown rice and miso soup; or a baked veggie, tofu and whole grain casserole; or a vegetable quiche with a whole grain crust, and light yogurt-wine sauce; or baked or broiled seafood with a green salad and brown rice or steamed veggies; or roast turkey with cornbread or rice and a salad. Have a glass of wine for digestion, heart health and relaxation.

—**Before Bed:** have a cup of chamomile tea or apple or papaya juice, or a cup of Red Star nutritional yeast broth; or a glass of aloe vera juice for regularity the next morning.

Recipes for anti-aging diets: •BLENDING EAST and WEST; •HEALING DRINKS; •SOUPS, LIQUID SALADS; •ENZYME-RICH FOODS; •SALADS; •MINERAL-RICH FOODS; •LOW FAT RECIPES; •HIGH FIBER FOODS.

Herb and Supplement Choices

• **Take anti-aging superfoods every day:** My favorites- Omega Nutrition VITALITY SUPER GREEN; NutriCology PROGREENS; Green Foods VEGGIE MAGMA; Rainbow Light HAWAIIAN SPIRULINA; Pines MIGHTY GREENS; Ethical Nutrients FUNCTIONAL GREENS; Monas CHLORELLA; Vibrant Health GREEN VIBRANCE; Futurebiotics VITAL GREEN tabs; Nature's Secret ULTIMATE GREEN tabs.

• **Boost your enzymes:** the length of life is tied to your food enzymes because they decrease your body's rate of enzyme exhaustion. My favorites - Enzymedica DIGEST, TRANSFORMATION PUREZYME (protease); Herbal Products & Development POWER PLUS; Rainbow Light ADVANCED ENZYME SYSTEM.

• **Boost antioxidants to stay disease free:** My favorites- MICROHYDRIN available at Healthy House; Alpha lipoic acid; Bee pollen-Royal Jelly; CoQ-10; Germanium; Carotenes; Vitamin C with bioflavonoids; Vitamin E; Glutathione; (OPC's) Oligomeric *Proanthocyanidins*; Selenium.

—**Best herbal antioxidants:** *Ginkgo biloba*; *Astragalus*; *Shiitake mushrooms*; *Reishi mushrooms*; *Cat's Claw*; *Arjuna*; *Pine bark*; *Grapeseed*; *Alfalfa*; *Hawthorn*.

• **Optimize your brain nutrients:** My favorites- NADH (Co-enzyme Nicotinamide Adenine Dinucleotide); Phosphatidylserine; Choline: (Just eating 2 TBS of lecithin a day can do the job!)

• **Adaptogen herbs keep immune response strong:** My favorites- *Panax Ginseng* (red, white and American ginsengs); *Siberian Ginseng* (*eleuthero*); *Noni*; *Schizandra*; *Suma*; *Gotu Kola*; *Fo-Ti* (*Ho-Shou-Wu*); *Cordyceps*; *Horsetail*; *Bilberry*.

• **Natural growth hormone:** Allergy Research BIOGEN GH or BIOGEN PRO (practitioners only); Liddell VITAL HGH.

Bodywork and Lifestyle Techniques

• **Advantages of regular exercise for anti-aging:**

–Exercise boosts circulation and oxygen use for energy.
–Exercise reduces the risk for heart attacks and cancer.
–Exercise fans the metabolic fires for weight control.
–Exercise reduces stress and tension, and relaxes you.
–Exercise stimulates hormone production.
–Exercise contributes to strength; Inactivity to fatigue.
–Weight bearing exercises trigger bone remineralization.
–Exercise helps agility and joint mobility.

• **Limit your use of microwaves.** Microwaving foods kills enzymes, an important tool for healing, detoxification, glandular functioning and estrogen metabolism.

• **Deep breathing is a powerful way to decrease stress and slow the aging process.** Deep diaphragm breathing lowers anxiety, relaxes and loosens muscles, and generates an inner feeling of peace and calm. Diaphragm breathing strengthens heart and lungs, AND encourages more restful sleep.

1) Inhale deeply through your nose. Try to fill your lungs.
2) Exhale slowly through your mouth.
3) Breathe deeply for 30 seconds to calm and center yourself during anxious moments. Breathing deeply for just one minute prevents the short breaths which negatively affect the oxygen-carbon dioxide content of your blood.
4) Breathe deeply to fill the lower part of your lungs. Notice the pop-pop feeling in your chest as unused lung pockets open up. Slowly exhale; your abdomen tightens.
5) As you breathe in, think of oxygen reaching and recharging all the cells of your body. As you exhale, imagine all the stress and tension leaving your body.

Can't find a recommended product? Call the 800 number listed in Product Resources for the store nearest you and for more info.

You Look Marvelous! Diet for a Body Beautiful

A beautiful body comes from within. Radiant skin, lustrous, lively hair, bright eyes and strong pink nails, all mirror a body in good health. Your appearance elements are also the surest signs of your nutritional condition. If your hair, skin and eyes need help, feed them the best nutrients. Good dietary care and habits show quickly. I find that most people experience noticeable appearance improvement in about three weeks.

Beautiful skin, for example, is more than skin deep. Your skin is your body's largest organ. Skin mirrors our emotional state and our hormone balance. The skin's protective acid mantle inhibits the growth of disease-causing bacteria. Skin problems reflect a stressed lifestyle almost immediately. (Allergies show up first on your skin.) Our skin is the essence of renewable nature...it sloughs off old, dying cells every day for a new start. Herbal nutrients are great for skin... they're packed with absorbable minerals, antioxidants, EFA's and bioflavonoids to cleanse, hydrate, heal, alkalize, and balance. Relaxation, nourishment and improved nutrition show quickly in skin beauty.

Your hair is another mirror of your health. Changes in hair are often the first indication of nutritional deficiencies. We all want it... thick, gorgeous hair. Your scalp has at least 100,000 hairs so you have a lot to work with. Hair consists of protein layers called keratin. In healthy hair, the cell walls of the hair cuticle lie flat like shingles, leaving hair soft and shiny. In damaged or dry hair, the cuticle shingles are broken and create gaps that make hair porous and dull. Hair problems are never isolated conditions. They are the result of more basic body imbalances.

Your eyes are not only the windows of your soul, but windows to body health as well. Your lifestyle profoundly affects your "eyestyle." No other sense is so prone to poor health conditions. Many drugs, (prescription, recreational and over-the-counter), react with your eyes. The worst offenders are cocaine, excessive use of chemical diuretics, sulfa drugs or tetracycline, aspirin, nicotine, phenylalanine and hydrocortisone. A happy liver is the key to healthy eyes. The most stressful eyesight situations are using a computer for most of your workday, and a sedentary lifestyle. Most eye-improving supplements need 2 to 3 months for effectiveness.

Are your appearance elements showing signs they need some TLC?

—**Check your hair:** Is it too dry or too oily? Is it brittle hair with split ends? Does it lack of bounce and elasticity? Do you have lots of falling hair (normal shedding is about 25 to 50 hairs a day? Do you have flaky deposits on your scalp?

—**Check your eyes:** Is your vision degenerating? Do your eyes become strained easily? Does your sight become worse as the day goes on? Do you get frequent headaches over your eyes? Do you get spots and floaters before your eyes?

—**Check your skin:** Is your skin and its acid mantle out of balance? with sores or spottiness? Does it look dry and cracked? Is it itching, chapped, always scaling? Is it too dry or too oily? Is it red and rashy? (all signs of an unbalanced acid mantle).

A diet for beautiful hair, skin and eyes also helps: *Chronic Acne, Hair Loss, Deteriorating Vision and Night Blindness, Dandruff, Fungal Skin Infections, Dry Skin, Age Spots, Easy Bruising, Chronic Skin Infections, Eczema and Psoriasis, Split, Brittle Nails, Glaucoma and Conjunctivitis.*

One Week Toxin Elimination Cleanse for Skin, Hair and Eyes

A brown rice cleanse is based on macrobiotic principles for body balance. A brown rice diet is cleansing, yet filling. You don't feel like you're on a cleanse at all, yet it does the trick. It's a diet that uses rice as a nutrient building food, and vegetables and vegetable juices as concentrated cleansing supplements. A brown rice diet is loaded with B-vitamins and essential fatty acids. It's full of potassium, natural iodine, and other minerals, so most people notice improvement in their hair, skin texture and nail growth. Most people experience about a 2 to 5 pound weight drop during this cleanse, and it's a great way to transition from an unhealthy diet into a better diet. Most people notice an improvement in vitality and energy levels right away, too.

The night before your brown rice cleanse...
A green leafy salad for dinner sweeps your bowels. Take an herbal enema the night before your cleanse.

The next day....
—**On rising:** take 2 fresh squeezed lemons, 1 TB maple syrup in 8-oz. of water; or a glass of aloe vera juice or apple juice.
—**Breakfast:** have watermelon juice (rich in natural silica); or apple/alfalfa sprout juice with Crystal Star SILICA SOURCE™ drops.
—**Mid-morning:** have or a skin tonic drink: juice 1 cucumber, 1 handful fresh parsley, 1 4-oz. tub fresh sprouts and sprigs of fresh mint. or have a green drink, like Mona's CHLORELLA or Crystal Star ENERGY GREEN™.
—**Lunch:** have a veggie juice like PERSONAL V-8 (page 569); or take Crystal Star CLEANSING & PURIFYING™ tea or DAILY DETOX by M.D. with 2 Transformation DIGESTZYME caps.
—**Mid-afternoon:** have a carrot juice; or an herb tea like nettles or green tea; or apple juice, or apple/alfalfa sprout juice; or have a superfood green drink, like Crystal Star ENERGY GREEN™ with 1 teasp. nutritional yeast and 1 teasp. wheat germ added.
—**Dinner:** have steamed brown rice and mixed steamed vegetables. Sprinkle with snipped, dry sea greens (like dulse or kelp). Use 1 TB flax or olive oil, and 1 TB Bragg's LIQUID AMINOS. Or make a high luster skin broth: In 2 ½ cups water, cook 2 cups chopped fresh mixed vegetables, add 1 teasp. miso and 2 TBS chopped dried sea greens. Add 4 TBS. sunflower seeds for a protein boost. Vegetable protein aids faster healing for damaged skin.
—**Before Bed:** have Crystal Star BEAUTIFUL SKIN™ TEA or Japanese green tea for skin support; or a pineapple/papaya, papaya or apple juice; or Red Star nutritional yeast broth for high B vitamins; or a cleansing booster drink like Crystal Star FIBER & HERBS CLEANSE™ caps or Nature's Secret ULTIMATE CLEANSE to stimulate the body to eliminate wastes rapidly.

The next 6 days:
Have 2 to 3 glasses of any blend of mixed vegetable juices throughout the day. Don't eat any solid food during the day. Have steamed brown rice and mixed vegetables for an early dinner each evening. Drink at least 6 to 8 glasses of pure bottled or mineral water throughout the day for best results.

Herb and Supplement Choices

• **During detox:** Take $^1/_4$ to $^1/_2$ teasp. ascorbate vitamin C crystals with any drink or juice 3 to 4 times daily throughout the elimination diet, for interstitial tissue and collagen formation.

—Take liquid acidophilus with any juice or drink - 1 teasp. 3 to 4 times daily throughout the elimination diet, for best assimilation and to keep the system alkaline.

• **Skin herbal support:** Crystal Star BEAUTIFUL SKIN™ CAPS - blemishes and skin maintenance; Nature's Apothecary SKIN SUPPORT - blood purifiers and mineralizers; Herbs Etc. DERMATONIC - stimulates waste elimination.

• **Smoothing/hydrating herbs for skin:** Crystal Star SKIN THERAPY #2™ CAPS; chamomile tea or CamoCare FACIAL THERAPY; lavender aromatherapy oil to reduce puffiness.

• **Skin vitamins and minerals:** Diamond HERPANACINE; Futurebiotics HAIR, SKIN & NAILS; MSM (Methyl Sulfonyl Methane) helps create softer & smoother skin and repairs damaged or scarred skin: MSM WITH MICROHYDRIN available at Healthy House.

• **Silica, a mineral for collagen support, reduces dry, wrinkled skin.** Eidon SILICA MINERAL SUPPLEMENT; Flora VEGESIL; Crystal Star SILICA SOURCE™.

• **Antioxidants are important for skin health:** Beta carotene protects against the sun's free radicals; Vitamin E protects against the lipid peroxidation caused by UV rays; Bioflavonoids improve vascularization of the skin.

• **Essential fatty acids:** helps skin dehydration and wrinkling: *Evening Primrose* oil 4000mg daily.

• **Enzyme support:** Protease heals skin disorders; Transformation PUREZYME.

Bodywork and Lifestyle Techniques

• **Get early morning sunlight** on the face and body every day possible, for natural A and D.

• **Rub the face with insides of papaya and cucumber skins** when you peel them for your juices. They are excellent for alkalizing acid waste and are a natural AHA treatment.

• **AHA's:** Noni of Beverly Hills BRILLIANT TREATMENT CREAM with 5% AHAs and vitamins B, C and E.

• **Make a skin beauty face tea:** chamomile and calendula flowers, lemon juice, rosehips and rosewater. Strain, and apply with cotton balls to the skin, or pour as a rinse through the hair, to add minerals and toning agents.

• **Enema:** Take an enema the first and the last day of your skin cleansing program to help release toxins and clear the skin. Or, have a colonic for a more thorough cleanse.

• **Dry brush for healthy skin:** Use a natural bristle brush. Start with the soles of your feet - brush vigorously making rotary motions and massage every part of your body - starting at the feet and work up to the neck.

• **Massage** your skin and scalp for circulation and tone.

• **Essential oil support:** Essential oils assist a skin cleanse: lavender, geranium, sandalwood and neroli. Use one or a combination of all three oils. Put a total of 15 drops essential oil in 2-oz of a carrier oil (such as jojoba) and rub on the skin.

• **Bathe:** High mineral bath. Add 1 cup Dead Sea salts, 1 cup Epsom salts, $^1/_2$ cup regular sea salt and 4 TBS. baking soda to a tub; swish in 3 drops lavender, 2 drops geranium, 2 drops sandalwood and 1 drop neroli oil.

Can't find a recommended product? Call the 800 number listed in Product Resources for the store nearest you and for more info.

Good Looks Restoration Diet for Skin, Hair and Eyes

A good diet is the first place to turn when you want to make real improvements in your appearance. Beautiful eyes, skin, hair and nails need a diet rich in fresh fruits and vegetables, and plenty of water. Beautiful skin, hair and eyes all depend on a healthy liver. Too much alcohol, caffeine and drugs put a heavy load on the liver and rob the body of B vitamins. All tissues need a rich, high oxygen blood supply, and plenty of mineral building blocks. Plants are the most absorbable way for the body to get them.

Watchwords for beautiful skin, hair, nails and eyes:

Soft smooth skin depends on vitamin A, vitamin C, mineral-rich foods, and vegetable protein foods for collagen and tissue strength. Eat potassium-rich foods if your skin is dry: leafy greens, spinach, bell peppers, bananas, broccoli, sesame and sunflower seeds, fish and sea greens. Eat cleansing foods if your skin tone is muddy: fresh fruit, vegetable and fruit juices, celery, cucumbers. Eat vitamin C, E, carotene-rich foods for better skin texture: sea foods and fresh greens. Eat cultured foods if your skin is spotty: yogurt, tofu and kefir. Eliminate red meats, fried, fatty and fast foods. Reduce caffeine, dairy foods and salty, sugary foods. They show up on your skin. Eat high fiber foods: fruits, vegetables and whole grains to maintain regularity, and healthy skin. Don't rely exclusively on fiber supplements for your fiber.

Turn your hair from drab to fab with vegetable or whole grain protein for maximum growth, and high carotene foods like broccoli, carrots and greens for "permanent" appeal. Eat these foods if your hair is brittle: Carrots, green peppers, lettuces, bananas, strawberries, apples, peas, onions, green peppers, cucumbers, sprouts, green tea. Have aloe vera juice in the morning if your hair is dry. Avoid saturated fats, sugars and processed, refined foods. They show up in hair texture.

Your eyes sparkle when you eat protein from the sea and soy foods (rich in omega-3 fatty acids), whole grains, low fat dairy foods, and eggs (full of zeaxanthin). Good vision vegetables are broccoli, sunflower and sesame seeds, leeks, onions, cabbage, cauliflower, corn, barley, blueberries, watercress. Eyes love vitamin A and high mineral foods: leafy greens (kale); sea greens, loaded with carotenoids and EFA's (2 dry TBS daily); orange and yellow veggies; broccoli, seafood and parsley. Reduce your sugar intake. Avoid chemicalized foods, especially fried and saturated fat foods, pasteurized dairy and red meats. These foods cause the body to metabolize slowly, use sugars poorly, and form crystallized clogs in your eyes.

Liver malfunction is a common cause of eye problems. Keep your liver happy with B-vitamins, high fiber foods that absorb excess bile and increase regularity; potassium-rich sea foods, chlorophyll-rich leafy greens and sea greens, enzyme-rich yogurt and kefir, and sulphur-rich eggs, garlic and onions.

When you're working on the appearance of your eyes, try to have a vision drink twice a week: Mix 1 cup carrot juice, $\frac{1}{2}$ cup eyebright tea, 1 egg, 1 TB toasted wheat germ, 1 tsp. rose hips powder, 1 TB honey, 1 tsp. sesame seeds, 1 tsp. Red Star nutritional yeast, 1 tsp. kelp granules.

The Daily Diet

—On rising: a glass of watermelon juice in summer; apple/cranberry juice in winter; and/or a superfood drink, like Transitions EASY GREENS with sea greens, or Crystal Star SYSTEMS STRENGTH™ drink. A low fat protein drink each morning has a dramatic effect on dry hair; Add 1 tsp. Red Star nutritional yeast for hair color; a glass of aloe vera juice like Herbal Answers ALOE FORCE juice for cleansing.

—Breakfast: have a glass of grapefruit juice, or Crystal Star BIOFLAV, FIBER & C SUPPORT™ drink; make a mix of the following hair and skin foods and take 3 TBS daily: wheat germ (oil or flakes), blackstrap molasses, nutritional yeast and sesame seeds. Sprinkle some every morning on your breakfast food - whole grain cereal or granola with yogurt and fresh fruit (especially bananas, strawberries, papaya and peaches); or oatmeal or whole grain pancakes, with a little maple syrup or honey.

—Mid-morning: have a cup of miso soup with sea greens snipped on top; or some yogurt with fresh fruit; or a green drink, such as Sun Wellness CHLORELLA or Crystal Star ENERGY GREEN™ drink.

—Lunch: have a green leafy salad, with cucumber, sprouts, bell pepper and lemon-oil dressing; or steamed vegetables with marinated tofu and brown rice or a baked potato; or a fresh fruit salad, with peaches, apricots and cottage cheese or yogurt cheese; or a seafood and spinach pasta salad with peas; or an avocado, low-fat cheese sandwich with lentil, or onion soup.

—Mid-afternoon: have a carrot juice or Green Foods CARROT ESSENCE drink; have a cup of refreshing herb tea, like chamomile or red clover tea, or Crystal Star BEAUTIFUL SKIN™ or HEALTHY HAIR & NAILS™ TEA; or a cup of ramen soup with noodles, or miso soup; and/or crunchy raw veggies with kefir cheese or yogurt cheese.

—Dinner: have a large dinner salad with red onions, cucumbers and sprouts, and whole grain muffins with kefir cheese; or a light beans and rice dish with a small green salad; or a broccoli, or asparagus quiche with onion soup; or baked or broiled seafood or fish with veggies and brown rice; or an oriental stir-fry with Chinese greens, rice and a light broth soup.

—Before bed: have a glass of papaya or apple juice; or Red Star nutritional yeast broth for relaxation and B vitamins.

Note: Drink plenty of pure bottled water every day for clear skin. Avoid red meats, refined sugars and flour, caffeine-containing foods, fried or fatty foods, foods with colorings and preservatives. All slow metabolism, use sugars and fats poorly, and encourage clogs to form. NO JUNK FOODS.

Recipes for looking marvelous: •BLENDING EAST and WEST; •HEALING DRINKS; •SOUPS, LIQUID SALADS; •ENZYME-RICH FOODS; •SALADS; •MINERAL-RICH FOODS; •LOW FAT FOODS; •HIGH FIBER FOODS.

Herb and Supplement Choices

• **Minerals are critical to hair health:** Crystal Star HEALTHY HAIR & NAILS™ tea; Horsetail extract; or Crystal Star SILICA SOURCE™ extract daily or Body Essentials SILICA GEL. Sea greens minerals are dramatic for hair growth: 2 TBS daily dried snipped sea greens or 6 kelp tablets daily; or Crystal Star IODINE-POTASSIUM™ caps 4 daily or Nature's Path TRACE-MIN-LYTE with sea greens.

• **EFA's for hair shine:** Evening Primrose oil 2000mg daily. Rub in Jojoba oil daily; Shampoos rich in EFA's-Hemp or Henna shampoo, Neem Oil and Babassu Palm shampoo.

• **Essential fatty acids are critical for skin:** Eat chia and sunflower seeds; Evening primrose oil 4000mg daily; Nature's Secret ULTIMATE OIL, Aloe vera gel; Barleans flax oil caps 3 daily. Zia ULTIMATE MOISTURE; Vitamin A & D 25,000/1,000IU.

• **Smoothing/hydrators for skin:** MSM, 1000mg daily; Cysteine 1000mg. PHYCOTENE MICROCLUSTERS, mixed carotenes from sea greens available at Healthy House. Make my sea plant rapid facial: sprinkle 1 tsp. kelp granules in a bowl. Blend with 1 TB aloe vera gel. Apply to face and neck; leave on 10 minutes, rinse.

• **Expand your eye power:** Crystal Star EYEBRIGHT HERBAL™ capsules 4-6 daily; Ginkgo biloba extract 2x daily.

• **Clarifying natural eye treatments** (use as an eyewash and take internally): Crystal Star EYEBRIGHT HERBAL™ tea; Sea greens caps for blurry vision; Raspberry tea bags or green tea bags for bloodshot eyes; Borage seed tea for sore eyes.

• **For "computer" eyes:** Press points under eyebrows; press points in inner corners of eyes; squeeze eyebrows; look up, down, right and left every half hour.

Bodywork and Lifestyle Techniques

• **Bodywork for hair:** Massage scalp each morning for 3 minutes to stimulate hair growth. Sunlight helps hair grow, but too much sun dries and damages. Wash hair in warm, not hot water. Rinse in cool water for scalp circulation.

• **A super hair tonic:** Mix 8-oz green tea and 8-oz. rosemary tea (fresh sprigs best). Strain; add 1 TB lemon juice, 1 TB white vinegar. Work through hair, leave on 1 minute. Rinse.

• **Hot oil treatment:** Mix olive oil with drops of essential lavender and rosemary oils; rub in hair. Leave on 5 minutes; rinse.

• **Bodywork to enhance a cosmetic diet:** Early morning sunlight on the body for vitamin D; Fresh air, rest and mild exercise to keep the circulation free and flowing; Dry skin brushing once a week for circulation and to slough dead cells.

• **Beautiful skin secrets:** Swirl 3 TBS honey in bath water for silky skin. Apply body lotion after your shower before you dry off for the most moisture to your skin.

• **My personal make-up remover:** Mix in a dark bottle, avocado, almond and sesame oils; very nourishing.

• **Kitchen cosmetic face lifts:** apply, leave on 30 minutes, rinse off. 1: Yogurt/lemon juice to balance pH and restore acid mantle. 2: Honey/almond/oatmeal scrub or Crystal Star LEMON BODY GLOW™ to exfoliate. Follow with blend of aloe vera gel and vitamin E oil. 3: Egg whites or Zia SEAWEED LIFT for skin tightening. 4: Honey/ red wine mix for AHA wrinkle treatment.

• **Eye relaxation techniques:** Blink to cleanse, lubricate and de-stress. Look right; look up; look left; look down; look diagonally up down and to the sides. Massage temples, pinch skin between the brows; then palm your eyes for 10 seconds. Bathe eyes in cool witch hazel, or chamomile tea.

Can't find a recommended product? Call the 800 number listed in Product Resources for the store nearest you and for more info.

248

A Healthy Pregnancy for Two

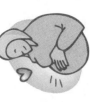

Start with pre-conception planning:

In America today, one in six married couples of child-bearing age has trouble conceiving and completing a pregnancy. Poor nutrition and stress seem to be at the base of most fertility problems. For men, conception is affected by a zinc deficiency, a fast food diet, chronic infections and too much alcohol. For women, conception inhibitors are anxiety, emotional stress, severe anemia and hormone imbalance. New research implicates hormone mimics from pollutants, and chemical residues in food and water to infertility in both sexes.

Note: If you're worried by early studies linking herbs like St. John's wort, ginkgo biloba and echinacea to infertility, know that the herbs were only tested in a test tube on hamster eggs. It is highly improbable that these herbs used in a living human would have the same effect. Herbs are processed as foods by our enzyme systems.... neutralizing, in the vast majority of cases, potential for toxicity.

A good diet is critical for successful conception:

Nature tries in every way possible to insure the survival of a new life. I've seen over and over again that a good diet and lifestyle is imperative for at least six months before trying to conceive for both partners.

—A **"virility nutrition"** program for men (up to 40% of the time, the man is the infertile one in conception problems) includes a short cleansing diet, then zinc-rich foods, healthy omega-3 fats, some meat, but mostly plant protein foods, minimal sweets and dairy foods, and plenty of whole grains. Natural vitamin E significantly improves sperm motility in men. The amino acid L-carnitine boosts sperm quality in subfertile men. Unless you're grossly overweight, don't go on a weight loss diet during preconception. Severe food limitation has a direct impact on the testicles. A man's fertility rise may take place in as little as 2 months after his diet improvements.

—A **"fertility nutrition"** program for a woman includes plenty of salads and greens, very low sugars, and a smaller volume of whole grains and nuts. Her diet should be low in saturated fats, but rich in essential fatty acids from sea greens and omega-3 oils. Eat fish and seafoods but avoid other meats during pre-conception. Unless organic, much of America's meat and poultry is antibiotic and hormone laced. Drink a cup of green tea every morning. A new study shows that women who drink a cup of green tea daily get pregnant faster! Important: Normalize your body weight to conceive! Overweight women increase their risk of developing toxemia or high blood pressure during pregnancy. Severely underweight women risk premature births or low birth weight babies. A woman's fertility rise may take 6 to 18 months after her diet change.

—Both men and women should limit their saturated fat intake to about 10% of the diet. Especially reduce sugary foods (sweeteners like aspartame are particularly hazardous for your unborn child) and meats that are regularly laced with nitrates and-or hormones, like red meats, and smoked, cured and processed meats. Be sure you're getting enough high C foods. There is a link between infertility and low vitamin C in both sexes.

—**Lifestyle habits are important.** Avoid or reduce your tobacco, caffeine, and alcohol. (Moderate wine is ok until conception.) Get light exercise, and morning sunshine every day possible. Apply alternating hot and cold compresses to the abdomen or scrotum to increase circulation to the reproductive areas. Massage therapy sessions, and deep breathing exercises are very beneficial.

See my eBook "Do You Want To Have A Baby?" for complete information for both men and women trying to conceive a child.

An Optimal Diet During Pregnancy

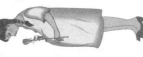

A woman's body changes so dramatically during pregnancy and childbearing that her normal daily needs change. Her body takes care of some of its needs through cravings. During this one time of life, the body is so sensitive to its needs that unusual cravings may be good for you. Every single thing the mother does or takes in affects her child. Good nutrition for a child begins before it is born, even before it is conceived. New research shows that when a child reaches adulthood, his or her risk for heart disease, cancer, and diabetes can be traced not only to heredity but to the eating habits of the parents. A nutritious diet helps build a healthy baby, minimizes the mother's discomfort, lessens birth complications and reduces excess weight gain that can't be lost after birth.

A good diet during pregnancy helps prevent miscarriage and high blood pressure, and supports your body against toxemia, fluid retention, constipation, hemorrhoids and varicose veins, anemia, gas, heartburn and morning sickness. A good diet after the birth is important for breast milk, reducing post-partum swelling, and for healing stretch marks.

Promise yourself and your baby that at least during the months of pregnancy and nursing, your diet and lifestyle will be as healthy as you can make it. A largely vegetarian diet of whole foods provides optimum nutrition. Base your pregnancy diet on nutritional power-houses.... whole grains, leafy greens, fish (avoid shark and swordfish, notorious for high mercury levels that can be dangerous to a developing fetus), turkey, eggs, legumes, nuts, seeds, green and yellow vegetables, nutritional yeast, bananas and citrus fruits.

Your Diet Keys: Eat small frequent meals instead of large meals.

1: **Protein requirements increase during pregnancy.** Quality protein prevents and cures toxemia. Most experts recommend 60 to 80 grams of protein daily during pregnancy, with a 10 gram increase every trimester. Focus on vegetable protein - whole grains, seeds and sprouts, with fish, seafood or turkey at least twice a week. Take a protein drink several times a week: Mix $1/2$ cup soy milk or rice milk, $1/2$ cup yogurt, $1/2$ cup orange juice, 2 tsp. nutritional yeast, 2 tsp. wheat germ, 2 tsp. molasses, $1/2$ tsp. vanilla, a pinch cinnamon.

2: **Have a fresh fruit or a green salad every day.** Add other fiber foods like whole grain cereals and vegetables for regularity.

3: **Drink plenty of healthy fluids.** Pure water and juices like pineapple, papaya, cranberry and apple juice throughout the day keep your system flowing. Carrot juice twice a week is ideal.

4: **Eat folacin-rich foods.** Spinach and other leafy greens, yams, sea greens, brown rice and asparagus boost healthy cell growth.

5: **Increase your essential fatty acids (EFA's).** Fish, spinach, arugula, especially 2 TBS dry sea greens for healthy brain and skin.

6: **Eat carotene-rich foods.** Carrots, squashes, tomatoes, yams, and broccoli for disease resistance.

7: **Eat zinc-rich foods.** Pumpkin and sesame seeds for good body formation.

8: **Eat vitamin C foods.** Broccoli, bell peppers and fruits for connective tissue.

9: **Eat bioflavonoid-rich foods.** Citrus fruits and berries for capillary integrity.

10: **Eat alkalizing foods.** Miso soup and brown rice combat and neutralize toxemia.

11: **Eat mineral-rich foods.** Sea greens, leafy greens, whole grains for baby building blocks; silicon-rich foods for bone, cartilage, connective tissue growth; brown rice, oats, green grasses, green drinks for collagen-elastin formation.

Important diet watchwords you should know during pregnancy and nursing:

—**Don't restrict your diet to lose weight.** Low calories often mean low birth weight for the baby.

—**Eat a wide range of healthy foods to assure baby access to all nutrients.** Avoid cabbages, onions and garlic. They can upset body balance during pregnancy. Broccoli, cauliflower, milk and chocolate aggravate colic in nursing babies. Avoid red meats.

—**Avoid chemicalized, smoked, preserved, colored foods.** Refrain from unnecessary drugs of all kinds and excess caffeine.

—**Avoid X-rays, chemical solvents, CFCs (hair sprays, cat litter).** A baby's system can't handle these things easily.

—**Avoid smoking and secondary smoke.** Your baby, like you, metabolizes the harmful cancer-causing residues of tobacco. The chance of low birth weight, SIDS and miscarriage is much more likely if you smoke. Smoker's infants have a mortality rate 30% higher than non-smoker's. Nursing babies take in small amounts of nicotine with breast milk, and become prone to lung infections.

—**Avoid alcohol** to reduce risk of Fetal Alcohol Syndrome, disabilities, mental retardation and motor-skill problems.

The diet in this chapter can improve the following pregnancy associated problems: *Morning Sickness, Gas, Toxemia, Fluid Retention, Miscarriage Risk, Varicose Veins, Hemorrhoids, Stretch Marks, Poor Lactation.*

About Breast Feeding

Mother's milk is best. Unless there is a major health problem, your breast milk should be the only food for your baby during the first six months of life... or up to a year for the most health benefits. Despite the claims made for fortified formulas, nothing can take the place of breast milk. The first thick, waxy colostrum is extremely high in protein, essential fatty acids needed for brain and nervous system development, and protective antibodies. A child's immune system is not fully established at birth, and the antibodies in breast milk are critical. They fight early infections and create solid immune defenses that prevent the development of allergies. Breast-fed babies have lower bouts of colic and other digestion problems than bottle-fed babies. Breast milk is loaded with bifidobacteria, beneficial micro-organisms that make up 99% of a healthy baby's intestinal flora — extremely important protection against salmonella food poisoning and other intestinal pathogens. The baby who is not breast fed loses Nature's "jump start" on immune response and may face health disadvantages that can last a lifetime.

Mother's milk is the best for giving your baby essential fats needed for proper development of the brain, nervous system, and eyes. A study in the Journal of Pediatrics shows that breast-feeding may even make your baby smarter throughout life, giving him or her an academic advantage! The determining factor seems to be the high content of DHA (docosahexaenoic acid) in breast milk, an essential fatty acid which comprises over 50% of the brain. DHA, vital to infant development, increases 3 to 5 times in the last trimester of pregnancy and triples again in the first 12 weeks of life.

If there is simply no way to breast feed your baby, goat's milk is a better alternative than either chemically-made formulas or cow's milk, both of which result in children with higher risk of allergies.

Recipes to help your pregnancy diet: • BLENDING EAST and WEST FOODS; • BREAKFAST and BRUNCH; • SOUPS, LIQUID SALADS; • ENZYME-RICH; • SALADS, HOT and COLD; • MINERAL-RICH; • HIGH FIBER RECIPES.

Herb and Supplement Choices

• *Take supplements carefully during pregnancy, even if your method is holistically oriented. Mega-doses of anything are not good for the baby's system. Dosage should almost universally be less (usually about half of normal), to allow for the infant's tiny capacity. Ideal supplements should be food-source complexes.*

• **Supplements that can help you during pregnancy:**

 —**Green drink:** a good nutrition "delivery system" during pregnancy. Crystal Star ENERGY GREEN™ drink mix; Body Ecology VITALITY SUPER GREEN; Morada Research Laboratories GOD'S GARDEN; Vibrant Health GREEN VIBRANCE.

 —**Prenatal:** start 8 weeks before birth; should contain 350 to 500mg magnesium. New Chapter PERFECT PRENATAL.

 —**Food source multi-mineral:** Nature's Path TRACE-MIN-LYTE; Crystal Star MINERAL SPECTRUM™.

 —**Folic acid:** Take 800mcg daily before the first three months of fetal development to prevent neural tube defects.

 —**Vitamin B-6:** for bloating, leg cramps and nerve strength.

 —**Bioflavonoids:** Over 50% of women who habitually miscarry have low levels of vitamin C and bioflavonoids. Take bioflavonoids 1000mg with vitamin C daily, or Crystal Star BIOFLAVONOID, FIBER & C SUPPORT™ drink, or BILBERRY EXTRACT, one of the single richest sources of herbal flavonoids.

 —**Kelp tablets:** about 6 daily, or Crystal Star IODINE/PO-TASSIUM SOURCE™ capsules.

 —**Natural vitamin E:** 200IU, or wheat germ oil capsules.

 —**EFA's:** (omega-3 rich flax oil, borage seed or evening primrose oils), for baby's brain development.

 —**Zinc:** 10-15mg daily for better brain formation.

Bodywork and Lifestyle Techniques

• **Get some mild exercise every day.** The best is a brisk walk for fresh air, oxygen and circulation.

• **Get some early morning sunlight** for half an hour every day possible, for vitamin D, calcium absorption and bone growth.

• **Get plenty of rest and adequate sleep.** Body energy turns inward during sleep for repair, restoration and fetal growth.

• **During the last trimester:** Rub vitamin E or wheat germ oil on your stomach and around vaginal opening each night to make stretching easier and skin more elastic. Begin to take extra minerals as labor approaches.

Note: If you practice reflexology, do not press the acupressure point just above the ankle on the inside of the leg. It could start contractions.

Can't find a recommended product? Call the 800 number listed in Product Resources for the store nearest you and for more info.

Healing Your Heart

Heart disease has been the leading killer of men in America for almost 100 years. Since 1984, it's also been the biggest killer of women. Today, the death toll is nearly half a million men and over half a million women each year. Of all the world's people, Americans are still in the highest risk category for heart disease. If you think today's medicine will protect you, think again. Even some doctors are beginning to believe that medical care for the heart is based on big bucks, not health. Drugs and surgical techniques to "protect" your heart are a booming business. Surgery alone costs Americans over $50 billion each year. (Incidentally, new studies show fish oil capsules after a balloon angioplasty can help prevent re-clogging….a big problem.)

Clearly, modern medicine has saved and extended lives. But is "heroic medicine" always the best choice when you aren't in danger of imminent death? Modern medicine was developed during war time when emergency treatment was the only way to deal with an emergency situation. So most medical procedures have a "battlefield mentality," prohibitively expensive, highly invasive, traumatic – often unnecessarily risky. By-pass surgery, the most popular surgical heart disease "solution," benefits less than 10% of heart patients. Many don't live 6 or 7 years after their first operation.

Studies over the last 2 decades show that many patients do significantly <u>worse</u> after heart surgery than patients who use other treatments. Most of us know someone for whom by-pass surgery or a pacemaker became the beginning of the end of a normal lifestyle. My own father-in-law was one of those. There is some good news: There has been a 28% reduction in U.S. heart disease deaths since 1987. Studies indicate this trend is largely the result of lifestyle changes to improve heart health, not high tech medical procedures or drug therapy.

It's critical for you to know the facts before making the decision to have surgery or take heart drugs. Drugs and surgery can carry serious risks. You may not be getting all the information you need because people with a big interest in the mega bucks of heart disease aren't telling you.

Let me say at the start that surgery, no matter how skilled or how advanced, is never the whole answer. Your doctor knows this, too. All heart surgery MUST be followed by permanent changes in diet and lifestyle for ongoing heart health. Here are some of the facts you should know:

1: <u>PACEMAKER IMPLANT SURGERY</u>, at $25,000 each, electrically-powered pacemakers are implanted just under the skin sending out electrical impulses to stimulate heartbeat. But electrical devices like cell phones, medical instruments, even shopping mall security equipment can interfere with a pacemaker, creating fluctuations in heartbeat that can lead to drowsiness, shortness of breath or blackouts. Of course, the pacemaker battery eventually wears out, so it must be continually monitored.

per, is for people with a slow heart rate. Battery-powered pacemakers are implanted just under the skin sending out electrical impulses to stimulate heartbeat. But electrical devices like cell phones, medical instruments, even shopping mall security equipment can interfere with a pacemaker, creating fluctuations in heartbeat that can lead to drowsiness, shortness of breath or blackouts. Of course, the pacemaker battery eventually wears

2: <u>ANGIOGRAMS</u>, at $11,000 each, help diagnose the severity of coronary artery disease. Liquid material visible to an X-ray is injected into the coronary artery, so doctors can locate blockages. The procedure itself can cause a stroke, heart attack, or death.

3: BYPASS SURGERY, the most popular, and the most expensive, heart disease "solution," actually benefits less than one-tenth of heart disease patients. Blocked portions of coronary arteries are bypassed with grafts taken from veins in the legs. But, veins of the leg are not designed to withstand the high pressure blood flow from the heart, so many patients don't live beyond 6 or 7 years after their first operation. Nearly 1 in 25 people die during the bypass surgery itself. Bypass surgeries can even lead to brain damage. Still, over 575,000 operations at over $45,000 per are performed each year.

4: BALLOON ANGIOPLASTY uses a balloon-tipped catheter to open up blocked arteries. It costs $15,000 per and causes a heart attack in 4% of people having the procedure. In 5%, the blockage is actually made worse. 35% of treated blockages return to their pre-op severity in less than a year. I personally know two people who had to have another angioplasty within a year after surgery.

Are new heart protecting drugs widely heralded in the media a better answer? Drugs like Zocor, Mevacor and Pravachol to lower cholesterol, still cause liver toxicity, stomach distress and vision impairment. They also deplete CoQ$_{10}$, an essential co-enzyme that strengthens the heart, by up to 50%. **Some heart "protecting" drugs can even cause a heart attack!**

Recent studies show that calcium channel blockers, the top selling blood pressure drugs, increase heart attack risk up to 60%! The research also shows that they raise the risk of suicide. In June of 1998, Roche laboratories pulled its new blood pressure drug, Posicor, off the market because of the high risk of fatal drug interactions. These risks are only some of calcium channel blockers' problems. In the long-term, the hazards may outweigh the benefits of these drugs. Newest findings suggest a link between these drugs and breast cancer.

Let's clear up a question I often hear about calcium channel blockers. Many of you are told by your doctors and pharmacists that your calcium channel blocker breaks up calcified deposits in the arteries... in other words that calcium is the villain. Then you hear from natural healers that calcium helps reduce blood pressure. It's the hero.

What's the real story about calcium and heart disease? Here's how calcium channel blockers work. They inhibit the entry of calcium into heart cells and smooth muscle cells of blood vessels. Without calcium, the cells cannot contract and the result is less blood pressure. But this goes against Nature because calcium is an important mineral for heart health! Calcium regulates the smooth activity of the heart muscle and inhibits heart spasms. Calcium also helps lower cholesterol. It is most beneficial when it is brought into the body with a balanced ratio of magnesium in foods like dark green veggies (or sea greens), whole grains, nuts, seeds, beans and organic poultry. Both calcium and magnesium need to be present for optimum absorption.

Magnesium is Nature's calcium channel blocker. Magnesium naturally blocks the entry of calcium into heart muscle and vascular smooth muscle cells, reducing vascular resistance and regulating blood pressure. Magnesium protectively balances out the negative effects of calcium overload on the heart.

Why do Americans fall victim to heart disease when most heart disease is 100% preventable through simple diet and lifestyle changes? **Is our 20th century lifestyle so bad that we are literally killing ourselves?** Perhaps.

Let's get to the heart of the matter.

First: There's still our sad American diet. Less than 25% of us get the recommended 5 servings of fruits and vegetables a day that protect against heart disease. Even worse, 25% of the "vegetables" we do eat in America are french fries- the most damaging for cardiovascular health! Low fiber is a big problem, despite all the media attention. The typical American eats less than one-third of the daily fiber recommended for cardiovascular health!

Second: There's our sedentary lifestyle. Lack of exercise makes us a wide open target for heart disease. Regular moderate exercise cuts risk for heart attack and stroke almost in half. Our computers have changed our lives at every level. New statistics from the National Institute of Health show an astounding 58% of adult Americans get no exercise at all!

Third: Americans are "stressed out," and our stress levels are rising. Most Americans feel overwhelmed on a regular basis. Financial or work-related stress in common. A recent survey find that over 25% of the baby boomers (at the peak of their careers and earning power) still feel out of control in their lives! Chronic stress attacks your entire cardiovascular system. It causes coronary arteries to constrict, blood pressure to soar and cholesterol to build on artery walls. It's no wonder our hearts are about to explode!

Fourth: Smoking constricts arteries and can cause blood pressure to skyrocket, too. Researchers estimate that 150,000 heart disease deaths would prevented each year if Americans just quit smoking!

Is heart disease contagious? It may be.

The infectious bacteria *Chlamydia pneumoniae*, (a species of the bacteria that causes the STD, Chlamydia) may be a factor in heart disease development. C. *pneumoniae* is a common cause of pneumonia, sinusitis and bronchitis – most people are infected by it 2 or 3 times during their lives. Here's where heart disease comes in. Blocked blood vessels are 20 times more likely to carry C. *pneumoniae* than unblocked vessels. C. *pneumoniae* also creates inflammation involved in atherosclerosis. A new clinical trial finds that antibiotic therapy reduces the number of heart attacks and deaths in hospital heart patients. If you are recovering from a heart attack or have coronary heart disease, a month long course of *Echinacea-Goldenseal* extract or Crystal Star's ANTI-BIO™ caps may flush out infectious bacteria trapped in blocked lymph glands and blood vessels.

Is gum disease tied to heart disease? Experts think so.

People with periodontal disease are 2.7 times more likely to have a heart attack than people with healthy gums! Gum disease allows toxic bacteria from excess plaque to enter the bloodstream, causing blood platelets to clump and accelerate atherosclerosis. The National Institutes of Health are now exploring the link between periodontal disease and heart attacks. If you already have gum disease or periodontitis, add CoQ10 to your daily healing program. It is a specific for teeth and gums, and your heart.

Diets to prevent heart disease can also improve: *Congestive Heart Failure, High or Low Blood Pressure, Cholesterol Build-Up, Atherosclerosis, Stress and Tension, Blood Clots, Phlebitis, Heart Palpitations. Excessive Bleeding, Poor Circulation, Hemorrhoids, Varicose Veins and Spider Veins.*

Rehabilitation Diet after a Heart Attack

The heart health diet below is for those of you who have survived a heart attack or major heart surgery. Coming back is tough. Sticking to a new lifestyle that changes the way you eat, exercise, handle stress and the details of your life is a challenge. Lifestyle changes are not easy, and they take time to accomplish. But they are an infinitely preferable choice for your quality of life, and must take place for there to be permanent results. Use the diet on this page as a blueprint for a healthier heart and arteries; it's proven successful against heart disease recurrence. It reduces dietary fats 30% or more, includes plenty of fish and seafood for Omega-3 oils, emphasizes mineral-rich foods, particularly potassium and magnesium for cardiotonic action, adds whole grains and vegetables for energy and stamina, has fiber-rich foods for a clean system, and subscribes to a little white wine before dinner for relaxation and digestion. *Note: Follow this diet for one to three months after an attack or surgery. Return to it any time as needed.*

Watchwords:

• Eat plenty of fish to balance blood viscosity with preventive effects for heart attacks. • Add a brisk, daily walk. • Do deep breathing exercises every morning. • Use dry skin brushing, alternating hot and cold hydrotherapy (page 463), and smaller meals with a little white wine to increase circulation. • Eat magnesium-rich foods, like wheat germ, tofu, bran, broccoli and potatoes for heart regulation. • Relax and have a good daily laugh. A positive mental outlook can do wonders for your heart and your well-being.

—**On rising:** have some grapefruit, apple or grape juice; or 2 lemons squeezed in a glass of water with honey.

—**Breakfast:** have fresh tropical fruits for extra potassium topped with a little yogurt; mix 2 TBS <u>each</u>: lecithin granules, toasted wheat germ, nutritional yeast, sesame seeds, molasses and flax oil. Take 2 teasp. every morning on yogurt, or sprinkle on pancakes, cereal, or whole grain toast. Add a little maple syrup, honey or apple juice to sweeten if desired.

—**Mid-morning:** have a green drink (page 569), or Monas CHLORELLA or Green Foods GREEN MAGMA, or Crystal Star ENERGY GREEN™ drink with 1 teasp. Bragg's LIQUID AMINOS; or a potassium drink (page 568), or Futurebiotics VITAL K; or fresh carrot juice; or a mint tea; or Crystal Star BIOFLAV. FIBER & C SUPPORT™ drink, or HEARTSEASE/ CIRCU-CLEANSE™ tea.

—**Lunch:** have baked onions, and a cup of miso soup with sea greens snipped on top; or a green salad with nuts, seeds, sprouts, and lemon/oil dressing; or baked tofu with brown rice and broccoli; or a baked potato with yogurt cheese, and a leafy salad; or a vegetable/grain or bean soup with a sandwich on whole grain bread; or a light seafood salad with spinach pasta for EFA's.

—**Mid-afternoon:** have a relaxing herb tea such as alfalfa/mint tea, or Crystal Star RELAX TEA™ with raw crunchy veggies or whole grain crackers and a soy, or veggie and yogurt dip; or a circulation booster drink: Mix 1 cup tomato juice, 6 TBS wheat germ oil, 1 cup lemon juice, and 1 TB nutritional yeast.

—**Dinner:** have a vegetarian casserole with whole grain pasta or brown rice, veggies, and a light sauce; or baked or broiled fish (especially salmon and tuna) or shellfish (especially oysters and scallops) with brown rice and steamed veggies; or a tofu and whole grain loaf with a green salad; or steamed or baked veggies with whole grain muffins or cornbread, and a little butter.

—**Before bed:** fresh fruits; or apple juice; or Red Star nutritional yeast broth, or hot Crystal Star SYSTEMS STRENGTH™ drink.

Herb and Supplement Choices

• **In an emergency:** 1 teasp. cayenne powder in water, or cayenne tincture drops in water may help bring a person out of a heart attack; or take liquid carnitine as directed. One-half dropperful Hawthorn extract every 15 minutes; or Crystal Star HEART STABILIZER extract available from Healthy House.

• **Tone the heart muscle:** NutriCology CoQ-10 with TOCOTRIENOLS (to help lower cholesterol). Vitamin C with bioflavonoids, up to 5000mg daily for interstitial arterial integrity-elasticity, and to prevent TIA's (little strokes). EVENING PRIM-ROSE oil 4000mg daily (EFA's help tone arterial muscle); Omega Nutrition ESSENTIAL BALANCE caps; Magnesium 800mg.

• **Improve blood flow:** Golden Pride FORMULA ONE oral chelation w. EDTA; Wakunaga KYOLIC SUPER FORMULA 106; Crystal Star GINSENG-REISHI extract, or Gingko Biloba extracts as vasodilators, 3x daily; Transformation PUREZYME; MICROHYDRIN, available at Healthy House.

• **Antioxidants clear the cardiovascular system:** Crystal Star HEARTSEASE-HAWTHORN caps, or HEARTSEASE-CIRCU CLEANSE™ tea; Grapeseed PCO's 300mg daily; Biogenetics BIO-GUARD; Metabolic Response Modifiers ALPHA-LIPOIC ACID; Spirulina or 2 TBS daily sea greens.

• **Cardiotonics for a stronger and steadier beat:** CoQ-10, 60mg 3x daily; Carnitine 1000mg daily; Cayenne-Ginger caps or Garlic capsules 6 daily; Siberian ginseng caps 2000mg or tea, 2 cups daily; Wheat germ oil caps for tissue oxygen.

• **Reduce blood stickiness to prevent a heart attack:** Bromelain 1500mg to increase fibrinolysis; Chromium picolinate or Solaray CHROMIACIN for arterial plaque and insulin resistance. Omega-3 fish or flax oils 3x daily.

Bodywork and Lifestyle Techniques

• **In an emergency:**
  —Bite down on the tip of the little finger to help stop a heart attack.
  —Apply hot compresses and massage chest of the victim to ease a heart attack.
  —Chewing an aspirin immediately following symptoms of a heart attack, may be able to reduce mortality through its ability to reduce arterial blockage.

• **Take alternate hot and cold showers** frequently to increase circulation.

• **Smoking constricts arteries and can cause blood pressure to skyrocket.** Researchers estimate that 150,000 heart disease deaths would be prevented each year if Americans just quit smoking! Is it time for you to quit?

• **Take some mild regular daily exercise.** Do deep breathing exercises every morning for body oxygen, and to stimulate brain activity.

Can't find a recommended product? Call the 800 number listed in Product Resources for the store nearest you and for more info.

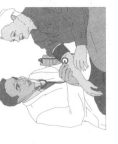

A Man's Healthy Heart Program

—**Emotional health is a major factor in men's heart problems.** Stress, anger, and overwork are now, (and probably have always been), major triggers of heart attacks for men. A Harvard School of Public Health study shows that men with the highest anger scores on personality tests are three times more likely to develop heart disease.

—**High blood pressure** often called "the silent killer," affects 1 in 3 of all U.S. adults. Men are more at risk for HBP than women until about age 55. High blood pressure is most dangerous for African American males. When blood pressure is high, the heart and arteries are over-worked, and atherosclerosis speeds up. Coronary heart disease is 3 to 5 times more likely in people with high blood pressure! Over-consumption of salt, a high stress lifestyle with little "downtime," and smoking are key factors in the development of high blood pressure.

—**Atherosclerosis** (hardening of the arteries) is strongly tied to a diet high in animal fat, especially from butter, red meat, ice cream and eggs, the very foods many men overeat! Atherosclerotic plaques on your arteries restrict blood flow to organs and tissues leading to heart attacks, strokes, even gangrene.

1) Men tend to overeat-especially fatty foods. A low fat, high fiber diet is essential for recovery from existing heart problems. Reduce fatty dairy foods like ice cream and rich cheeses. Cut back on red meat, especially pork. Eat seafood at least once a week. An 11 year study covering over 22,000 men found that eating seafood just once a week cuts men's risk of sudden cardiac death by 52%!

2) Use olive oil instead. You can't fry in olive oil, but fried foods are so bad for your heart that this is probably a plus. Olive oil boosts healthy HDL cholesterol levels and removes dangerous blood fats. Try Spectrum Naturals cold pressed extra virgin olive oil.

3) Men need more fiber! Fiber has been proven to reduce arterial plaque from atherosclerosis. Herbs are a good source of cleansing fiber for men. I recommend an herbal fiber rich drink mix daily like Crystal Star's CHOL-LO FIBER TONE™.

4) Add spices like garlic, onions, tumeric and cayenne peppers to your diet. Hundreds of clinical trials show garlic thins the blood, normalizes blood pressure, and reduces cholesterol and arterial plaque build-up. Both onions and garlic stimulate healthy circulation. Cayenne peppers strengthen all cardiovascular activity, and reduce blood pressure. Tumeric, an anti-inflammatory spice, helps decrease cholesterol and atherosclerosis. Boost circulation to thin "sticky blood" with Crystal Star HEARTSEASE-CIRCU-CLEANSE™ tea or Futurebiotics CIRCUPLEX.

5) Eat more SUPERGREEN foods, especially spinach, chard and sea greens, for magnesium therapy and EFA's. Magnesium is a key mineral for heart regulation. A magnesium deficiency can contribute to hypertension, irregular heartbeat, even heart failure!

6) Eat vitamin C rich foods like citrus fruits, broccoli or peppers. Low blood levels of vitamin C are linked to progressing atherosclerosis and to increased heart attack risk. A new study shows that men with no pre-existing heart disease who are deficient in vitamin C have 3.5 times MORE heart attacks than men who are not deficient in vitamin C.

7) Herbal stress busters are an excellent choice for men. They can reduce anxiety linked to high blood pressure and heart palpitations. Herbal nervines like kava kava, passionflower and scullcap calm acute stress reactions. Especially for men, I recommend Siberian ginseng, a primary adaptogen that builds body resistance to stress and restores nervous system health.

A Man's Healthy Heart Diet

Diet remains the single most influential factor in heart disease. You can carve a better future with your own knife and fork, than with a lifetime of dependence on drugs, pacemakers, or multiple surgeries. If you have more than one of the following heart disease markers, take the watchwords below "to heart."

Are you: more than 20 pounds overweight? sometimes impotent? frequently short of breath?
Do you have: pain upon exertion? cold hands and feet? frequent leg cramps? mental fuzziness? blurred vision? high blood pressure or diabetes? high LDL cholesterol?

1–Limit your coffee to 1 cup a day. Drink green tea every morning instead.
2–Lower your cholesterol by significantly reducing your intake of red meat, dairy foods and fried foods.
3–Reduce high phosphorus foods: soft drinks, beef, pork, and poultry. They promote negative calcium balance.
4–Raise your high fiber foods - whole grain breads and cereals, vegetable or whole grain pastas, and lots of fresh greens.
5–Raise your antioxidants with more vegetables. In tests, vegetarians have healthier hearts and arteries. The risk of stroke from clogged arteries decreases by over 35% for each increase of 3 fruit or vegetable servings per day.
6–Take a healthy artery drink twice a week. Some suggestions - Nature's Secret ULTIMATE FIBER, Crystal Star CHOL-LO FIBER TONE™ (low cholesterol means clearer arteries), Herbal Answers HERBAL ALOE FORCE.
7–Have a little wine at dinner; wine has an enzyme that breaks up blood clots. Eat smaller meals, especially at night.

<u>Can donating blood regularly prevent a heart attack for a man? Yes, it can!</u>
Men have twice as much iron in their bodies as women. Iron acts as a catalyst in cholesterol oxidation, linked to artery hardening and scarring. Recent studies show that men cut their risk for heart attack or stroke up to a third by reducing excess iron when they regularly donate blood.

<u>Does oral chelation reverse men's heart disease?</u>
Chelation therapy with EDTA has largely been ignored by mainstream medicine, but it has been used successfully for blood vessel diseases for over 40 years. Intravenous chelation with EDTA (a synthetic amino acid) binds to and flushes out arterial plaque that causes artery hardening. Intravenous chelation is a powerful but expensive therapy. Oral chelation is a good option for many people, especially men. It's cheaper and more convenient that IV chelation, yet still improves blood flow and may even reverse some vascular problems. Consider Golden Pride's oral chelation program, FORMULA #1 or Metabolic Response Modifiers CARDIO-CHELATE.

Recipes to help your healthy heart diet: • FISH and SEAFOODS; • ENZYME-RICH RECIPES; • HIGH FIBER • HIGH PROTEIN without MEAT; • DAIRY-FREE COOKING; • MINERAL-RICH RECIPES; • LOW FAT RECIPES

Herb and Supplement Choices

•**Normalize blood circulation:** Crystal Star HEARTSEASE-HAWTHORN™ capsules, or HEARTSEASE CIRCU-CLEANSE™ tea with butcher's broom; astragalus tea or ginseng-cayenne caps daily. Silica returns good circulation: Flora VEGESIL or Eidon SILICA as directed.

•**Oral chelation shows good results:** Golden Pride FOR-MULA 1 oral chelation therapy with EDTA; Enzymatic Therapy ORAL NUTRIENT CHELATES; Metabolic Response Modifiers CARDIO-CHELATE

•**Inhibit atherosclerosis:** Ginkgo biloba extract also relieves claudication; chromium picolinate 200mcg daily.

•**Lower cholesterol and triglycerides:** Ester C 3-5000mg daily with bioflavs keeps LDL cholesterol from being oxidized; Vitamin E 400IU w. selenium 200mcg daily also reduces intermittent claudication. Magnesium, 800mg daily to raise "good" cholesterol.

•**Liver support for fat metabolism:** Milk thistle seed extract for 3 to 6 months; Crystal Star GREEN TEA CLEANSER™; Enzymatic Therapy CO-ENZYMATE B-complex; Carnitine 1000mg; Niacin 500mg 2x daily with pancreatin 1400mg; Metabolic Response Modifiers ALPHA-LIPOIC ACID.

—**Good fats help your liver:** High omega-3 flax oil, 3x daily, or evening primrose oil, 4000mg daily for 2 months.

•**Lower homocysteine levels:** 1) B Complex, 100mg daily. Add 50mg extra of B_6 and 400mcg extra of folic acid; 2) Garlic, 1200mg a day maintains aortic elasticity; 3) Daily ginger prevents blood "stickiness;" 4) Red wine, a glass with dinner.

•**Antioxidants help remove artery plaque:** MICROHYDRIN 3 daily, from Healthy House; PCO's from grape seed or white pine 100mg daily; CoQ-10, 100mg daily; Phos-Chol 1000mg.

Bodywork and Lifestyle Techniques

—Lifestyle measures:

•Stop smoking. Keep your weight down. Relax. Meditation has proven to be good for your arteries.

•For arteriosclerotic retinopathy: reduce fats, especially saturated fats from meats in your diet. Reduce sugar intake to help normalize blood sugar balance. Take garlic capsules daily to help normalize blood pressure levels.

•Ginger or Cayenne/garlic capsules 4 to 6 daily, as an alternative to the much-touted aspirin therapy. Chronic aspirin use can have side effects, such as stomach irritation, ringing in the ears, and metabolic imbalance. If you choose to take aspirin, take it at low dosage. Small doses are just as effective.

—Bodywork:

•Take a brisk walk daily. Aerobic exercise helps raise HDL levels. Then, use a dry skin brush over the body to stimulate circulation.

•Take an alternating hot and cold shower to increase blood circulation.

•Stop smoking. Nicotine can be lethal as a blood vessel constricting agent.

•Eat smaller meals more often. NO large heavy meals.

Can't find a recommended product? Call the 800 number listed in Product Resources for the store nearest you and for more info.

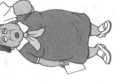

What about heart disease in women?

Over half a million American women die from cardiovascular disease each year... that's half of all women's deaths and 100,000 more deaths than men! Even more frightening, new studies reveal women receive less medical treatment despite having more cardiac symptoms than men. Heart disease for women is linked to high cholesterol, obesity or too little exercise as it is in men. **It is also clearly hormone-related.** There is no time that a woman's risk for heart disease is higher than during menopause. Risk for heart disease rises noticeably with every year a woman approaches menopause and continues to rise with age. Because of this, hundreds of thousands of prophylactic, hormone replacement therapy prescriptions are written every year by doctors trying to protect menopausal women from heart disease.

Yet, the use of hormone replacement therapy or ERT to protect against heart disease is highly debatable. There is no conclusive evidence that estrogen protects against heart disease. Hormone replacement therapy does not prevent heart attack for women who already have heart disease. In fact, a 1997 review from the International Meeting on Atherosclerosis concludes that the heart protective benefits attributed to estrogen may actually result from population selection bias or healthier lifestyles changes during the course of the studies. I don't think hormone replacement therapy, with its links to uterine and breast cancer, is the best answer as a preventive for heart disease. I think there are better solutions for preventing heart disease naturally that don't carry these risks.

If you're thinking about trying hormone replacement therapy to prevent heart disease, here are facts you should know:

1: The most commonly prescribed hormone replacement drug, Premarin, actually suppresses folic acid, contributing to high homocysteine levels, a known risk factor for heart disease.

2: Tests with some estrogen contraceptive pills actually increase a woman's risk of heart disease, heart attack, stroke and serious blood clotting problems.

3: Some reports suggest that SERMs (selective estrogen receptor modulators) like Evista may protect against heart disease. But Evista should not be taken by women with congestive heart failure. Evista also increases risk of serious blood clots in the legs, lungs or eyes, particularly if you're sedentary for long periods of time.

What are the biggest heart problems for women?

—**A heart attack is especially serious for a woman.** Statistics show that a woman is 50% **more likely** to die from a heart attack than a man! Women have heart attacks at older ages when they are in poorer health than men. A woman's arteries are less able to recover for the partial death of heart muscle caused by a heart attack, so a second heart attack is even more dangerous for women.

—**Congestive Heart Failure:** Over two million women suffer from CHF, where the heart is unable to efficiently pump blood. The risk for menopausal women with CHF for sudden cardiac arrest and death is up to 9 times higher than the general population! Symptoms to watch for: extreme fatigue and water retention (particularly bloated ankles). Consider WOMEN'S HEART PROTECTOR for CHF, available from Healthy House, and creatine 3000mg daily; or Natural Balance CREATINE 3000 to 5000mg daily as protection.

—**Dangerous Atrial Fibrillation:** Women with this irregular heartbeat are 90% more likely to die than those without. If you're affected by atrial fibrillation, a cardiotonic, herbal heart protector with arjuna and hawthorn like Crystal Star WOMEN'S HEART STABILIZER from Healthy House, or even Hawthorn extract itself, can help regulate heartbeat and strengthen your entire cardiovascular system.

—**Low DHEA levels** may be a marker for women with heart disease. Still, I advise caution when taking superhormones like DHEA. 25 milligrams a day (the level in health food stores) may be too high, and sometimes leads to irregular heart beat. DHEA is also a stimulant and blood thinner. It shouldn't be used in with blood thinning drugs, aspirin or thyroid medication.

Are You Having a Panic Attack or a Heart Attack?

Many women confuse panic attacks with heart attacks during menopause because their symptoms seem so severe. Menopausal heart palpitations and nighttime anxiety attacks are extremely common. When I first went into menopause, I remember waking up terrified that I was having a heart attack, but found out later it was a panic attack.

Heart attack symptoms are _different_ for women. Women are less likely to have intense chest pains during a heart attack, one reason researchers believe they are more reluctant to seek treatment. If you are having the symptoms below, seek medical attention immediately! Ignoring symptoms could mean risking your life. Here are the warning signs:

- **Pressure or pain in the center of the chest lasting more than a few minutes. Trouble talking or understanding speech.**
- **Numbness spreading to the face, neck or arms, usually on one side.**
- **Chest pain and severe headache with light-headedness, sweating, nausea or shortness of breath.**
- **Dimness or loss of vision, especially in one eye**
- **Unexplained sudden fatigue or back pain. Intense tooth, jaw or ear pain on one side.**

If you have the panic attack symptoms below, they will more than likely pass quickly. If symptoms persist, seek out a qualified health practitioner. Herbs offer relief from nighttime panic attacks. I keep heart stabilizing herbs like hawthorn, arjuna, ashwagandha and passionflowers by my bed at night for immediate relief.

- **Hyperventilating or feeling short of breath especially at night.**
- **Racing heartbeat, dizziness or feeling faint.**
- **Bolting upright out of bed in the early morning hours.**
- **Feeling like you're "going crazy" or losing control, or being full of fear that has no basis in reality and the fear interfering in the normal functioning of your life.**

A Woman's Healthy Heart Program

Diet is your best medicine against heart disease. Many food nutrients can prevent heart disease, even reverse existing conditions.

1: Sea greens act as total body tonics to restore female vitality during menopause. Sea greens are loaded with vitamins like D and K that help make steroidal hormones like estrogen and DHEA which protect against heart disease during menopause. Sea greens also dissolve fatty deposits in the cardiovascular system that cause heart disease. The natural iodine in sea greens occurs in a balanced ratio with potassium, calcium, magnesium and trace elements that regulate blood pressure and balance electrolytes. If you're worried about high blood pressure, sea vegetables actually relieve tension in blood vessels caused by too much salt. They help lower blood pressure! Nori has the least sodium of all sea vegetables.

2: Phytoestrogen foods like soy help maintain normal vascular function. Soy foods not only lower cholesterol, but along with herbs, soy is a rich source of phytoestrogens for female vitality and heart protection during menopause.

3: Take natural vitamin E (400IU) daily. Even though it's old news, vitamin E daily still cuts heart attack risk 77%. Soy foods are a good diet source of vitamin E AND phytoestrogens (see above). Animal studies find soy isoflavones can reduce arterial plaque.

4: Take a daily herbal heart tonic to protect against congestive heart failure, especially if you have reached menopause. Use a combination like Crystal Star HEART STAR HEART PROTECTOR for WOMEN, from Healthy House for 6 months as circulatory support.

5: CoQ-10, 100mg daily, strengthens the heart muscle and helps it work effectively. (CoQ$_{10}$ also protects against breast cancer.)

6: EFA's (essential fatty acids) are important to women's heart health, because they are critical for hormone balance, a big part of women's heart problems. EFA's help decrease the "stickiness" of blood platelets. Evening primrose oil, about 2000mg daily, provides top quality EFA's for women. Have cold water fish 3 times a week for heart-healthy omega-3 oils and EFA's. Salmon is one of God's gifts, a rich source of omega-3 fatty acids and vitamin E (farm-raised now so you don't have to worry about endangerment).

7: Eat potassium-rich foods for cardiotonic activity: The American Heart Association says that women with a diet high in potassium-rich foods have a 38% lower risk of a stroke. My favorites are sea greens, broccoli, bananas, leafy greens and brown rice.

Lower your homocysteine levels naturally.
A simple 4 point program shows results for women in 1 to 3 months.

—**B vitamins to the rescue.** A high intake of folic acid and B$_6$ lowers risk for heart disease 45% in women (Feb. 1998 Journal AMA). Take B Complex, 100mg daily. Add 50mg extra B$_6$ and 400mcg extra folic acid to help break down homocysteine.

—**Four garlic capsules** (1200mg a day) maintain aortic elasticity.

—**Daily ginger.** Some doctors advise taking aspirin to prevent a stroke or heart attack. The medical justification for this is that aspirin inhibits an enzyme that makes blood prone to dangerous stickiness. Ginger not only inhibits this same enzyme but it does so without aspirin's side effects like gastric bleeding. Use ginger regularly in cooking. Crystallized ginger is fine, too. Ginger also lowers cholesterol by "roto-rooter-ing" your circulatory system as it travels to your extremities.

—**Red wine especially contains plant estrogens,** antioxidants, and anticoagulant properties to help protect women from cardiovascular disease after menopause. Two to four glasses of wine a month have also been shown to prevent macular degeneration.

Herb and Supplement Choices

• **Heart protective herbs for menopausal women:** Crystal Star FEMALE HARMONY™, or Ginkgo Biloba extract helps prevent ischemia-caused fibrillation; Crystal Star WOMEN'S HEART PROTECTOR caps, from Healthy House; Vitex extract; Licorice root tea; Crystal Star GINSENG-LICORICE ELIXIR™ drops.

• **Heart disease preventives:** Folic acid to keep homocysteine levels down, with B-6 100mg and Country Life sublingual B-12, 2500mcg; or Stress B Complex 150mg; • Country Life RELAXER capsules and Country Life CALCIUM-MAGNESIUM-POTASSIUM capsules; Cayenne-Ginger caps or Solaray COOL CAYENNE 2 daily, or Heartfoods CAYENNE products.

• **Regulate heart action:** Heart regulating herbs usually work within 1 minute for simple palpitations. Hawthorn extract as needed (about 800mg daily); or Crystal Star HEART STABILIZER; Cayenne extract drops; Siberian ginseng extract drops; Crystal Star HEARTSEASE-HAWTHORN™ caps, a preventive. Magnesium 800mg daily. To deter atrial fibrillation: Rainbow Light CALCIUM PLUS, 4 daily; or Country Life CAL-MAG-BROMELAIN caps.

• **Reduce fatty deposits that cause some arrhythmias:** Berberine herbs, goldenseal root, Oregon grape root, or barberry. Add taurine 1000mg daily with vitamin C 2000mg daily.

• **Normalize circulation:** *Butcher's broom* tea (for 2 to 3 weeks); *Rosemary* tea; *Ginger* capsules 2 daily; *Peppermint-Sage* tea or Solaray CHROMIACIN 3x daily.

• **Antioxidants are preventives:** OPC's from white pine or grapeseed 100mg daily; Futurebiotics VITAL K daily; CoQ-10, 60mg 3x daily; MICROHYDRIN available from Healthy House; Vitamin E 400IU with selenium 200mcg. daily.

Bodywork and Lifestyle Techniques

–Bodywork:

• Plunge your face into cold water when arrhythmia occurs to stop palpitations.

• Avoid soft drinks. The phosphorus binds up magnesium and makes it unavailable for heart regularity.

• Springlife POLARIZERS help normalize against heart arrhythmias.

• Apply hot compresses and massage chest of the victim to ease a heart attack.

• Chewing an aspirin immediately following symptoms of a heart attack, may be able to reduce mortality through its ability to reduce arterial blockage.

• Take alternate hot and cold showers frequently to increase circulation.

• Smoking constricts arteries and can cause blood pressure to skyrocket, too. Researchers estimate that 150,000 heart disease deaths would be prevented each year if Americans just quit smoking! Is it time for you to quit?

• Take some mild regular daily exercise. Do deep breathing exercises every morning for body oxygen, and to stimulate brain activity.

• Consciously add relaxation and a good daily laugh to your life. A positive mental outlook does wonders for stress.

Can't find a recommended product? Call the 800 number listed in Product Resources for the store nearest you and for more info.

Diet to Lower High Blood Pressure

High blood pressure is a major problem in America's fast-paced, high-stress world. It is the leading health problem for women today. (Fewer than half have their blood pressure under control.) It causes 60,000 deaths a year and directly relates to more than 250,000 deaths from stroke. It silently steals your health and foreshadows cardiovascular disease that can steal your life. Most cases of high blood pressure are caused by atherosclerosis and exhausted kidneys - factors that can be brought under control by diet and lifestyle improvement. In fact, clinical studies show that people with hypertension who make good life changes fare much better than those on anti-hypertensive drugs. It is worth noting that vegetarians have less hypertension and fewer blood pressure problems.

Do you have high blood pressure? Check these signs:

—frequent headaches and irritability? chronic constipation? *(from calcium and fiber deficiency)*

—dizziness and ringing in the ears? frequent heart arrhythmias? flushed complexion? red streaks in your eyes? *(from auto-toxemia)*

—great fatigue along with sleeplessness? depression? kidney malfunction? *(from insulin resistance and poor sugar metabolism)*

—chronic respiratory problems? *(from excess mucous and wastes)*

—uncontrolled weight gain and fluid retention? *(thyroid imbalance from increased fat storage, too much salt, red meat, and lack of exercise)*

Eighty-five percent of high blood pressure is preventable without drugs.

1–Keep your body weight down. Go on a juice diet for 1 day every week for 2 months to reduce extra blood fats.

2–Control your salt use. (See Low Salt Diet, pg. 100). The key to salt balance is drinking plenty of water. When your body perceives low water, it responds by retaining sodium to reduce further water loss, starting a vicious cycle of cravings for salty foods and liquids that ends in high blood pressure. (Constantly taking diuretics for high blood pressure can aggravate this cycle.) Eliminate foods that provoke high blood pressure - canned and frozen foods, cured, smoked and canned meats, peanut butter, soy sauce, bouillon cubes and condiments, fried chips and snacks, dry soups.

3–Then follow the High Blood Pressure Diet on the next page: include lots of vitamin C, magnesium and potassium foods: broccoli, bananas, dried fruits, potatoes, seafood, bell peppers, avocados, celery, brown rice and leafy greens.

4–Eat smaller meals more frequently; consciously undereat. Avoid refined foods, caffeine, salty, sugary, fried, fatty foods, prepared meats, heavy pastries and soft drinks. All cause potassium depletion and allow arterial plaque build-up.

Can natural therapies lower blood pressure? Most people don't require medication to control their disease. Millions can reverse high blood pressure with simple diet and lifestyle therapy. 1997 Harvard Medical School research finds a low-fat diet may lower blood pressure as much as drugs. Meditation for 20 minutes, twice daily is as effective as drug therapy to lower blood pressure.

Diet to Lower High Blood Pressure

A diet change is the best thing you can do to control high blood pressure. The rewards are high - a longer, healthier life - and control of your life. Avoid antacids that neutralize natural stomach acid and invite your body to produce even more acid.

Watchwords: 90% of high blood pressure is thought to be the result of a calcium deficiency, usually accompanied by arterial plaque build-up. Make sure you're getting enough food source calcium in your diet.

—**On rising:** Have citrus juices, a potassium drink (pg. 568) or a high nutrient drink like All One VITAMIN-MINERAL drink, or Crystal Star BIOFLAV, FIBER and C SUPPORT™ drink.

—**Breakfast:** Make a mix of 2 TBS each: lecithin granules, toasted wheat germ, nutritional yeast, honey and sesame seeds. Sprinkle some on fresh fruit or mix with yogurt and add a teasp. New Chapter GINGER WONDER SYRUP; or have a poached or baked egg with bran muffins or whole grain toast, and kefir cheese or unsalted butter; or some whole grain cereal or pancakes with a little maple syrup.

—**Mid-morning:** A veggie drink (pg. 569) or Crystal Star ENERGY GREEN™ drink, or Green Foods GREEN MAGMA, Nutricology PRO-GREENS, Futurebiotics VITAL K, or Knudsens natural V-8 juice or peppermint tea: or a cup of miso soup with sea greens snipped on top, or low-sodium ramen noodle soup; and some crunchy raw veggies with kefir cheese or yogurt cheese dip.

—**Lunch:** Have one cup daily of fenugreek tea with 1 teasp. honey; then have a tofu and spinach salad with some sprouts and bran muffins; or a large fresh green salad with a lemon-flax oil dressing. Add plenty of sprouts, tofu, raisins, cottage cheese, nuts, and seeds as desired; or have a baked potato with yogurt or kefir cheese topping, and a light veggie omelet; or a seafood and vegetable pasta salad; or some grilled or braised vegetables with an olive oil dressing and brown rice.

—**Mid-afternoon:** Have a bottle of mineral water, a cup of peppermint tea, or any tea with Crystal Star GINSENG/LICORICE ELIXIR™ extract for sugar balance. Have a veggie green drink, V-8 juice, or carrot juice; or a cup of miso soup with a hard boiled egg, or whole grain crackers; or dried fruits, and an apple or cranberry juice.

—**Dinner:** Have apple, pear or papaya juice before dinner. Then have a baked vegetable casserole with tofu and brown rice, and a small dinner salad; or a baked fish or seafood dish with rice and peas, or a baked potato; or a vegetable quiche (such as broccoli, artichoke, or asparagus), and a light oriental soup; or some roast turkey and cornbread dressing, with a small salad or mashed potatoes with a little butter; or an Asian vegetable stir fry, with a light, clear soup and brown rice.

Note: A little wine is fine with dinner for relaxation, digestion and tension relief.

—**Before bed:** Have a cup of miso soup, or Red Star NUTRITIONAL YEAST broth, apple juice, or some chamomile tea.

Recipes for a high blood pressure diet: • HIGH FIBER FOODS; • SEAFOODS; • ENZYME-RICH RECIPES; • BREAKFAST FOODS; • PROTEIN without MEAT; • DAIRY FREE COOKING; • MINERAL-RICH RECIPES; • LOW FAT FOODS.

Herb and Supplement Choices

•**Regulate blood pressure:** Crystal Star HEARTSEASE H.B.P.™ caps or tea daily, or America's Finest GUGULIPID - HAW-THORN complex; Vitamin E therapy: Take 100IU daily for 1 week, then 400IU daily for 1 week, then 800IU capsules daily for 2 weeks. Add 1 selenium 200mcg, and 1 Ester C with bioflavs each time. Add PHYCOTENE MICROCLUSTERS available at Healthy House for accelerated uptake. Golden Pride FORMULA ONE oral chelation a.m. and p.m. with EDTA.

•**Tone your arteries with flavonoids:** Take HAWTHORN extract, especially for palpitations. Ginkgo Biloba extract for circulation; Cayenne-ginger caps 4 daily, or Wakunaga AGED GARLIC extract; Grifron MAITAKE caps; PCO's 300mg daily; Garlic caps 6 daily; Siberian ginseng extract caps, 2000mg.

•**Naturally reduce edema:** Crystal Star TINKLE™ caps; Dandelion extract drops in tea. If taking diuretics, take vitamin C 1000mg, potassium 99mg, and B-complex 100mg daily.

•**Reduce risk of a stroke:** MRI ALPHA-LIPOIC ACID; Crystal Star GREEN TEA CLEANSER™, Rainbow Light CALCIUM PLUS caps with high magnesium, 6 daily; Wakunaga KYOLIC SUPER FORMULA 106.

•**Reduce stress to control hypertension:** Nature's Secret ULTIMATE B daily with extra B$_6$ 100mg, and niacin 100mg 3x daily. Crystal Star RELAX CAPS™; CoQ$_{10}$ 60mg 3x daily; Country Life RELAXER caps with GABA; Suma caps 6 daily.

•**Boost your essential fatty acids:** Omega-3 fish or flax oils 3 daily; Evening Primrose Oil 3000mg daily.

•**Handle fats and dairy foods better:** Bromelain 1000mg. daily; Chromium picolinate 200mcg. daily for insulin resistance. Transformation LYPOZYME; Planetary TRIPHALA caps.

Bodywork and Lifestyle Techniques

•You have high blood pressure if you have a repeated reading over 150/90mmHg. If you have high blood pressure, monitor your progress often with a home or free drugstore electronic machine reading.

•**Avoid tobacco in all forms** to dramatically lower blood pressure. Smoking constricts blood vessels, making your heart work harder. Smoking also aggravates high blood sugar levels.

•**Avoid Phenylalanine** (especially as found in Nutra-Sweet) and over-the-counter antihistamines that aggravate high blood pressure.

•**Eliminate caffeine and hard liquor.** They can cause adrenaline rushes that make blood pressure soar. (A little wine at night with dinner can actually lower stress and hypertension.)

•**Exercise is important.** Take a brisk 30 minute walk every day, with plenty of deep lung breathing.

•**Relaxation techniques are important.** Massage and meditation are two of the best for hypertension.

•**Use a dry skin brush all over the body** frequently to stimulate better blood flow.

•**Reflexology point:** Pull middle finger on each hand 3x for 20 seconds each time, daily.

Can't find a recommended product? Call the 800 number listed in Product Resources for the store nearest you and for more info.

Diet to Lower High Cholesterol

Cholesterol is a fat-related substance essential to every body function. Poor metabolism and artery clogging foods lead to serious deposits in arterial linings, and to gallstones. There are two kinds of cholesterol: **HDL** (high density lipo-protein, or "good" cholesterol), and **LDL and VLDL** (low density and very low density lipo-proteins, or "bad" cholesterol). **Triglycerides** are a sugar-related blood fat that travels with cholesterol. High triglycerides cause blood cells to stick together, impairing circulation and leading to heart attack.

Oxidized LDL-cholesterol significantly contributes to accumulation of artery plaque. This progression is inhibited, and may even be prevented by taking PCO's (oligomeric proanthocyanidin complexes), a class of powerful antioxidant polyphenols that are rich in grape seed and white pine. *Note: High cholesterol levels do not seem to increase heart disease risk in people 70 and older; and some cholesterol-lowering drugs are actually harmful. Ask about yours.*

What level should your cholesterol be?

High cholesterol affects as many as 60 million Americans, and it is a major factor for coronary heart disease. Cholesterol screening is recommended for all adults, but test results can be complicated. Here's a rundown of what is tested in today's cholesterol screening and what it can mean for your health.

LDL (low density lipoprotein), the "bad" cholesterol, carries cholesterol through the bloodstream for cell-building, but leaves behind the excess on artery walls and in tissues. Ideal LDL levels are less than 130 mg/dL. Levels between 130 mg/dL to 159 mg/dL are borderline high. Levels 160 mg/dL and over are high. Pay close attention to your results here. High LDL cholesterol accumulated on arteries walls can eventually block the flow of blood to your heart or brain, resulting in a heart attack or stroke.

New research points out new concerns. Almost half of all heart disease patients have pattern-B LDL's, smaller and denser than normal LDL's. Pattern-B LDL's enter into blood vessels 40% faster than normal LDL's, so fat is deposited on artery walls faster than it can be removed. Studies show people with more than 25% of pattern-B LDL cholesterol have three times the normal risk of heart diseases – even when their total LDL count is normal! New cholesterol screening shows pattern-B LDL cholesterol levels.

HDL (high density lipoprotein), the "good" cholesterol, helps prevent narrowing of the artery walls by transporting excess LDL cholesterol to the liver for excretion as bile. Ideal HDL cholesterol levels are 60 mg/dL and above. Levels below 35 mg/dL are too low.

Triglycerides increase the density of LDL cholesterol molecules. Ideal triglyceride levels are less than 200 mg/dL. 200 to 399 mg/dL is considered borderline. Heart attack rate is twice as high if your triglyceride level is above 250. Levels 400 mg/dL and above are dangerous to health.

Total cholesterol levels: Should be less than 200 mg/dL. Levels 200 to 239 mg/dL are borderline high. Anything over 240 mg/dL is high and puts you at an increased risk for heart disease. Low cholesterol levels (below 180) affect 10% of Americans and can be dangerous, too. According to a new study done by the University of Washington, low cholesterol is a risk factor for hemorrhagic stroke! But beware.... Side effects of cholesterol-lowering drugs like Zocor, Mevacor and Pravachol include liver toxicity, stomach distress and vision impairment. According to a study in Journal of Clinical Pharmacology, these drugs also deplete CoQ_{10}, an essential co-enzyme that strengthens the heart and arteries, by up to 50%!

Is your cholesterol too high? Check these signs:

—Is your circulation poor? *(from plaque formation on the artery walls)*
—Do you get frequent leg cramps and pain?
—Do you lead a high stress lifestyle? Is your high blood pressure too high? *(from a diet too low in fiber)*
—Do you have bouts of difficult breathing? Are your hands and feet always cold?
—Is your skin and hair always dry? *(from a diet without enough essential fatty acids)*
—Do you get heart palpitations and dizziness alternating with periods of lethargy?
—Do you have multiple allergies and kidney trouble? *(from a diet too high in saturated fats and sugars)*

Watchwords:

1—Cholesterol in foods like eggs isn't the culprit. Eggs are a whole food, with phosphatides to balance the cholesterol. The big contributor to high blood cholesterol levels is saturated fat and over-eating. Focus instead on plant foods like red yeast rice and Red Star NUTRI-TIONAL YEAST. Vegetarians who occasionally eat eggs and small amounts of low fat dairy are at the lowest risk for arterial or heart disease.

2—A low fat, high fiber diet is still the key to reducing cholesterol. Reducing sugar is the key to lowering triglycerides. Fiber drinks and supplements really help... usually with noticeable benefits in 1 to 2 months. Two good drinks I recommend are Crystal Star CHOL-LO FIBER TONE™ drink and Green Foods BERRY BARLEY ESSENCE.

3—Foods that lower bad cholesterol: soy foods (with isoflavones), olive oil, whole grains like oats, high fiber foods like fresh fruits and vegetables, beans, yogurt and cultured foods, and yams.

4—Substantially reduce or avoid animal fats, red meats, fried foods, fatty dairy foods, salty/sugary foods, refined foods.

5—Eat smaller meals, especially at night. A little wine with dinner reduces stress and raises HDL's.

6—A morning cup of green tea (or Crystal Star GREEN TEA CLEANSER™), and a royal jelly/ginseng drink (or Beehive Botanical ROYAL JELLY/GINSENG caps) for a month makes a noticeable difference in cholesterol levels.

Recipes for a high cholesterol-lowering diet: • HIGH FIBER FOODS; • SEAFOODS; • ENZYME-RICH RECIPES; • BREAK-FAST FOODS; • PROTEIN without MEAT; • DAIRY FREE COOKING; • LOW FAT RECIPES; • SALADS, HOT and COLD.

Bodywork and Lifestyle Techniques

Bodywork:

•**Reduce your body weight.** Many overweight people have abnormal metabolism. If you are 10 pounds overweight, your body produces an extra 100mg of cholesterol every day.

•**Exercise is preventive medicine for cholesterol.** Even if you cut your fat, you need to exercise to lower your LDL's. Take a brisk daily walk or other regular aerobic exercise of your choice to enhance circulation and boost HDL.

•**Eliminate tobacco use of all kinds.** Nicotine raises cholesterol levels.

•**Practice a favorite stress reduction technique at least once a day.** There is a correlation between high cholesterol and aggression. Men who are the most emotionally repressive have the highest cholesterol levels.

Herb and Supplement Choices

•**Balance LDL to HDL levels (the real secret):** Crystal Star CHOL-EX™ caps, 3 daily, 2 months; Crystal Star GINSENG-REISHI extract. • Red yeast rice; Futurebiotics CHOLESTA-LO.

•**Support cardiovascular health:** Crystal Star HEARTSEASE-CIRCU-CLEANSE™ tea; Hawthorn extract 3x daily. Golden Pride FORMULA ONE oral chelation with EDTA. Source Naturals TOCOTRIENOLS 34mg.

•**Boost antioxidant intake:** CoQ$_{10}$ 100mg daily; Grapeseed PCO's 100mg daily; or BILBERRY extract 2x daily for PCO's; MICROHYDRIN available at Healthy House; Carlson E-ELITE soft gels; • Carnitine 1000mg. daily.

•**Good fats balance out bad fats:** Evening Primrose Oil 4000mg daily; Omega-3 rich flax oil capsules daily.

•**Raise HDL's:** Panax ginseng (protects the liver); Suma root; Solaray ALFA JUICE caps; Herbs Etc. CHOLESTERO-TONIC.

•**Lower LDL, VLDL and triglyceride levels:** Grifron MAITAKE mushroom caplets; Cayenne-Ginger capsules 2 daily; Garlic, or Garlic-Fenugreek seed caps 6 daily decrease bad cholesterol10%); Nutricology NAC (N-acetyl-cysteine) 500mg 2x daily; Chromium 200mcg for triglycerides.

•**Help the liver metabolize cholesterol:** Drink green tea or take Crystal Star GREEN TEA CLEANSER™, Milk Thistle Seed extract for 3 months; Dandelion root tea; Schiff ENZYMALL with ox bile daily. Solaray LIPOTROPIC 1000. Nature's Herbs CHOLESTEROL POWER; Planetary TRIPHALA caps.

•**Niacin therapy reduces harmful blood fats and benefits nerves.** (Not for use in cases of glucose intolerance, liver disease or peptic ulcer.) Flush-free niacin is OK. Dose: 1000mg daily; Bio-Resource LO-NIACIN with glycine 500mg if sugar sensitive.

Can't find a recommended product? Call the 800 number listed in Product Resources for the store nearest you and for more info.

Holistic Recovery and Recuperation

Long illness, severe injury, any surgery procedure or hospital stay, puts the body through tremendous physical and psychological trauma. Optimal nourishment at these times is necessary for faster and better healing, for cleaning out drug residues and overcoming their side effects, and for returning the body to health after the poor nutrition of most hospitals. (Why do hospitals have such terrible food? Hospital meals seem to aggravate illness rather than strengthen for defense against it.)

Your body has the power to heal itself, but its vital recuperative forces need extra nutritive help after injury or illness to do it. Low immune response after illness or surgery, poor appetite and reduced assimilation call for more concentrated nutrients than a normal diet provides. Once the system stabilizes and the body begins to supply its own healing powers, the increased support can be moderated to normal amounts. The body will begin to take over more and more of its own work, and begin replacing the nutrition it has lost.

Are you considering surgery or a long course of drug therapy?

Consider well, and know your options. There's a new epidemic in the new millennium.... doctor and drug-caused disease. Iatrogenic disease, literally "disease caused by doctors, hospitals or drugs" has hit the media radar screen in a big way. And rightly so... it's a snowballing problem in today's drug-oriented society. Up to 90% of us will take more than one course of prescriptions drugs. Two and one-half billion prescriptions are filled by U.S. pharmacies every year. That number is expected to skyrocket to 4 billion by the year 2005! The majority of us will spend some time in the hospital at some point in our lives. But prescription drugs can hurt as well as help, and you may leave the hospital sicker than you were when you checked in. Even worse, you might not leave at all!

Adverse drug reactions or interactions are estimated to be between the 4th and 6th leading cause of death in the United States — with a death toll of nearly 200,000 people each year. More than 2 million patients in U.S. hospitals per year are harmed by the side effects of drug therapies or other hospital treatments. Deepak Chopra, M.D. estimates that "the number of people that die in the U.S. as the result of medical treatment is equivalent to three 747 crashes, with fatalities, every two days." In fact, you're actually more likely to be injured or killed by a routine visit to a physician than in an automobile accident.

The latest figures show the rate at which patients pick up an infection while in a U.S. hospital has also increased... an astounding 36% in the last 20 years! 90,000 patients die each year as the result of hospital-acquired infection. If you have a serious immune disorder like AIDS, or cancer or are undergoing treatments which kill immunity like chemo or radiation, infections that are spread through hospitals can spell life or death. The financial cost is devastating at, conservatively, around $140 billion annually.

Are we taking a prescription for disaster?

Today's wonder drugs may not be so wonderful. Seventy-five percent of all adverse drug reactions (ADR's) are due to the inherent toxicity of the drug used. Of the 198 drugs the FDA approved between 1976-1985, 102 of them were found to have serious risks, including heart attack, heart failure, blindness, birth defects, severe blood disorders, and kidney and liver failure.

Amazingly, half of all people are prescribed medicines that interact, sometimes with deadly consequences. Further, while the elderly are prime targets for drug therapy and regularly take 2 or 3 different prescriptions at the same time, at least 250 available drugs should not be taken by older adults. Parkinson's symptoms, memory deterioration, injurious accidents, all thought to be the result of aging process, are regularly the result of drug therapy!

More worrisome: Today people can get their prescriptions easily over the web. Just fill out a short on-line questionnaire, and a powerful and potentially dangerous drug treatments arrive in the mail. Some state regulators have even found web sites advertising the highly controversial drug Viagra linked to as many as 130 deaths. Their slogan: "Need Viagra? No prescription? No problem!"

One company gave away frequent flyer points for American Airlines to doctors who prescribed the beta blocker drug, Inderal, to patients. Doctors who wrote 50 prescriptions for the heart drug could actually claim a FREE round trip ticket anywhere in the U.S. That company is still thriving today, with the largest number of prescriptions today written for its estrogen replacement drug derived from pregnant mare's urine. Even the medical studies are affected. A 1998 study in the New England Journal of Medicine reveals that an author's published opinion on the safety of a calcium-channel antagonist is strongly related to his or her financial ties to the manufacturer.

Does nutrition fit into the drug-mold for health?

If you thought medical schools had finally realized how important nutrition is to healing, think again. The average U.S. physician STILL only spends 2.5 hours in nutrition courses during their 4 years in medical school. Moreover, only 25% of medical schools require future doctors to take nutrition courses. The best research shows us that optimum nutrition is the BASIS of good health and disease prevention. New studies show that a wholesome diet and a healthy lifestyle can prevent up to 90% of all cancers. Experts affirm that most heart disease is 100% preventable with simple changes in diet and lifestyle. Yet, hospital food is notorious for nutritional deficiencies, and more than likely your doctor knows little or nothing about the healing power of nutrition.

The latest studies show that medical nutrition could save Medicare $1.3 Billion by 2002 by reducing hospital stays and complications for acute and chronic diseases of the elderly. One HMO hoping to cut down costs found that using herbs to replace certain drugs could save them between $500,000 and $750,000 in drug costs yearly. Another report shows that nutritional supplements could save another $20 billion in hospital costs. These savings could be realized specifically in the use of folic acid to prevent birth defects, multivitamins and minerals to prevent low birth weight infants, and vitamin E for coronary heart disease.

If nutrition is so important, then why aren't doctors learning more about it in medical school? As sad as it is to report this, it is in the financial interests of doctors and pharmaceuticals companies to keep you sick. Pharmaceutical companies gross over $122 billion a year (more than $1 million every hour) in sales. Doctors' incomes depend on performing surgeries, prescribing drugs and ordering lots of tests. Not to mention that pharmaceutical companies enchant physicians with gifts, free travel and free medical equipment. Drug companies spent an excess of $5,000 on individual doctors in 1988. The newest figures haven't been revealed, but those numbers are probably much higher.

You may be shocked by this information, but, obviously modern medicine isn't all bad. The ability to isolate microbes that cause infectious disease, and to create treatments that would kill those microbes without killing the patient, was a milestone in modern medicine. Still, even with the vast medical arsenal available to doctors today, they can only cure about one-fourth of the illnesses presented to them. A recent report by the U.S. Office of Technology Assessment shows only 10 to 20% of standard medical procedures are effective!

We're all searching for the right blend of medicine.

It's been a well-kept "grass roots" secret, but in response to the limitations of modern medicine, 63% percent of Americans in 1999 used some form of complementary or alternative medicine. That number is expected to rise dramatically as the results of new clinical trials on natural healing therapies become available. Four out of ten people also turn first to alternative medicine practitioners instead of conventional physicians. Harvard research shows more visits are being made to alternative healers than to conventional doctors. As a result, an increasing number of MDs are including holistic treatments, adopting some of the practices of natural medicine, in order to offer their patients the best of both worlds. More than half of all medical professionals also use some form of alternative medicine for their own self-care.

I feel we need both types of medicine to stay well in today's world. Our bodies are so complicated......with an incredibly complex immune system, thousands of enzymes, delicate fluid balance, and interlocking circulatory pathways. Multiply those things by the uniqueness of each person, and you can see why we need a wealth of choices for our health.

If you're affected by the pitfalls of modern medicine, natural therapies are ideally suited to help your body recuperate and regenerate. There is no question that although sometimes necessary, drug therapy (particularly long term) and surgical procedures take its toll on even the healthiest of persons. Take healing steps before and after your surgery to strengthen your system, alleviate body stress, and increase your chances of rapid recovery and healing. Rebalancing body chemistry, boosting nutrients, restoring foundation strength and immune response should be your focus for a healthy recovery.

Recuperation diets are effective for other problems where healing-strength nutrition is needed: *Anemia and Pernicious Anemia, Parkinson's Disease, Meningitis, Malnutrition from Eating Disorders like Bulimia and Anorexia, Rheumatic Fever, Infertility, Sterility, Sports Injuries and Muscle Atrophy, Poor Wound Healing.*

Holistic Healing from Surgery or Illness

Up to 40 million Americans have in-patient surgery for their health every year. However, as more and more Americans are going under the knife, I see a growing trend in health care that is frightening and disconcerting. Patients are rushed in and out of operating rooms, and then rushed out of the hospital with no tools on how to recover. Most doctors provide little or no information on how diet choices and supportive therapies can jumpstart healing from surgery and get you on the fast track back to health.

The body has the power to heal itself, but its vital recuperative forces need extra nutritive help after surgery to do it. The emphasis in this chapter is on rebuilding strength, regenerating healthy new tissue, and replenishing overall vitality. The recovery diets are high in protein and amino acids, depleted during body trauma and vital for new cell growth.

Note: An initial fast for cleansing is not the way to begin if your body is greatly weakened or under acute trauma, even though it probably harbors many drug residues. There is often so much depletion and stress, that a rigorous fast is self-defeating. Raw vegetable juices as additions to other foods, however, are an excellent means of purifying and normalizing the system.

Pre-op techniques strengthen your body for surgery. Start 2 to 3 weeks before your scheduled surgery.

Strengthen your immune system and supply your body with healing nutrients. Include daily:

—Extra vegetable protein. You must have protein to heal. Eat brown rice, other whole grains and sea greens.
—Vitamin C 3000mg with bioflavonoids and rutin for tissue integrity.
—B Complex 100mg with pantothenic acid 500mg for adrenal strength.
—A multivitamin/mineral with anti-oxidants, beta-carotene, zinc, calcium and magnesium for tissue repair.
—Take a full spectrum, pre-digested amino acid compound drink, about 1000mg daily.
—OPC's, pycnogenol or grape seed, 50mg 2x daily, as powerful antioxidants.
—Garlic caps, 4-6 daily, an antibiotic that enhances immune function. (Discontinue 2-3 days before surgery.)

Strengthen your ability to heal. Include daily:

—Bromelain 750mg twice daily (with Quercetin 250mg if you expect inflammation).
—CoQ-10, 100mg 2x daily and/or germanium 150mg capsules, 2x daily - as free radical destroyers.
—CHLORELLA 15 tablets, 1 packet of powder, or Crystal Star ENERGY GREEN™ drink for chlorophyll.
—Centella asiatica (gotu kola) capsules, 2 caps 2x daily for nerve tissue strength.
—Crystal Star GINSENG SIX SUPER™ tea, 2x daily for recuperation strength.
—Vitamin K for blood clotting. Food sources: leafy greens, blackstrap molasses, alfalfa sprouts.
—Take a potassium juice (page 568), a potassium supplement liquid, or a protein-mineral drink daily.

A healing/mending program like this gives the body super nutrition for a limited time-temporarily increasing calories, protein, even fats to provide concentrated raw materials for serious nutritional deficiencies.

Note 1: The medical community uses information and testing results from synthetic, rather than naturally-occurring vitamin E sources, like wheat germ and soy. Thus, many doctors insist that no vitamin E be taken four weeks prior to surgery in an effort to curb post-operative bleeding. I have not found this to be a problem with natural vitamin E, but suggest that you consult your physician if you are in doubt.

Note 2: Immediately prior to surgery, take a pinch of ginger powder (or 8 - 10 drops ginger extract) in water to relieve nausea after surgery. Don't take garlic 2 to 3 days before surgery (it's a slight blood thinner).

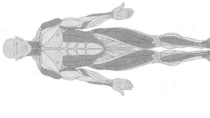

<u>Accelerate healing after surgery.</u> Start Post-Op healers immediately when you come home.

<u>Eat a very nutritious diet. Include frequently:</u>

–AloeLife ALOE GOLD drink, diluted as directed in one 8-oz. glass daily.

–A potassium broth (page 568), or a vegetable drink (page 569).

–A protein drink: Nature's Life SUPER-GREEN PRO-96, ALL ONE multi drink or Transitions EASY GREENS.

–Plenty of fresh fruits and vegetables. Have a green salad every day.

–Daily sushi (at least 6 pieces), or sea greens for vitamin B_{12} and new cell growth.

–Brown rice and other whole grains with tofu for protein complementarity and more B vitamins.

–Yogurt and other cultured foods for friendly intestinal flora.

Herbal combinations can contribute a great deal to the success of surgery — nurturing, normalizing, supporting, healing. **Specific systems that herbs can heal:**

• Cardiovascular System and Blood Vessels - hawthorn, garlic and ginkgo

• Respiratory System - mullein and coltsfoot

• Digestive System - chamomile and lemon balm

• Glandular System - panax ginseng

• Bowel/Urinary System - corn silk for the bladder; yellow dock for the bowel

• Reproductive System - women: black cohosh, false unicorn root. men: saw palmetto and damiana

• Nervous System - oats and St. John's wort

• Musculo-Skeletal System - aloe vera, oatstraw, sarsaparilla

• Skin - sea vegetables, nettles, red clover, and calendula, St. John's wort oil or cream for scarring

• Immune System - nettles, cleavers, red clover

• Drug and Liver detoxification - milk thistle seed

Recovery and Recuperation Diets

Note: Certain foods may interfere with medications. Dairy foods and iron supplements interfere with some antibiotics. Acid fruits (oranges, pineapples and grapefruit) may inhibit the action of penicillin and aspirin. Avocados, bananas, cheese, chocolate, colas and fermented foods interfere with monoamine oxidase (MAO), an anti-depressant, hypertension drug. Avoid fatty foods before and after surgery; they slow nutrient assimilation.

Clean the body and vital organs to counteract infection. Include daily for one month:

—High potency, multi-culture compound such as Prevail INNER ECOLOGY, or UAS DDS-Plus with FOS with meals.
—Crystal Star LIV-ALIVE™ capsules, tea or extract.
—Crystal Star GINSENG/REISHI MUSHROOM extract to clear toxicity and provide deep body tone.
—Bovine cartilage capsules 6 daily, or colloidal silver, 1 teasp. for 1 week, then $^1/_2$ teasp., to fight infection.
—Enzyme therapy such as Transformation PUREZYME or Prevail VITASE.
—Fresh carrot juice, vegetable juice or herbal tea daily.

Build up the body tissues. Include daily for one month:

—Crystal Star SYSTEMS STRENGTH™ drink, and BODY REBUILDER™ with ADR-ACTIVE™ caps.
—Vitamin C with bioflavonoids and rutin 500mg only, with pantothenic acid 1000mg.
—Carnitine 250mg with CoQ-10, 60mg 3x daily as antioxidants.
—Zinc 30-50mg, Futurebiotics VITAL K potassium, or Flora VEGE-SIL to help rebuild tissue.
—Co-enzymate B complex sublingual, 1 tablet 3x daily, or Country Life sublingual B_{12}.
—Enzymatic Therapy LIQUID LIVER capsules, or Crystal Star CHLORELLA-GINSENG extract.
—Herbal Answer's ALOE FORCE SKIN GEL or Crystal Star ANTI-BIO™ gel to heal skin and scars.

Other recovery and recuperation information:

—If you are taking antibiotics, take them with bromelain 150mg for better effectiveness, and supplement with B Complex, Vitamin C, Vitamin K and calcium.
—If you are taking diuretics, add Vitamin C, potassium and B complex, to strengthen kidneys.
—If you are taking aspirin, take with vitamin C for best results.
—If you are taking antacids, supplement with Vitamin B_1 and/or calcium.
—If your surgery involved bone and cartilage, take Crystal Star MINERAL SPECTRUM™ capsules 4 daily.
—If you smoke, add Vitamin C 500mg, E 400IU, beta-carotene 50,000IU and niacin 100mg.
—If you are considering chelation therapy, remember that it works in your body like a magnet collecting heavy metals and triglycerides. It is not recommended if you have weak kidneys; too many toxins are dumped into the elimination system too fast, causing stress on a healing body. Consider FORMULA 1 by Golden Pride or Metabolic Response Modifiers CARDIO-CHELATE.

Rapid Recovery Diet for Recuperation and Regeneration

Use this diet for about 4 weeks. It supplies an abundance of vitamins, minerals, trace elements, essential fatty acids and proteins to rebuild a weakened body. It has generous amounts of fresh fruits, vegetables and juices for gentle cleansing, to encourage release of drug residues and toxic wastes while promoting rapid regeneration of new tissue. It includes plenty of protein-rich foods for repair, complex carbohydrates and healthy fats for energy, cultured foods for friendly intestinal flora, and chlorophyll greens for blood building. Small, frequent simple meals are recommended instead of large heavy meals, so that the body can assimilate nutritive elements easily and efficiently.

—**On rising:** have a protein drink like All One VITAMIN-MINERAL drink or Unipro PERFECT PROTEIN in pineapple/papaya juice.
—**Breakfast:** have some yogurt with fresh fruit; then a whole grain cereal with wheat germ, sesame seeds and kefir on top; or baked, poached or scrambled eggs with cottage or kefir cheese and whole grain toast; or a small omelet with veggies or a low-fat raw cheese filling; or buckwheat pancakes or oatmeal with honey, maple syrup or molasses.
—**Mid-morning:** take a potassium drink (page 568) 3 times a week; on alternate days Monas CHLORELLA or Green Foods GREEN MAGMA with 1 teasp. each nutritional yeast and wheat germ added, or Crystal Star SYSTEMS STRENGTH™ drink with 1 teasp. Bragg's LIQUID AMINOS added; or have some miso soup with sea greens snipped on top; or whole grain baked chips or veggie chips with yogurt cheese or kefir cheese dip; or a dried fruit / fresh fruit blend with raisins, figs, apples and grapes.
—**Lunch:** have brown rice with baked tofu and steamed veggies; or a roasted, organic turkey sandwich with mayonnaise, or avocado on whole grain bread; or beans and rice with fresh salsa; or a seafood salad with whole grain or spinach pasta; or a protein salad with sprouts, sea greens, nuts and seeds; or a baked potato with a spinach and mushroom salad, and green dressing.
—**Mid-afternoon:** a glass of fresh carrot juice; or a cup of strengthening herb tea, such as dandelion root, Siberian ginseng, or Crystal Star GINSENG SIX™ Super Tea, or FEEL GREAT™ tea; or Knudsen RECHARGE electrolyte replacement drink, and yogurt with nuts and seeds, or fresh fruit; or a green drink (page 569) with 2 teasp. unsprayed bee pollen added.
—**Dinner:** have a brown rice casserole with tofu and steamed veggies, some baked chicken or fish, and a cup of miso soup; or roasted, organic turkey with baked yams and a green salad with yogurt dressing; or a vegetable quiche or pizza on a chapati crust; or a light spinach pasta with a low-fat sauce, and green salad; or a high protein dinner stew and salad with lemon-yogurt dressing; or a hearty seafood-vegetable stir-fry with brown rice; or a large open-face dinner sandwich and a light soup.
—**Before bed:** have 1 teasp. Red Star nutritional yeast in hot water; or a relaxing herb tea, like chamomile or mint; or a small bowl of oatmeal with maple syrup or honey.

Note: A glass of wine at dinner is fine for digestion. Drink plenty of pure water (8 glasses every day) for good hydration, and to keep drug residues and toxins flushing out of the body.

Recipes to help your healing diet: •**FISH and SEAFOODS;** •**ENZYME-RICH RECIPES;** •**SOUPS - LIQUID SALADS** •**HIGH PROTEIN without MEAT;** •**CULTURED FOODS;** •**MINERAL-RICH RECIPES;** •**SALADS, HOT and COLD.**

Facial Surgery Healing Program

We all want to look great at every age. The plastic surgery industry is booming! Face lifts are now the most commonly performed procedure in cosmetic surgery — fifty-three percent of total surgery procedures are for Americans between 51 and 64 years of age.

PRE-OP: daily - 2 to 3 weeks before surgery: No aspirin or alcohol 1 week before or 2 weeks after surgery. They increase bleeding tendency and reduce healing ability.

—Bromelain 1500mg and Evening Primrose oil caps 2000mg
—Royal Jelly/Siberian ginseng combination (best in an extract or tea)
—Ester C - 5000mg with bioflavonoids 500mg
—Vitamin K, sea greens and-or plenty of alfalfa sprouts
—Crystal Star ZINC SOURCE™ extract, IODINE-POTASSIUM and GINSENG 6 SUPER capsules
—Brown rice and a green salad every day

POST-OP: pre-suture removal, daily for 1 week: (Apply ice packs every hour to reduce swelling for 3 days)

—Crystal Star ANTI-FLAM™ capsules as needed, for pain relief or swelling
—Bromelain 750mg. with quercetin 250mg 2x daily, to reduce bruising
—Transformation PUREZYME 3-5 caps <u>between</u> meals to reduce any inflammation and promote rapid healing
—Co-Q10, 60mg 3x daily, for enzyme therapy tissue repair
—Centella Asiatica capsules (gotu kola), for nerve damage repair and reducing numbness
—Ester C - 5000mg w. bioflavonoids for new collagen production, tissue tightening, capillary healing
—Evening Primrose oil caps 2000mg daily, for essential fatty acids
—Royal Jelly-Siberian ginseng combination, for amino acids (protein for healing)
—Vitamin K, sea greens or plenty of alfalfa sprouts, (for bruising and bleeding)
—Brown rice and a green salad every day, for B vitamins (skin) and chlorophyll healing (blood)

POST-OP: post-suture removal, daily for 3 weeks:

—Bromelain 1500mg with Ester C - 5000mg with bioflavonoids daily; Evening Primrose oil caps 2000mg
—Apply Crystal Star BEAUTIFUL SKIN™ gel, PHYCOTENE CREME from Healthy House; aloe vera, for scar and scab healing
—Royal Jelly-Siberian ginseng tea combination; CoQ10, 60mg 2x daily and gotu kola capsules for nerve restoration
—Brown rice and a green salad every day. Add sea vegetables for skin tone and texture

2 Months later:

—Use a seaweed-aloe vera gel mask if you have had a full face lift: 1 tsp. kelp granules in 1 TB aloe vera gel.

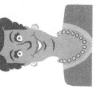

Scar Healing Diet after Facial Sugery

Surgery and major medical treatments are always traumatic on the body. Preparing your body before surgery and following a good post-op program makes an enormous difference. After an initial recovery period, your body may be ready for a short 3 to 7 day elimination diet to clean out drug residues and toxic waste, especially if they are still adversely affecting your well-being. Follow this less intense, but still highly nutritious diet to continue rebuilding energy and immune defenses.

This is a tissue restorative diet so it must be high in vitamin C foods and beta-carotene, as anti-infectives and to supply new collagen and interstitial tissue production. It is rich in B vitamins to lessen trauma and stress on the body, build blood and metabolize proteins. It is high in minerals for good digestion and basic body building blocks. Minerals are critical to tissue repair. A scar healing diet must be high in oxygenating foods to create an environment where infection cannot flourish.

—**On rising:** continue with a good high protein or vitamin/mineral drink, as in your initial healing diet; and/or take 1 TB blackstrap molasses in juice or Crystal Star BIOFLAV. FIBER and C SUPPORT™ drink.

—**Breakfast:** have some yogurt with fresh fruit, nuts or seeds; or whole grain granola with yogurt or kefir topping; or an omelet, soft boiled or scrambled egg with whole grain toast or English muffins and butter; or oatmeal or buckwheat pancakes with maple syrup; or fresh fruit with vanilla soy or almond milk or kefir or kefir cheese.

—**Mid-morning:** take at least one potassium drink or green drink, Monas CHLORELLA, Wakunaga KYO-GREEN, or Crystal Star ENERGY GREEN™ drink each day, with 1 teasp. Bragg's LIQUID AMINOS; or have an herb tea, like Crystal Star FEEL GREAT™ or GINSENG SIX™ Super tea; or licorice root, or Siberian ginseng tea. Add $\frac{1}{4}$ teasp. royal jelly to any tea for an extra healing boost; or a cup of ramen soup with sea vegetables, and baked veggie chips.

—**Lunch:** have a tofu and brown rice casserole; or a veggie-seafood salad; or a baked yam with a green salad and lemon-oil dressing; or black bean or lentil soup; or a leafy salad with sea greens and wheat germ sprinkled on top, and a lemon dressing.

—**Mid-afternoon:** have fresh fruit with low-fat cheese or kefir cheese; and a circulation tea like ginkgo biloba tea; or Knudsen RECHARGE electrolyte replacement, or Crystal Star SYSTEMS STRENGTH™ drink; or a bottle of mineral water.

—**Dinner:** have baked or grilled fish, with brown rice pilaf and a green salad; or an oriental stir-fry with miso soup, sea greens and brown rice; or a vegetable - seafood quiche or casserole; or a light spinach or artichoke pasta with a light vegetable or seafood sauce; or a vegetable or seafood soup with a leafy green salad.

—**Before Bed:** have a cup of Red Star nutritional broth, or a relaxing herb tea, like Crystal Star PILLOW TIME™ or RELAX™ tea.

Recipes to help your scar healing diet: •FISH and SEAFOODS; •ENZYME-RICH RECIPES; •SOUPS - LIQUID SALADS •HIGH PROTEIN without MEAT; •CULTURED FOODS; •MINERAL-RICH RECIPES; •LOW FAT RECIPES

Herb and Supplement Choices

• **To clean the body and vital organs:** Sonne Liquid Bentonite in the morning; acidophilus complex 3 times daily with meals; Crystal Star LIV-ALIVE™ CAPS or LIV-ALIVE TEA™.

• **To normalize glands:** wild cherry bark or burdock tea; Crystal Star ADRN-ACTIVE™ caps; B-complex 100mg daily.

• **To build healthy body tissue:** MSM 1000mg daily; vitamin E 400IU 2x daily, Enzymatic Therapy LIQUID LIVER with GINSENG, Flora VEGE-SIL caps or Body Essential SILICA GEL; vitamin B-12 internasal or sublingual; Crystal Star BODY REBUILDER™ CAPS, or SYSTEMS STRENGTH™ drink.

• **To replenish depleted mineral building blocks:** Eidon POTASSIUM (liquid), Crystal Star ENERGY GREEN DRINK™ and MINERAL SPECTRUM™ caps; Nature's Path TRACE-LYTE with sea greens.

• **To encourage wound and body trauma healing:** ascorbate vitamin C with bioflavonoids, up to 5000mg. daily; or Crystal Star BIOFLAV , FIBER and C SUPPORT DRINK™, Transformation PUREZYME 3-5 caps between meals; bromelain caps 1500mg, and Germanium 150mg daily.

• **To rebuild immunity:** HAWTHORN or ECHINACEA 100% extracts; vitamin A 25,000IU, Sun Wellness CHLORELLA tabs 15 to 20 daily (or granules), high potency digestive enzymes such as Transformation DIGESTZYME or Herbal Products and Development POWER-PLUS ENZYMES, and immune stimulating herbs such as Crystal Star HERBAL DEFENSE TEAM™ formulas, and IRON SOURCE™ caps or extract.

Note: As your body takes over its own work and strength returns, decrease the dosage and number of supplements.

Bodywork and Lifestyle Techniques

• **Take early morning sun baths every day possible** for vitamin D and tissue/bone building.

• **Take a brisk walk every day for circulation and tissue oxygen.** Go ocean walking and/or swimming when you can. Do deep breathing whenever you can.

• **Avoid all junk foods.** They fill you up, but deprive you of much needed nutrition at a critical time.

• **Get a massage therapy treatment** at least twice a month to align body energy and clear obstructions.

• **Take an oxygen energy bath** at least once a week (see page 464).

• **Apply aloe vera gel** on scars and lesions.

Can't find a recommended product? Call the 800 number listed in Product Resources for the store nearest you and for more info.

Diets for More Brain Power

The human species has done a 180° turn in the last millennium. Today we rely on brain a lot more than brawn. (Some of us worry that our brains didn't quite realize this big shift was going on because our brains feel so overworked and overcrowded.) The truth is, memory problems and mental fogginess reflect nutritional deficiencies or deep body imbalances more than brain capacity.

The brain is incredibly sensitive, and it is so active that it highly sensitive to nutrient deficiencies. Drugs and stimulants like alcohol, caffeine and tobacco accelerate its activity for a short time, but then actually depress it. Fluoride, aspartame (Nutrasweet), aluminum and MSG have been implicated in the destruction of brain cells. Sometimes we can literally see a food like sugar act on the brain in terms of anger, irritability or depression. A diet high in refined sugar actually decreases the blood sugar available to the brain. Saturated fats lead to mental fogginess; heavy starches induce lethargy. Severe deficiencies or overloads can even cause mental illness. Clinical tests show that two-thirds of mental health problems are based in poor diet.

Stress is one of the most severe deterrents to brain health. If too much of the stress hormone (cortisol) is produced in the brain, mental function declines. Chronic stress, tobacco, heavy alcohol and marijuana all inhibit the brain's release of vasopressin, which results in impaired memory, attention and reaction time.

The brain is also our primary health maintenance organ. When it is well-nourished long enough, even grave mental problems can straighten themselves out. The right nutrients stabilize emotional reactions and temperament. Optimal nutrition can even reverse aging signs like deteriorating alertness, poor balance and muscle coordination.

I'm a big believer in brain food. Mental acuity, concentration, memory and creativity all depend on the quality of nourishment you give your brain. Diet also controls neurotransmitters for learning, sleep, and I.Q. Your brain can use nutrients with far more synergistic effects than those same nutrients in other areas of the body. Clinical trials show that your brain's neurotransmitter levels can be significantly increased by a single nutritious meal!

Brain nutrients affect brain performance rapidly because many nutrients go to the brain first. Sometimes the results are spectacular. Research on the brain vs modern computers showed that the brain, with its tens of billions of neurons, was a million times more powerful than a computer!

Important diet tips for brain power:

1: EFA's... essential fatty acids... Nearly half the weight of the brain is EFA's, (essential fatty acids, the "good" fats which are vital components of cell membranes in the body.)

- **Add more EFA's from the sea.** Cold water fish like tuna or salmon boost brain power. Or use 1 TB of flax seed oil daily.
- **Sea greens are valuable sources of EFA's.** Add 2 TBS dried, snipped sea greens like sushi nori, kelp or dulse to your diet. I like them on rice, salads, soups, casseroles or pizzas, or in miso soup. Or, have 6 pieces of sushi a week (great for your hair and nails, too).

2: Antioxidants.... all those fatty acids in the brain are very vulnerable to stress and free radical assault. Although the brain makes up only 2 ½% of our body weight, it uses 25% of our available oxygen, more than 25% of available glucose and 20% of our blood supply!

• **Phosphatidylserine** supplements sharpen memory, improve concentration, even fight brain diseases like Alzheimer's. Dosage is around 1000mg a day. You can also get phosphatides from food sources like lecithin or brewer's yeast.

• **Ginkgo Biloba** enhances blood flow to the brain. Ginkgo Biloba, a powerful antioxidant as well as a source of EFA's, has a well-documented history of improving brain conditions ranging from short-term memory loss to dementia.

• **Ginseng** boosts brain power. Studies reveal that ginseng allows people to work longer and harder at mental tasks, with less mistakes. I recommend a combination of ginsengs. Herbal nutrients work better as a team.

• **Kava Kava,** a traditional Polynesian social drink, works for relaxed energy. It certainly elevates mood and relieves stress, but I wouldn't rely on it to improve concentration or mental acuity. (Don't use kava and alcohol together.)

• **Royal Jelly,** the sole food of the queen bee, is a rich source of B vitamins and EFAs which nourish your brain. It also contains acetylcholine, a key antioxidant nutrient linked to healthy brain function.

• **Gotu Kola,** a brain and nerve tonic, improves learning, poor concentration and memory. More than ginkgo, its nerve repair and restorative ability is useful for anxiety- stress reactions without caffeine-like side effects. Like ginkgo, gotu kola improves circulation to the brain. It is effective as a tea for children with hyperactive attention deficit disorder.

• **Rosemary,** rich in antioxidants, is a powerful central nervous system stimulant that has been used to enhance memory for centuries. Shakespeare refers to "rosemary for remembrance" in Hamlet. Greek students today, as they have for millennia, take rosemary wine to study for tests. Use essential aromatherapy oil of rosemary to sail through mental work. Just apply 1-2 drops on the temples.

3: Minerals... provide significant bio-chemical ingredients for brain neuro-transmission, the key to your brain's communication with your body. Electrolytic potassium, magnesium, calcium, iodine, zinc and trace minerals chromium, boron, manganese and molybdenum are all important for brain health. Minerals are critical to brain function; yet today they're far more likely to be deficient in the diet than vitamins, amino acids or enzymes, especially in diets that lack whole foods.

4: B-vitamins, choline, tyrosine and tryptophan... synthesize neurotransmitters. If you're noticing slower, poorer memory, or less mental sharpness than you're used to, consider boosting your brain's levels of these nutrients.

• **B vitamins are essential in forming the myelin sheath,** a shield substance that insulates neuron connections so they can transmit messages effectively. Alzheimer's symptoms like memory loss, emotional instability and reduced attention span regularly accompany B vitamin deficiencies.

• **Choline,** a B-complex family member, is one of the few nutrients that is able to penetrate the blood-brain barrier, so it passes directly into the brain cells. Choline can enhance memory and revitalize your brain so that you feel energetic all over. Studies at M.I.T. show that choline is effective in treating bi-polar illness, Alzheimer's and tardive dyskinesia. Food sources of choline: egg yolks, meat, and fish. Lecithin is a good supplement source of choline from soybeans or sunflower seeds.

• **Tyrosine**, an amino acid, increases the production of dopamine and norepinephrine, neurotransmitters that buffer the effects of stress on your glands and nerves. Tyrosine improves mental alertness and quick response, eases anxiety and helps to relieve tension. It also protects your brain from the shock of extreme stress. Food sources: whole grains, soybeans, legumes, dairy products, fish and meat. If you take it as a supplement, about 500mg daily is a normal dose.

• **Tryptophan**, an amino acid, influences the neurotransmitter serotonin, which makes you more relaxed. Tryptophan helps your thinking stay clearer and eases the effects of stress. Food sources: brown rice, corn, turkey, legumes and most dairy foods.

5: Calcium and magnesium... help stabilize and protect brain membranes. Magnesium helps manufacture ATP, energy for the cells, and is essential for the enzymes that produce neurotransmitters. Magnesium even helps prevent migraine headaches. Calcium boosts the potential of nerve and muscle cells so that they can communicate through electrical impulses.

Does your brain power need a boost?

• Do you feel mentally foggy, spacy or slow? Have you lost the ability to concentrate?
• Do you frequently have unexplained depression, gloominess or bad moods?
• Have you lost the ability to remember well or for a reasonable length of time?
• Do your muscles respond more slowly than usual? Is your muscle coordination poor?
• Do you feel anxious or paranoid?
• Do your nerves feel raw and on edge no matter how much sleep you get?
• Are you often tired for no physical reason? Do you cry unexpectedly and often for no explained reason?

The best way to get good, long term, mental enhancement is to feed and use your brain. Cheerfulness, optimism and relaxation increase brain function. Studies show classical music is especially good. Experts tell us we can actually expand the size of our brains with challenging concentration activities such as memory games, chess, and crossword puzzles by promoting new projections from existing nerve cells. Reading, writing and new experiences also stimulate enhanced thought.

Breathe energy into your brain. Brain breathing is one of the best ways I know to energize your mind. Your brain requires three times more oxygen than the rest of your body. Oxygen is essential to the production of energy and the heart of metabolism. Without oxygen, the energy of the food you eat could not be released to you. One expert, Philip Rice, M.D., a delinquent child specialist, said "Fifty-five percent of the delinquent behavior in children can be attributed to oxygen starvation." (See page 285 for Paul and Patricia Bragg's BRAIN BREATHING exercises.)

This diet improves several areas of poor brain, motor and memory function: *Stress Reactions like Anxiety and Nervous Tension, Depression, Schizophrenia and other Psychosis, Mental Retardation and Down Syndrome, Mental Exhaustion and Burnout, Alzheimer's and Parkinson's Diseases, Senility from Premature Aging, Epilepsy Seizures, Chronic Insomnia, Autism and Hyperactivity in Kids, Narcolepsy.*

Brain Power Booster Diet

You can eat with your brain in mind. The brain has a large appetite. The following diet to improve mental activity is rich in brain foods - supplying potassium, amino acid protein precursors, B-vitamins for choline, and complex carbohydrates for glycogen production. It is low in fats and gooey foods that clog, and free of refined foods that cause blood sugar imbalance. It emphasizes small frequent meals instead of heavy meals that siphon brain fuel and energy away for digestion.

This diet is structured for fast brain response. Oxygen is a key nutrient. The brain uses 20% of the body's oxygen supply. Good blood flow from the liver and spleen keep brain oxygen high. Focus on oxygenating foods, like wheat germ, Omega-3 oils, nuts, seeds, sea foods and soy foods.

—**On rising:** have green tea; or take ALL 1 VITAMIN-MINERALS, Barleans BARLEANS GREENS, Omega Nutrition VITALITY SUPERGREEN, NutriCology PRO-GREENS or Crystal Star ENERGY GREEN™ drink in juice, with 1 teasp. Bragg's LIQUID AMINOS added.

Note: Now is a good time to take brain boosting supplements. See supplements section at the end of this diet for suggestions.

—**Breakfast:** have some low-fat yogurt with fruit, and 1 teasp. each: wheat germ, lecithin granules, sesame seeds, and Red Star nutritional yeast; or whole grain cereal or pancakes with either maple syrup, apple juice, vanilla soy milk, or honey and fresh fruit; or a poached, baked, or soft boiled egg with whole grain toast or English muffin and a little butter; or oatmeal with maple syrup.

—**Mid-morning:** have a green drink (pg. 569), a potassium drink (pg. 568) or Monas CHLORELLA or Crystal Star SYSTEMS STRENGTH™ drink; or an herb tea like gotu kola or Crystal Star CREATIVI-TEA™, or RAINFOREST ENERGY™ tea; or low-fat yogurt with nut and seed toppings; or miso soup with sea greens snipped on top and whole grain chips or crackers; or an apple and water.

—**Lunch:** have a fresh green salad with sprouts and brown rice; or 6 or more pieces of sushi; or baked/ broiled seafood with miso soup or other light broth; or a seafood salad with whole grain pasta; or a roast turkey salad or sandwich or any veggie sandwich on whole grain bread, with a little mayonnaise and low-fat cheese; or tofu with steamed veggies and brown rice or millet or bulgar.

—**Mid-afternoon:** have a energizing herb tea, such as Crystal Star MEDITATION™ tea for calm mental energy, or HIGH ENERGY TEA for outgoing energy, or a ginseng or rosemary tea; and/or a low-fat yogurt with fruit or nuts; or crunchy raw veggies with a low-fat dip and a small bottle of mineral water; or some fresh fruit with low-fat cheese or soy cheese.

Note: Now is another good time to take brain boosting supplements - to keep you alert for the rest of the day.

—**Dinner:** have steamed veggies with tofu and brown rice or other whole grain, or vegetable pasta; and baked or broiled seafood with a fresh green salad or light soup; or baked, broiled or roasted chicken or turkey with a green salad and light dressing; or a light vegetable quiche or vegetarian pizza on a chapati or pita crust; or an oriental stir-fry with brown rice and a light soup.

—**Before Bed:** Brain rest is a big part of brain health. Have a relaxing cup of hot herb tea, like chamomile, or Crystal Star RELAX™ tea; or a cup of hot Red Star yeast broth for relaxation and B vitamins.

Recipes to help your brain power diet: •BREAKFAST and BRUNCH; •BLENDING EAST and WEST; •LOW FAT and VERY LOW FAT RECIPES; •FISH and SEAFOODS; •MINERAL-RICH RECIPES; •HIGH PROTEIN without MEAT.

Herb and Supplement Choices

•**Antioxidants for brain energy:** MICROHYDRIN, from Healthy House, dramatically increases oxygen uptake to brain cells; Glutathione 100mg daily; Alpha Lipoic Acid (neutralizes toxins, recycles glutathione); CoQ$_{10}$, 60mg 2x daily (with vitamin E 400IU and selenium 200mcg); NADH 10mg daily; wheat germ oil, two teasp. daily offer as much available oxygen to the body as an oxygen tent for 30 minutes; germanium 50mg daily; ACL (acetyl-L-carnitine) up to 2500mg daily.

•**Keep electrical-nerve connections healthy:** Ginkgo biloba extract; take $^1/_4$ teasp. each: Glutamine powder and glycine powder; magnesium 800mg daily; evening primrose oil caps 2000mg. daily, cayenne or ginger-cayenne caps daily.

•**Keep circulation flowing, nervous system healthy:** lecithin, choline 600mg (If choline levels are low, try Huperzine A 50mg to allow levels to rise); Omega-3 fish or flax oils, Siberian ginseng extract, and B-Complex 100mg daily.

•**Feed the brain with minerals:** potassium: Futurebiotics VI-TAL K, Eidon LIQUID POTASSIUM, or Crystal Star SYSTEMS STRENGTH DRINK™; magnesium and zinc; iodine from kelp or Crystal Star IODINE THERAPY™; Nature's Path TRACE-MIN-LYTE with sea greens.

•**Nourish your brain with EFA's:** Ginseng brain nutrients: Crystal Star GINSENG 6™ SUPER caps, or MENTAL INNER ENERGY™. New Chapter SUPERCRITICAL DHA; Royal jelly caps; Gaia Herbs GINKGO/GOTU KOLA SUPREME.

•**Sharpen your memory:** Crystal Star MENTAL CLARITY™ caps, CREATIVI-TEA™, or MEDITATION™ teas; Diamond-Herpanacine DIAMOND MIND caps; Super Nutrition EINSTEIN'S FAVORITE; Planetary Herbs BACOPA-GINKGO (fast results).

Bodywork and Lifestyle Techniques

•**Exercise oxygenates your brain to deal with stress.** Studies show that deep breathing and exercise are better than drugs at reducing anxiety. Deep brain breathing oxygenates and can step up your physical, mental and spiritual capabilities.

—**The Bragg Super Power Breath exercise: Repeat 5 times**
  1: Stand erect with feet apart for good balance.
  2: Slowly inhale through your nose and mouth, and raise your hands overhead — pushing downward with your diaphragm and expanding your chest.
  3: Bend forward as if to touch your toes and exhale at the same time through your mouth.
  4: Again slowly inhale through your nose and mouth and return to the standing position with hands raised overhead. Draw in air to the full capacity of your lungs.

  Note: See Paul & Patricia Bragg's SUPER POWER BREATHING FOR SUPER ENERGY book for more.

•**Try TM for TLC.** Transcendental meditation has been proven to help you reach a state of restful alertness to reduce stress.

•**A rosemary stuffed sleep pillow** is excellent for memory center improvement.

•**Oxygenate** with a daily, arm-swinging $^1/_2$ hour walk.

•**An alternating hot and cold shower** can bring additional blood to the brain almost immediately.

•**Avoid sugar and refined foods.** They affect the brain first.

•**Avoid aluminum products,** such as deodorants with aluminum chlor-hydrate, and aluminum pots and pans.

Can't find a recommended product? Call the 800 number listed in Product Resources for the store nearest you and for more info.

Alzheimer's and Parkinson's Healing Diet

The number one fear of older Americans isn't heart disease or cancer... it's Alzheimer's. **Alzheimer's disease** is a progressive condition that attacks the brain, forming neurofiber tangles and plaques that result in dementia symptoms—impaired memory, decreased intellectual and emotional function, and ultimately complete physical breakdown. It's a devastating, relentless assault that's rising at a rapid rate in industrialized countries worldwide. In the U.S., 10% of the population over sixty-five suffers from some form of dementia. Alzheimer's itself now affects 4 million Americans at a cost of over $100 billion in nursing care and lost wages of family members. By 2050, 14 million more Americans will fall victim to the disease.

Alzheimer's disease progresses slowly. Memory loss and disorientation are the first signs, but eventually there is almost complete loss of physical function and reversion to childhood helplessness. Contributing causes may include genetic factors, but like most degenerative diseases, environmental exposure to harmful chemicals, aluminum or inorganic silicon are likely. Some Alzheimer's victims are really victims of too many drugs, or have severe nutritional deficiencies. Although orthodox medicine has been unable to make a difference in Alzheimer's, natural therapies have been successful in slowing the deterioration of brain function.

Parkinson's disease, often a risk factor for Alzheimer's, is the progressive deterioration of specific nerve centers in the brain. The disease changes the balance of acetylcholine and dopamine, two brain chemicals essential for transmission of nerve signals. The altered balance of these two neurotransmitters results in a lack of control of physical movements, characterized by a slowly spreading tremor, muscular weakness and body rigidity. Normal posture becomes stooped, walking becomes shambling, motion is trembling and lifespan is shortened. The victim, whose thinking processes often remain normal, feels frozen, unable to move voluntarily. Parkinson's affects men and women equally, usually between the ages of 50 and 75. Although the direct cause of Parkinson's is unknown, it is believed that a neurotoxin causes oxidative damage to the basal ganglia that control muscle tone. L-dopa, the drug of choice for Parkinson's, has hallucinatory side effects and causes leg cramps. Natural therapy helps re-establish normal biochemistry.

Are there early signs of Alzheimer's or Parkinson's disease?

—Is there a noticeable loss of ability to think clearly or remember familiar names, places or events?
—Is there loss of touch with reality, impaired judgement, confusion, difficulty in completing thoughts or following directions?
—Are there clear, unexplained personality or behavior changes? Is there unexplained depression?
—Is there a slight tremor in the hands with numbness and tingling in the hands and feet? Does the head shake as well?
—Is there slight dragging of the feet, pronounced with stress or fatigue? Has movement become increasingly difficult?
—If movement is lethargic, has speech also become slow and difficult to follow?
—Has the face lost expression (because of muscle rigidity)? Is there slight drooling? Is vision noticeably impaired?

Alzheimer's-Parkinson's Nutritional Healing Diet

Good nutrition can produce noticeable improvement in Alzheimer's and Parkinson's patients. Nutritional deficiencies are regularly present in both conditions. Some experts think lack of B-vitamins may even be one cause of Alzheimer's. An antioxidant-rich diet with plenty of fruits and vegetables can slow disease progression. Significant evidence over the last several decades shows that higher aluminum levels are found in the brains of those with Alzheimer's and Parkinson's. Cooking utensils, deodorants and your water supply should be checked for aluminum (aluminum may occur naturally in water, but it's added as alum). Preserved foods like relishes or condiments, antacids that are regularly taken, and baking powder are other aluminum culprits. Calcium citrate supplements may increase aluminum absorption. Magnesium and silica help block aluminum absorption.

Use the following starter diet for 2 to 3 weeks to cleanse and alkalize. Use organically grown foods when possible. Then, follow a modified macrobiotic diet (pg. 206) for 3 to 6 months until condition improves. Antioxidant-rich foods are critical. More than any other food group they slow the progression of both Alzheimer's and Parkinson's. Eat smaller meals more frequently. Keep meat protein low. Eliminate alcohol, caffeine and refined sugars. Especially avoid fatty, fried foods. Both too much fat and too many total calories are associated with Alzheimer's and Parkinson's. Drink plenty of water, ideally, eight 8-oz glasses daily.

Live cell therapy from green drinks and chlorella has been notably successful in reducing symptoms. Take vegetable drinks (pg. 569) at least twice a week, or use Monas or Sun Wellness CHLORELLA once a day.

—**On rising:** take an antioxidant juice: grape, grapefruit, lemon and cherry (for bioflavonoids), or orange, a source of selenium.
—**Breakfast:** have cranberry, grape, papaya or aloe vera juice, mix in 1 TB Crystal Star BIOFLAVONOID, FIBER & C SUPPORT™ drink for antioxidants; or have fresh cherries, bananas, oranges or strawberries with yogurt, and sprinkle on 2 tsp. of the following nut mix: sunflower seeds, lecithin granules, Red Star nutritional yeast and toasted wheat germ.
—**Mid-morning:** have an antioxidant-rich vegetable juice: 1) Carrot, kale, parsley and spinach, sources of beta-carotene; or 2) Kale, garlic, parsley, green pepper and spinach, sources of vitamin C, vitamin E and selenium (to slow progression).
—**Lunch:** have a large green leafy salad with lemon/oil dressing; and/or a hot miso broth or hearty veggie soup with marinated tofu or tempeh in tamari sauce (for soy estrogen balance). Add Red Star NUTRITIONAL YEAST to any choice.
—**Mid-afternoon:** have a glass of fresh carrot juice or fresh apple juice. Add 1 TB of a green superfood like Crystal Star SYSTEMS STRENGTH™ drink; Nutricology PRO-GREENS or Wakunaga KYO-GREEN; or Vibrant Health GREEN VIBRANCE.
—**Dinner:** have steamed brown rice and mixed steamed vegetables. Sprinkle with sea greens for absorbable minerals and EFA's, 2 TBS flax or olive oil, 1 TB. Bragg's LIQUID AMINOS, 1 tsp. liquid lecithin and 1 TB. nutritional yeast, sources of choline (a direct precursor of acetylcholine, the key neurotransmitter for memory) and B-complex (low levels linked to Alzheimer's).
—**Before Bed:** have a cup of green tea or Crystal Star GREEN TEA CLEANSER™, rich in brain antioxidants.

Recipes for Alzheimer's-Parkinson's diet: •MINERAL-RICH RECIPES; •CONDIMENTS and SEASONINGS; •FISH and SEAFOOD; •ENZYME-RICH RECIPES; •LIGHT MACROBIOTICS; •HIGH FIBER RECIPES; •CULTURED FOODS.

Herb and Supplement Choices

• **Reduce glyco-protein amyloid strings:** Transformation PUREZYME, powerful protease, 3 to 5 capsules; Ethical Nutrients Magnesium-Malic acid. Country Life Phosphatidyl Choline 5000-10,000mg. Zinc 30mg daily for amyloid plaques.

• **Antioxidants overcome oxidative damage to the brain:** Healthy House MICROHYDRIN; NutriCology ANTIOX FORMULA II; Country Life SUPER 10 ANTIOXIDANT.

• **Critical EFA's for nerves and brain:** Evening primrose oil 4-6 daily; DHA 200mg daily or Neuromins DHA as directed; Barleans lignan-rich flax oil 3x daily.

• **Enhance memory retention:** Huperzine-A, 50mcg, 2 daily. Phyto-hormones from herbal sources like ginseng and royal jelly; Crystal Star MENTAL INNER ENERGY™ caps, or CREATIVI-TEA™ 2x daily; Beehive Botanicals ROYAL JELLY-GINSENG caps. Ginkgo biloba extract, 60mg 3x daily stabilizes symptoms.

• **Nourish the brain:** Crystal Star BRAIN DEFENSE™ caps and SILICA SOURCE™ or Flora VEGE-SIL to prevent aluminum build-up; Biotec CELL GUARD w. SOD; YS ROYAL JELLY/GINSENG blend (with bee pollen and propolis). Chelation therapy cleans up arterial pathways - Metabolic Response Modifiers CARDIO-CHELATE.

• **Preserve brain cells with amino acid therapy:** NADH - 10mg in the morning before eating. Phosphatidylserine 100mg 3x daily or choline 650mg, for 3 months, or DHA for 3 months (nature's calcium channel blocker); Lysine 1000mg daily; Acetyl-L-Carnitine 500mg 2 daily; CoQ-10, 200mg daily.

• **Rebuild nerve strength to ease tremor:** Crystal Star RELAX CAPS™ 2 or STRESSED OUT™ extract to ease shakiness (helps within an hour); DLPA 500-750mg.

Bodywork and Lifestyle Techniques

• **Enema:** An enema during an Alzheimer's/Parkinson's cleansing program can help release toxins. A catnip enema once a month during healing helps liver/kidney function.

• **Exercise:** A brisk daily walk lowers the risk of developing Alzheimer's and is a good choice for Parkinson's therapy.

• **Exercise for brain cells:** Keep your brain active and challenged with mentally creative activities. Use hot and cold hydrotherapy showers for brain and circulation stimulation.

• **Relaxation techniques:** Chiropractic treatment, massage therapy, acupuncture and acupressure have notable success in reversing early Parkinson's and are helpful for Alzheimer's.

• **Moderate wine drinking** appears to boost brain activity AND deter Alzheimer's.

• **Flower remedies:** Natural Labs FORGETFULNESS for memory lapses and wandering thoughts, lack of alertness and attentiveness, and amnesia.

• **Try to limit prescription and over-the-counter drugs.** A Johns Hopkins study shows many Alzheimer's patients are really victims of too many drugs - most taking more than 6 different drugs simultaneously. 25% of the medications were either unsafe or ineffective; side effects from both drug interactions and the inappropriate medication affected brain neurotransmission. Most harmful were pain killers and sleeping pills that leached acetylcholine from brain tissues, and diuretics which leached potassium needed by the brain.

While it is sometimes necessary to take medication, drugs are so powerful that I feel it is critical for older people (indeed everyone) to be well informed about the drugs they are taking - dosage, side effects and interaction with other drugs.

Can't find a recommended product? Call the 800 number listed in Product Resources for the store nearest you and for more info.

Healing Diet for Depression and Schizophrenia

Depression is the most common adult psychiatric disorder, and it's on the rise worldwide. Depression is both a mental and emotional state, and affects women more than men. It's closely tied to disease. (Over 80% of terminal cancer patients have a history of chronic depression.) A common expression of depression I hear is the feeling of being in a box that you can't escape. Underlying origins for depression: 1) Great loss, as of a spouse or child; 2) Bottled-up anger and aggression turned inward; 3) Negative emotional behavior, often learned as a child to control relationships; 4) Biochemical imbalance involved with amino acid and other nutrient deficiencies; 5) Drug-induced depression. (Many prescription drugs create nutrient deficiencies that aggravate mood disorders.)

Manic depression (bipolar disorder), not to be confused with major depression, affects 2 million people in America today. It is characterized by two distinct phases: 1- a "manic" phase marked by intense hyperactivity, speaking abnormally fast, inflated self-confidence, impulsive behavior (like overspending or promiscuousness) and sleeplessness (a person with this disorder may go days without sleeping at all!); 2- a deep depression phase marked by excessive crying or sleeping, and more than likely suicidal thoughts.

The phases alternate from day to day, even hour to hour. Hallucinations and delusions make it difficult to distinguish from schizophrenia. The drug of choice for manic depression is Lithium, often used at near toxic doses, hard on the thyroid and kidneys.

Schizophrenia is a disabling psychosis whose symptoms include auditory or visual hallucinations, delusions, paranoia, depression and compulsive self-destructive behavior. Personal relationships are abnormal; work is almost impossible. The schizophrenic usually withdraws emotionally and socially. Anti-psychotic drugs to treat schizophrenia have serious drawbacks. Some patients develop a near catatonic state. Over 70% of patients taking antipsychotic drugs develop tardive dyskinesia, which almost totally isolates them socially. TD sufferers experience involuntary bizarre grimacing, chewing and twitching, and great difficulty speaking and eating. Research reveals that natural therapies are successful in treating schizophrenia and in reversing TD. Avoid yohimbe in herbal supplements; it may aggravate schizophrenia.

Are there early signs of depression or schizophrenia? We all get the blues from time to time, but if you have five of the following eight symptoms for at least a month, you may have major depression or psychosis.

–Unusually poor appetite with weight loss or unusually increased appetite with weight gain.
–Insomnia or sleeping excessively (hypersomnia). Low energy – great tiredness. Very low brain activity.
–Hyperactivity (going a mile a minute) then doing almost nothing for days in almost total social withdrawal.
–Loss of interest or pleasure in usual activities, usually decrease in sexual drive.
–Feelings of worthlessness, self-reproach or inappropriate guilt with recurrent thoughts of death or suicide.
–Dramatic emotional swings, often leading to violent outbursts. Paranoid delusions or hallucinations detached from reality.
–Diminished ability to think or concentrate. Or scattered and chaotic thoughts like random shotgun fire.

Improving Body Chemistry against Mood Disorders

While heavy drugs and psychotherapy have been the mainstays of conventional treatment for mental disorders like severe depression, manic depression (bipolar disorder) and schizophrenia, more and more studies show that natural therapies are startlingly effective in reducing symptoms, enhancing quality of life, even in reversing mental illnesses.... without the devastating side effects of drugs. *Note: Megadoses of some vitamins can produce adverse effects; consult with a natural health professional about the right therapies for you.*

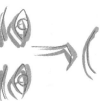

Watchwords for a diet to control schizophrenia and depression:

—Nutrition is a key to the brain's behavior. Nutrient deficiencies are almost always involved in mood disorders.

1: Get plenty of healthy protein (about 15% of your total calorie intake) to minimize depression. Amino acids in protein foods help build healthy neurotransmitters for coping skills. Include protein from seafoods, sea greens, rice, sprouts, soy foods, nuts, seeds, organic turkey and chicken, eggs and low fat cheeses to control depression-related tissue destruction. Protein foods like soy, cheeses and turkey are also rich in the amino acid L-tryptophan to help build serotonin, essential for overcoming depression and stress reactions.

2: Add Omega-3 rich foods from cold water fish or flax seed. Include seafood, especially salmon and tuna, at least 3 or 4 times a week. Omega-3 fatty acids help the brain neurotransmitters norepinephrine and serotonin perform their mood stabilizing functions. Omega 3 fatty acids in fish oil help relieve bi-polar disorder by balancing serotonin levels to stabilize mood.

3: Have a green salad every day. Have at least 4 other servings of high mineral vegetables and whole grains daily. You'll automatically be eating foods rich in calcium, potassium, iron, magnesium and B vitamins that are usually low in a depressed person's body.

4: Add a superfood daily for "extra strength" nutrition. Some good superfoods to choose from: Crystal Star SYSTEMS STRENGTH™, Nutricology PRO-GREENS or Wakunaga KYO-GREEN, or YS ROYAL JELLY WITH GINSENG.

5: Drink plenty of water each day. Dehydration is often linked to depression. Heavily treated water may harm neurotransmitters.

—If you are taking MAO inhibitor drugs, you must control your diet with care: avoid alcohol, cheese, red meat, yeast extract and broad beans - foods rich in tyrosine. Eliminate all preserved, refined and junk foods. Avoid sugary foods and caffeine - they wreak havoc on blood sugar levels clearly involved in psychotic behavior.

—Researchers from Albert Einstein medical school find vitamin C therapy, at a level of 2-6 grams daily, improves schizophrenia for one-third of patients who failed to respond to antipsychotic drugs. One patient became completely normal within two weeks of vitamin C therapy!

—Schizophrenia's symptoms are similar to a B-3 (niacin or niacinamide) deficiency. Researchers from Canada find that as many as 95% of people with acute schizophrenia can return to normal within two years of niacin therapy at a level of 3000 mg. daily. 65% of chronic schizophrenics, the most difficult to treat, return to normal within ten years of the therapy.

—If long-term antipsychotic drug therapy has already resulted in tardive dyskinesia, high dose vitamin E therapy shows new promise. Vitamin E, as a potent antioxidant, decreases free radical assault on brain tissue caused by antipsychotic drugs. In one study, 400 to 1200 IU of vitamin E daily reduced TD symptoms by a remarkable 43%!

Diet Plan to Control Schizophrenia and Depression

During your healing diet, avoid refined sugars, caffeine, red meats, foods with additives and preserved foods. Eliminate arginine foods like peanut butter and nuts. They can be toxic to a schizophrenic's brain. Avoid foods that create toxic build-up – preserved lunch meats, foods with coloring added, and most important, pesticide-sprayed fruits and vegetables. Pesticides are full of environmental estrogens which may disrupt the delicate hormone balance of the brain. Eat organically grown foods whenever possible.

—**On rising:** take a "brain balancing tonic:" in apple or orange juice to control a morning sugar drop: 1 teasp. each: glycine powder, rice milk or soy milk powder, protein powder, and Red Star nutritional yeast; or a protein/amino drink, such as Monas CHLORELLA, Wakunaga KYO-GREEN, or Crystal Star SYSTEMS STRENGTH™.

—**Breakfast:** an important meal: (include $^1/_3$ of daily nutrients); have oatmeal with yogurt and fresh fruit; or poached or baked eggs on whole grain toast with butter, kefir cheese or yogurt cheese; or whole grain cereal or pancakes with apple juice, rice milk, almond milk or soy milk, fruit, yogurt, nuts or fruit sauce; or tofu scrambled "eggs" with bran muffins, whole grain toast and a little butter.

—**Mid-morning:** have a green drink (page 569), Green Foods GREEN MAGMA with 1 teasp. Bragg's LIQUID AMINOS, or Crystal Star ENERGY GREEN™ drink as a liver nutrient; Have an adrenal tonic twice a week to prevent stress reactions that precipitate major depression: a glass of carrot juice with a pinch of sage and 1 teasp. Bragg's LIQUID AMINOS; or a sugar balancing herb tea, such as licorice, dandelion, or Crystal Star SUGAR STRATEGY LOW™ tea; and some crisp, crunchy vegetables with kefir or yogurt cheese.

—**Lunch:** have a fresh salad, with cottage cheese or soy cheese, nut or seed toppings, or sprinkle on 2 TBS of a mix of brain foods: lecithin granules, Red Star nutritional yeast, toasted wheat germ, pumpkin seeds - and use a lemon-canola oil dressing; or have a high protein sandwich on whole grain bread, with avocados, low-fat cheese; or a bean or lentil soup with tofu or shrimp salad or sandwich; or a seafood and whole grain pasta salad; or a vegetarian pizza on a chapati crust with low fat cheese.

—**Mid-afternoon:** have a hard boiled egg with sesame salt, and whole grain crackers with yogurt dip; or a licorice herb tea, such as Crystal Star GINSENG/LICORICE ELIXIR™ in water; or another green drink, such as Vibrant Health GREEN VIBRANCE with spirulina; or yogurt with toasted wheat germ, nuts and seeds.

—**Dinner:** have some steamed veggies with tofu, or baked or broiled fish and brown rice; or an oriental stir fry with seafood and vegetables; or a vegetable Italian pasta dish with verde sauce and hearty soup (add green beans for pancreatic support); have niacin-rich vegetables like broccoli, carrots, potatoes and corn; or a Spanish beans and rice dish, or paella with seafood and rice; or a veggie quiche or a small mushroom and spinach salad. Gradually add vegetable proteins, gluten-free grains (like brown rice, millet and amaranth), fish (like salmon, tuna, halibut), and sunflower seeds. Turkey is a good, calming tryptophan source for manic depression and schizophrenia.

—**Before bed:** have a cup of Red Star nutritional yeast broth or miso broth; or papaya juice with a little yogurt.

Recipes to help schizophrenia and depression: •HEALING DRINKS; •BREAKFAST and BRUNCH; •SALADS HOT and COLD; •MINERAL-RICH RECIPES; •SUGAR-FREE SWEETS; •SEAFOODS; •BLENDING EAST and WEST.

Herb and Supplement Choices

Note: Be aware that the two major classes of antidepressant drugs seem to block the effect of herbal nervines. St. John's wort is contra-indicated if you are taking PROZAC.

• **Relieve depression, improve your mood:** Crystal Star DEPRESS-EX™ extract or caps; NADH 10mg daily with St. John's Wort, a natural MAO inhibitor. Kava Kava caps 2 daily (not with alcoholic drinks). Ginkgo Biloba or Hawthorn extract for a feeling of well-being. Magnesium 800mg 2x daily. Rhodiola Rosea caps, effective herbal serotonin booster for depression. For bad moods, add 5-HTP 50mg at night.

• **EFA's lift mood, nourish the brain:** DHA 200mg, 2 daily; Source Naturals FOCUS DHA,3 daily; Evening Primrose Oil 4000mg daily; Nature's Secret ULTIMATE OIL; Crystal Star IODINE SOURCE™ drops; Biotec PACIFIC SEA PLASMA, or kelp tabs 8 daily for ocean EFA's.

• **Amino acid therapy:** SAMe 400mg daily (important in synthesizing brain chemicals); Glutamine 3000mg daily; Country Life MAXI-B with taurine, or MOOD FACTORS capsules as needed; DLPA 1000mg as needed; GABA 2000mg to mimic valium without sedation.

• **Nerve tonics and relaxers:** Crystal Star RELAX™ caps for nerve repair; Gotu Kola for nerve support; Morada Research NERVOUS SYSTEM nerve food; Country Life sublingual B-12, 2500mcg every other day for 2 months; Vitamin C with bioflavonoids, 3000mg daily helps withdrawal from chemical dependencies. B-complex 150mg with extra B-6 250mg daily.

• **B vitamins are key:** Stress B-complex 150mg; extra B_6 500mg and folic acid 800mcg daily, Real Life Research TOTAL B; Premier GERMANIUM w. DMG.

Bodywork and Lifestyle Techniques

• **Get some exercise every day,** especially brisk walking or jogging. Exercise is an antidepressant nutrient in itself.
    • **Take ocean walks** for sea minerals; a visit to a mineral-rich spring and spa are also effective.
    • **Do deep brain breathing exercises.** (See page 285.)
    • **Before you resort to PROZAC,** (with more side effect complaints than any other drug) ask your doctor about massage therapy, hypnotherapy or biofeedback. These techniques have success in overcoming chronic depression.

• **Try acupuncture.** Research from the University of Arizona finds acupuncture reduces or eliminates symptoms for 64% of depressed women- success rates that rival current anti-depressant drugs AND psychotherapy!

• **Plan an interesting daily schedule** so you don't drift and lose the days to inertia.

• **Chronic depression increases risk of osteoporosis.** Sunlight therapy - get some on the body every day possible for vitamin D.

• **Removing amalgam fillings** significantly improves symptoms for people with bipolar disorder. Add garlic 6 caps daily to boost benefits because it helps detox mercury in amalgam.

• **Try sleep deprivation:** 67% of people with no apparent cause for their depression benefit. A single sleepless night can wash away depressive symptoms.

• **Aromatherapy has undeniable mood elevating effects.** Just apply a little lavender oil to the temples. For the best results, close your eyes; concentrate on your breathing and the aroma for at least 5 minutes.

Can't find a recommended product? Call the 800 number listed in Product Resources for the store nearest you and for more info.

292

Overcoming Addictions

Do you need to clean out drug or alcohol toxins?

Americans have an expensive river of chemicals coursing through our national veins. We take almost twenty billion dollars worth of prescription drugs every year. Ten million Americans are officially classified as addicted to alcohol. One-third of Americans are heavy drinkers, consuming more than 15 drinks a week, accounting for 95% of the alcohol sold in the U.S. At a cost to taxpayers of nearly $300 billion dollars a year, some see it as the nation's number one health problem. It's a disease, leading to other health problems, not a character flaw. (For example, over-the-counter pain relievers now carry a liver damage warning for people who drink 3 or more drinks a day.) As with other addictive practices, alcohol abuse is marked by stress and depression, low self confidence, and by nutritional deficiencies. The use of "recreational" drugs is a problem at every level of today's society. Experts believe, however, that the most serious addictions are to prescription drugs. More than one million people a year (up to 5 percent of hospital admissions) are a result of bad reactions to prescription drugs. (See pg. 271.)

Clearly, modern drugs play lifesaving roles in emergency situations and they can help numerous health problems, especially short term; but most people begin taking drugs to alleviate boredom and fatigue, or to relieve physical or psychological pain. A detox program can be a significant weapon for releasing drugs and alcohol from your body, but withdrawing after long use can produce harsh effects. I highly recommend the supervision of a health professional for an addictions cleanse, especially if the dependency has been long term. Sometimes, the best way is to wean yourself gradually from the addictive substance while you carry on your addiction cleanse.

Feelings of dis-ease that drugs or excessive alcohol alleviate are merely warning signs of deeper internal imbalances. Alcohol abuse especially may be brought on by stress and marked by depression. Drugs and alcohol can aggravate an original health problem and add to the poisons in your body. Drug detoxification is a process of releasing the stored residues, at the same time changing lifestyle habits so that you are no longer dependent on them. It is critical to fortify your body enough to give it the power to resist returning to the addictive substance. Only a well-nourished body can offer both your body and mind sufficient sense of well being and strength to melt the relapse urges and desires.

Do you think you might be addicted?

—Do you only feel happy and relaxed after having a drink or taking an antidepressant or mood elevating drug?
—Do you relieve stress with a drink or a drug every day? Do you get headaches that feel like a continual hangover?
—Does your stomach protrude but you are thin everywhere else? *A sign of liver enlargement and inflammation.*
—Do you have esophagus impairment, reflux after eating, high blood pressure, or pancreatitis? Are your stools pale?
—Is your skin sallow? Your lower eyelid yellow? The whites of your eyes dingy? Do you sweat a lot? *Signs of liver exhaustion.*
—Have you lost your appetite? Have you gotten noticeably, or unusually thin? Do you have a marked intolerance for fatty foods?

—Is your digestion always bad? Do you have a metallic taste in your mouth? Are you drowsy after meals? *In the overwhelming number of cases, habitual drug and alcohol users suffer from chronic subclinical malnutrition, and from multiple depletions of critical nutrients. Vitamins, minerals, amino acids, fatty acids and enzymes are all impoverished, some by 50 to 60 percent.*

—Are you often foggy mentally? Have you become sensitive to certain foods? Or to household chemicals? Do you crave sweets? Is your blood sugar usually low? Do you ever get dizzy or black out? *Signs of rampant hypoglycemia from alcohol or drug overload.*

—Do you feel shaky and sweaty? Do you often get a "wired," nervous feeling, sometimes with heart palpitations? *This type of central nervous system overload is a sign of addiction.*

—Do you have frequent memory loss? *Short term memory loss is one of the first signs of alcohol abuse; damage to the brain is another.*

—Are you unusually anxious, even paranoid? Do you lose your temper or get in a bad mood easily? Do you feel depressed and cry a lot without any real reason? *Typically late symptoms of alcohol abuse.*

—Is there pain on your right side or under your right shoulder blade? Do you get stomach or muscle cramps frequently?

—Are you continually tired? *Extreme fatigue usually results from poor liver health, adrenal exhaustion or thyroid malfunction.*

—Is your immune response low? Do you seem to have a cold or flu all the time? *All drugs weaken normal immunity over time.*

What does it feel like to withdraw from drugs or alcohol?

Withdrawal symptoms are the same as addiction symptoms, only worse and more frequent. Breaking destructive habits is hard. Your body reacts when a substance it thinks it depends on is removed. The initial withdrawal phase is the most difficult part of an addiction detox and can last from a day or two to a week or more. You'll get chronic headaches, usually with diarrhea as your body tries to release toxins faster, and a lot of irritability. Some people experience hallucinations, disorientation or irrational thinking. Some go into depression. You'll probably lose sleep, and your sleep will be interrupted during the night. Most people in withdrawal are sensitive to light and noise, hot and cold flashes, and sweating.

But every day gets easier. Look at each episode of discomfort as a little victory on the road to recovery. One of the laws of the universe is that we don't have to fight the same battle twice. As your body dislodges and removes more toxins day by day, you have the satisfaction of knowing (if you don't add any more) that they are gone for good.

Some benefits you'll notice as your body responds to an addiction cleanse:

• **Your mood lifts as your nerves heal. Natural mood enhancers, like** *St. John's Wort* **and** *Kava Kava,* **help in the weaning process.**

• **Memory and thinking improve. Take** *Ginkgo Biloba* **extract for a month to help speed up your brain processes.**

• **Your skin becomes clearer—less muddy; your eyes become brighter.**

• **Digestion for most people improves right away.**

• **Immune response noticeably improves, usually within a month.**

Diet to Help Overcome Alcohol Addiction

Purposely making major life style improvements is sometimes the cause of the problem to curb the craving for alcohol's effects. A high-stress, fast-paced, jet-lag lifestyle overloads your biochemical detox systems so that you get a steamroller effect on the "morning after." A hangover should be gone by five o'clock the next day. If it isn't, you probably have alcohol poisoning. A severe hangover is alcohol poisoning with dehydration thrown in. Your body can't work adequately unless you give yourself a break. The real idea is to reduce alcohol consumption below your toxicity level.

The best medicine for changing body chemistry. This step works at reducing alcohol's damage to your body and brain, but the suggestions in this chapter are effective natural means of

Alcohol detox watchwords:

1: **Drink 8 glasses of water each day of your cleanse.** Dehydration is a hallmark of alcohol abuse. Water flushes alcohol and drugs from every corner of your body. Include healthy herb teas, too.

2: **Take green superfoods like spirulina, chlorella and barley grass.** They're rich in chlorophyll, phytochemicals, antioxidants, vitamins, minerals, enzymes, and more. Superfoods help nourish your body, build immunity and stave off cravings.

3: **Love your liver.** No alcohol detox program works without liver regeneration. A short liver cleanse (pg.162) can thoroughly clean out alcohol residues. Drink cranberry juice to protect your liver.

4: **Reduce sugar cravings.** Follow the HYPOGLYCEMIA DIET in this book for 3 months. Take a daily protein drink, like Solgar WHEY TO GO to balance body chemistry and replace electrolytes quickly. Add 1 TB lecithin granules or flax oil to control fatty liver.

5: **Think B-vitamins, EFA's, protein and minerals** for a solid nutrition base, especially magnesium-rich foods like wheat germ, sea greens, Red Star nutritional yeast, whole grains, brown rice, green leafy veggies, potatoes, low-fat dairy foods, eggs and fish.

6: **Avoid fried foods, sugary or heavily spiced foods and caffeine.** They aggravate alcohol craving. Sodas speed up alcohol release in the blood. Fructose (not table sugar) helps your body burn alcohol.

7: **Take Red Star nutritional yeast broth or miso soup every night** for B vitamins and to curb cravings at night (the worst time).

8: **Re-stabilize your body with high fiber foods** like brown rice and vegetables to soak up alcohol. Add antioxidant foods like cruciferous veggies and soy foods to help detoxify.

9: **Don't take "hair of the dog" drinks;** they drag out a hangover. Eat crackers and honey at bedtime instead to burn up and soak up alcohol. If your hangover doesn't go away, take a catnip, chlorophyll or coffee enema to clear out toxins.

10: **To stave off a killer headache,** drink several glasses of water or a glass of aloe vera juice at bedtime and in the morning.

11: **Help chase your hangover with antioxidants.** Drink plenty of orange juice, tomato juice, or Knudsen's VERY VEGGIE SPICY juice. Make a rapid hangover elimination drink: Mix tomato juice, green and yellow onions, celery, parsley, hot pepper sauce, rosemary leaves, fennel seeds, basil, water, and Bragg's LIQUID AMINOS. Drink straight down.

12: **Alcohol and the herb kava are sedative-depressants.** If you take kava for depression or tension, don't drink alcohol for at least 6 hours after taking it. You'll get highly intoxicated.

Step-by-Step Addictions Healing Diet

—**On rising:** have a protein drink like All One VITAMIN-MINERAL drink, or Nutricology PRO-GREENS, or Unipro PERFECT PROTEIN in pineapple/papaya or pineapple/coconut juice. A superfood-aloe vera drink gives energy and controls morning blood sugar drop: add 1 tsp. each to aloe vera juice: spirulina, bee pollen granules, nutritional yeast; or use 1 TB of a superfood mix: Crystal Star ENERGY GREEN™ Drink; Arise & Shine POWER UP; Green Foods GREEN MAGMA.

—**Breakfast:** Make a mineral mix: 1 tsp. each: sesame seeds, toasted wheat germ, bee pollen granules, nutritional yeast. Sprinkle some on yogurt and fresh fruit, or whole grain cereal or granola topped with apple juice or kefir, or baked, poached or scrambled eggs with cottage or kefir cheese; or have a small omelet with veggies or a low-fat raw cheese filling; or buckwheat pancakes or oatmeal with honey, maple syrup or molasses.

—**Mid-morning:** have fresh carrot juice 3 times a week; on alternate days, Super V-7 veggie juice: 2 carrots, 2 tomatoes, handful each spinach and parsley, 2 celery ribs, $^1/_2$ cucumber, $^1/_2$ bell pepper. Add 1 TB green superfood like Crystal Star ENERGY GREEN™, Transitions EASY GREENS, or Green Foods GREEN MAGMA; or have some miso soup with sea greens snipped on top; or baked veggie chips with kefir cheese dip; or a dried fruit / fresh fruit blend with yogurt cheese.

—**Lunch:** have brown rice with baked tofu and steamed veggies; or a fresh protein salad with sprouts, nuts and seeds. Snip on sea greens, 1 tsp. nutritional yeast, 1 tsp. flax or olive oil, 1 tsp. lemon juice and Bragg's LIQUID AMINOS; or beans and rice with fresh salsa; or a seafood salad with spinach pasta; or a baked potato with a spinach and mushroom salad for EFA's; or 6 pieces of sushi with ginger.

—**Mid-afternoon:** have a glass of fresh carrot juice; or a cup of strengthening herb tea, such as dandelion root, Siberian ginseng, or Crystal Star GINSENG SIX™, FEEL GREAT™, or HIGH ENERGY™ tea; or Knudsen's RECHARGE electrolyte replacement drink, and yogurt with nuts and seeds, or fresh fruit; or a hard boiled egg with light mayonnaise or kefir cheese, or whole grain crackers with low-fat cheese; or a green drink (page 569) with 2 teasp. unsprayed bee pollen added.

—**Dinner:** have brown rice and steamed vegetables with chopped onions, nutritional yeast, snipped shiitake mushrooms, tofu and steamed veggies; or some baked chicken or fish, and a cup of miso soup; or roasted, organic turkey with baked yams and a green salad with yogurt dressing; or a vegetable quiche or pizza on a chapati crust; or a light spinach pasta with a low-fat sauce, and green salad; or a high protein dinner stew and salad with lemon-yogurt dressing; or a hearty seafood-vegetable stir-fry with brown rice; or a large open-face dinner sandwich on whole grain bread and a light soup.

—**Before bed:** have 1 teasp. Red Star r.utritional yeast in hot water; or a relaxing herb tea, like chamomile or peppermint; or a small bowl of oatmeal with maple syrup or honey; or have a cup of miso soup with 1 TB sea greens and 1 teasp. sushi pickled ginger root.

Recipes to help your healing diet: HEALING DRINKS; •FISH and SEAFOODS; •ENZYME-RICH RECIPES; •HIGH FIBER RECIPES; •HIGH PROTEIN without MEAT; •CULTURED FOODS; •MINERAL-RICH RECIPES.

Herb and Supplement Choices

• **Support your detox:** Crystal Star WITHDRAWAL SUPPORT™ caps 3 months, with REISHI-GINSENG extract, or Country Life SHIITAKE/REISHI COMPLEX; Curb cravings-boost energy: Siberian ginseng extract drops in angelica root tea, or Crystal Star MENTAL INNER ENERGY™ caps.

• **Ease withdrawal:** NutriCology BUFFERED C POWDER 3 tsp. daily on an empty stomach or Alacer EMERGEN-C with bioflavonoids $^1/_2$ teasp. in water, with B-complex 100mg, zinc 30mg, and 5-HTP - 50mg. Angelica-scullcap tea eases withdrawal and controls cravings. Dandelion-burdock-ginger tea with honey quells nausea. Taurine 500mg for nerve health.

• **Improve brain communication:** Crystal Star CALCIUM SOURCE™ extract, a rapid calmer; add spirulina 500mg daily; *Scullcap-black cohosh* tea calms nerves; *Kava kava* calms nerves (but also magnifies intoxication levels).

• **Liver support shortens withdrawal significantly:** MRI GLUCOTIZE (controlled release alpha lipoic acid); Crystal Star LIV-ALIVE™; add *Milk Thistle Seed* 120mg extract (6 months).

• **Curb alcohol cravings:** take supplements below daily with meals for a month: Glutamine, 3000mg daily reduces craving; Time Release Niacin 1000mg daily; Tyrosine 1000mg.

• **Shore up for critical deficiencies:** Vitamin C, up to 10,000mg daily (or until stool turns soupy); Evening primrose oil 1000mg daily for EFA's; B-complex, 100mg 2x daily (B-vitamin deficiency increases desire for alcohol). Critical enzymes for alcohol detox are zinc dependent - Zinc 50mg 2x daily. Passionflower-hops tea controls craving and regulates blood sugar. Cayenne-ginger capsules settle stomach and relieve headaches.

Bodywork and Lifestyle Techniques

• **MEN:** The liver controls hormone balance. Excessive drinking especially affects men and their estrogen levels through liver damage; abuse often means enlarged breasts, reduced sex drive and beard growth, and shrunken testes.

—Although it states the obvious, avoid the places, people and circumstances that sharpen your desire to escape through alcohol. This usually means a major life change and may seem impossible. But it almost always starts the road to lasting success and is often the only way.

—**Bodywork:**

• **Acupuncture and massage therapy realignment** help curb craving for alcohol.

• **Improved body fitness and system oxygen are important.** Aerobic exercise like a daily walk reinforces your supplement therapy.

• **Get outside in the fresh air -** the more oxygen in the lungs and tissues, the better.

• **Apply cold compresses to the head** before and after a long hot shower to wash off toxins coming out through the skin. (You won't believe what a difference this makes.) Or, take alternating hot and cool showers to stimulate circulation and eliminate blood alcohol.

• **Take a sauna for 20 minutes.** Scrub skin with a dry skin brush.

Can't find a recommended product? Call the 800 number listed in Product Resources for the store nearest you and for more info.

Diet to Help Overcome Drug Addictions

Drug abuse in one form or another has become a fact of modern life. Our high stress lifestyles deplete energy reserves, motivating many people to seek a quick "voltage" fix to overcome fatigue and relieve tension or boredom. If you use drugs, sugar, alcohol or caffeine as fuel for your body, you're creating multiple nutritional deficiencies. This depletion sets off a chain reaction which results in stress and craving for nutrients, the process is repeated in a futile effort to satisfy increasing need, and addiction eventually occurs.

For most people, this is just the beginning, because drug-caused malnutrition and reduced immunity swiftly lead to hypothyroidism, fatigue syndromes like Hashimoto's, or other auto-immune diseases like mononucleosis, hepatitis, or HIV related infections. Even if these serious disorders are avoided, the consequences are high. Drug abusers and potential drug abusers are always either sick or coming down with something. As soon as one cold, sore throat, bout of "flu," or bladder infection is treated, a new one takes its place. Work is impaired, job time is lost, and family and social life greatly affected.

Nutritional support is the key to recovery from addictions. The overwhelming majority of habitual drug and addictive substance users suffer from malnutrition, metabolic upset and nutritional imbalances. When these conditions are corrected, the need to get high by artificial means is sharply diminished. The following diet can establish a solid nutrition foundation for rebuilding a depleted system. It is designed to revitalize metabolic deficiencies quickly. It is rich in vegetable proteins, high in minerals (especially magnesium to overcome nerve stress), with Omega-3 oils, vitamin B and C source foods, and antioxidants. Regeneration takes time - often up to a year to detoxify and clear drugs from the bloodstream.

Drug detox watchwords:

1: **Eat magnesium-rich foods** - green leafy and yellow vegetables, citrus fruits, whole grain cereals, fish, legumes.

2: **Eat potassium-rich foods** - oranges, broccoli, green peppers, seafoods, sea vegetables, bananas, tomatoes.

3: **Eat chromium-rich foods** - nutritional yeast, mushrooms, whole grains, seafoods, peas. Increase alkalinity with fresh foods.

4: **Cravings and withdrawal symptoms intensify when you eat foods like meats, milk products, refined flours and sugars.** Include slow-burning complex carbohydrates from whole grains and fresh vegetables, and vegetable protein from soy, grains and sprouts.

5: **The brain is dependent on glucose as an energy source.** Drug withdrawals often mean blood glucose levels drop with the consequent results of sweating, tremor, palpitations, anxiety and cravings. Eliminate sugars, alcohol and caffeine from your diet.

6: **Enzymes are important:** include fresh foods for plant enzymes (and take Transformation DIGESTZYME) to stabilize body chemistry.

7: **Superfoods that work for a drug detox:** Chlorella, called "the un-poisoner" has powerful detoxifying capabilities; Body Ecology VITALITY SUPER GREEN with *royal jelly* and *evening primrose oil*; Crystal Star SYSTEMS STRENGTH™ (especially for prescription drugs); Nutricology PRO GREENS with EFA's; Nature's Path TRACE-MIN LYTE with sea greens; All One VITAMINS & MINERALS (green phytobase) .

8: **Eat some vegetable protein at every meal** to keep cravings controlled.

Your daily diet:

—**On rising:** take a "superfood" drink for energy and to control morning blood sugar drop: 1 teasp. each in apple or orange juice: glycine powder, spirulina granules, sugar-free protein powder, nutritional yeast; or Vibrant Health GREEN VIBRANCE or Unipro PERFECT PROTEIN; or a mineral drink, like Crystal Star SYSTEMS STRENGTH™ drink.

—**Breakfast:** make a concentrated food mineral mix to shore up mineral depletion: 1 teasp. each: sesame seeds, toasted wheat germ, unsulphured molasses, bee pollen granules, and nutritional yeast. Sprinkle some on any of the following breakfast choices - fresh fruit with yogurt or kefir cheese topping, or oatmeal or hot kashi pilaf with a little yogurt and maple syrup topping, or a whole grain cereal, muesli or granola with apple juice or fruit yogurt, or a poached or baked egg on whole grain toast with kefir or yogurt cheese.

—**Mid-morning:** have a green drink (page 569), or Monas CHLORELLA or Green Kamut Corp. GREEN KAMUT drink, or Crystal Star ENERGY GREEN™ drink; and/or a whole grain muffin or corn bread with a little butter, kefir cheese or yogurt spread; and a small bottle of mineral water.

—**Lunch:** have a fresh veggie salad with cottage cheese, topped with nuts, seeds and crunchy noodles; or a high protein sandwich on whole grain bread, with avocados, low-fat cheese, and leafy greens; or some oriental fried rice and miso soup with sea greens; or a seafood salad with a black bean or lentil soup; or a vegetarian pizza on a whole grain or chapati crust.

—**Mid-afternoon:** have a glass of fresh carrot juice; or a strengthening herb tea, like dandelion root, Siberian ginseng, or Crystal Star GINSENG SIX™, FEEL GREAT™, or HIGH ENERGY™ tea; or a hard boiled egg with light mayonnaise or yogurt, and whole grain crackers; and another bottle of mineral water, or herb tea, like Crystal Star HIGH ENERGY™ tea.

—**Dinner:** have a vegetable casserole with tofu, or chicken and brown rice; or a broccoli or mushroom quiche or whole grain crepes with a light sauce and a green salad; or a Spanish paella with seafood and rice, or a Mexican beans and rice dish; or an Oriental stir-fry with noodles and vegetables, and miso soup; or a whole grain pasta with steamed vegetables and a green salad; or a large open-face dinner sandwich on whole grain bread and a light soup.

—**Before bed:** have 1 teasp. Red Star nutritional yeast in hot water; or a relaxing herb tea, like chamomile or peppermint; or a small bowl of oatmeal with maple syrup or honey; or have a cup of miso soup with 1 TB sea greens and 1 teasp. sushi pickled ginger root; or apple or papaya juice.

Recipes for your drug detox diet: • FISH and SEAFOODS; • ENZYME-RICH RECIPES; • SOUPS - LIQUID SALADS • HIGH PROTEIN without MEAT; • CULTURED FOODS; • MINERAL-RICH RECIPES; • SANDWICHES.

Herb and Supplement Choices

• **Normalize body chemistry:** Crystal Star GINSENG 6™ SUPER tea, WITHDRAWAL SUPPORT™ caps; MICROHYDRIN available at Healthy House; acidophilus for friendly G.I. flora; chromium to rebalance sugar levels; Enzymes- Transformation DIGESTZYME; Rainbow Light ADVANCED ENZYME SYSTEM.

• **Clean out drug residues:** Crystal Star HEAVY METAL™ or DETOX™ capsules 4 daily; Monas CHLORELLA 1 tsp. daily; M.D. Labs DAILY DETOX tea; Vitamin C crystals - up to 10,000mg daily, with niacin 1000mg 3x daily.

• **Detoxify the liver:** MRI GLUCOTIZE (controlled release alpha lipoic acid) Crystal Star LIV-ALIVE™ tea, or GREEN TEA CLEANSER™ with milk thistle seed extract for 2 months, and B-complex 150mg daily.

• **Curb cravings, boost circulation:** ginkgo biloba extract; Glutamine 2000mg. Crystal Star GINSENG-REISHI extract;

• **Increase energy:** Crystal Star GINSENG SIX™ Super Energy caps, or Siberian ginseng; astragalus extract.

• **Rejuvenate neurotransmitters:** Enzymatic Therapy THY-ROID/TYROSINE caps; 5-HTP, 50mg 2x daily; Country Life RE-LAXER (GABA with taurine).

• **Minimize withdrawal discomfort:** *Rosemary* tea; Crystal Star RELAX™ caps; *gotu kola* caps; DLPA 750mg for cravings and depression; *Oatstraw* tea for sleeplessness and anxiety; *Chamomile* for stress, scullcap for nerves, *ginkgo biloba* for memory loss; Full spectrum amino acids for stabilizing, 1000mg daily.

—**Withdrawal help for specific drugs:** Methionine for heroine; Tyrosine and Siberian ginseng for cocaine; CoQ-10 up to 300mg for prescription drugs; lithium orotate 5mg for uppers and depressants; B-complex 150mg for LSD.

Bodywork and Lifestyle Techniques

• *Note: Strong drugs, from LSD to hard alcohol to nicotine to heroin, can put you at higher risk for Alzheimer's disease due to microvascular blockage and cerebral dementia.* See my book DETOXIFICATION for a complete cleanse.

—**Bodywork:**

• **Enema:** especially important when detoxing from drugs - take an enema the first and second day of your detox. Irrigate: Or have a colonic for a more thorough colon cleanse.

• **Exercise:** every day if possible, to help movement of toxins out of the body - it also brings oxygen to the cells. Exercise also helps reduce the stress of detoxing from addictions. Take a walk every day of your cleanse, breathing deeply.

• **Biofeedback, chiropractic, massage therapy, yoga and acupuncture techniques** have a high success rate in overcoming drug addictions.

• **Guided imagery:** give your body active encouragement. Guided imagery is a relaxation technique to use frequently during an addictions detox. Imagine each gram of the addictive substance dislodging itself from your tissues, floating into your bloodstream and into your bladder or bowel for elimination. Make sure you visualize it leaving your body.

• **Nicotine increases craving for drugs** by stripping the body of stabilizing nutrients. Use Natural Labs ADDICTIONS.

• **Lobelia extract drops every half hour** can sometimes help normalize from an overdose situation.

• **Apply tea tree oil, or B&T CALI-FLORA GEL to heal ulcers** in the nose from cocaine or other sniffer drugs.

• **Deep breathing exercise:** Do deep breathing exercises on rising, and in the evening on retiring to clear the lungs.

Can't find a recommended product? Call the 800 number listed in Product Resources for the store nearest you and for more info.

Strengthening the Male Body

Today's fast paced, high stress lifestyle almost demands that men be Supermen. A man must be strong physically during workouts and sports, supportive emotionally in relationships, balanced under stress, mentally creative and quick, and sexually keen and virile. Diet and exercise are the main pillars supporting a man's health and energy. Both are woefully lacking in the modern American man's life. Poor farming methods and processed foods have made us one of earth's most nutritionally deficient nations. Our hectic, yet sedentary lives don't allow for exercise unless a very conscious effort is made.

Lack of exercise for a man is as great a health risk as high nutrient in itself for the male system. Men need exercise for women. Heart muscle and tone can be lost if exercise is not a regular part of a man's life. To maintain a healthy level of fitness, a man should exercise at least three times a week for 20 to 30 minutes each time. His chosen exercise should raise his heart rate at least 65 to 70% of its capacity - to the point of breathlessness for 5 minutes. A fit male body needs vigorous tain low body fat.

Male metabolism needs more fiber, protein and complex carbohydrates than a woman, but not high fats. His diet should include animal proteins in moderation, like occasional eggs, chicken, turkey, low-fat dairy foods, and sea foods. Amino acid rich foods like seafoods, green superfoods, bee products and wheat germ provide easily convertible proteins. Zinc-rich foods like sea foods and sea greens encourage prostate and reproductive system health. Men also seem to thrive on more cooked than raw foods for the stability of more solid nutrients. Those in whole grains, beans, rice and soy products offer longer endurance and increased sensitivity.

blood pressure, high cholesterol, or even smoking. Exercise is a weight control and general health to a greater degree than regular part of a man's life. To maintain a healthy level of fitness, erals and enzymes for optimum performance and to help main-

Do you know about the male "Superhormone Revolution?"

It's sweeping the US today. The media is flooded with mass advertising for hormone supplements, like Human Growth Hormone, Testosterone Replacement Therapy (TRT) and ANDRO. Every day, we are tempted to try new and different hormones or combinations of hormones called "hormone cocktails." They're an incredibly profitable business and advertised as anti-aging aids for long life-span and renewed sexual vitality.

But before taking the step to take superhormones, take a step back: Just loading up on hormones may not be the answer to men's lifestyle disorders. Hormones are tricky- even dangerous -substances to work with. Tiny amounts can cause big reactions- both good and bad. They may be marketed as supplements rather than drugs, but we need to regard superhormones with respect and caution. From what we know so far, taking supplemental hormones is perhaps appropriate for an acute situation or to address a short-term need. Long term use seems to do more harm that good. A better choice, especially for healthy men with normal hormone levels, might be foods or herbs that contain plant hormones.

The diets in this chapter help several male problems: *Prostate or Testicular Inflammation, Difficult Urination, Recovery after Prostate Surgery. Thymus and Lymphatic Imbalance, Adrenal Exhaustion, Impotence.*

An update on the most popular male superhormones.

TESTOSTERONE: Do you have a low testosterone? Low testosterone affects an astounding 1,000,000 American men! Yet in a recent survey, 68% of men cannot name a single symptom caused by low testosterone. Only 15% named low sex drive as a symptom of low testosterone; 6% named fatigue; 3% named a decrease in muscle mass; and less than 1% linked low testosterone to men's osteoporosis. Clearly, many men are in the dark about how hormone imbalances affect their health. Low testosterone can cause low energy, depression, muscle loss, poor sexual performance, impotence or low sex drive, and slowed growth of facial or body hair.

Today, more physicians prescribe testosterone replacement therapy (TRT) for men with low testosterone or as they approach "andropause," the male equivalent of menopause. Some studies show TRT greatly improves these symptoms for men. In addition, research done by Dr. Jens Moller reveals the use of testosterone may help heal gangrene, benefit diabetes and reduce angina attacks.

However, testosterone drugs, regardless of source or delivery system, can be dangerous for many people. Men with hormone-related problems like prostate enlargement (a major problem for up to 50 percent of men by age fifty), cancers of the prostate and testes, or liver disease should definitely avoid TRT drugs. In addition, excess testosterone can deplete heart protective HDL cholesterol, and may lead to overly aggressive behavior and acne. Some experts find that testosterone drugs actually cause testicle shrinkage! TRT may also convert into estrogen in men, causing side effects like breast growth and bloating. Note: TRT can affect the action of insulin or anticoagulant drugs. Be sure to advise your physician of any drugs you're taking before starting TRT therapy.

Can you boost testosterone with herbs? Ginseng is the only source of plant testosterone known. In a 1996 study published in Panminervia Medica, men who took four grams of ginseng daily for three months experienced an increase in sperm count and testosterone levels. Another study reports better penile function and libido in men on ginseng therapy. I highly recommend a ginseng compound for men for more sexual satisfaction and daily energy. Crystal Star MALE GINSIAC™ extract is a good choice.

ANDRO (*Androstenedione*), is a by-product of the steroid hormone DHEA, synthesized in a lab from the seeds of the Scotch Pine. Although most of us know about ANDRO because of Mark McGwire, ANDRO has been around a long time. In the 1970s, top East German athletes used ANDRO as a testosterone-based steroid to boost their Olympic performances. Today, ANDRO is marketed for athletes who want to increase muscle mass or accelerate recovery from injuries. It is also promoted as a safer Viagra substitute for men (and women) who want to recharge libido.

Does ANDRO work? For men (or women) with a clear testosterone deficiency Andro has clearly been shown to boost libido. ANDRO is a direct precursor to testosterone and has a powerful effect on sex drive. In some studies, ANDRO supplements have increased a man's testosterone supply up to three times the normal level! If you think you have low testosterone, get a professional hormone panel. Most doctors can give them. I called the ANDRO manufacturers directly. They can give you directions on where to get a test. Ph. 800-545-9960. I know the people personally. They can give you good information about ANDRO.

Is ANDRO safe? It's definitely a powerful hormone stimulant, so it shouldn't not be taken casually. We know very little about its long-term effects on health and hormone balance.

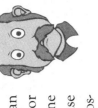

Some of the effects from ANDRO we do know: In some men, ANDRO boosts testosterone levels too much and too fast, causing too much testosterone production, as well as aggressive behavior and acne. The conversion of androstenedione to estrogen is known to accelerate aging in both men and women. A study in the June 1999 Journal of the American Medical Association finds that ANDRO may not always increase blood levels of testosterone as previously believed, but can actually convert into estrogen. This especially concerns men, ANDRO's target market! Excess estrogen in men's bodies can increase risk for pancreatic cancer and heart disease. It also can cause side effects like enlarged breasts or water retention! (For women, ANDRO may cause facial whiskers, chest hair growth or voice deepening.) After long-term ANDRO use, your body may perceive too much hormone and shut down normal testosterone production (as happens with melatonin). Teens, be warned- abnormally high testosterone levels in kids can stunt growth and cause permanent heart and liver damage. Don't take ANDRO if you have hormone-related problems like prostate enlargement or prostate or testes cancer. ANDRO should not be taken by people with acne, liver disease or Cushing's syndrome.

Are there safer alternatives to ANDRO? Consider the herb tribulus terrestris. In India, tribulus has been used since ancient times to enhance libido and as a treatment for impotence in men. Athletes are attracted to its benefits of increased strength and stamina. Trimedica TRIBULUS TERRESTRIS is a good choice or ENDURA OPTIMIZER by Unipro/Ethical Nutrients.

HUMAN GROWTH HORMONE (hGH) is produced by the pituitary gland which promotes bone growth and regulates height. It is available only by prescription, and daily injections cost an astounding $8,000-16,000 a year! hGH treatment has some benefits. It may help very, very short children with growth hormone deficiency to grow for a time. (A 16-year study in the British Medical Journal reveals growth hormone may not improve these children's growth rates over the long-term.) hGH also reduces tissue-wasting caused by advanced AIDS, improves skin elasticity and reduces wrinkles. Further, it seems to increase muscle mass and bone density, decrease body fat, and stimulate a sense of well being in elderly men.

But before you rush to your doctor to get your hGH prescription, know its cautions: hGH is linked to carpal tunnel syndrome and aching joints (similar to "growing pains" in youth); hGH can increase diabetes risk; and some hGH users develop abnormal bone or tissue growth. One of the most frightening reports is the story of a professional athlete who took the hGH to improve his performance and had to have massive skin grafts because his bones literally grew through his skin!

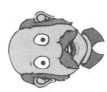

Can you boost growth hormone levels naturally? It's the best way to reap the benefits without the drawbacks. Weight training can boost hGH, increasing both mass and strength of bones and muscle. The amino acids arginine and glutamine also affect hGH release. A 1995 study shows that L-glutamine supplements, 2000mg per day slightly increase hGH release. Arginine promotes an increase of hGH, especially when injected intravenously. A full spectrum amino acid complex like Anabol Naturals AMINO BALANCE in conjunction with weight training may provide the best results.

Experts that I've spoken to at Allergy Research have developed a new, safer way to supplement hGH superhormone. Growth hormone microdoses, monitored by a health practitioner, appear to offer the same benefits with fewer health risks! Allergy Research Group BIOGEN PRO is a microdilution of growth hormone that is absorbed through the tissues of the mouth.

Andropause

Men's hormone changes have been much less publicized and researched than women's, but hormone disruption is as much a part of a man's life as it is a woman's. Some men are more attuned to their hormonal fluctuations than others. Some recognize clear monthly changes in their energy levels, mood, work and sports performance. Blood levels of testosterone do fluctuate dramatically at different times in life- from 250 to 1,200 nanograms, and these changes affect a man's performance, mood and sexuality. While a man's hormone rhythms are less dramatic than a woman's, testosterone levels start to decline around age 40, falling up to 10% each decade. This phenomenon called "andropause" is now recognized by eight in ten family physicians as a real condition that affects quality of life for men. Many physicians now recommend TRT, or testosterone replacement therapy for andropausal men.

The needs of the male body increase as a man approaches andropause. Men need a high energy diet to keep active as they grow older, plenty of nutrients to retain sexual potency, and proteins to maintain muscle mass. If you're in andropause, consider natural therapies as an effective way to renew vitality. Men I've talked to who are using them report better energy, increased stamina and more sexual satisfaction.

Are you in andropause? Signs to watch for:

—Is your energy unusually low lately? Is your work output or sports performance less than you're used to?
—Have you lost height? Are your shoulders slightly hunching? (a sign of early osteoporosis) Get a side view in your mirror.
—Has your beard or head hair growth slowed? Is your chest hair getting sparse but ear hair increasing?
—Have you lost muscle mass? Has your strength or endurance decreased?
—Is your urination frequent and/or difficult, especially at night? (a sign of an enlarged prostate)
—Are your erections less strong or less frequent? Is your sex drive lower than normal for you?
—Are you anxious about your well-being and your future?

Natural therapies renew male vitality. Diet improvements (even if your diet is okay) are essential:

1: Reduce fried foods, caffeine and sugar, red meats and fatty dairy foods (full of disrupting hormones). All deplete the adrenals and drain male energy.

2: Don't go too far. An extremely low fat diet is disastrous for andropausal health. Recent studies find it may reduce testosterone levels almost to preadolescent levels — not good news for an older man! Include healthy fats from seafood instead, and lean, hormone-free turkey and chicken regularly. Flax seed oil is a healthy oil to use in salad dressings. (Use about 1 TB.)

3: Increase your intake of zinc to renew sexual potency. Zinc, highly concentrated in semen, is the most important nutrient for male sexuality. Eat high zinc foods like liver, oysters, nutritional yeast, nuts and seeds. Add zinc-rich spirulina to your superfood list. Try Ethical Nutrients ZINC STATUS (checks for zinc deficiency and is a supplement).

—Take care of your prostate.

Many men don't realize how much they can relieve prostate problems without drugs. The pharmaceutical industry isn't going to tell them! In Europe, botanical medicines are the first-choice treatments for men instead of drugs. European physicians believe that for the majority of prostate problem, drugs are unnecessary! Some prostate drugs, like Proscar, can cause impotence and decreased libido. Herbs like saw palmetto and pygeum show excellent results in wide clinical trials without these side effects.

Here's why: As men grow older they tend to accumulate more of the rogue testosterone, dihydrotestosterone (DHT), which causes cells to multiply and the prostate to enlarge. Numerous studies show that saw palmetto reduces the symptoms of BPH by blocking DHT, inhibiting the enzyme 5-alpha reductase related to prostate enlargement. Consider Crystal Star PRO-X™ FOR MEN or Morada Research Laboratories PROSTATE to help reduce prostate enlargement and dribbling urine. (Usually improvement in 48 hours.) Check your alcohol intake. Heavy drinking can lead to prostate problems and impaired erections. Dr. Howard Peiper's book Natural Solutions For Sexual Enhancement, says "alcohol, especially beer, elevates levels of DHT in the body and can be a contributing factor in sexual dysfunction." DHT elevation is linked to testosterone decline and elevation of female hormones.... definitely undesirable for men. (See page 311 for a good prostate health diet and more info.)

—Build muscle mass.

Take a high protein drink every morning to build muscle mass and stamina. Unipro PERFECT PROTEIN has branch-chain amino acids, leucine, isoleucine and valine - ideal for building muscle protein. Before you turn to a drug-based growth hormone supplement, consider L-glutamine 3000mg to 4000mg daily. It helps your pituitary stimulate your own growth hormone - for some men dramatically. Add a glutamine fortified body builder like Nutritional Tech. GLUTA-PRO, to improve muscle tone.

—Renew sexual potency.

Try the Ayurvedic herb *tribulus terrestris*, or *Epimedium* (horny goat weed) to boost libido and impotence in men. Athletes like its benefits of increased strength and stamina. Try Trimedica TRIBULUS TERRESTRIS, or Pinnacle HORNY GOAT WEED, or Crystal Star MALE PERFORMANCE™ caps with a long history of success for enhancing the sexual experience.

—Don't forget regular exercise.

It's a vital component of male sexuality. It makes your body stronger, function better and endure longer. In one study, 78 healthy, but sedentary men were studied during nine months of regular exercise. The men exercised 60 minutes a day, three days a week. Every single man reported significantly enhanced sexuality, including increased frequency, performance and satisfaction. Rising sexuality was even correlated with degree of fitness improvement. The more fitness the men were able to attain, the better their sex life!

—Feed your adrenals.

Men need healthy adrenals to keep active and energized as testosterone levels begin to decline. I've talked to many men over 40, working stressful jobs with major family responsibilities who just can't keep it up anymore because their adrenals are shot from years of abuse. If you tend to eat fast foods on the run, drink a lot of coffee and get little sleep you're setting your body up for an adrenal crash. Adrenal exhaustion for men sometimes precipitates depression and severe stress reactions. Crystal Star •ADRN™ extract has a long history of success in restoring a man's energy and vitality.

What about environmental hormones and male hormone problems?

New evidence is substantiating the dangers of estrogen-imitating chemicals and pesticides on men as well as women. An unusually large number of male babies (both animals and human) are showing up with male feminization (small testicles, low sperm count, and miniature penises), a trend many scientists believe is directly related to chemicals in our environment. The dramatic rise in prostate cancer deaths over the last 50 years is another wake-up call to change our environment for health.

While the rate of prostate cancer has doubled since World War II, male sperm counts have fallen by half - a trend that has led to speculation that America's current environment and lifestyle interferes with a man's ability to make sperm. Semen analysis tests over the last few decades show undeniably that total sperm count as well as sperm quality of the U.S. male population is deteriorating. In 1940, the average sperm count was 113 million per ml. In 1993 that value had dropped to 65 million. Total amount of semen has fallen dramatically, from 3.5 ml in 1940 to 2.74 ml in 1993. Today men have only about 39% of the sperm counts they had in 1940. For the first time in America's history, one in six married couples of childbearing age has trouble conceiving and completing a pregnancy.

Pollutants used to be considered strictly estrogenic, like poly-chlorinated bi-phenols (PCBs), dioxin and agricultural pesticides. But new reports reveal that androgens in pollutants (substances that mimic male sex hormone) are much more widespread than previously thought. Vanderbilt University School of Medicine found that of ten pollutants, 5 were androgenic while only 2 were estrogenic. Men can really benefit from adding more dietary fiber from whole grains, fresh fruits and vegetables that can bind to and eliminate hormone-disrupting pollutants lodged in their bodies.

What about male impotence? Do we live in the Age of Viagra?

Impotence affects 52% of U.S. men between 40 and 70 years of age. Viagra, one of the first designer drugs to be marketed directly to the public, is promoted as a love aid for impotent men. Its phenomenal success (between 3 and 4 billion prescriptions each year so far) says a lot about the state of male bodies today. Viagra's manufacturer is developing faster acting versions of the drug. Other drug companies are developing a Viagra rival to tempt both the male and female libido. The fact that it is a powerful, potentially dangerous drug has been vastly understated in the public advertising.

Viagra enhances the mechanism needed for erection, relaxing smooth muscles and increasing circulation to the penis. It is useful for some cases of impotence caused by spinal cord injuries, diabetes or radical prostatectomies.

But does Viagra mean better sex?

Three years into the Viagra craze we see that enhancing sexuality through drug chemistry is not what we thought it was. It's much more in terms of danger, and much less in terms of help for impotence. Side effects and risks surfaced almost immediately. At this writing there have been over 130 Viagra-related deaths- from massive cardiac arrest, stroke, cardiovascular complications or drug interactions. Although the company that manufactures Viagra maintains it's safe if used properly, the reports speak for themselves.

Can natural therapies help if you're impotent?

Unless you have a clear medical condition, better libido results not from a pill, but from a good lifestyle program. Many sexual difficulties often begin in the dining room, from stress and a poor diet, not the bedroom.

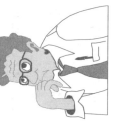

Atherosclerosis, clearly related to diet, can block blood supply to the penile artery, and is the primary cause of impotence in nearly half of men over 50! Diabetes, smoking, overuse of alcohol or sedatives, and anti-depressant drugs or high blood pressure medicines regularly cause impotence.

It is almost universally recognized today that impotence and low libido are overwhelmingly physical, rather than psychological, conditions. The main problem is at the dinner table, not in the bedroom. A recent study on male impotence showed that over 80% of the men in the test had atherosclerosis. This hardening of the arteries had damaged the blood vessels (including the penis blood vessels) to the extent that the men could not sustain an erection.

Atherosclerosis is caused by a high-fat, cholesterol-rich diets. A high-fat diet may also lead to diabetes or latent diabetes, injuring the nerves that stimulate an erection. Too much fat abnormally elevates prolactin from the pituitary gland, suppressing hormones responsible for good sexual function. The first step toward a better sex life is to get saturated fats out of your diet. Low fat, largely vegetarian meals, with lots of fresh foods and whole grains, provide plenty of complex carbohydrates, proteins and soluble fiber to build and regulate health, while avoiding cholesterol and reducing fat to 20% or less of daily calories.

Physical improvements happen quickly. Within a few hours of eating a low-fat meal, circulation to all organs increases. Prolactin levels fall in just a few days on a low-fat diet. Atherosclerosis begins to reverse. Weight is usually lost and libido rises. However, an extremely low fat diet is disastrous for andropausal health. It may reduce testosterone levels almost to preadolescent levels – bad news for an older man!

Sexual function depends on healthy glands and organs to produce sex hormones. Herbs work through the glands to rebalance and nourish. Herbs enhance and enrich sexual feelings and activity, but they do not overwhelm or instigate it, like some drugs. Ginkgo biloba improves circulation, increases vascular strength and reverses atherosclerosis impotence. In one study, ginkgo was 30% more effective than drug injections with 50% of patients showing regained potency. Take the whole herb extract, about 15 drops under the tongue, 2 or 3 times a day.

What about vasectomies?

Science has long debated whether a vasectomy, the contraceptive procedure which severs or seals off the vessel that carries sperm from the testes, increases the risk of prostate cancer in men. New studies on two large groups of men, show that vasectomies do increase risk of prostate cancer. In one study of 73,000 men, 300 of the men developed prostate cancer between 1986 and 1990. The men with vasectomies had a 66% greater risk of prostate cancer than the men without vasectomies. In a separate study, vasectomies increased the risk of prostate cancer by 56%. As sperm builds up in the sealed-off vas deferens after a vasectomy, the body re-absorbs the cells. This confuses the immune system, making it less alert to tumor cells. Sometimes the body's immune defenses try to mount a response against its own tissue. A vasectomy also affects testicle secretions and lowers prostatic fluid. When the natural movement of sperm and hormones is artificially prevented, a host of male health problems result.

A Quick Fresh Foods Detox for Men

For gland, hormone, prostate or sexual potency problems, a short 3-day fresh foods cleansing diet is recommended to clean out sediment or calcification, and to alkalize the body. The diet is very high in vegetable and whole grain fiber for alkalizing, is full of plant enzymes, essential fatty acids and zinc sources. Use only unsaturated oils in this diet. Always wash commercial produce thoroughly to reduce harmful pollutant residues and buy organic whenever possible. The produce sections in health food stores are like gold, not just in terms of taste and local freshness but in the concept that good food really is good medicine!

—**On rising:** take 2 lemons or 2 teasp. cider vinegar in water with 1 teasp. maple syrup each morning, or a cup of green tea; and a vitamin/mineral drink, such as ALL ONE MULTIPLE VITAMINS & MINERALS, Nutricology PRO-GREENS or Crystal Star SYSTEMS STRENGTH™ drink.

—**Breakfast:** take a glass of organic apple juice or have fresh-cut apples; or a potassium drink (pg. 568) with 1 teasp. Bragg's LIQUID AMINOS; make a mix of 2 TBS each: lecithin granules, wheat germ, Red Star nutritional yeast, pumpkin seeds, and oat bran. Sprinkle 1 or 2 TBS onto a whole grain cereal, or mix into yogurt every morning;

—**Mid-morning:** have a glass of fresh carrot juice; and/or a vegetable mineral drink, such as Green Foods GREEN MAGMA, or Crystal Star ENERGY GREEN™, or a cup of chamomile tea with whole grain crackers and raw vegetables with yogurt cheese.

—**Lunch:** have a green drink (page 569) or Sun Wellness CHLORELLA, or make an enzyme juice with pineapple-alfalfa sprouts and add 1 teasp. spirulina powder. Or have light solid food such as a green leafy salad with a lemon/oil or Italian dressing (include celery, avocados, nuts and seeds); or a cup of miso soup, with Chinese rice noodles and sea greens; or a tofu and brown rice casserole with steamed veggies; or a lentil or black bean soup with whole grain crackers.

—**Mid-afternoon:** have another glass of organic apple juice or 2 apples; or a cup of white oak bark or chamomile tea with Crystal Star ADRN™ extract drops added. Make fresh veggie or tofu dip, add in 2 handfuls pumpkin seeds and spread on whole grain crackers or celery.

—**Dinner:** before dinner, have a cup of water with 1 dropperful Crystal Star GINSENG-LICORICE ELIXIR™ or any good ginseng tea; have some steamed veggies with brown rice or couscous; or a baked or broiled fish or seafood with a small salad; or a large dinner salad with brown rice, yogurt or vinaigrette dressing, toasted nut/seed toppings; or a baked potato with an tamari-olive oil dressing, and a green leafy salad; or a vegetable casserole or quiche with whole grain crust; or a spinach pasta salad, hot or cold with seasoned steamed veggies.

—**Before bed:** have a pineapple/papaya juice, or pineapple/coconut juice; or a cup of chamomile or alfalfa/mint tea; or a cup of Red Star nutritional yeast broth (1 teasp. in a cup of hot water); or a cup of herb tea, such as Crystal Star RELAX TEA™.

Recipes to help your quick cleanse diet: •DETOXIFICATION FOODS; •HEALING DRINKS; •SOUPS, LIQUID SALADS; •ENZYME-RICH FOODS; •SALADS, HOT and COLD; •MINERAL-RICH • LIGHT MACROBIOTIC EATING.

Male Andropause Diet

The needs of the male body are profound. These needs increase as a man approaches andropause. Men need a high energy diet to keep active as they grow older, an ample supply of nutrients to retain sexual potency, and proteins to maintain muscle mass. Add more high energy foods like complex carbohydrates from whole grains, legumes, and fresh fruits and vegetables. Add a superfood drink each afternoon like Crystal Star ENERGY GREEN™ drink to reduce any craving for high fat junk foods. Ethical Nutrients FUNCTIONAL GREENS is another good choice.

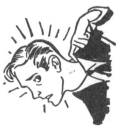

Watchwords:

1: Eat smaller, more frequent meals. Overeating can suppress hormone production.

2: Add soy foods (tofu, tempeh, soy milk, etc.) to your diet for hormone normalizing isoflavones.

3: Drink green tea to flush out fats that harbor hormone disrupting chemicals.

4: Drink in moderation. Heavy drinking can lead to prostate problems and impaired erections.

5: Wash produce to reduce hormone disrupting pollutant residues. Use Healthy Harvest FRUIT & VEGETABLE RINSE.

6: Limit dairy foods and meats (especially beef and pork), notorious for hormone-disrupting chemicals. Chicken is also an offender; buy hormone-free poultry - Petaluma Poultry ROSIE the ORGANIC CHICKEN, Diestel and Coleman Natural Products.

7: Limit your use of microwaves. Microwaving foods kills enzymes. Enzymes are important for gland and hormone metabolism.

—**On rising:** Herbal fiber reduces cholesterol and eliminates fatty build-up that contributes to impotence. Crystal Star CHOL-LO FIBER TONE™ takes about 3 months; or a high protein drink such as Unipro PERFECT PROTEIN in juice.

—**Breakfast:** make a mix of 2 TBS each: sunflower seeds, pumpkin seeds, toasted wheat germ. Sprinkle some each morning on toasted oat cereal (wild oats have helped increase frequency of intercourse and orgasm for men for millennia), pancakes or granola. Top with maple syrup, molasses, apple juice or yogurt; add poached or baked eggs with whole grain toast or muffins.

—**Mid-morning:** have a fresh carrot juice, or small bottle of mineral water; or a green drink like Monas CHLORELLA, Nutricology PRO-GREENS or Crystal Star ENERGY GREEN™; and a cup of noodle ramen soup with sea greens snipped on top.

—**Lunch:** have some fish or seafood with brown rice and a small salad; or a chicken, avocado and low-fat cheese sandwich or salad; or a whole grain, high protein salad or sandwich with lots of nuts, seeds, tofu or yogurt, and lentil or black bean soup.

—**Mid-afternoon:** have some low-fat cottage cheese with nuts and seeds, and whole grain crackers; or a dried fruit and nut mix with a bottle of mineral water; or a hard boiled egg with a tea like ginseng tea (use about 1 dropperful panax ginseng extract in water; or try a ginseng/ royal jelly blend in water); or Nature's Path TRACE-LYTE drink for electrolyte minerals.

—**Dinner:** have an Italian whole grain pasta or polenta dish with a seafood stew; or a roast turkey and whole grain stuffing meal, with steamed vegetables and a fresh salad; or fresh baked seafood or salmon with brown rice and peas.

Note: A little wine at dinner helps relaxation, digestion, and release from stress.

—**Before bed:** have a cup of Red Star nutritional yeast broth; or a cup of Crystal Star CUPID'S FLAME TEA™ with honey.

Herb and Supplement Choices

• **Revitalize the male body:** For hormone balance: Glutamine 200mg daily for growth hormone; Crystal Star MALE PERFORMANCE™ for 3 months; Siberian Ginseng extract; Crystal Star GINSENG-LICORICE ELIXIR™; Nature's Secret BEYOND ENDURANCE; Crystal Star ENERGY GREEN™.

• **Essential fatty acids normalize production of steroid hormones:** EVENING PRIMROSE OIL 2000mg daily; Twin Lab MAX-EPA; Nature's Secret ULTIMATE OIL; Omega Nutrition ESSENTIAL BALANCE OIL, caps and liquid.

• **For low sperm count:** Carnitine 2000mg daily helps sperm cells "swim" to their destination; B$_{12}$ 6,000 mcg. daily.

• **Hormone tonics for more energy:** Crystal Star ADRN™ extract with FEEL GREAT™ caps; Rainbow Light ADAPTO-GEM caps; YS ROYAL JELLY-GINSENG blend (with bee pollen and propolis); Panax ginseng-Damiana caps.

• **Male virility:** *Yohimbe* extract; *Tribulus terrestris* caps; *Ginkgo biloba* extract; *Panax ginseng-Sarsaparilla*; *Horny Goat Weed.*

• **Boost hormone production:** Crystal Star MALE GINSIAC™ extract with fresh panax ginseng roots and potency wood; Golden Pride REJUVENATE FOR MEN; CoQ-10, 60mg 3x daily improves physical performance.

• **Boost nutrient intake:** Life Essence ONE 'N ONLY; Country Life MAX FOR MEN; Nature's Herbs MALE VITE; Cal-mag-zinc 4 daily; zinc, 75 to 100mg. with vitamin E 400IU and selenium, 200mcg daily for reproductive system support; Magnesium 750 mg; Ascorbate vitamin C 3000mg. daily with CoQ 10, 60mg 3x daily; Omega-3 fish oils, 3 daily for unsaturated fatty acids and circulation.

Bodywork and Lifestyle Techniques

• **Environmental estrogens in hormone-injected food animals, herbicides and pesticide affect male sperm counts.** Avoid hormone-injected meats and dairy foods, and herbicide-sprays to avoid environmental estrogens (see page 345).

• **Exercise** can increase sex drive. Regular exercise such as dancing, walking and swimming stimulates circulation and increases body oxygen.

• **Early morning sunlight on the body and genitals** every day possible for general sexual health and to help prevent prostate problems.

• **Massage therapy re-establishes unblocked meridians** of energy and increases circulation.

• **Deep abdominal breathing** - (see page 472.)

• **Yoga stretches every morning.**

• **Alternating hot and cold hydrotherapy showers** each morning for circulatory/organ health.

• **Smoking disrupts hormone activity.** The cadmium contained in cigarette papers interferes with the utilization and absorption of zinc

• **Check your prescription drugs;** some have the side effect of impaired sex drive. Prolonged recreational drug use also inhibits sperm production. Heavy metal or radiation damages sperm and chromosome structure.

Can't find a recommended product? Call the 800 number listed in Product Resources for the store nearest you and for more info.

Plumbing Problems - a Diet for Prostate Health

<u>Your prostate can be your worst friend. Your prostate can be your libido's worst enemy.</u>

The little doughnut-shaped gland that lies below a man's bladder is a source of big problems for many men. Disorders usually begin after age 35, and recent studies show that almost 60% of men between the ages of 40 and 60 have BPH (benign prostatic hyperplasia). By 70, it's over 70% and by age 80, over 80%.

The prostate's job in life is to secrete a fluid/enzyme mixture for sperm health and motility. As middle age approaches, the prostate often enlarges, strangling the urethra, and causing the BPH symptoms of frequent urination, trouble starting urination, weak flow and the feeling that the bladder isn't empty afterwards. This discomfort can magnify during lovemaking. While BPH is not cancer, an enlarged prostate can eventually completely block the flow of urine, an obviously life-threatening condition. Even if the problem never reaches that state, you should take care of it immediately. The inability to fully empty the bladder along with the pressure build up can result in a painful bladder infection, and dangerous inflammation of the kidneys.

Obesity, and hormonal changes such as increased estrogen levels and altered testosterone levels, are at the root of the problem. Research shows that prostate health is linked to the decline of testosterone production. Enlargement seems to be caused by an enzyme, testosterone reductase, that interacts with testosterone and produces di-hydro-testosterone, a hormone form also involved in male pattern baldness. When testosterone is not converted into this metabolite form, the prostate continues its youthful functions and does not enlarge.

<u>Worried about prostate problems? With BPH, the disease is basically the symptoms. Here are early signs:</u>

—**Inflamed, swollen, infected prostate gland (under the scrotum and testes)**
—**Frequent, painful desire to urinate with dribbling urine; incontinence in severe cases**
—**Feverish feeling (because of inflammation); lower back and leg pains**
—**Impotence, loss of libido, and/or painful ejaculation**
—**Low immune response; unusual insomnia and fatigue**

Drugs like PROSCAR and PROS-GUARD report side effects of decreased sexual potency and libido - in some cases it is stifled entirely. But benign prostate problems respond well to nutritional and herbal support. In fact, for many men, natural therapy for prostate problems works better than the most powerful prostate drugs on the market.

<u>Watchwords should be:</u> less fat, more fiber, stay fit. Limit antihistamines; their overuse impairs liver and prostate function.

First: take a *saw palmetto* herbal combination. I recommend PROX™ FOR MEN capsules by Crystal Star (*with saw palmetto, pygeum Africanum bk., licorice, gravel rt., juniper, parsley, potency wood, goldenseal, uva ursi, marshmallow, ginger, suma, capsicum and hydrangea rt.*). Symptom improvement is often quite rapid —within 48 hours.

The Prostate Healing Diet

A healthy prostate depends on a healthy diet. A high fat, high cholesterol diet puts a man at greatest risk. So does a diet with too little fiber (men should get about 35 to 45 grams of fiber daily). Increase your fiber from green salads, fresh fruits, whole grains and steamed vegetables for better elimination. Too much alcohol and caffeine affect prostaglandin balance that controls the inflammation process. Lack of essential fatty acids and zinc are also involved. Add whole grains, soy foods, sea foods and sea greens (2 TBS daily) for EFA's and zinc. Avoid red meats, caffeine, hard liquor, carbonated drinks, especially beer, during healing. Limit spicy foods that irritate your bladder. Avoid tobacco, fried, fatty and refined foods forever. Use the diet here for 1 to 3 months. It lays down the groundwork for maintaining male system health and immune response.

Watchwords: Make a prostate health mix of bee pollen granules, toasted wheat germ, pumpkin seeds, oat bran, nutritional yeast, sesame seeds, and crumbled dry sea greens; take 2 TBS daily over rice, miso soup or a salad every day. Drink 6 glasses of water or cleansing fluids daily. Have a green drink (pg. 569) every day and take your chosen supplements twice a day with green tea during healing.

—**On rising:** take 2 TBS cranberry concentrate (or cider vinegar), and honey in water every morning for two weeks to cleanse sediment; then take ALL ONE VITAMIN/MINERAL or Crystal Star SYSTEMS STRENGTH™ drink for iodine and potassium, or Nature's Plus SPIRUTEIN protein drink, or make a soy protein drink and add 1 TB molasses, 1 tsp. spirulina, 1 tsp. lecithin granules.

—**Breakfast:** make up a prostate health mix of 2 TBS each: bee pollen granules, toasted wheat germ, pumpkin seeds, oat bran, nutritional yeast, sesame seeds, and crumbled dry sea greens; Sprinkle some daily over low fat whole grain granola, or mix into yogurt and add fresh fruit if desired; or poached, or baked eggs with whole grain toast; or whole grain pancakes with maple syrup or almond butter (vitamin E); or pineapple/coconut, or pineapple/papaya-juice, and a bowl of fresh fruits.

—**Mid-morning:** have an apple or other fresh fruit; or some crisp raw veggies with kefir cheese or yogurt cheese; or some whole grain crackers or corn chips and a veggie/yogurt dip; and/or a green drink, or Sun Wellness CHLORELLA drink.

—**Lunch:** have some marinated, baked tofu and millet or brown rice, and a light soup; or a vegetable protein or roast turkey sandwich on whole grain bread with a cup of light soup; or a hearty but low-fat Mexican beans and rice meal; or a seafood and shellfish stew or hot salad with pasta; or a vegetarian pizza on a chapati or whole grain crust.

—**Mid-afternoon:** have a cup of chamomile or ginseng, or Crystal Star MEDITATION™ TEA; and some whole grain crackers or chips with a tofu or yogurt dip or spread; or some low-fat cheese and fresh fruit.

—**Dinner:** have an Italian meal with spinach pasta (EFA's), a light seafood sauce, and green salad; or a Chinese stir fry with brown rice and miso soup with sea greens snipped on top; or a hearty soup or stew with lentils or black beans and whole grain bread with yogurt or kefir cheese; or a veggie or seafood quiche or omelet or frittata with a fresh herb sauce, and green salad.

—**Before bed:** have some Red Star nutritional yeast broth in a cup of hot water; or chamomile or Crystal Star RELAX TEA™.

Recipes to help a prostate healing diet: •LIGHT MACROBIOTIC EATING; •HEALING DRINKS; •BREAKFAST; •SOUPS, LIQUID SALADS; •ENZYME-RICH FOODS; •SALADS, HOT and COLD; •MINERAL-RICH •HIGH FIBER.

Herb and Supplement Choices

• **Reduce inflammation and pain:** Crystal Star PRO-X™ caps 6 daily, (or extract for 1 month), then 4 daily for 1 month; Crystal Star RELAX™ caps to ease urination; EVENING PRIMROSE oil 4000mg daily for 1 month, then 2-4 daily for 1 month with bee pollen caps 2 daily, and ANTI-BIO™ caps 4 daily for 1 month. Enzymedica PURIFY or Bromelain for fast healing.

—**Follow-up:** Crystal Star MALE PERFORMANCE™ for regeneration, and IODINE/POTASSIUM™ caps, or kelp tabs 10 daily for prevention; GINSENG/LICORICE ELIXIR™ to guard against prostate cancer. Take vitamin E 400IU; or white oak bark tea, or Melatonin .3mg at night to reduce size.

• **Flush sediment and congestive residues:** Vitamin C crystals, $^1/_2$ tsp. every hour to bowel tolerance for 2 weeks, then $^1/_2$ tsp. 4x daily for 2 weeks, then 3000mg daily for 1 month; Glycine 1000mg for sediment control; Transformation PUREZYME to dissolve lesions. *Uva Ursi* tea, *Una da Gato* caps; *Nettles* extract or *Horsetail-Nettles* tea to reduce prostate swelling rapidly. GABA to relieve frequent urination.

• **Soothe pain with EFA's:** *Evening Primrose oil* 4000mg daily; Barleans lignan-rich flax oil 3x daily; Y.S. ROYAL JELLY; Nutricology PRO GREENS with EFA's; Crystal Star ANTI-FLAM™ caps 2 as needed.

• **Preventive supplements:** Zinc - about 50 to 75 mg daily; an EFA like *Evening Primrose Oil* 4000 daily; Bee pollen (4 TBS. or 10 capsules daily) or royal jelly (2 teasp. daily) to balance endocrine activity; Vitamin E 400IU with selenium 200mcg daily, an antioxidant mineral that attacks free radicals and is essential for sperm production. Sea greens for selenium and PHYCOTENE MICROCLUSTERS available at Healthy House.

Bodywork and Lifestyle Techniques

• **Sexual intercourse during prostatitis irritates the prostate and delays recovery.** After recovery, sex life should be normal in frequency with a natural climax.

• **Hot and cold sitz baths** shows some success for some men. See page 465.

• **Use chamomile tea enemas** (pg. 571) once a week during healing as an acid neutralizer. Or take warm chamomile sitz baths for 20 minutes at a time morning and evening.

• **Apply ice packs to reduce pain.**

• **A brisk daily walk helps.**

• **Warm baths soften and relax.**

• **Massage therapy re-establishes unblocked meridians** of energy and increases circulation.

• **Deep abdominal breathing** - page 472.

• **Yoga stretches every morning.**

• **Exercise** is vital to male hormone health.

• **Get morning sunlight on the body** every day possible, on the genitalia for men.

• **Smoking disrupts hormone activity.**

• **Muscle Testing (Applied Kinesiology),** is useful for determining which hormonal herbs or supplements are specific to your problem. Once you learn the simple technique (see a nutritional consultant, a holistic chiropractor, a massage therapist), you can easily do it at home to decide which products are right for you.

Can't find a recommended product? Call the 800 number listed in Product Resources for the store nearest you and for more info.

Renewing Female Health and Balance

A healthy female system works in an incredibly complex balance. It is an individual model of the creative universe. A woman is usually a marvelous thing to be, but the intricacies of her body are easily, causing pain and poor function. From child-bearing age to pre-menopause, and menopause, to post-menopause, many women are affected by hormone imbalances are involved in a myriad of health problems sion, low libido and infertility. Hormones help regulate monthly cycle. Tiny amounts can cause big reactions, both world is not easy. Every day, we are bombarded with manpollutants, hormone drugs and hormones injected in our most of us can benefit from. Using lifestyle therapy to rethan regulating hormones by injection which sometimes entirely. I find natural, hormone balancing therapies after birth, a D & C, or an abortion allow your body to achieve its own hormone levels and bring itself to its own balance at its deepest levels.

delicately tuned; they can become unbalanced or obstructed ing age to pre-menopause, and menopause, to post-menopause, and fluctuations that rattle their lives. Female hormone including: fibroids, endometriosis, headaches, PMS, depreseverything from energy flow, to inflammation, to a woman's good and bad. Maintaining hormonal balance in today's made hormones — from widespread hormone-mimicking foods. A hormone balancing lifestyle program is something balance hormone ratios gently harmonizes your body, rather stops natural hormone production by the endocrine glands trauma, stress or serious illness, or after a hysterectomy, child-

Drugs, chemicals and synthetic medicines, standing as they do outside the natural cycle of things, often do not bring positive results for women. These substances usually try to add something to the body, or act directly on a specific problem area. The gentle, but effective nutrients in whole foods (and herbs as concentrated foods) are identified and used by our body's own enzyme action. They encourage the body to do its own work, and recover its own balance. Nutritional therapy nourishes in a broad spectrum, like the female essence itself. A woman's body responds to it easily without side effects. I find that most women know their own bodies better than anyone else, and can instinctively pinpoint foods within a diet range that are right for her personal renewal. Relief and response time are often quite gratifying.

Hormones, incredibly important and potent substances, seem to be at the root of most women's problems. Even in tiny amounts they have, as any woman can tell you, dramatic effects. Many female ailments are caused by too much estrogen production, such as fibrocystic breast disease, endometriosis, PMS, and heavy, painful menstrual periods. The growth and function of the breasts and uterus are controlled by estrogens and prolactin which are produced by the ovaries and pituitary gland. A diet too high in fats raises these hormones to disease-forming levels. In women, the whole reproductive system is affected.

A healthy endocrine system is a must for solving female problems because the glands are the deepest level of the body processes. Good nutrition and nourishment for the glands can "change the world" for a woman. Many hormones are protein based, so that a diet high in vegetable proteins and whole grains, with some lecithin and nutritional yeast on a regular basis, is very important to effective gland and hormone health.

What About Environmental Hormones?

Hormone disrupters are so commonplace in modern culture that there is no way to avoid them. Hormone disrupters come from pollutants, drugs, hormone-injected meats and dairy products, plastics, pesticides, and hormone replacement drugs. (The hormone replacement drug for women, Premarin, is the number two selling drug in America!) Only in the last five years has anyone realized how common environmental estrogens are in today's world. Nearly 40% of pesticides used in commercial agriculture are suspected hormone disrupters. Compounding the problem, these chemicals increase in potency 160 to 1600 times when they combine inside your body from several different sources, like from hormone-injected meats and pesticide-sprayed produce.

Since the Earth's waterways are connected, pollutants containing disrupting hormones reach your food supply wherever you live. And it's just the beginning. Genetically altered foods are booming. In the year 2000, 70% of foods on grocers shelves are already genetically modified. We have no clear understanding of how THEY will factor into the hormone-chemical-pollutant quotient (see page 130). The problem is becoming mind-boggling. In 1999, the Environmental Protection Agency implemented a congressionally mandated plan to test 87,000 compounds for their effect on the reproductive systems of humans and animals.

Reports show the devastating effect of these pollutants on wildlife. Pallid sturgeons, found only in the Mississippi river, are now condemned to extinction. Decades of exposure to PCB's (polychlorinated biphenyls) and DDT (dichloro-diphenyl-trichloroethane) have resulted in NO species births for 10 years. Turtle studies at the University of Texas find that even when environmental factors like heat, are controlled for a male outcome, female or intersex turtles hatch instead after just a small amount of PCB's are painted on the eggs.

The effects of estrogen disruption mean maintaining female hormone balance is clearly a challenge.

Estrogen-mimicking pollutants may even be changing the face of human evolution. Hormone disrupters affect the entire system of our glands and hormones. They alter the development of our own hormones— disrupting hormone balance at its core. They compete for hormone receptor sites and bind to them in place of natural hormones, causing major fluctuations in hormonal levels.

Science is just beginning to accept, even though naturopaths have known for some time, that man-made estrogens can stack the deck against women by increasing their estrogen levels hundreds of times. Although science still tells us there is no significant difference between man-made and natural hormones, it seems apparent from the evidence of thousands of women, that even if a lab test can't tell the difference, our bodies can. Nearly HALF of African-American girls and 15% of Caucasian girls now begin to develop sexually by age 8, a clear indicator of hormone disruption. There is grim news about estrogenic chemicals and human fetuses, too. Male and female hormones must remain in balance in an embryo for sexual organs to develop normally. Exogenous estrogens can upset the normal balance, resulting in children with stunted male sex organs or with both sets of sex organs.

There is a link between pesticides and breast cancer. Pesticides are stored in body fat areas like breast tissue. Pesticides like PCB's and DDT affect the glands and hormones the way too much estrogen does. One study shows 50 to 60% more DDE and PCB's in women who have breast cancer than in those who don't. Some researchers think that the reason older women are experiencing a higher rate of breast cancer may be that they had greater exposure to DDT before it was banned.

The dramatic rise in breast cancer is in ratio to the accumulation of organo-chlorine residues in the environment. Israel's recent history offers a case study. Until about 20 years ago, both breast cancer rates and contamination levels of organo-chlorine pesticides in Israel were among the highest in the world. An aggressive phase-out of these pesticides has led to a sharp reduction in contamination levels, followed by a dramatic drop in breast cancer death rates.

Significant rises in breast and uterine fibroids, polycystic ovary disease, endometriosis and pelvic inflammatory disease are also associated with chronic exposure to estrogen mimics.

Is there any way to reduce your exposure?

—First: Cut back on fat! Hormone disrupters accumulate in body fat. This is why a high fat diet is a major risk factor for long term exposure to them, and why it may lead to increased risk for hormone-driven cancers.

—Second: Eat sea greens like wakame, nori and dulse regularly. Algin, a gel-like substance in sea greens, protects against chemical overload (often involved in breast cancer) by binding to chemical wastes so they can be eliminated safely from the body.

Are the new designer estrogens, the SERMs (selective estrogen receptor modulators), estrogen disrupters?

SERMs are a part of the new revolution in hormone replacement drugs. It's not about hot flashes anymore because women are finding out they can handle them on their own with herbs and foods, as they have for centuries. SERMs were developed to fight what are perceived as menopausal diseases like osteoporosis, heart disease, even Alzheimer's disease, without increasing breast and uterine cancer risk, like traditional HRT drugs (see pages 326-328 in this chapter).

Designer estrogen SERMs seem promising at first glance. Some reports suggest that Evista (the most widely prescribed SERM) may prevent breast cancer without increasing risk for other cancers, and may protect against heart disease. Further, studies show Evista does increase bone density in women with osteoporosis. But Evista comes with its own set of drawbacks. Evista may not prevent fractures, the very problem women fear most, and it does not prevent bone loss in the spine. Twenty-five percent of patients in one study reported more hot flashes, a sign of estrogen disruption, while using Evista. Evista also increases risk for serious blood clots in the legs, lungs and eyes - especially for sedentary women. Its effects on circulation are so powerful many women discontinue therapy because leg cramps caused by the drug are so severe.

Scientists are even concerned that Evista may increase risk for Alzheimer's disease because it seems to act as an anti-estrogen in the brain (hot flashes may be a sign of falling hormone levels in the brain). In Alzheimer's, where estrogen appears to provide protection, anti-estrogen activity in the brain is obviously not desirable. Evista should not be taken by women with a history of congestive heart failure (faced by many women after menopause), pregnant women or individuals with active cancers. Drug-resistance to Tamoxifen (an anti-breast cancer drug) may develop if you take Evista because the two drugs are so closely related.

We may have more knowledge about our bodies than we did 50 years ago, but we still don't understand hormones well. Although doctors are ecstatic about SERMs, these drugs still work at the hormone level and may disrupt delicate hormone balance. Phytohormone-containing herbs like wild yam, red clover and dong quai are really natural SERMs, which safely control menopause symptoms and may even help protect women from diseases like osteoporosis or heart disease after menopause.

I believe herbs are still a better choice for hormone balance.

Many of the phytoestrogen containing herbs, like black cohosh for instance, are not just natural (instead of chemical) direct estrogens. As living medicines, they can work intelligently with your body. In many cases, these herbs don't compete for receptor sites or have a direct estrogenic activity in the body. In fact, they work mainly as adaptogens which balance glandular activity and normalize body temperature fluctuations. They do what herbs always do best no matter what the problem is ..... they are body normalizers.

Is hormone replacement therapy always necessary after a hysterectomy?

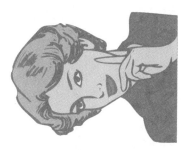

More than a half million American women have hysterectomies every year. The surgery is major, sometimes requiring a month or more of recovery time, but still, 1 in 4 women will have their uterus removed by the time they're 60. 1 in 1,000 women actually die as a result. Endometriosis, uterine fibroids, or heavy periods are common reasons for a hysterectomy. The surgical removal of a woman's uterus or ovaries (or both) can mean major disruptions in hormonal health, premature menopause and usually a lifelong prescription of hormone replacement drugs. In many cases, natural therapies can help a woman avert surgery and help her body normalize naturally. Vitex extract and natural progesterone creams help manage heavy, abnormal bleeding.

Herbs are also an excellent choice to boost hormone production by the adrenal glands if surgery has already been done. By supporting endocrine health, rainforest herb Maca can control hysterectomy-induced symptoms like depression, low libido, constipation and hot flashes. An added bonus: Maca is rich in absorbable calcium, magnesium and silica, important for bone strength. Natural Balance INNERGY is an energizing formula with herbs like tribulus and maca known for balancing hormones and increasing libido.

The diet is rich in nourishment for the glands with plenty of iodine and mineral-rich foods to help the following conditions: *Breast and Uterine Fibroids, Hormone Imbalances, Infertility, Endometriosis, PMS, Cramping and Menstrual Difficulties, Menopausal Symptoms, Osteoporosis Risk, Vaginal and Skin Dryness, Cysts, Polyps and Benign Tumors, Adrenal Exhaustion.*

Do you need a gland cleanse?

Your glands (and their hormone secretions) are involved with almost every body function and biochemical reaction. They're critical to good health, especially as you age. The comment "you're as young as your glands" has merit. Hormones, like adrenaline, insulin, and thyroxine, are chemical messengers exerting wide-ranging effects. Hormones affect our moods, energy levels, mental alertness and metabolism. Glands, hormones and the brain are affected first by nutritional deficiencies, pollutants, chemicalized foods and synthetic hormone mimics. Lack of minerals, for instance, something most Americans live with today, undermines the health of almost every gland and organ. The chronic stress loads that most Americans live under have a direct effect on hormone balance. We can see this easily in low levels of steroidal hormones produced by our "stressed-out" adrenals.

Is your body showing signs that it needs a gland cleanse?

- –unexplained bloating or weight gain caused by sluggish metabolism (indicating impaired thyroid activity)
- –unstable blood sugar reactions like unexplained moodiness or hyperactivity (indicating unbalanced insulin levels)
- –chronic poor digestion (may mean low enzyme output from a congested pancreas)
- –sallow skin color; poor skin texture (often means a sluggish liver and poor gallbladder activity)
- –chronic fatigue yet the inability to sleep through the night (may indicate adrenal exhaustion or pineal imbalance)
- –almost constant colds or flu bouts, even out of high risk seasons (glands are always affected by chronic respiratory infections)

Get the best results from your gland cleanse:

1: Trace minerals and protein are important for gland function. Add green superfoods to your diet for gland function. Add green superfoods to your diet for most rapid results.
2: Long periods of stress exhaust the whole gland system. Herbal adaptogens like ginseng noticeably improve the way your body handles stress. Add herbs like panax and Siberian ginsengs, suma, gotu kola, dong quai and ashwagandha to your healing program.
3: Eat smaller meals. Overeating can suppress hormone production.
4: Limit dairy foods and meats (especially beef and pork), notoriously high in hormone-disrupting chemicals. Chicken is also an offender. I hear from women who have a 1 : 1 reaction with breast swelling from eating chicken injected with hormones. Look for hormone-free poultry at health food stores - Petaluma Poultry ROSIE THE ORGANIC CHICKEN, Diestel and Coleman Natural Products.
5: Wash produce thoroughly to reduce hormone disrupting pollutant residues. Use Healthy Harvest FRUIT & VEGETABLE RINSE.
6: Add soy foods (tofu, tempeh, soy milk, etc.) to your diet for hormone normalizing isoflavones.
7: Drink green tea to flush out fats that harbor estrogen-disrupting chemicals.
8: Eat cruciferous veggies like steamed broccoli and cauliflower to help flush excess estrogens out.

This cleanse helps many female imbalance conditions: *Infertility; PMS Symptoms; Menstrual cramping and Inter-period Spotting; Hypothyroidism (Hashimoto's); Endometriosis; Ovarian Cysts; Breast and Uterine Fibroids; Adrenal Malfunction; Recovery after Hysterectomy or Abortion.*

A Woman's Fresh Foods Detox Diet

A fresh foods cleansing diet is recommended to clear your body of toxins and allow it a brief rest before beginning a new way of eating to nourish your glands. A cleanse of this type for women also generates clearer skin, a more even temperament, fewer allergies, sweeter breath, softer hair and brighter eyes as clogging toxins and congestion leave the body.

Note: The glands are affected first by dehydration. Drink 8 glasses of water a day during your cleanse. Eliminate caffeine during your cleansing diet for the best improvement of female problems; limit caffeine after your cleanse for preventive health. Avoid red meats, hard alcohol (too much concentrated sugar), carbonated sodas and tobacco.

The night before your gland cleanse...

—Take a gentle herbal laxative: Crystal Star LAXA-TEA™; M. D. Labs DAILY DETOX Tea, with Gaia Herbs DAILY DETOX extract.

—**The next day:** if possible, depending on the season, for the first day of your juice cleanse, go on a watermelon juice only cleanse. Drink throughout the day to rapidly flush and alkalize. If watermelon is not available, start with the following:

—**On rising:** take lemon juice in water with 1 tsp. maple syrup; or a glass of aloe vera juice with herbs and 1 tsp. Red Star nutritional yeast flakes; or Crystal Star CLEANSING & PURIFYING TEA™.

—**Breakfast:** take 2 teasp. of cranberry concentrate in water with 1 teasp. honey; or Crystal Star BIOFLAV., FIBER & C SUPPORT or Ethical Nutrients TRIPLE BALANCE drink for estrogen balancing; or fresh fruit with yogurt and toasted wheat germ.

—**Mid-morning:** apple or carrot juice with 1 TB green superfood, like Vibrant Health GREEN VIBRANCE, or 1 tsp. sea greens; or V-8 juice (page 569), or Knudsen's VERY VEGGIE juice with 1 teasp. Bragg's LIQUID AMINOS; and some raw celery or cucumber sticks with kefir cheese or yogurt cheese, and a small bottle of mineral water.

—**Lunch:** have a bowl of miso soup with sea greens snipped on top. Sprinkle with 1 tsp. Red Star nutritional yeast for B vitamins; or have a green salad with sprouts, carrots and lemon/oil dressing and sea greens snipped on top.

—**Mid-afternoon:** have a green drink, with 1 teasp. Bragg's LIQUID AMINOS; or a veggie juice like Personal Best V-8 (page 569), or a high vitamin/mineral drink like ALL ONE for balance; have some raw crunchy veggies (especially broccoli and cauliflower) with an all-vegetable dip or soy spread; and a balancing herb tea, such as Crystal Star FEMALE HARMONY TEA™.

—**Dinner:** have a Mineral Rich Broth: Simmer 30 minutes: 3 carrots, 1 cup parsley, 1 onion, 2 potatoes, & 2 stalks celery. Strain and add 1 TB Bragg's LIQUID AMINOS; or a green salad with yogurt dressing and green tea.

—**Before Bed:** have an apple-alfalfa sprout juice; or a glass of papaya-pineapple juice to enhance enzyme activity; or 1 tsp. cranberry concentrate in chamomile tea; or a cup of Red Star nutritional yeast broth for B vitamins; or Crystal Star RELAX TEA™ for easier sleep.

Recipes that can help your detox diet: •DETOXIFICATION and CLEANSING FOODS; •HEALING DRINKS; •SOUPS, LIQUID SALADS; •ENZYME-RICH FOODS; •SALADS, HOT and COLD; •LIGHT MACROBIOTIC EATING.

Herb and Supplement Choices

•**For female hormone balance:** Crystal Star FEM-SUP-PORT™ extract, or FEMALE HARMONY™ caps or tea, or Crystal Star PRO-EST BALANCE™ herbal progesterone roll-on (rapidly effective). Add *Vitex* or *black cohosh* extract; or take Imperial Elixir ROYAL GINSENG for WOMEN.

•**For women with abnormal periods:** *Vitex* extract or Rainbow Light VITEX-BLACK COHOSH complex; or Moon Maid Botanicals PRO-MENO wild yam cream, or Crystal Star PRO-EST BALANCE™ wild yam cream.

•**Hormone tonics for more energy:** Crystal Star FEEL GREAT™ and ADRN-ACTIVE™ formulas; Planetary SCHIZAN-DRA ADRENAL SUPPORT; Crystal Star HEAVY METAL CLEANSE™ if you are regularly exposed to toxic pollutants.

•**Essential fatty acids normalize hormone production:** *Evening primrose oil,* 3000mg daily; Barleans OMEGA TWIN FLAX/ BORAGE COMBO and ESSENTIAL WOMAN; Nature's Secret ULTIMATE OIL; Omega Nutrition OMEGA PLUS caps.

•**For hormone boosting after hysterectomy or during menopause:** Royal Jelly-Red Ginseng combo; Rainforest herb Maca; Trimedica TRIBULUS TERRESTRIS.

•**Hormone support nutrients:** Calcium-magnesium 2000mg daily, iron, 20mg; B-complex 100mg. Note: If you are taking synthetic hormones, they can destroy vitamin E in the body, increasing risk for heart disease. Add vitamin E 400IU daily to counteract this.

•**For adult acne or hair growth on face, chest and chin:** *Saw palmetto* extract 160 mg, 2x daily. (Do not use if trying to become pregnant or if on hormone therapy.)

Bodywork and Lifestyle Techniques

•**Enema:** Take a liquid chlorophyll enema the first day of your gland cleanse to help release toxins out of the body. Or have a colonic irrigation to deep cleanse the glands.

•**Exercise:** Exercise is a cleansing nutrient in itself because it changes body chemistry. 1) Take a regular 20 minute "gland health" walk every day. 2) Do yoga stretches every morning. 3) Get morning sunlight on the body every day possible, on the arms for women. 4) Do deep breathing - page 472.

•**Environmental:** Avoid environmental pollutants as much as possible. Glands feel the damaging effects first.

•**Acupressure points:** Stroke the tops of both feet for 5 minutes each to stimulate hormone secretions.

•**Massage therapy:** reestablishes unblocked meridians of energy and increases circulation.

•**Essential oil support:** To assist your gland cleanse, use one or more, bergamot, chamomile, eucalyptus and lavender oil in a combination. Put a total of 15 drops essential oil in 1-oz of a carrier oil (such as jojoba) and rub on the skin.

•**Bathe/Sauna:** A relaxing mineral bath - add 1 cup Dead Sea salts, 1 cup Epsom salts, $^1/_2$ cup regular sea salt and $^1/_4$ cup baking soda to a tub; swish in 3 drops lavender oil, 2 drops chamomile oil, 2 drops marjoram oil and 1 drop ylangylang.

•**Smoking disrupts hormonal activity.**

•**Muscle Testing** (Applied Kinesiology), is useful for determining which hormonal supplements are specific to your problem. Once you learn the simple technique (see a nutritional consultant, a holistic chiropractor, or a massage therapist) you can easily do it at home to decide which products are right for you. For more information, see pg. 466.

Can't find a recommended product? Call the 800 number listed in Product Resources for the store nearest you and for more info.

320

Preventing PMS Naturally

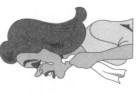

PMS is by far the most common women's health complaint.

Experts say a whopping 90% of all women between the ages of 20 and 50 experience some degree of PMS. Symptoms like headaches, acne, food cravings, bloating, constipation or diarrhea, and mood swings can make them feel out of control all month! Over 150 symptoms have been documented. The hormone shift in estrogen/progesterone ratios during the menstrual cycle is the major factor in PMS symptoms. (Women report the most symptoms in the two week period before menstruation, when the ratios are the most elevated.) The modern woman's lifestyle seems almost made-to-order for stress and imbalance. Low brain serotonin, excess estrogen, prostaglandin imbalance, and a diet loaded with sugar and caffeine are all implicated in PMS.

Still, PMS seems to be partially a consequence of the modern woman's emancipation. In times past, women were a silent, long-suffering lot, who felt that female disorders were just part of being a woman. Women were not out in the high profile workplace with men; they could go to bed and suffer alone. In addition, our diets consisted of more whole and fresh foods than they do today.

While most women try to "grin and bear" the aggravation of PMS, up to 10% have symptoms serious enough for them to seek professional help. But drugs and chemical medicines, standing as they do outside a woman's natural cycle, usually do not bring positive results for women. Indeed the medical establishment, with its highly focused "one-treatment-for-one-symptom" protocols has not been successful in addressing PMS. For example, contraceptive drugs, regularly given to reduce symptoms, make PMS worse for some women. Antidepressant drugs like Prozac, the new rage for PMS treatment, mean insomnia and shakiness for many patients. Natural treatment is much more gratifying. It emphasizes a highly nutritious diet, herbal tonifiers, and naturally-derived vitamins to encourage the body to provide its own balance for relief.

PMS symptoms tend to get worse for most women in their late thirties and beyond. They are often magnified after taking birth control pills, after pregnancy, and just before menopause because of hormone imbalances. But, with such a broad spectrum of symptoms affecting every system of the body, there is clearly no one cause and no one treatment. A holistic approach is far more beneficial, and self care allows a woman to tailor treatment to her own needs.

The Natural Keys To Controlling P.M.S:

Menstruation is a natural part of our lives. PMS is not. Women can take control of PMS naturally and effectively. Natural therapies work well for most women because they address the full spectrum of factors involved. A woman can expect a natural therapy program for PMS to take at least two months, as the body works through both ovary cycles with nutritional support. The first month, there is a noticeable decrease in PMS symptoms; the second month finds them dramatically reduced. Don't be discouraged if you need 6 months or more to gently coax your system into balance. Even after many of the symptoms are gone, continuing the diet recommendations, and smaller doses of the herb and vitamin choices makes sense toward preventing PMS return.

1: Essential fatty acids balance prostaglandins. Prostaglandins are vital hormone-type compounds that act as transient hormones, regulating body functions almost like an electrical current. Foods like ocean fish, olive oil, and herbs like Evening Primrose, normalize prostaglandins by balancing your body's essential fatty acid supply. Too much saturated fat from meats and dairy foods inhibits prostaglandin balance and proper hormone flow. Arachidonic acid in animal fats tends to deplete progesterone levels and strain estrogen/progesterone ratios. EVENING PRIM-ROSE OIL 3000mg daily, especially along with a broad spectrum herbal balancing compound like Crystal Star FEMALE HARMONY (see below), shows excellent results for many women.

2: Love your liver to balance estrogen and progesterone levels. Lower your fat intake and reduce dairy foods to help your liver do its job. A high-fat diet hampers liver function. Many dairy foods are a source of synthetic estrogen from hormones injected into cows. At the very least, switch to non-fat dairy products. Estrogen is stored in fat; non-fat foods don't contribute to estrogen stores. Focus on high quality vegetarian protein to improve estrogen metabolism. On PMS days, avoid dairy products altogether. A cup of green tea, or a green tea blend like Crystal Star GREEN TEA CLEANSER™ each morning can go a long way toward relieving organ congestion and detoxifying the liver. Non-fat yogurt is a good choice because it also contains digestive lactobacillus. Reduce caffeine to one cup of coffee or less a day. Caffeine tends to deplete the liver and lowers B vitamin levels, contributing to anxiety, mood swings, and irritability. Fifteen to 30% of women with breast tenderness during PMS find relief by stopping caffeine use. A little wine is fine, but avoid hard liquor to control PMS. Strong alcohol compromises liver function by lowering B vitamin levels, reducing its ability to break down excess estrogen. Consider MILK THISTLE SEED extract or a dandelion tea daily.

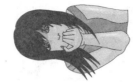

3: Enhance your thyroid to reduce PMS. Estrogen levels are controlled by thyroid hormones. If the thyroid does not have enough iodine, insufficient thyroxine is produced and too much estrogen builds up. Sea greens are a good choice for thyroid balance because they are rich in potassium and iodine. Two tablespoons daily in a soup or salad, or over rice, or six pieces of sushi a day, are a therapeutic dose. Or try Crystal Star POTASSIUM/IODINE™ caps, Bernard Jensen LIQUI-DULS, or New Chapter OCEAN HERBS.

4: Phytohormone-rich herbal compounds help balance body estrogen. Phyto-estrogens are remarkably similar to human hormones. They help raise body estrogen levels that are too low by stimulating the body's own hormone production, or by attaching to estrogen receptor sites. Remarkably enough, plant estrogens can also lower estrogen levels that are too high. Even though they are only $1/400\text{th}$ or less of the strength of the body's own circulating estrogens, they are able to compete with human estrogens for receptor sites. When the weaker estrogens attach to receptors, the net overall effect is a lowering of the body's estrogen levels. Phytohormone-rich plants like soybeans and wild yams, and hormone-rich herbs like black cohosh, panax ginseng, licorice root and dong quai, have a safety record of centuries. A broad-spectrum herbal combination like Crystal Star FEMALE HARMONY™ tea or capsules, or Herbal Magic FEMSTRUATION may be taken as a stabilizing resource for keeping the female system female, naturally. Whole, wild yam creams also show success against PMS as transdermal sources for estrogen/progesterone ratio balance.

A Woman's PMS Prevention Diet

Improve your diet to control PMS. Women with severe PMS symptoms eat 60% more refined carbohydrates, 280% more sugars, 85% more dairy products, and 80% more sodium than women who don't get PMS. Avoid highly processed (fast and junk) foods, and dairy foods during PMS. A low fat, vegetarian diet with regular seafood clearly diminishes symptoms. Add soy foods like miso, tempeh and tofu, and cruciferous veggies to reduce excess estrogen linked to PMS. This diet focuses on nourishing the adrenals, for balanced hormone secretions. Keep the diet low in salt and sugar. Eat plenty of cultured foods, like yogurt and kefir for friendly flora. Eat brown rice often for B vitamins. Eat smaller meals often for blood glucose balance. If you're like most women, you'll thrive on fresh fruits and vegetables and brown rice, with limited yeasted breads and beans. Caffeine foods should be limited; red meats, tobacco and hard alcohol should be avoided. Drink 6 glasses of water daily to keep the system flowing and fats flushed out. Have a small bottle of water with any of the meals in the following diet.

—**On rising:** take ALL ONE VITAMIN/MINERAL drink or Solgar WHEY TO GO protein; or a fruit smoothie with 1 tsp. spirulina added.

—**Breakfast:** make a mix of 2 TBS each lecithin granules, Red Star yeast, flax seeds, and wheat germ. Sprinkle some on whole grain cereal, fresh fruit or yogurt, poached or baked eggs, or oatmeal with a little maple syrup; or have a fresh fruit smoothie with prunes and apples; or have some tofu scrambled "eggs," with toasted pita bread; or rice pilaf with tamari sauce.

—**Mid-morning:** try a mood swing, anti-constipation blender drink: 2 cups fresh peaches, chunked; 2 frozen bananas, chunked and 1 cup apple juice; or alfalfa/mint tea; or a cup of miso or ramen noodle soup with sea greens and rice cakes.

—**Lunch:** have some steamed veggies with rice, tofu and a light tamari dressing; or a salad with baked, marinated tofu and greens, and a lemon-oil vinaigrette; or a seafood salad with brown rice or veggie pasta; or a light oriental soup and salad, with sea greens and crunchy noodles; or a baked potato with yogurt or kefir cheese, a green salad and green tea; or hot soup.

—**Mid-afternoon:** have a green drink, like Monas CHLORELLA, Green Foods GREEN MAGMA, or Crystal Star ENERGY GREEN™ with 1 teasp. Bragg's LIQUID AMINOS; or a refreshing herb tea such as Crystal Star FEMALE HARMONY™ or RELAX TEA™; or some whole grain crackers with kefir cheese, or soy spread; or have some dried fruits with a little low-fat cheese or cottage cheese dip; or a hard boiled egg with a little sesame salt, some whole grain crackers and mineral water.

—**Dinner:** have baked or grilled fish with a light sauce, brown rice, and sautéed veggies; or an oriental meal, with miso soup and sea greens, rice pasta, and Chinese greens; or have an oriental vegetable stir-fry with miso soup and brown rice; or a veggie or seafood quiche with a whole grain crust; or a small omelet with a low-fat filling; or a light Italian meal with spinach or artichoke veggie pasta and baked vegetables; or a baked potato or steamed broccoli or cauliflower with low-fat cheese.

Note: A light white wine at dinner is fine for digestion and relaxation.

—**Before bed:** have a glass of mineral water, or a relaxing herb tea, such as peppermint tea or Crystal Star GOODNIGHT™ TEA.

Recipes that can help your PMS diet: •BREAKFAST and BRUNCH; •BLENDING EAST AND WEST; •FISH and SEAFOOD; •ENZYME-RICH FOODS; •SALADS HOT and COLD; •LOW FAT RECIPES; •DAIRY-FREE; •MINERAL-RICH.

Herb and Supplement Choices

•**Normalize hormone fluctuations:** Crystal Star's 2-month program is highly successful: FEMALE HARMONY™ capsules 2 daily each month, with EVENING PRIMROSE oil 6 daily the 1st month, 4 daily the 2nd month. Before your period, drink green tea or Crystal Star GREEN TEA CLEANSER™ each morning as a mini detox. Take TINKLE TEA™ for 5 days for pre-period edema. Use PRO-EST BALANCE™ roll-on or ANTI-SPZ™ caps, 4 at a time for cramping. During your period use FLOW EASE™ tea, or CRAMP BARK COMBO™ extract as needed. (LYSINE/LICO-RICE™ gel for PMS mouth sores.)

•**Relieve estrogen build-up:** Crystal Star IODINE/POTAS-SIUM caps; or Futurebiotics HERBAL HARMONY; Mood Maid PRO-MENO wild yam cream; vitamin E 400 IU daily. Rebalance hormone levels with Burdock tea 2 cups daily.

•**Relieve cramping:** Chamomile tea; Ginger tea or New Chapter DAILY GINGER extract drops in water; Transitions PRO-GEST CREAM - rub on abdomen; Homeopathic Mag. Phos.; Calcium/magnesium caps to relax the uterus.

—**Pelvic applications for cramps:** Ice packs; Ginger compresses on pelvic area; New Chapter ARNICA GINGER gel.

•**Ease mood swings:** 5-HTP, 50mg; Crystal Star DEPRESS-EX™ caps; Now SAMe caps. Nature's Secret ULTIMATE B; GABA 2000mg daily; Crystal Star RELAX CAPS™, Vitamin C up to 5000mg daily to neutralize heavy metal toxins.

•**Relieve excessive flow:** Bayberry caps 4 daily; Cranesbill/red raspberry tea; Vit. C 3000mg w. bioflavonoids or •Bilberry extract (bioflavonoids); vitamin K 100mcg.

•**Relieve lower back pain:** Barleans Omega-3 rich flax oil 3 daily; quercetin 1000mg and bromelain 1500 mg.

Bodywork and Lifestyle Techniques

•**A good massage or shiatsu session** before your period releases clogging mucous and fatty formations. Massage breasts and ovary areas to relax reproductive organs.

•**Exercise** is a must for female balance. Exercise improves the way your body assimilates and metabolizes nutrients, especially hormones. It changes food habits, and decreases craving for alcohol or tobacco. It boosts beta endorphin levels in the brain. It improves circulation to relieve congestion. It encourages regularity for rapid elimination of toxins.

•**Stretching-relaxation exercises** such as yoga with deep breathing and tai chi help. Acupuncture and reflexology are also effective.

•**End your daily shower with a cool rinse** to stimulate circulation and relieve lymph congestion.

•**Meditate to banish PMS.** Harvard studies show 57% improvement for women with PMS who meditate twice daily for 15-20 minutes.

•**Be sparing with your schedule during premenstrual days.** Give yourself some slack, take some time to read, listen to music and relax.

•**Light is linked to PMS.** Get out in the sunshine at least 20 minutes a day.

•**Stop smoking,** and avoid second-hand smoke. Nicotine inhibits hormone function.

Can't find a recommended product? Call the 800 number listed in Product Resources for the store nearest you and for more info.

Menopause - Updating Your Choices

There is a big difference between just surviving menopause and being prepared for it - knowing what to expect and what can help you adjust. Menopause is intended by nature to be a gradual reduction of estrogen by the ovaries with few side effects. In a well-nourished, vibrant woman, the adrenals and other glands pick up the job of estrogen secretion to keep her active and attractive after menopause. This phenomenon increases with age as nature compensates for menopause... as well as for hysterectomy side effects.

There are 25 million menopausal women in America in the year 2000. As of this writing, synthetic hormones are the most prescribed drugs in the U.S., of any kind. Science tells women that the arrival of menopause increases the risk of heart disease and osteoporosis as estrogen and progesterone levels change.

But is this really true? Certainly, menopause does effect the balance of important minerals, like calcium and magnesium, and vitamins like E and B complex. These pressures are some of the reasons so many physicians prescribe Hormone Replacement Therapy, or HRT, for menopausal women.

Hormones are a megabucks business today. Whether natural or synthetic, there's a whirlwind of controversy around all of them. Newly aging baby boomers are driving the billion dollar dance. As they cross the 50 yard line of life, new facts of life are staring them in the face. The boomers are demanding new answers and lots of change.

Clearly, people don't age the way they used to. Our physical labor is less, we don't live our lives outdoors as much. For the most part, we have better health care, and more knowledge about how to care for our bodies than we did fifty years ago. But we still don't understand hormones very well at any age. Hormones have widespread effects many of which are poorly understood, and they are tricky substances to work with. Tiny amounts can cause big reactions, both good and bad.

Menopause may actually be Nature's way of lessening hormone production to protect women from hormone-driven cancers like breast and uterine cancer. There is a general misconception that estrogen is lost at menopause. But estrogen is not lost - production is simply reduced by 50 to 60%. Nature, in its wisdom, curtails estrogen enough to preclude pregnancy and menstruation, but not enough to stop estrogen protections, or the female essence. Women continue to manufacture estrogen after menopause, supplying it from steroidal substances in the body. Adrenal and pituitary glands help pick up estrogen production to keep the female system female.

If you are in your 40's or 50's, and are about to be confronted with the great Hormone Replacement Therapy choice, consider carefully before you agree. Of the women in menopause today, about half start synthetic hormone replacement, but only half of those stick with it because of the side effects or fear of cancer risk.

I don't believe hormone replacement is the right course for most women. I listen to thousands of women around the country as I speak about menopause. The overwhelming vote is that there are numerous problems, side effects and unknowns about hormone replacement drugs that tamper with the deep hormone levels of a woman's body. Unless you have specific, extenuating circumstances, a natural menopause with herbal support, is the best way. Even women who don't have a symptom-free menopause, say they feel younger and more energetic when they address their menopausal changes the gentle, natural way.

Will we ever know enough to feel safe taking synthetic hormones? Information about hormone replacement becomes critical as evidence increases about the side effects and frightening risks of taking them. Many women are never told that they don't have to take estrogen replacement forever. Nor are they told to reduce dosage gradually if they do stop to allow their bodies to adjust, so that menopause symptoms don't return and body elasticity is not lost. If they need hormone replacement at all, many women only need it for a year or less. I know this is true of women who choose plant hormones for menopause symptoms.

In addition, increased cancer risk from using synthetic hormones is validated by the latest clinical studies. The threat of both breast cancer and uterine cancer is dramatically escalated, and the risk becomes greater as a woman ages.

The medical community and the drug companies, for whom synthetic hormones are an incredibly profitable business, continue to justify hormone replacement risks because of the perceived advantages to osteoporosis and heart disease. Many physicians believe Hormone Replacement Therapy is the most effective way to prevent osteoporosis and heart disease no matter how good you feel.

Yet, recent research shows that the benefits of HRT for these two diseases are not validated over the long term. There is no proof that less estrogen **causes** heart disease or osteoporosis. Let's remind ourselves again that decreasing estrogen (especially estradiol) production during menopause may be Nature's way of **protecting** women from hormone-involved diseases like breast and uterine fibroids, endometriosis, and breast, ovarian or uterine cancers.

In fact, the use of synthetic estrogen as protection against heart disease is highly debatable, and it does not reverse osteoporosis. Nor does synthetic estrogen mean that calcium deposits **in the bone.** It only slows down the leaching of calcium **from the bone.** I believe the risks for heart disease and osteoporosis can be better addressed by diet improvement, exercise and certain herbal supplements.

To be fair, there is debate even among the medical community about the connection between estrogen and heart disease. The primary impetus for the estrogen/heart disease claim followed a *New England Journal of Medicine Nurses' Study,* a report long on statistical abstraction and short on clinical evidence. The authors of the study admit that the question is highly debatable. The only long-term, epidemiologic study in the United States, the *Framingham Study,* found no coronary benefit from estrogen. A contrary study by Dr. Jerilynn Prior lists 16 references disputing the claim that estrogen provides cardiovascular benefits.

<u>**Considerations about hormone replacement therapy:**</u> Many drug substances are called natural hormones today. Let's clarify. Only our bodies produce completely natural human hormones. Other types of hormone substances fall into three categories: synthetic, synthesized or whole plant complexes.

* **Synthetic hormones** are made by chemical or biochemical synthesis, such as the partial estrogen, "ethynol estradiol," completely man-made. Other synthetic estrogens used in hormone replacement drugs include dienestrol, estradiol, esterified estrogens and estropipate. Each of the pseudo-estrogens or partial estrogens has shown a clear link to the increased risk of breast cancer. (Estrogen replacement alone is no longer practiced except for women who have undergone hysterectomies because it is so closely linked to cancer of the uterine lining.) Today, synthetic HRT uses a combination of estrogen and progesterone, as in the drug Provera.

* **Synthesized hormones** are made by rearranging molecules from separate chemical groups, or simpler compounds. The constituents of natural substances are recombined. DHEA supplements, for instance, are produced by the synthesis of a steroidal saponin (diosgenin) from wild yams. "Natural" progesterone creams are made with synthesized progesterone.

* **Whole plant hormones** are naturally present in the plant. In nature, nutrients are never isolated. Many plants contain phytosterols that trigger varying levels of hormonal activity. Plant hormones behave like, and are remarkably similar to human hormone activity and can even be taken up by human hormone cell receptors. Examples of herbs containing phytoestrogenic compounds include: black cohosh, dong quai, wild yam, licorice, red clover, hops and fennel. Legumes like soybeans, black beans and flax, are also active plant estrogen compounds.

The latest on Hormone Replacement Therapy?

No drawbacks have been reduced. Many have increased. Common side effects of taking synthetic estrogen that you won't like:

1) **HRT artificially continues menstruation, spotting and cyclical bleeding.** HRT can cause incomplete shedding of the uterine lining. Australian studies reveal that 85 percent of women taking HRT complain about withdrawal bleeding, worse than their former periods. If there is persistent bleeding, then there increased risk of endometrial cancer.

2) **HRT increases risk of breast and bone cancer even when progesterone is added.** Endometrial cancer is still a risk, too, although some studies show decreased risk when progesterone is added to estrogen. The Centers for Disease Control reported in 1991 that for a women on HRT for ten years the risk of cancer of the uterus or breast goes up **30 percent.**

3) **HRT increases appetite, causes fluid retention, aggravates mood swings and localizes fat deposits on the hips and thighs.** Many women eventually get PMS-like symptoms, including depression and agitation.

4) **Hormone replacement can destroy Vitamin E in the body, actually increasing the risk of heart disease** and also liver disease.

5) **HRT increases uterine and breast fibroid growth.** Estrogen-dependent fibroids, and menstrual migraines stay actively stimulated.

6) **HRT users report a drop in sex enjoyment and an increase in nervous tension.** Mood swings may worsen. Some women develop depression and hot flashes. A 1988 Swedish study reports that while an estrogen-progesterone combination was more helpful in controlling hot flashes and sweating than estrogen alone, positive mental outlook decreased.

7) **HRT should not be used by women with high blood pressure, breast or uterine fibroids,** high cholesterol, chronic migraines, or endometriosis. Some hormone driven cancers stem from poor liver function where the liver does not process estrogens safely. Avoid synthetic estrogen if you have a history of breast, bone or uterine cancer, or thrombosis. Both gallbladder and liver disease increase with use. Do not use if you have diabetes, or during pregnancy.

8) **Long term consequences are unknown.** There are no long term studies of women that offer reliable, unbiased data. Scientists are counting the current generation of HRT users as an experiment in progress.

Note: Studies don't reflect the different ways that HRT acts in individual women. Women have widely different diets, weight, liver function, enzyme activity, age, alcohol sensitivity, estrogen levels and metabolism. Some women feel better on HRT, some don't see any effects and some are worse with the drug.

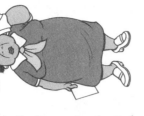

Do women have credible hormone replacement alternative to drugs? Yes, they do. Plant hormones can be a better answer. A 1996 Journal of Medical Ethics of Cambridge University Medical School concluded that plant-derived estrogen (estriol) "is an effective, economical and acceptable alternative to equine estrogen." Many doctors agree.

The best option, in my opinion, is a combination of phytohohrmone (estriol) rich herbs that can help a broad spectrum of a woman's needs during menopause. Plant hormones provide ample support with fewer long-term risks for women. In addition to the safety factor, my experience has been that none of the man-made hormones work as well as natural, plant-derived hormones from herbal combinations, especially over the long term.

Plant hormones offer a gentle, effective way to stimulate a woman's own body to produce amounts of estrogen and progesterone that are in the right proportion for her needs as menopause progresses. They can help control hot flashes, tighten sagging tissue, lubricate a dry vagina and normalize circulation. In addition, phyto-hormone-rich herbs help uterine and organ tone by improving circulation, acting as system tonics for women - generally keeping the female system female.

We know that plant hormones are remarkably similar to human hormones. Phytoestrogens and phytosterols have hormonal effects and behave like hormones as they lock into human cell receptors. Yet, plants are taken in naturally by the body as foods, through the enzyme system, not as drugs working outside the system. Phytohormone-rich herbal compounds are effective, yet safe and gentle. At only $1/_{400th}$ **or less** of the potency of synthetic or circulating estrogen, plant estrogens do not have the unpleasant side effects of increased appetite, fluid retention, heavy periods and cellulite deposits caused by synthetic hormones. Yet they can offer menopause symptom control for a woman who is not producing enough estrogen on her own.

Naturally-occurring flavonoids in many phyto-hormone rich herbs **also** exert a similar balancing effect on hormone secretions. Much like the body's own estrogen and progesterone hormones, plant flavonoids help elevate good cholesterol HDL's and keep arterial pathways clear.

The full medicinal value of herbs for hormone activity is in their complexity and balance, not in their concentration or strength.
A single herb contains dozens of natural chemical constituents working together with little danger of toxicity.

A balanced combination of plant hormone-rich herbs works even better - addressing a broader range of needs, yet still with whole plant gentleness and absorbability.
A common view held in Europe today among research experts involved with medicinal plants is that the benefits of a medicinal plant cannot be explained by one constituent, but involve a synergistic effect from diverse compounds. The American Cancer Society even advises that food sources (and we have to remember that herbs are foods) are the best, most absorbable sources of nutrients, providing potential cancer protection benefits not offered by synthetic or isolated supplements.

Pay attention to these four critical areas to sail through menopause naturally:

1: Adrenal gland health is critical to an easy menopause.

Adrenal stress symptoms are similar to menopausal symptoms - nervous tension, mild to severe depression, irritability, fatigue, and unpredictable mood swings. Stressful living and poor eating habits mean many women reach their menopausal years with prematurely worn out adrenals. Depleted adrenals cannot help a woman achieve her new hormone balance after menopause.

As I travel around the country, talking to women about more natural ways to deal with menopausal symptoms, it's almost the first question I ask when a woman complains of dramatic symptoms. Excessive hot flashes, and extreme fatigue are the first two things I hear, so it's a pretty safe bet that she has swollen, exhausted adrenals. Results are quick for many women. Changing your habits to support long term adrenal health will almost certainly result in eliminating unpleasant menopausal symptoms.

Are your adrenals exhausted? Three or more yes answers should alert you.

—Do you lack energy or alertness? Do you have unexplained moodiness, crying spells and guilt?
—Do you have severely cracked, painful heels? Do you have nervous moistness of hands and soles of feet?
—Do you have brittle, peeling nails or extremely dry skin?
—Do you have frequent heart palpitations or panic attacks?
—Do you have severe reactions to odors, or certain foods? Do you have chronic heartburn and poor digestion?
—Do you have chronic lower back pain (adrenal swelling)?
—Do you have hypoglycemia and cravings for salt or sweets?
—Do you have high incidence of yeast or fungal infections?

1. Stress is toxic to the adrenal glands. Adrenal exhaustion can keep you locked in a low-energy/high-stress loop. Herbs are some of the best therapy I know for revitalizing swollen, exhausted adrenal glands.
—For acute stress reactions: consider herbal nervines like *scullcap*, *St. John's wort*, *kava*, *passionflower*, *oatstraw*, *chamomile* or *valerian*.
—For chronic stress: use herbs like *black cohosh*, *ashwagandha*, *Siberian ginseng*, *sarsaparilla and gotu kola*.

2. Your glands keep you active and attractive. Revitalize your adrenal health with sea greens!
—Sea vegetables act as total body tonics to restore female vitality during menopause. Add sea greens to your diet like nori, wakame, dulse, kombu and kelp (2 TBS. daily, snipped into salads and soups). Sea vegetables are a rich source of fat-soluble vitamins like D, K which assist with production of steroidal hormones like estrogen, and DHEA in the adrenal glands that support the female body during menopause. New studies indicate that up to 40% of the U.S. population is deficient in Vitamin D. Eating sea veggies is a great way to shore up a Vitamin D deficiency.

2: Is your thyroid low? Do you think you might be suffering from Hashimoto's disease?

Today, low thyroid (hypothyroidism) is a common problem, aggravated by the strain pollutants in our environm Since World War II, an above average number of people have thyroid problems. Researchers speculate that the env that came into our culture during and after the war (some not well-tested for safety) affected thyroid health. To million people, most of whom are women between 45 and 65.

Almost one in ten women over the age of 65 has early-stage hypothyroidism clearly linked to Hashimoto's! P mune disorder where the immune system suddenly attacks healthy tissue. It's the most frequent cause of low thyroid, a of enlarged thyroid (goiter) in America. Iodine depletion from X-rays or low dose radiation (like mammograms) may be a prime fact development. Hashimoto's is related to disorders like diabetes, adrenal exhaustion, Grave's disease and vitiligo. At its worst, Hashim completely destroy the thyroid gland. Natural treatments for Hashimoto's focus on rebalancing glandular health, reducing symptoms and norma izing immune response.

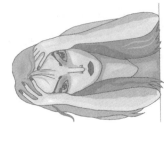

Do you have signs of low thyroid? Three or more yes answers should alert you.

- great fatigue and muscular weakness (especially in the morning)
- hormonal imbalances (like PMS, delayed or absent menstruation)
- bloating, gas and indigestion immediately after eating; unusually high LDL "bad" cholesterol levels
- unusual depression, usually with markedly reduced libido; noticeable memory loss
- unexplained hair loss in women, often accompanied by breast fibroids
- unexplained obesity, with frequent constipation; puffy face and eyelids, unusually dry or itchy skin
- unusual sensitivity to cold; poor immune response
- appearance of goiter (swelling of the thyroid gland)
- low selenium levels

You can boost your thyroid levels safely and naturally.

1. Avoid table salt (use an herb salt instead), but eat plenty of iodine-rich foods. Sea greens because of their high minerals, especially iodine, are the fastest way to nourish an underactive thyroid. I recommend 2 TBS daily over rice, soup or a salad. Also consider sea foods, fish, mushrooms, garlic, onions and watercress.

2. A largely fresh foods, immune-boosting diet full of fruits and vegetables should be your mainstay diet. Take a potassium drink (pg. 568) several times weekly. (Also see superfoods below.)

3. Avoid "goitrogen" foods that prevent your body's use of iodine, like cabbage, turnips, peanuts, mustard, pine nuts, millet, tempeh and tofu. (Cooking these foods inactivates the goitrogens.)

4. Eat vitamin A-rich foods: yellow vegetables, eggs, carrots, dark greens, raw dairy.

5. Avoid refined foods, saturated fats, sugars, white flour and red meats.

3: Have you had bladder control problems since you began menopause?

More than 11 million women have bladder control problems. Bladder control problems begin to affect women during menopause. The majority of women over 75 have bladder control disorders, but incontinence is not just a problem of the elderly. Over 45 percent of women between the ages of 20 and 50 suffer from incontinence at some point in their lives. Experts say that because estrogen helps keep the lining of the bladder and urethra strong, declining estrogen levels in menopause cause the bladder muscles to weaken. When this happens, pressure from coughing, laughing, running upstairs, lifting or even getting a hug can push urine through the weakened muscle. Called "stress incontinence," it's relatively common, but many women are too humiliated to talk about it with a health professional, and nobody wants to spend their adult years in diapers, the remedy most professionals offer.

Regain bladder control with natural therapies.

1. **What you eat and drink makes a difference.** How you eat does, too. Eat small meals more frequently, rather than large meals.
   —Caffeine foods, like coffee, tea, cola, or chocolate make urine control difficult. Caffeine acts as a powerful diuretic and should be avoided. Also avoid alcoholic beverages which can over-relax bladder muscles and cause leakage problems.
2. **Lifestyle therapy works.** Consider biofeedback or acupuncture; both show success for bladder control problems.
   —Drink lots of water. Dehydrated women have more incontinence than women who drink enough fluids. Highly concentrated urine irritates the bladder and may cause muscle spasms. Do toning Kegel exercises daily, simple exercises that help strengthen the urethra muscles to reduce stress incontinence. Tighten pelvic-floor muscles for 10 seconds, then relax for ten seconds.
3. **Herbal therapy shows promise for bladder control problems.** —A bladder control, tissue strengthening and toning formula like Crystal Star BLDR-K CONTROL™ is highly recommended. *I personally know many people who have reduced or reversed "stress incontinence," by using this combination.*

4: Have you grown facial hair but lost head hair since menopause?

Extremely common conditions for menopausal women, female pattern baldness is a disconcerting problem involving genetics, vitamin-mineral uptake and stress. The slow-down in estrogen production affects the functioning of hair follicles, resulting in the head hair loss and facial hair growth women hate. Excess dihydrotestosterone (DHT) in women can cause hair follicles to become dormant as in men. Balanced thyroid hormone production is critical to normal hair growth. Hypothyroidism leads to coarse, lifeless hair which easily falls out. Hyperthyroidism causes soft, thinning hair and hair loss.

   1. **Sea greens make a big difference** - Women notice improved hair growth and texture in 3 to 4 weeks. Take 2 TBS daily of dry chopped sea greens, and eat lots of sushi. Reduce animal fats to unclog hair follicles; add soy foods for plant protein (hair is 97% protein!).
   2. **So do supplements** - Take Evening Primrose Oil 4000 mg daily; and Crystal Star CALCIUM SOURCE™ or a cal/mag/zinc combination with high magnesium daily. Take B-complex 100mg with extra B-6 daily and sublingual B-12, 2500mcg every other day.
   3. **Apply herbs** - Mix fresh, blender-ground ginger with aloe vera gel and apply to hair; leave on 15 minutes. Apply a tea of rosemary or nettles to help prevent falling hair. Apply 2 TBS hot olive and wheat germ oils for 30 minutes to stimulate hair growth.

Women's Hormone Balancing Menopause Diet

If you're on a raging hormone roller coaster, with hot flashes, mood swings, vaginal dryness and low libido, check out this diet for the natural way to "keep the change!" Compose your diet of 50% fresh foods for the best enzyme benefits. Limit dairy foods and meats, especially beef and pork, high in hormone disrupting chemicals. Reduce sugars and alcohol. (A little wine with dinner is fine.) Avoid caffeine. It taxes the adrenal glands, and upsets hormone levels. Steam and bake foods - never fry. Especially eat cold water fish like salmon and tuna for EFA's and to cut heart disease risk. To reduce hot flashes, add soy foods like miso and tofu and avoid spicy foods. Balance estrogen levels by boosting boron foods, like green leafy veggies, fruits, nuts, and legumes. (Boron also helps harden bones.) Most menopausal symptoms stem from exhausted adrenals and reduce poor liver function where estrogen is not being processed correctly. Whole grain fiber, fresh fruits and veggies regulate estrogen levels and reduce mood swings. Eat calcium-rich vegetables and soy foods. Eliminate carbonated drinks loaded with phosphates that deplete calcium. Avoid junk-filled, chemical-laced foods.

—**On rising:** take a protein drink like Nutricology PROGREENS or Crystal Star BIOFLAV, FIBER & C SUPPORT™ with cranberry; or lemon juice in water with 1 tsp. honey. Add 2 teasp. Red Star nutritional yeast for best results.

—**Breakfast:** add a ginseng-royal jelly-honey blend (Y.S. makes one) to hot tea water ; make a mix of 2 TBS each: toasted sesame seeds, sunflower seeds, wheat germ and lecithin granules. Sprinkle some each morning on yogurt and/or fresh fruit, or oatmeal, a whole grain cereal or rice pilaf. Top with apple juice, 1 TB. maple syrup, or molasses if desired.

—**Mid-morning:** have a green drink (page 569), Monas CHLORELLA with EFA's or Crystal Star ENERGY GREEN™ with sea greens. and/or a cup of miso or noodle ramen soup with sea veggies snipped on top.

—**Lunch:** have an onion or black bean soup with a carrot and raisin salad; or baked or broiled seafood with a green leafy salad with sprouts and celery; or a baked potato or yam with a low-fat yogurt dressing and a small green salad; or some steamed veggies with rice, tofu and light tamari dressing; or a salad with baked, marinated tofu and greens, and lemon-oil vinaigrette; or a seafood salad with brown rice or veggie pasta; or a light oriental soup and salad, with sea greens and crunchy noodles.

—**Mid-afternoon:** have low-fat cottage cheese with nuts and seeds and rice cakes; or a dried fruit and nut mix with a bottle of mineral water; or a hard boiled egg with a refreshing herb tea like spearmint tea, or hibiscus sangria, (See Book Two: The Healing Recipes).

—**Dinner:** have a broccoli or asparagus quiche with a chapati crust; or a stir-fry with Chinese greens, shiitake mushrooms, and tofu, or miso soup with sea greens; baked or grilled fish with a light salsa, brown rice, and sautéed veggies; or a baked rice and veggie casserole with yogurt sauce; or a light Italian meal with spinach or artichoke pasta, baked veggies and low-fat cheese.
Note: A little wine at dinner is nice for relaxation, digestion, and release from stress and inhibitions.

—**Before bed:** have papaya-pineapple juice to enhance enzyme activity; or 1 teasp. cranberry concentrate in chamomile tea; or a cup of Red Star nutritional yeast broth for B vitamins; or Crystal Star RELAX TEA™ for easier sleep; or a mint tea.

Recipes to help your menopause diet: •**BLENDING EAST and WEST;** •**FISH and SEAFOODS;** •**SOUPS, LIQUID SALADS;** •**ENZYME-RICH FOODS;** •**SALADS, HOT and COLD;** •**MINERAL-RICH RECIPES;** •**CULTURED FOODS.**

Herb and Supplement Choices

•**For hot flashes:** Crystal Star's highly successful program: 1-EST-AID™ caps 4-6 daily the first month, 2 daily for 2 months, to control hormone imbalances; 2-CALCIUM SOURCE™ caps for bone weakness accompanying estrogen changes; 3-Evening primrose oil caps 4000mg daily to handle mood swings. 4-EASY CHANGE™ caps or roll-on for the years of the change; 5-ADR-ACTIVE™ or FEMALE HARMONY™ caps for a feeling of well-being. 6-Add GINSENG 6 SUPER™ caps or tea for energy; and MILK THISTLE SEED extract to help normalize estrogen levels.

—**More suggestions:** Transitions For Health WOMEN'S PHASE II and PRO-GEST CREAM as directed; Transitions for Women HOT FLASH FORMULA, or Moon Maid PRO-MENO wild yam cream; Ester C with bioflavs 4x daily, Futurebiotics MENOPHASE I and II; Imperial Elixir DONG QUAI 3000; Vitex extract.

•**Normalize body fluctuations:** Bioflavonoids, structurally similar to body estrogen, like Ethical Nutrients SUPER FLA-VONOID-C; Vitamin E 800 daily; CoQ10 200mg daily.

•**For sleep disturbances:** One gram niacinamide at bedtime to stimulate serotonin; Natural Balance RHODIOLA ROSEA; 5-HTP, 100mg or Crystal Star NIGHT CAPS™.

•**Elevate mood - increase energy:** Ginkgo biloba extract; Siberian ginseng extract; Nature's Secret ULTIMATE B; Stress B-complex 100mg; Country Life MAXINE capsules daily.

•**Iodine therapy for thyroid-metabolism balance:** Sea greens, 2 TBS daily or sushi daily to your diet; take Crystal Star IODINE/POTASSIUM caps or New Chapter OCEAN HERBS; or Bernard Jensen LIQUI-DULS; or Nature's Path TRACE-MIN-LYTE; or Kelp tabs 8 daily.

Bodywork and Lifestyle Techniques

•**Exercise regularly** outdoors to get the advantages of natural vitamin D for bone health. A daily brisk walk keeps the system flowing.

•**Do deep stretches on rising** and each evening before bed. Yoga for body toning.

•**Weight training 3 times a week,** along with aerobic exercise is a perfect way to keep skin from sagging. Weight training helps you keep the muscle while you lose the fat. In a natural menopause, when estrogen levels drop naturally, so does some body fat and excess fluids.

•**Get a massage therapy treatment once a month** for energy restoration, a body tune-up and a feeling of well-being.

•**Smoking contributes to breast cancer, emphysema, osteoporosis, wrinkling and early menopause.** Now is the time to quit!

•**Twenty minutes in a sauna daily** significantly cuts night sweats for menopausal women.

Can't find a recommended product? Call the 800 number listed in Product Resources for the store nearest you and for more info.

Healing Your Liver

Be good to your liver. A healthy liver is the key to a healthy life! The health of every body system depends to a large extent on the vitality of the liver. It is a powerful chemical plant that converts everything we eat, breathe and absorb through the skin into life-sustaining substances. The liver is a major blood reservoir, and a key organ of detoxification, filtering out toxins at a rate of over a quart of blood per minute. It synthesizes and secretes bile to digest fats and prevent constipation. The liver is a vast storehouse for vitamins, minerals, and enzymes that it releases to build healthy cells. It is the major organ of metabolism for proteins, fats and carbohydrates. It also produces natural antihistamines to keep immunity high. Fortunately, since we live in an increasingly toxic world, the liver has amazing regenerative powers. A complete liver renewal program takes from three months to a year.

Liver exhaustion and damage interfere with all of these vital functions. Since the common American diet is high in calories, fats, sugars and alcohol, with unknown amounts of toxic substances in the form of preservatives, pesticides, and nitrates, almost everybody has liver malfunction to some extent. Slight liver damage appears as low energy, poor digestion, allergies, constipation, age spots, headaches and hair problems. Major problems occur after many years of abuse, when the liver is so exhausted it loses the ability to detoxify. Fortunately the liver seems to possess almost miraculous powers of recovery. Even in life-threatening situations, such as cirrhosis, hepatitis, acute gallstone attacks, mononucleosis, and pernicious anemia, the liver can be cleansed and rejuvenated, and major surgery or even death averted.

Is your liver exhausted?

Your liver is an amazing organ, but protecting your liver from toxic overload and exhaustion is not easy. In the United States, liver disorders, largely a result of a lifestyle that includes lots of toxins, are responsible for more than 50,000 deaths annually. Liver exhaustion symptoms to look for are:

—Liver disease such as cirrhosis or chronic hepatitis, or unusually high cholesterol levels
—Unexplained fatigue and headaches
—Thick, coated tongue (yellowish or white), usually accompanied by chronic constipation
—Jaundice or yellowish tint to the skin, eczema, psoriasis, acne rosacea or several age spots
—Gas or discomfort that worsens after a fatty meal. (The liver is responsible for fat metabolism.)
—A man who is thin everywhere else but who has a protruding stomach often has an enlarged liver
—Frequent cold and flu infections, and a high incidence of allergic reactions

Many gland and organ problems can be remedied by keeping a healthy liver: *Weight and Cellulite Control; Gallbladder Health and Gallstones, Menstrual and PMS Difficulties, Endometriosis, Breast and Uterine Fibroids, Male Impotence, Female Infertility, Drug and Alcohol Abuse, Hepatitis, Herpes, Shingles, Osteoporosis, Spots Before the Eyes, Spleen Malfunction. Kidney Disease, Jaundice.*

Liver and Organ Healing Diet

Many problems can be solved or prevented by a short liver cleanse once or twice a year. The following diet may be used in toxic situations for rapid improvement. Start with this 3-day nutrition plan: Focus on fresh plant foods: 1) high chlorophyll plants for enzymes; 2) fruits and vegetables for fiber; 3) cultured foods for probiotics; 4) eight glasses of water a day for system flushing; 5) Add $1/4$ teasp. vitamin C crystals to each drink you take. It's a natural chelator of heavy metal toxins that deteriorate liver function.

The evening before your healing cleanse: take a cup of miso soup with sea greens.
The next day....

—**On rising:** take 1 lemon squeezed in cranberry juice; or 2 TBS. cider vinegar in water with 1 teasp. maple syrup.
—**Breakfast:** take a potassium drink (page 568) or carrot-beet-cucumber juice, or Crystal Star SYSTEMS STRENGTH drink™ in organic apple juice. Add 1 teasp. spirulina, 1 teasp. nutritional yeast and 1 teasp. lecithin granules to any drink.
—**Mid-morning:** take a green veggie drink (page 569); or take a green superfood like Wakunaga KYO-GREEN, Crystal Star ENERGY GREEN or NutriCology PRO-GREENS with EFA's.
—**Lunch:** have a glass of fresh carrot juice and a small bowl of Rejuvenative Foods VEGI DELITE cultured vegetables.
—**Mid-afternoon:** have a cup of peppermint tea, pau d'arco tea, or Crystal Star LIV-ALIVE TEA™, or another green drink.
—**Dinner:** have carrot juice or a mixed veggie juice; or miso soup with sea greens; or Rejuvenative Foods VEGI DELITE cultured vegetables.
—**Before Bed:** take another glass of organic apple juice, pineapple/papaya or cranberry juice. Add 1 teasp. honey or 1 teasp. royal jelly.

Follow with a diet of 100% fresh foods for the rest of the week. (Don't forget - 8 glasses of water through the day.) Keep fat low in your nutrition plan. It's crucial to liver regeneration Avoid red meats, caffeine, alcohol, refined starches and dairy products during all healing phases. Reduce sugars, saturated fats and fried foods permanently.

Liver health and support foods:

•**Vegetable fiber foods absorb excess bile and increase regularity:** beets, artichokes, radishes and dandelions are because they promote the flow of bile, the major pathway for chemical release from the liver.
•**Potassium-rich foods:** sea foods, sea greens, dried fruits.
•**Chlorophyll-rich foods:** leafy greens, sea greens.
•**Enzyme-rich foods:** yogurt and kefir, yogurt cheese and kefir cheese, and cultured vegetables.
•**Sulphur-rich foods:** eggs, garlic and onions, cabbages, broccoli and cauliflower.

Recipes that can help your liver diet: •**DETOXIFICATION FOODS;** •F
and COLD; •**SOUPS - LIQUID SALADS;** •**HEALING DRINKS;** •**CULT**

• ENZYME-RICH RECIPES; • SALADS, HOT
RED FOODS; • MINERAL-RICH RECIPES.

• Ta
cleanse plants are

• Take se
easier detoxif

• Massage the
sage during your c

• Overheating by t
pg. 571 in this book.

• Good liver lifestyle practices:
  —Eat smaller meals, minimize late night eating.
  —Get adequate, regular sleep.
  —A daily brisk aerobic walk.
  —Overusing either saccharin foods or acetaminophen drugs
  can cause liver toxicity.

ature is effective. See

Herb and Supplement Choices

• **Gently cleanse the liver:** SAMe 800mg daily with Crystal Star LIV-ALIVE™ caps 6 daily and tea, 2 cups daily, with Crystal Star BITTERS & LEMON CLEANSE™ extract each morning. Alpha Lipoic Acid 300-600mg daily; Enzymatic Therapy LIVA-TOX or Nature's Apothecary LIVER CLEANSE. Ascorbate vitamin C 500mg every hour during cleansing stage, then 3000mg daily.

• **Enhance liver vitality:** Pau d'Arco tea; Reishi or Maitake mushroom extracts; Bupleurum extract (especially if immune compromised); Royal jelly 2 teasp. daily; Nutricology GERMANIUM 150mg; Crystal Star GINSENG/REISHI extract; Crystal Star GINSENG/LICORICE ELIXIR™ an ongoing liver tonic.

• **Enzyme support:** Transformation DIGESTZYME; Herbal Products POWER-PLUS ENZYMES.

• **Probiotics normalize liver function:** Natren TRINITY; UAS DDS-PLUS with FOS; Prevail LIVER FORMULA caps.

• **Prickly herbs heal your liver:** Take one or a combination of the drops in water 3x daily: MILK THISTLE SEED extract in aloe vera juice; ARTICHOKE extract; DANDELION ROOT extract; BURDOCK ROOT extract.

• **Bitters herbs boost liver and bile:** Crystal Star GREEN TEA CLEANSER™; barberry-turmeric capsules; Gaia SWEETISH BITTERS; dandelion extract drops; Turmeric-cardamom-lemon peel added to any drink.

• **Boost liver antioxidants:** Enzymatic THYMU-PLEX; Carnitine 1000mg; Beta-carotene 100,000IU, or PHYCOTENE MICROCLUSTERS from Healthy House; CoQ$_{10}$ 200mg daily; PCO's from grapeseed or white pine 100mg daily.

Can't find a recommended product? Call the 800 number listed in Product Resources for the store nearest you and for more info.

336

Gallstone Flush Diet

The gallbladder helps digest fats by producing bile (a compound of cholesterol, bile pigments and salts). In the United States, high bile cholesterol levels are the main cause of gallstones, with most stones (80%) composed of cholesterol and varying amounts of bile salts, bile pigments and inorganic calcium salts. When bile in the gallbladder becomes supersaturated with cholesterol, it combines with other sediment matter present and begins to form a stone. As the stones enlarge, the gallbladder becomes inflamed, causing severe pain that feels like a heart attack, and, in some cases, it can be life threatening if left untreated. Stones can also block the bile passage, causing pain and digestive harm. A stone may grow for 6 to 8 years before symptoms occur. Continued formation of gallstones is dependent on either increased accumulation of cholesterol or reduced levels of bile acids or lecithin.

Signs that you may be at risk for gallstones: Ultrasound provides a definitive diagnosis.

–Do you have periods of nausea, vomiting, fever and intense abdominal pain that radiates to the upper back? *(signs of gallbladder inflammation; 95% of people suffering from cholecystitis have gallstones.)* If you have these symptoms, seek medical help immediately.
–Are you more than 30 pounds overweight? *(Gallstone risk increases three to seven times if you are.)*
–Do you have high cholesterol levels? *(They contribute to increased gallstone risk.)*
–Do you get enough vitamin C? *(Vitamin C plays a key role in the breakdown of cholesterol.)*
–Are you a yo-yo dieter? *(The Annals of Internal Medicine finds that women whose weight fluctuates by 10 to 20 lbs. at a time have a 31% higher risk of developing gallstones. When weight fluctuated more than 20 lbs. at a time, gallstone risk was 68% higher!)*
–Do you have chronic heartburn, gas and pain after eating? *(especially fried foods, eggs and cow's milk)*

Do you need a gallstone cleanse?

High risk factors: poor diet with high cholesterol, obesity, certain drugs, age, and Crohn's disease. Blood cholesterol lowering drugs that contain fibric acid derivatives like clofibrate and gemfibrozil increase levels of bile cholesterol. Dietary factors like high blood sugar, high calorie and saturated fat intake which lead to obesity are also involved. A predisposing factor for gallstones is excessive sugar consumption. (Do not use highly sweetened protein powder drinks.) About 20 million Americans have gallstones, or gallbladder cholecystitis (acute gallbladder inflammation); 75% of them are women. Yo-yo dieting increases risk of gallstones.

Gallstones are far easier to prevent than to reverse. The key to prevention of gallstones is diet improvement. The primary gallstone culprit is a diet high in saturated fats, especially from red meats and dairy products. A vegetarian, high fiber diet is the best choice. Artichokes, pears and apples are good choices. Vegetable proteins from foods like soy, oat bran and sea greens help prevent gallstone formation. Reduce your intake of animal protein, especially eggs and dairy foods (casein in dairy foods increases formation of gallstones). Yogurt and kefir are OK. Avoid fried foods and sugary foods altogether if you are at risk for gallstones.

The Nine-Day Gallstone Flush Plan

Traditional gallbladder cleansing flushes have been very effective in passing and dissolving gallstones. Depending on the size of the stones and the length of time they have been forming, the flushing programs may last from 3 days to a month. Have a sonogram <u>before</u> embarking on a flush to determine the size of the stones. If they are too large to pass through the bile and urethral ducts, they must be dissolved first, using the Crystal Star STN-EX™ herbal program for 1 month, or a surgical procedure. Important note: In the acute pain stage, all food should be avoided. Only pure water should be taken until pain subsides.

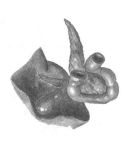

Three-day Olive Oil and Lemon Juice Flush:

—**On rising:** take 2 TBS olive oil and juice of 1 lemon in water. <u>Sip through a straw if desired.</u>
—**Breakfast:** have a glass of organic apple juice.
—**Mid-morning:** take 2 cups of chamomile or cascara tea.
—**Lunch:** take another glass of lemon juice and olive oil in water; and a glass of fresh apple juice.
—**Mid-afternoon:** have 2 cups of chamomile or cascara tea.
—**Dinner:** have a glass of carrot-beet-cucumber juice; or a potassium drink (page 568).
—**Before bed:** take another cup of chamomile tea.

Follow with a 5 day Alkalizing Diet:

—**On rising:** take 2 TBS cider vinegar in water with 1 teasp. honey; or a glass of grapefruit juice.
—**Breakfast:** have a glass of carrot-beet-cucumber juice, a glass of aloe vera juice, or a potassium drink (page 568).
—**Mid-morning:** have 2 cups of chamomile tea, and a glass of organic apple juice.
—**Lunch:** take a vegetable drink with Transitions EASY GREENS, or Crystal Star ENERGY GREEN™ drink, or AloeLife FIBERMATE drink, a small green salad with lemon-olive oil dressing and a cup of dandelion tea.
—**Mid-afternoon:** have 2 cups of chamomile tea, and another glass of apple juice.
—**Dinner:** have a small green salad with lemon-oil dressing; and another glass of apple juice.
—**Before bed:** 1 cup chamomile tea, aloe vera juice or dandelion tea.

End with a One-day Intensive Olive Oil Flush:

At 7 p.m. on the evening of the 5th day of the alkalizing diet, mix 1 pint olive oil and 10 juiced lemons; take ¹/₄ cup every 15 minutes until used. Lie on the right side for best assimilation.

Important note: Although I have personally seen several gallstone sufferers use the 9 day program on this page pass gallstones without surgery, I recommend it only under the supervision of a qualified health professional. The liver and gallbladder are interconnecting, interworking organs. Problems with either affect both. Before undertaking a Gallstone Flush to pass gallstones, have an ultrasound test to determine the size of the stones. If they are too large to pass through the urethral ducts, other methods must be used.

Herb and Supplement Choices

• <u>Increase bile solubility to reduce cholesterol levels:</u> Enzymatic Therapy coated peppermint oil caps- PEPPERMINT PLUS; Crystal Star BITTERS & LEMON CLEANSE™ extract helps dissolve bile solids; Herbal Answers ALOE FORCE JUICE daily, with MILK THISTLE SEED extract added to each glass.

• <u>Enzyme therapy:</u> Rainbow Light ADVANCED ENZYME SYSTEM or Transfromation LYPOZYME; Two acidophilus caps like UAS DDS-PLUS with FOS before meals; Vitamin C with bioflavs, up to 3000mg daily.

• <u>Bitters herbs increase bile flow and help expel small stones:</u> Dandelion root tea, 3 cups daily; Gaia SWEETISH BITTERS extract; Taurine 1000mg helps keep bile thinned.

• <u>Help dissolve stones:</u> Chamomile tea, 5-7 cups daily for a month to dissolve stones; or Gaia FENNEL/WILD YAM SUPREME; Crystal Star STN-EX™ caps w/ lemon juice and water.

• <u>Prevent stone formation:</u> Solaray ALFAJUICE caps. Fiber supplements reduce risk of stones - Rainbow Light EVERYDAY FIBER SYSTEM; All One WHOLE FIBER COMPLEX.

• <u>Reduce excess blood sugar to keep stones from forming:</u> Spirulina caps between meals, with B complex 100mg helps stabilize blood sugar; add Biotin 600mcg; Glycine caps and Chromium picolinate 200mcg daily regulate blood sugar; Gymenna sylvestre capsules, 2 before meals.

• <u>Lipotropics control and regulate cholesterol overload:</u> Choline-Inositol 2 daily; Phosphatidyl choline 500mg daily, or Solgar PHOSPHATIDYL-CHOLINE triple strength; with Omega-3 flax seed oil 3x daily; Vitamin A 25,000IU & D 1000IU. Methionine tablets before meals; Solaray LIPOTROPIC 1000; Vitamin E 800IU with selenium 200mcg daily.

Bodywork and Lifestyle Techniques

• <u>Take coffee, garlic or catnip enemas</u> every 3 days until relief. (A new study shows coffee lowers risk of gallstone disease - for some men 2 cups a day reduces risk by 30 to 40%.) See enemas pg. 571 for instructions.

• <u>Eat small meals</u> more frequently. No large meals.

• <u>Apply castor packs or cold milk compresses</u> to the abdominal area.

• <u>A sedentary lifestyle is a major high risk factor.</u> Get mild regular exercise and reduce body fat to keep gallstones away. Tests show that for men 2 to 3 hours of light jogging per week can reduce gallstone formation by as much as 40%.

• <u>Early morning sunlight</u> will boost your cleanse with natural vitamin D.

• <u>Acupuncture and acupressure</u> have been successful for gallbladder disease.

• <u>Massage therapy:</u> to stimulate circulation.

• <u>Bathe:</u> Take several long hot baths during a liver cleanse for faster, easier detoxification. Add to your bath 5 drops fennel, 5 drops lemon and 5 drops rosemary essential oils.

• <u>Heat therapy:</u> A sauna every day possible to induce sweating and faster elimination.

Can't find a recommended product? Call the 800 number listed in Product Resources for the store nearest you and for more info.

Hepatitis Healing Program

Infectious hepatitis is largely a disease caused by a risky lifestyle - almost 90% of intravenous drug users are infected. Others at risk include dental and medical workers, and over 25% of people receiving blood transfusions. There are several types of viral hepatitis. Type A: (infects 200,000 Americans each year) a viral infection passed through blood and feces; Type B: (infects about 1 million Americans each year) a sexually transmitted viral infection carried through blood, semen, saliva and dirty needles; sometimes develops into chronic hepatitis; Type C: (infects 4 million Americans each year) a post-transfusion form. Type D: caused by Epstein-Barr virus and cytomegalovirus; Non-A, Non-B: higher mortality viruses passed through transfusion blood products, which frequently develop into chronic hepatitis.

Severity of hepatitis ranges from chronic fatigue to serious liver damage, and even to death from liver failure, cirrhosis or liver cancer. Natural therapies have had outstanding success in hepatitis cases, both in arresting viral replication, and in regeneration of the liver.

Do you think you might have hepatitis? All forms of hepatitis are characterized by at least 3 of the following signs.

—unexplained great fatigue
—flu-like exhaustion and diarrhea
—enlarged, tender, congested abdomen (indicating liver sluggishness)
—loss of appetite to the point of anorexia
—unexplained nausea, sometimes vomiting
—dark urine, gray stools
—skin pallor or jaundice usually accompanied by histamine type itching on stomach or arms
—depression; skin jaundice
—cirrhosis of the liver, perhaps from bouts of mononucleosis or alcoholism

Liver Cleanse for Hepatitis

I have personally seen and followed the improvement of several people who have used the emergency liver detoxification program in this chapter. Each had been told by their physicians that they were at terminal status. None were young, and abuse had been going on for years. Each felt he had nothing to lose by commitment to an alternative healing program. As far as I know, all are still walking around today. Drink six to eight glasses of bottled water every day, to encourage maximum detoxification.

It doesn't happen overnight, but you can have every confidence that if there is any chance at all, the liver will find its way to a healthier state, even after severe drug or alcohol abuse. When the crisis has passed, a program of 6 to 9 months on a liver healing diet should be undertaken.

Hepatitis Healing Nutrients:

—For 2 weeks: Eat only fresh foods: salads, fruits, juices, bottled water (see below). Take a glass of carrot/beet/cucumber juice every other day. Take a glass of lemon juice and water every morning. Take Sun Wellness CHLORELLA granules daily.

—Then for 1 to 2 months: Take carrot-beet-cucumber juice every 3 days, and papaya juice with 2 teasp. spirulina each morning. Eat lots of vegetable proteins, with steamed vegetables, brown rice, tofu, eggs, whole grains and yogurt. Avoid red meats.

—Then for 1 more month: Take 2 glasses of tomato juice with wheat germ oil-nutritional yeast-lemon juice every day. Take a daily glass of apple-alfalfa sprout juice. Focus on vegetable proteins, cultured foods like Rejuvenative Foods VEGI DELITE, fresh salads and complex carbs for strength. Avoid refined, fried, fatty foods, sugars, heavy spices, alcohol and caffeine during healing.

Hepatitis Healing Diet:

—On rising: take 1 teasp. acidophilus like JARRO-DOPHILUS +FOS in juice or water; and fresh lemon juice or cider vinegar in a glass of water with 1 teasp. honey.

—Breakfast: take a glass of carrot-beet-cucumber juice, aloe vera juice, or a potassium drink (pg. 568).

—Mid-morning: take a green drink (pg. 569) with 1 teasp. of spirulina or Sun Wellness CHLORELLA granules and $^1/_2$ teasp. ascorbate vitamin C crystals (about 2500mg.) added; or a superfood like Body Ecology VITALITY SUPERGREEN or Crystal Star SYSTEMS STRENGTH™ drink.

—Lunch: take another green drink (pg. 569), or Green Kamut Corp. GREEN KAMUT, or Crystal Star ENERGY GREEN™ drink, Green Foods WHEAT GERM EXTRACT, or Nutricology PROGREENS with EFA's, with $^1/_2$ teasp. acidophilus complex and $^1/_2$ teasp. ascorbate vitamin C crystals.

—Mid-afternoon: take another glass of lemon juice and water; or a glass of papaya juice with $^1/_2$ teasp. vitamin C crystals added; and/or a cup of Crystal Star LIV-ALIVE TEA™.

—Dinner: take another green drink (suggestions above) with $^1/_2$ teasp. vitamin C crystals; and/or pineapple-papaya juice with $^1/_2$ teasp. acidophilus powder added.

—Before Bed: take another glass of lemon juice and water with 1 teasp. honey added; or a glass of aloe vera juice with $^1/_2$ teasp. spirulina powder added; or a cup of Crystal Star LIV-ALIVE TEA™; and/or a cup of Red Star nutritional yeast broth for B vitamins, body relaxation, and next day strength.

Note: Count on 2 weeks for emergency detox measures; 1-3 months for healing the liver, and rebuilding blood and body strength.

Recipes that can help your healing diet: •HEALING DRINKS; •ENZYME-RICH RECIPES; •SOUPS - LIQUID SALADS •SALADS, HOT and COLD; •CULTURED FOODS; •MINERAL-RICH RECIPES; •LOW FAT RECIPES

Herb and Supplement Choices

• **Cleanse the liver of toxins:** Source Naturals Alpha Lipoic acid 400mg daily or MRI GLUCOTIZE; Jarrow SAMe 200, 600mg daily; Crystal Star LIV-ALIVE™ capsules 4 to 6 daily, with LIV-ALIVE™ tea 2 cups daily for 1 month. Reduce dose to half the 2nd month. Take Ascorbate Vitamin C crystals, up to 10,000mg daily in water, to bowel tolerance for 1 month; Enzymatic Therapy LIVA-TOX, with THYMU-PLEX caps for thymus strength. Liver detox teas: Oregon grape-Red clover tea; Pau d' arco-Calendula tea.

• **Inhibit viral replication:** *Echinacea-St. John's wort therapy* for lymphatic support: alternate 4 days of echinacea extract and 4 days of *St. John's wort* extract. Nutribiotic GRAPEFRUIT SEED extract 10 drops 3x daily for 1 month in juice.

• **Heal liver tissue:** Phosphatidyl-choline caps, 1000mg daily; Solaray LIPOTROPIC PLUS caps; Rainbow Light LIVA-GEN extract with ADVANCED ENZYME SYSTEM formula; or Transformation PUREZYME caps. L-carnitine 2000mg daily; vitamin E 400IU daily; Nutricology GERMANIUM 150mg daily.

• **Normalize liver with tonics:** Nutricology NAC (N-acety-cysteine) 500mg 3x daily; Crystal Star GINSENG-LICORICE ELIXIR™ drops; Maitake mushroom extract caps; or dandelion root extract, or astragalus extract or lobelia extract drops in tea; or bayberry-cayenne capsules, 6 daily to control inflammation. Crystal Star ANTI-HST™ caps for histamine reactions for 1 month. Reduce to half 2nd month.

• **For long term liver support:** Trimedica MSM 1000mg; MILK THISTLE SEED extract and Crystal Star BITTERS & LEMON CLEANSE™ each morning for 3 months. Beta carotene 150,000IU daily, with B-complex 150mg, and Country Life sublingual B-12, 2500mcg and extra folic acid 800mcg.

Bodywork and Lifestyle Techniques

• **Overheating sauna therapy** for liver and kidney detoxification is effective (see page 462). Take a sauna every day of the cleanse to induce sweating and faster toxin elimination.

• **Get plenty of bed rest,** especially during the acute infectious stages.

• **Take early morning sunbaths** every day possible.

• **Use chlorophyll implants** twice weekly for the first two critical weeks of healing to detoxify.

• **Avoid all alcohol, amphetamines, cocaine, barbiturates, or tobacco** of any kind.

• **Use hot castor oil packs** over the liver area.

• **A coffee enema** (1 cup coffee to 1 qt. water) may be taken to flush released wastes (See page 571 for method.)

• **Apply Nutribiotic GRAPEFRUIT SEED** extract to lesions.

Can't find a recommended product? Call the 800 number listed in Product Resources for the store nearest you and for more info.

Boosting Sexuality and Libido

Can we re-light the spark? This chapter can help you fan the passion flames and keep your sexual fires going.

At the turn of the millennium Americans are living longer and, for the most part, living healthier. Today, scientists tell us that living to 100 or 120 in a disease-free state is entirely possible! Already, over half of Americans have more than one full career in their lifespan. Many of us are just beginning to live out our dreams in the second part of our lives. I know that's what's happening to me.

At the turn of the century, we want renewed youth and vigor to be a real part of the second half of our lives. Weight loss has been our national obsession since the sixties. At any given time, over 25 million Americans are seriously dieting. Almost 60% feel they SHOULD be dieting. We want to look great at every age, too. The plastic surgery industry is booming! Face lifts are now the most commonly performed procedure in cosmetic surgery accounting for 54% of all surgery procedures for Americans between ages 51 and 64.

Reclaiming youthful sexuality in the second part of our lives may be the last piece of the vitality puzzle. We think our modern era is the only one beset with libido-lowering elements. There is no question that our nutrient-poor, high fat diets, over-use of drugs and stimulants, and high-pressure lifestyles leads to low energy and lack of time for love. But the reality is that humanity in every era has felt the need for sexual help. After all, this part of our lives is at the most basic, elemental center of our being.

Can you rewind your sexual clock?

Of course you can! It's largely a myth that people lose their sexuality in later years, that sexual performance declines, or that sexual response is poor. A survey by the National Council on Aging reveals that fully half of Americans over 60 have sex at least once a month - and one quarter of those say they'd like to have it more often! I think sex gets better as you age.

Sexual vibrancy at any age means paying attention to your attraction package — not just to impress the opposite sex, but to show yourself as you look in the mirror that you've "still got it." Looking good is a big confidence builder.... and confidence is sexy. Although we may want to look young, most people over 50 don't want to look like they did in their 20's. Instead, studies show people want to look like they do now, only better. The markers for sexuality have changed, making for some interesting phenomena.

　—**For women it's a case of "want to" instead of "have to."** As women mature with more confidence and become more financially independent, men see them more as sexual partners rather than sexual objects.

　—**People tend to marry later,** know themselves better and know much more the kind of person they want to be with.

　—**There is less of young women marrying much older men for money. But more of older women marrying younger men for adventure.**

　—**Divorce in later life has become more common, accepted, and "no-fault."** For many, late-life divorce isn't the result of fights or jealousies as it might have been before fifty, but rather a sea change in one's goals and interests, and the wish to share them with someone who has the same. Most people speak glowingly of their later-life second, even third marriages as more romantic and sexually fulfilling than their first.

The change in American sexuality came onto mainstream radar with the advent of Viagra. It showed us a lot about ourselves:

–how much sexuality is a part of our later lives.

–how many problems there are in later life sexuality.

–most worrisome, the dangers of the new designer drugs used to sell them.

Viagra was one of the first designer drugs to be marketed directly to the public through advertising. It was and is promoted as a love aid for impotent men. The fact that it is a powerful, potentially dangerous drug has been vastly understated in its advertising.

More than a year into the Viagra craze we see that enhancing sexuality through drug chemistry is not what we thought it was. It's much more in terms of danger and much less in terms of help for impotence.

But the marketing worked. It's something America does to perfection. Viagra reached $1 billion in sales in just its first year (making a clear statement about how American men feel about their bodies today).

Viagra copycats and superhormones like DHEA and new and different hormones or combinations of hormones like cosmetics, beauty aids for long life-span and renewed sexual vitality.

Before making the decision to take superhormones, dangerous, substances to work with. Tiny amounts can tell you who is going through menopause. They may seem respect and caution. While there may be times when taking supplemental hormones is appropriate, a better choice, especially for people with normal hormone levels, might

ANDRO are flooding the world markets, tempting us to try called "hormone cocktails" for better sex. They're advertised take a step back and consider: Hormones are tricky- even cause big reactions- both good and bad as any woman can to be beauty aids, but we need to regard superhormones with be subtle, safe foods or herbs that have worked for centuries.

I always say the natural way is best...

Great sex doesn't come from a pill. It comes from a good lifestyle program. Natural remedies treat the whole person not just physical mechanisms involved in sexuality.

Herbs have been associated with love potions for thousands of years. Can some herbs really enhance libido and sexual performance? Today's studies show that, once again, science is validating herbal tradition. In fact, it turns out that certain herbs may have a great deal of influence on sexual response and performance in people. Herbs don't turn men into supermen or make women love slaves, but they can be a good remedy choice when there are sexual function problems or even to enhance healthy sexuality.

The aphrodisiac miracle foods of yesteryear are now seen as critical nutrients that may be missing in our bodies. Many of us are overfed and undernourished.

The "heart" of sexuality is that men and women are different. In fact, they are polar opposites at the basic, sexual level. The differences dramatically affect sexual response. We need to consider what each sex really needs to develop the best solutions.

344

Are hormone-like chemicals in your environment affecting your sexuality?

Hormone disrupters affect the reproductive health of both men and women. They affect your entire endocrine system, all the communication system of your glands, hormones and cellular receptors in your body. They wreak havoc on sexuality and fertility, and now are so commonplace in modern society that there is no way to completely avoid them. Hormone disrupters are found in pollutants, drugs, hormone-injected animal foods, plastics, and pesticides- things most of us are exposed to every day.

Pesticide sprayed foods are especially dangerous. Nearly 40% of pesticides used in commercial agriculture are suspected hormone disrupters. So, many of the pesticides used to produce your food contain hormone-like substances, exogenous estrogens and androgens (the major male and female hormones), that spell disaster for your sexual health.

Here's how...

–1. Hormone disrupters can alter the production and breakdown of your own hormones and the function of your hormone receptors- disrupting hormone balance at its developmental core.

–2. Hormone disrupters compete for hormone receptor sites in the body and can bind to them in place of natural hormones, causing major fluctuations in hormonal levels, affecting everything from sexuality and fertility to total body energy and health.

Some of the male problems we know are linked to environmental hormones.

1. prostate disease 2. testicular cancer 3. undescended testes, small penis size 4. infertility- Since 1960, the number of men with fertility problems who sought consultation has risen 32%! 5. poor semen quality or low sperm count- Sperm counts have decreased an average of 50% over just the past half-century!

Some of the female diseases associated with chronic exposure to environmental hormone mimics.

1. breast and reproductive organ cancer 2. fibrocystic disease of the breast and/or uterine fibroids 3. polycystic ovarian syndrome 4. endometriosis or pelvic inflammatory disease 5. infertility

You may be especially exposed to hormone disrupters if: you live in a high agricultural area; you eat a high fat diet – fatty areas of your body store these chemicals; you eat hormone-injected dairy foods or meats regularly

Is there any way to reduce your exposure? Limit consumption of fatty dairy products and meats which are notoriously high in hormone disrupting chemicals. Incorporate a detoxification program to help your body eliminate congested wastes and chemicals residues. Buy organic foods which are not sprayed with harmful hormone-disrupting chemicals whenever you can. Especially eat cruciferous veggies like broccoli to help flush excess estrogen from pollutants out of your body.

Sexuality Diet for Men

Men break down tissue; They expend energy, as in the discharge in sex. They need denser foods, more concentrated proteins and three times the volume of complex carbohydrates (like whole grains) as women. A man's sex drive and function is largely dependent on testosterone, sensory stimulation and a good blood supply to the erectile tissue, factors that rely on good nutrition and exercise.

Men are most often worried about their ability to achieve and maintain an erection, with the frequency they can have intercourse, and the length of their recovery period after intercourse. Men are capable of retaining their sexual virility well into their 80's. Growing older is not synonymous with inevitable sexual decline. Eighty-five percent of all impotence problems are physical, involving heart problems, drug actions and interactions, sexually transmitted diseases, prostate disorders, nerve diseases like MS, hormone disruption (sometimes caused by environmental estrogens), alcohol and tobacco. Even very young men are affected. It's a sad fact that in America today, one in six married couples of child-bearing age has trouble conceiving and completing a successful pregnancy.

Can a change in diet really affect a man's sexuality?

Impotence now affects 52% of men between 40 and 70 years of age. In about one quarter of physiological origin impotence, the problem is the dining room, not the bedroom! For these cases, normalizing libido is simply a matter of improving a poor diet. Junk food, saturated fats, high sugars, hard liquor, chemical and processed foods are key factors in a man not feeling "up to it."

Low zinc probably plays the largest nutrient role in low libido. Zinc is clearly the most important nutrient for male sexual function. Zinc is very concentrated in semen. Ejaculation significantly diminishes body zinc stores. Researchers speculate that a man's body may respond to depleted zinc stores by reducing sexual drive to conserve them. Chronic stress can wipe out zinc stores. Prescription and over-the-counter drugs can lower zinc levels. Antacids, acid blockers, alcohol, diuretics and cortisone are all zinc reducers. Adding more zinc-rich foods like oysters, nuts, seeds, legumes and liver is a good way to restore sexual vitality.

Are you zinc deficient? If you answer yes to several of these questions, you may have some degree of zinc deficiency.

–Is your appetite poor? Do you have a diminished sense of taste and smell?
–Do you have adult acne? Do you have dry, cracked, chapped lips on a regular basis?
–Do you get frequent colds, flu or ear infections? Do cuts or wounds heal slowly?
–Is your hair color dulling or going prematurely gray?
–Do you have prostate disease like BPH or prostatitis? Do you suffer from impotence or erection problems?
–Do your eyes tear excessively when exposed to bright light? Do you have macular degeneration or cataracts?

Problems that this diet can help: *Low Libido, Impotence, High Blood Pressure, Overweight, Chronic Stress Reactions, Prostate Inflammation, Hemorrhoids, Adrenal Exhaustion, Gland and Hormone Imbalances.*

A Man's Diet for Low Libido or Impotence

The diet on this page contains the nutrients that reinforce male energy, strength, vigor and stamina. The diet focuses in particular on heart and circulatory needs, because arterial clogging affects erectile tissue and often leads to impotence. Key nutrient "superfoods" rapidly rebuild the body for better sex. It can be used as a health insurance policy against many health problems facing men today.

__Watchwords:__ 1) Eat zinc source foods: seafoods and sea greens, nuts, seeds, beans and other legumes. 2) Dopamine (L-Dopa) is intimately associated with sex drive in men. One 16-oz. can of fava beans has almost a prescription dose! 3) Add mineral-rich foods like shellfish, greens and whole grains; EFA's from flaxseed and sea greens. 4) Eat fiber-rich foods like legumes, fruits and vegetables to avoid atherosclerosis of the penis. 5) Drink alcohol in moderation. Heavy drinking can lead to reduced erections. Drink plenty of water and mineral water throughout the day to keep the body light and flushed.

—**On rising:** Herbal fiber reduces cholesterol and eliminates fatty build-up that contributes to impotence. Crystal Star's CHOL-LO FIBER TONE™ takes about 3 months; or try a high protein drink such as Unipro PERFECT PROTEIN in juice.

—**Breakfast:** make a mix of 2 TBS each: sunflower seeds, pumpkin seeds, and toasted wheat germ. Sprinkle some each morning on toasted oat cereal (wild oats have been known to increase frequency of intercourse and orgasm for men for millennia), pancakes or granola. Top with 1 TB maple syrup, molasses, apple juice or yogurt; add poached or baked eggs with whole grain toast or muffins.

—**Mid-morning:** have a fresh carrot juice, or small bottle of mineral water; or a green drink (pg. 569), Sun Wellness CHLORELLA, Nutricology PRO-GREENS or Crystal Star ENERGY GREEN™; and a cup of noodle ramen soup with sea greens snipped on top.

—**Lunch:** have some fish or seafood with brown rice and a small salad; or a chicken, avocado and low-fat cheese sandwich or salad; or a whole grain, high protein salad or sandwich with lots of nuts, seeds, tofu or yogurt, and a lentil or black bean soup.

—**Mid-afternoon:** have some low-fat cottage cheese with nuts and seeds and whole grain crackers; or a dried fruit and nut mix with a bottle of mineral water; or a hard boiled egg with a tea like ginseng tea (use about 1 dropperful panax ginseng extract in water; or try a ginseng/ royal jelly blend in water); or Nature's Path TRACE-LYTE drink for electrolyte minerals.

—**Dinner:** have an Italian whole grain pasta or polenta dish with a seafood stew; or a roast turkey and whole grain stuffing meal, with steamed vegetables and a fresh salad; or fresh baked seafood or salmon with brown rice and peas. A little wine at dinner helps relaxation, digestion, and release from stress and inhibitions.

—**Before bed:** have a cup of Red Star nutritional yeast broth; or a cup of Crystal Star CUPID'S FLAME TEA™ with honey.

Note: Avoid junky, chemicalized, fast foods and pre-prepared foods. Because of their need for stability and shelf life, these types of foods are the most likely place to get heavily sprayed produce, and hormone or antibiotic injected meats. Especially avoid red meats full of saturated fats, fried, fatty and salty foods. Eat small meals more frequently, rather than large meals.

Recipes to help a man's libido diet: • FISH and SEA FOODS; • BREAKFAST and BRUNCH; • HIGH PROTEIN without MEAT; • COMPLEX CARBOHYDRATES; • HIGH FIBER RECIPES; • MINERAL-RICH • HEALTHY PARTY FOODS.

Herb and Supplement Choices

• **Revitalize the male system:** Ginseng and ginseng-like herbs are tonics for male sexual virility. Imperial Elixir AMERICAN GINSENG tabs (woodsgrown). Ginseng increases the weight of the seminal vesicles, sperm count and motility. It also enhances nitric oxide synthesis (like Viagra) which regulates muscle tone of blood vessels and controls blood flow to the penis: Ethical Nutrients TRUE ENERGY; Optimal Nutrients OPTI-POTENT POTION; Catauba or Potency wood, (*muira pauma*) 4000mg; Crystal Star LOVE MALE™ caps, MALE GINSIAC™ or LOVING MOOD FOR MEN™ extracts, MALE PERFORMANCE™ long term help.

• **EFA's boost healthy seminal fluids:** Highest potency royal jelly 60,000-120,000mg daily; Heart Foods KEEP IT UP tabs; Ginkgo Biloba for erectile dysfunction (In a recent study, ginkgo was actually more effective than drug injections. 50% of patients showed regained potency, compared to 20% using injection.); Unipro B₁₅ DMG liquid or tablets; Premier GERMANIUM with DMG. Zinc 50mg 2x daily with Vitamin E 400IU.

• **For a stronger erection:** Liquid niacin before intercourse; Arginine 3000mg 45 minutes before sex for more penile blood flow (not if you have herpes); Carnitine 2000mg 2x daily; Trimedica TRIBULUS TERRESTIS; Pinnacle HORNY GOAT WEED; Natural Balance COBRA; Crystal Star PRO-EST PROX™ roll-on for longer erections.

• **For low libido:** Pipsissewa (older men); 5-HTP 100mg an hour before sex); Histidine 500m with B-6 and niacin.

• **More frequent erections:** Yohimbe caps 750-1000mg to stimulate testosterone (Do not take yohimbe if you take diet products with phenylpropanolamine, or have heart, kidney, liver disorders). Country Life SUPER STRENGTH YOHIMBE.

Bodywork and Lifestyle Techniques

• **Environmental estrogens in hormone-injected food animals, herbicides-pesticides affect male sperm counts.** Avoid hormone-injected meats and dairy foods, and herbicide-sprays to avoid environmental estrogens (see page 345). Heavy metals and radiation can damage sperm structure.

• **EXERCISE.** Most men have no idea how closely regular exercise is linked to their libido. In one study, 78 healthy, but sedentary men were studied during nine months of regular exercise. The men exercised for 60 minutes a day, three days a week. Every man in the study reported significantly enhanced sexuality, including increased frequency, performance and satisfaction. The rise in sexuality was correlated with how much each man's fitness improved!

• **Acupuncture and hypnotherapy** are useful for impotence related to stress or psychological problems. In a Turkish study of 29 men, 20 of them overcame impotence after receiving acupuncture treatments.

• **If you smoke, quit!** Smoking just 2 cigarettes a day can inhibit an erection by restricting capillary blood flow. Cadmium in cigarette papers interferes with the utilization and absorption of zinc. A 1994 study of 4,400 Vietnam vets showed a 50% higher rate of impotence in smokers compared to non-smokers.

• **Get some early morning sunlight on the body and genitals** every day possible for general sexual health and to help prevent prostate problems.

• **Check your prescription drugs;** some have the side effect of impaired sex drive. Prolonged recreational drug use also inhibits sperm production and can affect erections.

Can't find a recommended product? Call the 800 number listed in Product Resources for the store nearest you and for more info.

Sexuality Diet for Women

Women build up tissue; they receive energy, then convert and enrich it to create life. They need less protein than men, and a smaller volume of complex carbohydrates for conception and fertility.

For women, sexuality comes down to hormones - those incredibly important, potent substances at the root of most women's problems. Hormones are the basis for all metabolic activity. Some have almost immediate effects, some have a delayed reaction. Even a minute imbalance or deficiency can contribute to low libido or vaginal dryness, the main sexual problems women face. Sadly, large surveys in the U.S. and Europe confirm this. Statistics find that as many as 50% of adult women have lost interest in sex or have difficulty becoming aroused. While men are worrying about what turns them on, women are more aware of what turns them off.

Is your libido low?

–Have you gained unusual weight (low thyroid and metabolism) or lost your normal energy (adrenal exhaustion)?
–Have you become dissatisfied with the path your life is taking? Are you depressed?
–Do you feel unattractive? Do you think you've lost your looks as you've aged?
–Have you been under a lot of emotional stress for a long period of time? Is your personal relationship unhappy?
–Is there unusual tension in your job? Have you resorted to too many prescription (or pleasure) drugs to get through your day?
–Has your diet deteriorated to fast foods on the run? Are you getting exercise every week?
–Was your childhood marked by physical abuse or great trauma? (sometimes the feelings don't surface for years)

Why are women's sex drives at an all-time low?

First: Adrenal exhaustion, one of the main reasons for waning libido, is at epidemic levels in America today, especially for women after menopause. When a woman's adrenals are functioning well, they pick up the job of estrogen secretion to keep her active and attractive after menopause. High stress lifestyles and poor eating habits mean many women reach their menopausal years with prematurely worn out adrenals, a fact that usually translates into less energy for lovemaking.

Are your adrenals exhausted? Here's an easy adrenal health self-test: It's a common diagnostic performed by most chiropractors, massage therapists and naturopaths. Use a home blood pressure testing kit.

1. Lie down and rest for 5 minutes. Take a blood pressure reading. Your systolic blood pressure should be below 120 and your diastolic blood pressure should be below 80 to be at optimal levels for health.

2. Stand up and immediately take another blood pressure reading. If your blood pressure drops below normal levels, your adrenals are probably functioning poorly. The amount of drop is usually in ratio to the amount of adrenal dysfunction.

Note: If your blood pressure drops to 90/60 or below, you may feel faint, dizzy or light-headed. Consider consulting a health professional.

A Woman's Adrenal Health Program. Sometimes, just nourishing your adrenals can revitalize a tired sex drive.

—Take vitamin C to help convert cholesterol to adrenal hormones.

—Eat vitamin B-rich foods like brown rice, or take a B Complex vitamin.

—Eat zinc-rich foods, like brown rice, sunflower and pumpkin seeds, nutritional yeast, bran, and oysters for stress reactions.

—Eat magnesium-rich foods, like leafy vegetables, almonds, avocado, carrots, citrus, lentils, and salmon to counteract depression.

—Take 500mg daily of the amino acid tyrosine to rebuild the body's natural store of adrenaline and increase libido.

—Take adrenal-boosting herbs like ginseng, sarsaparilla, parsley, sage, sea greens or garlic; or Crystal Star ADRN-ACTIVE™.

Second: Women with an underactive thyroid may also have low libido. (if you think a low thyroid might be your problem, see women's section, page 330 for signs and symptoms.)

Third: Vaginal dryness is a common libido problem after menopause. During reproductive years, estrogen stimulates the cells lining the vagina to maintain proper moisture. But during menopause, the vaginal lining may become thin and dry due to reduced circulating estrogen. That's when intercourse becomes painful (a definite turn-off for women). Some women also experience susceptibility to vaginal infection. Herbs can often come to the rescue.

—For immediate relief, I recommend applying vitamin E oil, or taking an oral extract of *licorice rt.* and *dendrobium* (Crystal Star's WOMEN'S DRYNESS™) to produce more fluid in the membranes. Panax ginseng and aloe vera also help the body produce fluid. In Ayurvedic healing, Shatavari (*Asparagus racemosus*) is a sexual tonic for women with vaginal atrophy.

Are there aphrodisiacs for women? If you've lost your interest in sex, check out the natural answers to low sexuality.

Many herbs show remarkable results for turning a woman's attention to love... even enhancing the sexual experience itself. Herbs with aphrodisiac properties for women work differently than those for men. Their activity is rather to nourish and tone rather than to stimulate. Action is much deeper in the body, slower, gentler and longer lasting, almost like the sexual experience itself.

—*Avena sativa* (wild and green oats): In a recent study done by the Institute for Advanced Study Of Human Sexuality, 300mg of wild oats extract three days a week led to a dramatic increase in multiple orgasms for women!

—*Tribulus terrestris* (puncture vine), an herb native to India and Africa increases sex drive without the side effects of traditional hormone drugs like weight gain (estrogen) or masculinization (testosterone). In one study, $2/3$ of women treated with tribulus report renewed sexual interest! It's also effective for menopause symptoms like hot flashes, depression and anxiety.

—Tonic herbs like *ashwagandha* and *Siberian ginseng* help low libido due to nervous exhaustion or over-work because they strengthen the glands and build resistance to stress.

—A *dong quai/damiana* combination can restore female hormone harmony and stimulate sex drive. Damiana is a mild aphrodisiac which works by increasing neurotransmitter messages, making a woman more sensitive to touch. It is a specific to treat frigidity in women. Dong quai, often called "the female ginseng," is considered the queen of all female tonic herbs by the Chinese.

A Woman's Diet for Low Libido or Infertility

This diet is full of key nutrient "superfoods" to rapidly rebuild the body for better sex, vigorous conception, and healthier babies.

Watchwords:

1) Increase soy foods for a mild, natural estrogenic effect. In a recent test, women who ate the equivalent of one cup of cooked soybeans daily showed an increase in the number of cells lining the vaginal walls, offsetting vaginal drying and irritation.

2) Eat foods rich in EFA's: sea foods, leafy greens, whole grains, nuts, legumes and seeds.

3) Taking vitamin E internally helps improve blood supply to the vaginal walls. Increase intake of foods with vitamin E like soy foods, wheat germ, seeds, nuts and vegetable oils for more body moisture and beta carotene foods like apricots, mangoes and carrots.

4) Boost adrenal energy with vitamin B foods like brown rice and sea greens.

5) Eat magnesium-rich foods, like almonds, leafy greens, avocado, carrots, citrus fruits, lentils, and salmon to counteract depression and anxiety.

6) Foods from the sea nourish an underactive thyroid for increased libido. Foods that enhance female libido: fennel, celery, parsley, high lignan flaxseed oil and shiitake mushrooms.

7) Two or three alcoholic drinks can delay orgasm in women or decrease its intensity. Drink plenty of water instead.

—On rising: take ALL-1 VITAMIN-MINERAL drink, or a high protein drink such as Nature's Plus SPIRUTEIN in juice.

—Breakfast: Mix 2 TBS each: toasted sesame seeds, sunflower seeds, toasted wheat germ and lecithin granules. Sprinkle some on yogurt or fresh fruit, rice cakes or whole grain cereal. Top with apple juice, maple syrup, molasses, vanilla soy milk or almond milk.

—Mid-morning: have a fresh carrot juice, or a small bottle of mineral water; or a green drink (pg. 569), Monas CHLORELLA, Wakunaga KYO-GREEN with EFA's, or Crystal Star ENERGY GREEN™; and/or a cup of miso or noodle ramen soup with sea greens.

—Lunch: have a leafy green salad with a light soup and corn bread; or a seafood or broccoli quiche with a green leafy salad; or a fresh fruit salad with cottage cheese or yogurt.

—Mid-afternoon: have some low-fat cottage cheese with nuts and seeds, and whole grain crackers; or a dried fruit and nut mix with a bottle of mineral water; or a hard boiled egg with an herb drink such as ginseng tea (use about 1 dropperful panax ginseng extract in water; or try a ginseng/royal jelly/honey blend in water.

—Dinner: have a fluffy omelet with vegetables and a green salad; or a stir-fry with Chinese greens and mushrooms, and baked tofu, or miso soup with sea veggies; or a whole grain pasta and vegetable casserole with yogurt/chive sauce.

—Before bed: have a cup of Red Star nutritional yeast broth; or a cup of Crystal Star CUPID'S FLAME TEA™ with honey.

Note: Avoid junky, chemicalized, fast foods and pre-prepared foods. These are the most likely foods to be heavily sprayed (produce), or hormone or antibiotic injected (meats) because they need a long shelf life. Especially avoid saturated fats, fried and salty foods. Eat small meals more frequently, rather than large meals.

Recipes to help a women's libido diet: •BLENDING EAST and WEST FOODS; •BREAKFAST and BRUNCH; •FISH and SEA FOODS; •LOW FAT FOODS; •HIGH PROTEIN without MEAT; •MINERAL-RICH; •HEALTHY PARTY FOODS.

Herb and Supplement Choices

•**Libido enhancers:** Crystal Star LOVE FEMALE™ caps for 3 days before a special weekend; Peruvian Maca 2 daily; Nutramedix INVOGOREX; Futurebiotics MAXATIVA for women; Country Life MAXINE'S INTIMA FOR WOMEN; Dong Quai/Damiana extract; Histidine 500mg with B-6 100mg; Yohimbe 500mg caps for a tingle. (See page 348 for contraindications.); Enzymatic Therapy THYROID/TYROSINE.

•**Enhance orgasm:** Enzymatic Therapy KAVATONE or 2 Cayenne-ginger capsules, or 4 Ginseng/Damiana caps; Montana Big Sky LOVING MOOD, or •Crystal Star CUPID'S FLAME™ tea or GINSENG 6 SUPER tea or caps; 100mg niacin - 30 minutes before sex to enhance sexual flush, mucous membrane tingling and the intensity of the orgasm.

•**Increased vaginal fluids:** Crystal Star WOMEN'S DRYNESS™ extract as needed; Vitamin E 800IU daily with highest potency royal jelly 60,000 to 120,000mg. 1 teasp. daily; or Alive ROYAL JELLY vials boost acetylcholine for sexual response; For immediate relief: Apply natural •vitamin E oil, sesame seed oil, aloe vera gel or Moon Maid VITAL VULVA.

•**Tonify the female system with adaptogen herbs:** Crystal Star FEEL GREAT™ caps, 2-3 caps daily; Transitions PROGEST cream, or Crystal Star PRO-EST BALANCE™ roll-on. Imperial Elixir GINSENG/ROYAL JELLY.

•**Essential fatty acids improve skin tone, and lubricate your body internally and externally:** EVENING PRIMROSE OIL 3000 mg daily; Nature's Secret ULTIMATE OIL.

•**For depression-related libido problems:** St. John's wort, or 5-HTP to increase serotonin; Ginkgo Biloba improves low libido in women caused by anti-depressant drugs.

Bodywork and Lifestyle Techniques

•**Sexual enhancement for a big weekend.** Both men and women can both benefit from taking herbal combinations for a week before a romantic getaway or private "date night."

• **Get regular daily exercise:** walking, slow jogging, bicycling, swimming and dancing.

•**Get plenty of quality rest and sleep.** Consciously work to avoid stressful situations. A little vacation together can do wonders, even if it's only a long, quality time weekend doing something you both like.

•**Avoid tranquilizers, anti-depressants,** Aldomet (for high blood pressure), hard alcohol and drugs that suppress hormones. These all suppress desire and sexual ability, too.

•**Aromatherapy** is one of the best ways to stimulate a loving mood. Aromatherapy oils have deep subconscious effects on our feelings, triggering memory, lifting emotions and altering attitudes. Essential oils have been used for thousands of years to enhance the sexual experience and to lure lovers. Sexuality-enhancing aromatherapy oils especially nice for women are ylang ylang, rose, clary sage, neroli and rosewood. I like to use an old fashioned aromatherapy burner, but a few drop of your favorite oil sprinkled on a pillowcase will do just fine.

Can't find a recommended product? Call the 800 number listed in Product Resources for the store nearest you and for more info.

352

Reduce Stress - Boost Energy

Are you stressed out? Is your energy at an all-time low? Stress is the universal enemy of modern mankind. Many people seem to be under stress most of the time. Over 20 million Americans have stress-related health problems! Up to 95 percent of visits to health care professionals are stress-related. Everyone is affected by varying degrees of stress.... people who work in polluted atmospheres, people who work with machines or instruments demanding constant attention, people who travel coast to coast regularly, people with boring jobs, etc. Stress causes useless fatigue; at its worst, it is dangerous to health. Prolonged stress drains our energy and creates a load of body imbalances. Profound stress, like that caused by job loss or the loss of a loved one takes a serious physical toll.

Stress is usually at the heart of heart disease. It is a major cause of chronic fatigue, insomnia, headaches, hypoglycemia, arthritis and compromised immunity. Degenerative diseases like cancers and diabetes are stress-related. Stress irritates body tissues in the form of gastritis, ulcers, cystitis, colitis and psoriasis. It irritates our mental processes in the form of moodiness, burn-out, overuse of drugs, depression and panic attacks. The common cold can be brought on by stress. Stress can even lead to baldness! Financial obligations, kaleidoscopic job pressures, seeking work in an mercurial job market, family demands, emotional problems, health concerns, and lack of rest and leisure can overwhelm even a stable, well-adjusted nature.

As our 21st century civilization races forward, Americans today are running harder and harder to stay in the same place. We try to get as much done as we can in as short a time as possible. Sometimes we try to do as many things as possible at the same time! Experts tell us that a certain amount of stress is healthy, that facing challenges and difficulties helps us grow and reach our potential, even adding spice to our lives.

What exactly is stress?
People tell me that stress makes their body shrivel up and head for cover. Actually the opposite is true. Stress directly depletes the adrenal glands, which become inflamed and swell. In prolonged cases, the adrenals cannot raise blood sugar for energy and hypoglycemia results. In severe cases, like Addison's disease, the adrenals swell to the point of hemorrhage and tissue death may result.

Most of us know stress as the "fight or flight" concept — a basic response to perceived danger. But as stress has loomed larger in our lives, modern medical science has redefined stress more definitively. Today, there's specific and nonspecific stress, external and internal stress, emotional and biological stress, and physiological and environmental stress.

Can almost anything trigger a stress response?
Yes.... just about everything triggers stress. The number of recognized "stressors" is sweeping and include: environmental disturbances like air pollution, plant pollens, toxic reactions to metals, or chemical halogens like chlorine and fluoride; physical trauma like infections, fractures, cuts, burns, parasite invasions, allergies, food sensitivities, or malnutrition (more common than one might think in America); even strong emotional reactions. Psychosocial stress, an umbrella covering almost every aspect of human life, is also recognized today. This doesn't count our personal stressors.

What happens during a stress response?
Experts identify three distinct stages as your body tries to adapt:

Stage 1: Alarm Reaction. This is the traditional "fight or flight" response. Your adrenal glands kick into action, releasing a flood of hormones that give you a burst of energy. Your heart rate and blood pressure increase. Your blood sugar rises as the liver releases stored sugar into your bloodstream. Your muscles tense; you start to sweat. Your immune system gets ready; blood-clotting mechanisms rev up. You're primed for quick action if needed. If the perceived danger passes, your alertness calms down and your pulse gradually returns to normal.

Stage 2: The Resistance Stage. If stress continues, your body starts to mobilize itself for a longer fight. The adrenal glands draw on nutrient reserves to provide longer-term energy, producing corticoid hormones to adapt to the stress. This mechanism works for a while, but it uses up nutrient and energy reserves if the stress continues. Cell-damaging free radicals form in greater numbers; the adrenal glands, cardiovascular and immune response systems become exhausted from maintaining a constant state of arousal.

Stage 3: The Exhaustion Stage. If your stress is unrelenting, your body's nutrient and energy reserves become even more depleted. Stress becomes serious. With nothing more to draw on, your adrenal glands fall into a state of exhaustion, perpetually releasing the hormones adrenaline, noradrenaline and cortisol, a futile coping effort that drastically diminishes your body's ability to deal with any stress at all. Adrenal exhaustion affects all body systems and places a great load on our organ systems, especially the heart, blood vessels, pancreas (hypoglycemia is a common result), and leads to other gland malfunction, like low sexual energy. If your diet is also poor, then your body's nutritional storehouse has almost no raw materials to draw on for normalizing itself; serious damage may take place to your kidneys, liver, intestinal tract, bones and immune system.

Are you stressed out?
Mild anxiety, unease, periodic nervousness or panic are symptoms of severe stress which upset body chemistry. Highly anxious people have trouble getting enough sleep — the very thing that most quickly improves their ability to deal with stress. Dealing with stress first, can often improve other problems automatically.

–Have you lost interest in things you used to find enjoyable?
–Do the corners of your eyes sag? Do you look noticeably older? Is your brow furrowed?
–Have you become short-tempered or easily angered? Easily bored or nervous?
–Are you tired or sad all the time? Do you have frequent insomnia?
–Do you have chronic head and neck aches? Chronic upset stomach?
–Is your blood pressure high? Do you get heart palpitations?
–Are you susceptible to frequent allergic reactions, especially skin disorders?
–Does your chest feel tight? Do you have trouble taking in enough air?

Can your body cope with stress? Can you transform stress into spice?
The stress process can be turned around. We can dramatically strengthen our body's ability to adapt to stress so that it doesn't undermine our physical and mental health. It's the extremes that get us into trouble.... when stress is unusual or long-lasting.

You're the doctor. Here's my lifestyle program to improve the quality of your life.

The same stress that makes one person sick can be an invigorating experience for another. The goal isn't to avoid all stress, but to maintain a high degree of health to survive stress well. You may need to reorganize your lifestyle. Major problems usually require major change. Poor health cannot be blamed entirely on stress. We fall prey to stress because of poor health. The balanced nutrition, exercise, and relaxation program in this section, gives your body tools to mount a healthy response to stress.

Food is your Pharmacy© for relieving stress.

1—**Your diet is your key to a stress free life.** Adrenal health is critical. If your adrenal glands are exhausted, they need nourishment, or you'll never recover your energy. Feed your adrenals with foods like sea greens (page 102) and green drinks (page 569) and superfoods like YS ROYAL JELLY/GINSENG blend (add to tea), Crystal Star SYSTEMS STRENGTH™ drink, Nutricology PRO-GREENS with EFA's, and Barleans BARLEANS GREENS drink.

2—**During periods of intense stress your body needs more nutrients.** A nourishing diet stops emergency borrowing by your body of protein, minerals, vitamins and fats to cope with extra stress. Even when certain nutrients are drawn down to give you bursts of extra energy, they can be restored quickly.

3—**Protein is critical in a stress reduction diet.** As stress increases, protein needs increase. Extreme, unyielding stress uses up a lot of protein. Adding clean protein from seafoods, sea plants, rice, sprouts, soy foods, nuts, seeds, organic turkey and chicken, eggs and low fat cheeses helps stop stress-related tissue destruction. Amino acids in protein foods help build healthy neurotransmitters which affect mood and coping mechanisms. For example, the amino acid L-tryptophan (in soy, cheeses and turkey) helps build serotonin, essential for overcoming anxiety, depression and insomnia. Add magnesium-rich foods from green vegetables and whole grains. Have fresh carrot juice and fresh fish or seafood at least once a week.

4—**Do you eat foods high in sugar and fat to get energy when you're under stress?** Today, most of these foods are full of chemicals and heavily refined. They degrade your bio-chemical balance, actually elevating stress. Eat B vitamin-rich foods like brown rice and whole grains. Make an anti-stress mix of nutritional yeast, toasted wheat germ, sunflower seeds, and molasses - take 2 TBS daily in food. Take miso soup before bed to relax.

5—**Do you use caffeine to boost your energy when you're under stress?** Caffeine increases stress symptoms of nervousness, irritability, headaches and heart palpitations. Reduce caffeine intake. Drink green tea instead for energy and antioxidants.

6—**Do you drink alcohol to feel better when you're under stress?** Alcohol escalates your adrenal hormone output, interfering with sleep cycles and normal brain chemistry. Take a glass of wine before dinner. No liquids with meals. Drink bottled water.

7—**How you eat may be as important as what you eat** because it affects how you metabolize your food. Eat in a relaxing environment, not when you're upset, distracted or on the run.

The diets in this section help many stress-related problems: *Anxiety, Depression, Stress Headaches, Migraine Headaches, Chronic Fatigue, Insomnia, Mental Burn-Out, Lower Back Pain, Neuralgia and Neuritis, Drug and Alcohol Dependency, Obsessive-Compulsive Behavior Patterns.*

Anti-Stress Diet

Begin with a 3-day liquid diet to clear your body of chemicals and pollutants that aggravate stress. (See page 148.) Follow with 1 to 2 days of all-fresh foods to rebalance your body's chemistry (pH). Add plenty of supergreen foods like chlorella, barley grass, green kamut, etc. for molecular proteins and chlorophyllins that can be absorbed directly into cell membranes to start rebuilding your body and give you energy. Then add whole grains, root vegetables and potatoes to boost serotonin for more emotional stability. Then add protein foods to help you think and react quickly, and feel more energetic.

—**On rising:** take a glass of 2 fresh squeezed lemons, 1 TB maple syrup and 8-oz. of water.

—**Breakfast:** (1st day) have a nutrient-dense Kick-Off Cleansing Cocktail: juice 1 handful fresh wheat grass or parsley—extremely rich in chlorophyll and antioxidants, 4 carrots, 1 apple, 2 celery stalks with leaves, $^1/_2$ beet with top; add whole grain granola or oatmeal with yogurt or apple juice on top; brown rice with sea greens; or a poached egg.

—**Mid-morning:** have a glass of fresh carrot juice or fresh apple juice. Add 1 TB of a green superfood like Crystal Star ENERGY GREEN™ drink mix or Vibrant Health GREEN VIBRANCE.

—**Lunch:** have a Salad-In-A-Glass: juice 4 parsley sprigs, 3 quartered tomatoes, $^1/_2$ green or red pepper, $^1/_2$ cucumber, 1 scallion, 1 lemon wedge. Add brown rice and steamed veggies or baked tofu, or a green salad with cottage cheese and bottled water.

—**Mid-afternoon:** have a cup of chamomile or green tea and celery sticks with kefir cheese.

—**Dinner:** a warm, mineral electrolyte broth: **for two bowls,** chop and cover with water in a soup pot, 4 carrots, 2 potatoes with skins, 1 onion, 3 stalks celery with leaves, 2 broccoli stalks, $^1/_2$ head cabbage and 1 handful fresh parsley. Simmer covered 30 minutes; strain, discard solids and drink liquid. (Or use Nature's Path TRACE-MIN-LYTE electrolyte drink with sea greens.) Or have a sea food dish, cous-cous, brown rice or spinach pasta with a light cheese sauce. And have Super Soup, with antioxidants and immune boosters: for two bowls, chop and cover with water in a soup pot, 1 cup broccoli, 1 leek (white parts) 2 cups peas, $^1/_2$ cup scallions, 4 cups chard leaves, $^1/_2$ cup fennel bulb, $^1/_2$ cup fresh parsley, 6 garlic cloves, 2 tsp. astragalus extract (or $^1/_4$ cup pieces astragalus bark), 6 cups vegetable stock, a pinch cayenne, 1 cup green cabbage, $^1/_4$ cup sea greens. Bring ingredients to a boil, simmer10 min. Let sit 20 minutes.

—**Before bed:** have a warm Red Star nutritional yeast broth or miso soup with sea greens snipped on top.

Don't forget water in your anti-stress program. Low water intake leads to dehydration. Dehydration contributes to stress because brain functions that depend on electrical energy become less efficient. Stress mobilizes primary nutrients and water out of body reserves. Basically, dehydration causes stress and stress causes further dehydration. Drink 8 glasses of water every day.

Recipes for your anti-stress program: •BREAKFAST and BRUNCH; •PROTEIN without MEAT; •SOUPS, LIQUID SALADS; •ENZYME FOODS; •SALADS; •MINERAL-RICH FOODS; •SANDWICHES; •HIGH FIBER FOODS.

Herb and Supplement Choices

• **Nerve relaxers and restorers:** Crystal Star RELAX™ caps and tea as needed, STRESSED OUT™ extract 2 to 3x daily; Deva Flowers ANXIETY drops; Black Cohosh extract drops.

• **Calm your mind:** Bach RESCUE REMEDY drops; Kava Kava extract or • Herb Pharm PHARMA-KAVA drops.

• **Rebuild and regenerate nerves:** Crystal Star MENTAL IN-NER ENERGY™ extract with ginseng and kava kava; Gotu kola or ginseng-gotu kola caps 4 daily; Siberian ginseng extract; Reishi mushroom extract; Bee pollen, 2 teasp. daily; Country Life MAXI B complex with taurine daily, or B complex 150mg with extra B-6 250mg daily; or Flora NERVE GUARD drops; Ester C 3000mg daily with bioflavonoids and rutin.

• **Minerals are dynamic nerve nourishers:** Nature's Plus MAGNESIUM-POTASSIUM-BROMELAIN caps; Rainbow Light CALCIUM PLUS with high magnesium; Crystal Star MINERAL SPECTRUM with sea greens; Nature's Path TRACE-MIN-LYTE daily. Morada Research NERVOUS SYSTEM nerve food.

• **EFA's repair nerves:** Evening primrose oil caps 4000 daily; EGG YOLK LECITHIN 3x daily, excellent results. Omega Nutrition ESSENTIAL BALANCE caps 3 daily, or DHA 200mg daily with magnesium 400mg 3x daily; Royal jelly 2 tsp. daily. Biotec PACIFIC SEA PLASMA, 8 daily.

• **Amino acids boost brain energy:** SAMe 400mg daily; Glutamine 1000mg daily; Country Life MOOD FACTORS caps or Anabol Naturals AMINO BALANCE; Tyrosine 500mg; DLPA 1000mg; GABA 1000mg to mimic valium without sedation.

• **Feed your adrenals:** Crystal Star ADR-ACTIVE™ caps, GIN-SENG/LICORICE ELIXIR™ drops; Planetary SCHIZANDRA adrenal support; Country Life RELAXER tabs for fast relief.

Bodywork and Lifestyle Techniques

• **Massage therapy once a month.** Hypnotherapy, aromatherapy, and shiatsu have all shown effective results against stress. Take baths with baking soda or sea salt.

• **Techniques** like yoga, meditation and massage therapy are wonderful for the nerves.

• **Quiet your mind** with deep, rhythmic breathing exercises every day.

• **Take a brisk walk** with deep breathing every day for body oxygen. Walk your dog.

• **Don't smoke.** Nicotine constricts the blood vessels, causing increased stress.

• **Go on a short vacation.** Take a long weekend. It will do wonders for your head.

• **Take a rest and relaxation period** every day. Listen to soft music. Meditate. Do 3 minutes of neck rolls.

• **Get early morning sunlight** on the body every day possible for purifying vitamin A and vitamin D.

• **Apply warm ginger compresses** to lower spine and stomach to stimulate systol/diastol activity.

• **Lose weight and stop smoking.** Tobacco and obesity both aggravate nerve disorders and tension.

• **Wear acupressure sandals** for a short period every day to clear reflexology meridians.

• **Aromatherapy nerve relaxer:** lavender oil. Or rub St. John's wort oil on the temples.

• **Relax your brain.** Gardening, crossword puzzles, hobbies, artwork, etc. can all relieve tension and anxiety.

• **Laughter is the best relief of all.** Have a good laugh every day.

Can't find a recommended product? Call the 800 number listed in Product Resources for the store nearest you and for more info.

Diet to Heal Your Headaches

Headaches don't fit into neat little diagnostic boxes. There have them. Natural remedies work extremely well for most headaches. Migraines are more than just bad headaches. They're a migraines, 75% of them women. Changes in estrogen levels migraine headaches for many women. Many vascular headache ods. Indeed, sometimes these work when nothing else does.

seem to be as many kinds and pathologies as there are people who aches because they normalize body chemistry (acid-alkaline balance). Upwards of 30 million Americans suffer from total body assault. Upwards of 30 million Americans suffer from during PMS, menopause or while using contraceptive drugs mean reactions can be successfully addressed by natural healing methods. Nutrition awareness is a must for preventing migraine headaches.

Analyze your headache:

—**Stress-anxiety headaches:** Pain over the eyes and eyestrain, a dull ache in the forehead and temples, inability to sleep, irritability, accompanied by neck aches and muscle tension.

—**Tension headaches:** Muscle contraction headaches of the scalp and back of the head, usually caused by stress or fatigue. They may last for hours or days and your head feels like it's in a vise. Most people find it hard to sleep. Tension headaches respond well to treatments like massage, relaxation techniques like acupressure, alternating hot and cold showers, and cold compresses.

—**Migraines:** Migraines mean constriction/dilation of brain, scalp and face blood vessels, lasting anywhere from 4 hours to two days, recurrent several times a month. Classic migraines are preceded by an aura, sudden sensitivity to smell and light, and visual problems; halos around lights; nausea and vomiting, made worse by light and movement; intense, lasting pain, usually on one side of the head; diarrhea, chills and fever. Common migraines have no aura, but much the same visual disturbances, changes in taste and smell, weakness and confusion as well as pain and fluid retention. **Migraines are also hormone-related.** Anxiety attacks, visual disturbances and temporary loss of taste or smell are all signs that a hormone-related migraine headache is imminent.

—**Cluster headaches:** Cluster headaches are clustered in time, two or more sudden, extremely painful headaches a day over the eyes or forehead. They usually affect men (connected to testosterone imbalance). There are no advance warning signs. Pain is severe and localized; blood vessels are dilated with irritated adjacent nerves; there are nasal histamine reactions as well as sensitivity to light and restlessness.

—**Sinus-neuralgia headaches:** Congestion and inflammation of the nasal sinuses. Some people feel as if their head is going to explode. If accompanied by neuralgia, a sinus headache becomes doubly painful.

1—Food allergies and intolerances are by far the biggest triggers for migraine headaches. **Avoid these known migraine triggers:** Pickled fish and shellfish, aged and smoked meats and other nitrate foods, aged cheeses, red wines, avocados, caffeine, chocolate, pizza, sourdough bread, sodas and refined sweeteners, MSG, soy sauce, citrus, peanuts, tomatoes.

2—**Other types of headaches also have trigger foods:** • Additive and chemical-laced foods; • Salty, sugary or wheat-based foods; • Excessive caffeine foods (withdrawal can be a precipitator); • Dairy foods, especially cheese; • Condiments, sulfites, MSG; • Too much alcohol, beer, wine; • Sodas (phosphorus binds up magnesium)

3—Use caffeine: At the first signs of migraine type headache: take 1-2 cups of strong coffee to prevent blood vessel dilation, or a glass of carrot-celery juice. Apply cold black tea bags to the eyes for 15 minutes. Or even just have a cup of black coffee.

4—Eat pain preventers: • High magnesium foods reduce throbbing: leafy greens, fresh sea foods and sea greens, nuts, whole grains, molasses. • Vitamin C rich foods: pineapple for bromelain, broccoli, peppers, sprouts, cherries. • Turkey for serotonin. • Almonds- 12 to 15 when you have a headache are enough for the salicin kick in.

Building Strength Against Stress and Tension

Go on a short 24 hour juice fast (pg. 570) to remove congestion - drink lots of water and lemon, veggie drinks (pg. 569) or potassium drinks (pg. 568). Follow the next day with an alkalizing diet: apples and apple juice, cranberry juice, sprouts, salads and some brown rice. Then follow the diet below for a month. The diet is alkalizing. Whole grains and vegetable proteins are abundant. Vitamin B rich foods, and high mineral foods with magnesium and iron help rebuild nerves. Salt and condiments are restricted. All processed and refined foods are omitted because they add to stress, and depletion of the adrenal glands.

—**On rising:** take a glass of lemon/honey/water, or other fresh fruit juice; and a vitamin/mineral drink such as All One MULTIPLE VITA-MINS & MINERALS or Crystal Star SYSTEMS STRENGTH DRINK™. Drink green tea daily or Crystal Star GREEN TEA CLEANSER™ as a preventive.

—**Breakfast:** have fresh fruit, like grapes, papaya, apples or grapefruit with yogurt and 1 teasp. each nutritional yeast, unsulphured molasses and toasted wheat germ to restore body balance; or have oatmeal or granola with the above mix and maple syrup.

—**Mid-morning:** have fresh carrot juice with $^1/_4$ teasp. sage powder; or a potassium broth or green drink, (pg. 569) with Bragg's LIQUID AMINOS; or red raspberry leaf herb tea; and some crunchy fresh veggies with a vegetable or kefir cheese dip.

—**Lunch:** have a broccoli quiche with a whole grain crust; or a large romaine or other leafy salad, with sprouts, celery, toasted sea greens and wheat germ; or a vegetable sandwich on whole grain bread; or marinated, baked tofu with brown rice; or a tuna or salmon salad or sandwich with green mayonnaise and lemon; or a whole grain or vegetable pasta salad, hot or cold.

—**Mid-afternoon:** have whole grain crackers, chips or raw vegetables with kefir cheese or a veggie dip; or some yogurt or kefir with fresh fruit; and a refreshing herb tea, like spearmint or lemongrass tea, or Crystal Star RELAX™ tea.

—**Dinner:** have baked, or grilled fish with a small green salad; or a large dinner salad with toasted almonds, seeds, wheat germ and yogurt dressing; or a seafood salad with baked potato or brown rice; or some steamed veggies with tofu and brown rice; or baked salmon with asparagus or peas and rice; or roast turkey with herb dressing.
Have a little white wine before dinner to relax and aid digestion.

—**Before bed:** take 1 teasp. miso or Red Star nutritional yeast in a cup of hot water for B vitamins and relaxation.

Recipes to help prevent headaches: •BREAKFAST and BRUNCH; •DAIRY-FREE COOKING; •HEALING DRINKS; •ENZYME-RICH FOODS; •HEALING DRINKS; •MINERAL-RICH FOODS; •LOW FAT FOODS; •HIGH FIBER FOODS.

Herb and Supplement Choices

• **Relieve tension headaches:** Crystal Star STRESSED OUT™ extract; Bromelain up to 1500mg -acts like aspirin without stomach upset; Enzymatic Therapy KAVA-TONE caps; Valerian-Wild Lettuce or Scullcap extract drops; Homeopathic Hylands Calms Forte; Gaia Herbs INFLA-PROFEN extract.

• **Control the pain:** For Migraines: Crystal Star MIGR-EASE™ caps (often works when nothing else does); Ginkgo biloba extract caps 6 daily; MICROHYDRIN, from Healthy House, especially for migraines. Crystal Star MIGR™ extract with feverfew, or Gaia Herbs MIGRA-PROFEN™ caps. DLPA 1000mg for natural endorphins. For Cluster Headaches: Take 1 ginger capsule at first sign of visual disturbance. Then take Crystal Star STRESSED OUT™ extract, with ASPIR-SOURCE™ caps for frontal lobe pain (usually results within 25 minutes). Rub •CAPSAICIN cream on temples or take Capsicum-Ginger capsules 4 daily,

• **Enhance nerve health:** Mineral-rich herbs provide bio-chemicals for neurotransmission. Crystal Star RELAX™ caps 2 as needed (relief felt in about 25 minutes). Nature's Plus QUERCETIN PLUS 500mg 2x daily with magnesium 500mg 2x daily, to prevent nerve twitching. Herbal Magic RELAXA HERBAL; Medicine Wheel STRESS EASE.

• **Magnesium-B-vitamin therapy:** Magnesium citrate 800mg daily with Country Life MAXI-B/taurine; Niacin therapy: 100mg as needed daily to keep blood vessels open.

• **Use balancing tonics:** Guayaki YERBA MATÉ green tea, an almost immediate tonic for stress headaches; Ginkgo Biloba extract capsules 6 daily; Country Life RELAXER caps.

• **Add EFA's:** Evening Primrose Oil 23000mg; rub Chinese WHITE FLOWER oil or TIGER BALM on forehead and temples.

Bodywork and Lifestyle Techniques

Note: If you have a history of heart problems, ask your doctor before taking migraine medicines that constrict blood vessels.

• **Take a brisk walk.** Breathe deeply. The more brain oxygen, the fewer headaches.

• **If you work under fluorescent light,** make sure bulbs don't flicker... it can bring on a blinding headache.

• **Ice it.** Apply an ice pack on back of the neck and upper back. Add a hot foot bath and pain reduction is dramatic.

• **Almost immediate results for migraines:** a coffee enema to stimulate liver and normalize bile activity; a bowel movement may relieve vomiting.

• **Aromatherapy for headaches:**
–Apply lavender oil on temples.
–Apply peppermint oil on temples.
–Apply eucalyptus for sinus headaches.

• **Effective physical therapies:**
–Chiropractic manipulation
–Acupuncture and acupressure
–Massage therapy
–Biofeedback/relaxation training
–Deep breathing exercises
–Fresh air and exercise
–Magnet therapy is effective for migraines.

• **Reflexology therapy:** 1) Apply pressure to inside base of the big toe 3 times for 10 seconds each time. 2) Massage temples for 5 minutes. Breathe deeply. Do 10 neck rolls. 3) Pull ear lobes for 5 seconds. Rub all around ear shell. 4) Hold hand open, palm down; massage flesh between thumb and forefinger with other hand. Pain should recede immediately.

360

Can't find a recommended product? Call the 800 number listed in Product Resources for the store nearest you and for more info.

Healing Fatigue Syndromes

Immune breakdown diseases are the plagues of our modern era. Immune exhaustion syndromes like candida, chronic fatigue syndrome, Hashimoto's, fibromyalgia and lupus are at a crisis point. They affect a woman's delicate body balance most. They are way under-diagnosed and they're reaching epidemic proportions. Most of us don't have very much to fight with. It's a big reason we're having so much trouble with our health care system today. I believe we're looking at medicine from the wrong end of the telescope. Modern medicine is only concerned with sickness. All drugs are formulated for, and marketed to, someone who is sick. All lab testing is done on infected, sick cells. We never look to see how a drug might affect healthy cells, or someone who is not sick.

Conventional medicine has been unable to cure or even to make a difference, in immune breakdown diseases. Here's why: genetic scientists and immunology experts tell us that each person has a unique immune system, that it springs from our unique DNA make-up and works uniquely for us. It's easy to see how impossible it would be to manufacture a drug that would work for everyone.... or even more than one person.

Maintaining strong immune response in today's world mental pollutants, the excessive stresses of modern all a challenge to your immune defenses. Drugs in your pect: Make no mistake, drugs can't normalize or nourish that, through your body's enzyme activity. Drugs work ference against a harmful process that's happening in your ful events in order to arrest a serious conclusion.

is becoming a constant battle. Daily exposure to environmental lifestyles, chemicalized foods, and new virus mutations are medicine cabinet, even modern medical "miracles" are suspect: you. Only your own immune powers, or your food can do exactly the opposite from foods. They run powerful interbody in order to stabilize it. They disrupt a cascade of harm-

The problem for your immune system is that drugs keep the interference process going. Over the long term, they tend to work against your body, hitting its delicate balance with a disruptive hammer. (That's one of the reasons you might have gotten good results from a drug at first, and poorer results as time went on.) Your body, especially your immune system, keeps trying to normalize itself- but it can't. As the disruption process goes on over time, with an overload of antibiotics, antacids, immunizations, and steroid drugs, your body gets further and further from normal. (As an example, Americans take over 85 million aspirin alone every single day.) Finally your immune response doesn't know what is normal. It cannot distinguish harmful cells from healthy cells- and ends up attacking the wrong elements, or everything, in confusion.

Chronic fatigue syndromes act like recurring systemic viral infections, viruses that often go undetected because their symptoms mimic simple illnesses like colds, flu, or acute, but less debilitating, mononucleosis. Following the acute stages these retro-viruses penetrate the nuclei of immune system T-cells where they are able to survive and replicate indefinitely. Multiplication of the virus and recurring symptoms appear with a rupturing of the organism and its release into the bloodstream. This can occur at any time, but almost always arises when a person is under stress or has reduced immune response due to a simpler illness such as a cold or cough.

Overcoming Candida Yeast Infection

Candida infection is rampant in American society today - mostly for women who try to be "wonder women," to do it all, and in the effort, severely compromise their immune response. Researchers see new ties between Candida overgrowth and many seemingly unrelated problems, like sexually transmitted diseases in both men and women, and ear infections and hyperactivity in children.

I've worked with Candida and leaky gut syndrome for over 2 decades. No program to overcome Candida yeasts will work for long without serious lifestyle and diet changes. Herbal medicines provide critical body support to restore your immune system. Candida albicans is a strain of yeast which inhabits the gastrointestinal and genito-urinary tracts. It is not normally harmful, but when immune response is weak, Candida flourishes by voraciously feeding on the excessive sugars in the American diet, infecting the entire body.

Candida is strongly tied to a body out of balance; it is caused largely by a lot of refined foods in your diet (especially junky, low nutrient foods), too much alcohol, too little rest and over-use of medications like antibiotics, birth control pills and steroid drugs that encourage fungal growth because they depress immunity. Most sufferers have the classic symptoms of extreme fatigue, digestive upsets like diarrhea, gas and bloating, and chronic vaginal yeast infections.

Leaky gut syndrome is usually a result of chronic exposure to candida yeast toxins which damage the intestinal lining. Yeast toxins and waste products then "leak" out through the impaired intestinal walls and infect surrounding tissue. Leaky gut syndrome compounds candida infection because it introduces yeast toxins to the rest of the body. Leaky gut is the link to the depression, headaches, joint and connective tissue inflammation, and irritable bowel syndrome that candida sufferers experience.

Is your lifestyle promoting Candida? 1) Poor diet - especially excessive intake of sugar, starchy foods, yeasted breads and chemicalized foods. 2) Repeated use of antibiotics—long use of antibiotics kills protective bacteria (that keep candida under control). 3) Hormone medications like corticosteroid drugs and birth control pills. 4) A high stress life, too much alcohol, too little rest.

Do you have a Candida infection?

Most of the orthodox medical world still chooses not to recognize, diagnose or treat Candidiasis seriously. It's no wonder since three out of the four main contributors - overuse of antibiotics, excess consumption of sugar, mercury dental fillings and birth control pills come from medical practice. Low success rates and a lack of understanding mean that the alternative professions of naturopathy, homeopathy, chiropractic and massage therapy deal with most cases. Their energy and dedication have dramatically advanced current knowledge about Candidiasis and its companion diseases, to shorten healing time, lessen overkill, and to recognize the overriding psychological aspects of the disease.

Candida may infect virtually any part of the body. The most commonly involved sites include the nail beds, skin folds, feet, mouth, sinuses, ear canal, belly button, esophagus, intestine, vaginal tract and urethra. Candida also infects deep internal organs. Likely sites of infection include the thyroid and adrenal glands, kidneys, bladder, bowel, esophagus, uterus, lungs and bone marrow.

Do you see the signs of a candida infection?

—Do you have recurrent digestive problems, gas, bloating or flatulence?
—Do you have rectal itching, or chronic constipation alternating to diarrhea?
—Do you have a white coating on your tongue (thrush)?
—Have you been unusually irritable or depressed? Do you have unexplained frequent headaches, muscle aches and joint pain?
—Do you feel sick all over, yet the cause cannot be found? Are the symptoms worse on muggy days?
—Has your memory been noticeably poor? Are you finding it hard to concentrate or focus your thoughts?
—Do you have chronic vaginal yeast infections or frequent bladder infections?
—If you are a woman, do you have serious PMS or other menstrual problems? Do you have endometriosis?
—If you are a man, do you have abdominal pains, muscle pain, prostatitis, or loss of sexual interest?
—Do you have chronic fungal infections like ringworm, jock itch, nail fungus or athlete's foot?
—Do you have psoriasis, eczema or chronic dermatitis? Are you bothered by erratic vision or spots before the eyes?
—Do you catch frequent colds that take many weeks to go away?
—Are you oversensitive to chemicals, tobacco, perfume or insecticides? Do you crave sugar, bread, or alcoholic beverages?
—Have you recently taken repeated rounds of antibiotics or corticosteroid drugs for a month or more, like Symycin, Panmycin, Decadron or Prednisone, or acne drugs?

Note: Not everyone can detect if they have Candida overgrowth. Candida can mimic the symptoms of over 140 different disorders. For instance, chronic fatigue syndrome, salmonella, intestinal parasite infestation and mononucleosis exhibit similar symptoms, but are treated very differently. Get a candida test before starting a healing program to save time and expense. Call Antibody Assay Labs (1-800-522-2611), for a blood test that includes both candida immune complexes and candida antibodies. For information on electrodermal candida screening, call Harmony Health Systems (770-345-6614).

The longer you wait to begin a candida detox and healing program, the harder the job becomes. Start now if you think you have candida. Here's what you'll be doing on a candida cleanse:

1: **Killing the candida yeasts:** The diet and supplement program will kill the yeasts. Avoid antibiotics, corticosteroid drugs and birth control pills, unless there is absolute medical need, so you don't get re-infected.

2: **Eliminating the dead yeasts from your body:** The cleansing diet and cleansing products will release the dead yeasts and their waste from the body. Enemas or colonics will expedite their removal.

3: **Rebuilding your normal systemic environment and immune defenses:** The program will strengthen your digestive system by enhancing its ability to assimilate nutrients. Afflicted organs, especially the liver, and glands will be strengthened. Metabolism will normalize and probiotic supplementation will promote friendly bacteria in the gastrointestinal tract.

Getting rid of a candida yeast infection is tough. If you have candida, you've probably already found out, conventional anti-fungal therapy for Candida delivers only temporary results. Drug therapy for candidiasis uses Nystatin, Ketaconazole and other antifungal products to try and kill the yeast invader. But this method only relieves the ill effects of candidiasis while the drug is being taken. It doesn't address the root of the problem, body chemistry imbalance, so there's almost always a candida relapse. Many of the drugs further suppress the immune system. An effective program must not only kill the yeasts but also strengthen the body's own immune defense mechanisms to keep candida under control. Empowering your immune response is the real key to overcoming candida. Natural therapies work far better because body balance is what they do best.

Here's a natural candida therapy program with a tried and true success rate:

• **For the first 6 weeks, you must eliminate all foods that Candida albicans thrives on.** I have structured a diet that starves the yeast but still nourishes your body with essential nutrients to re-establish normal balance. See the next page for full details and information.

• **Kill the yeasts and eliminate them from the body with herbal and enzyme therapy.** An herbal formula containing pau d'arco bark and garlic is a powerful anti-fungal remedy. Consider Crystal Star's CAND-EX™ Caps, 4 caps daily for 3 months, or Rainbow Light CANDIDA CLEANSE. (Both contain herbal yeast killers, anti-parasite factors, "friendly flora" support, and plant enzymes). Proteases assist our immune systems in the job of hydrolyzing (destroying) fungal, bacterial, viral and parasitic organisms. Plant protease, such as Transformation PUREZYME help strengthen the body's defense against Candida.

• **Keep candida in check by boosting friendly bacteria.** Antibiotics deplete friendly G.I. bacteria. Besides probiotics and enzyme supplements, cultured vegetables replenish friendly bacteria. Try Rejuvenative Foods RAW SAUERKRAUT or KIM CHEE.

• **Clear up vaginal yeast infections caused by candida with natural anti-fungals.** Herbs like *tea tree oil* work better than over-the-counter drugs like tioconazole (Monistat) or clotrimazole (Gyne-Lotrimin), which have a backfire history, allowing yeasts to develop drug-resistant strains. Instead try TEA TREE OIL suppositories by Thursday Plantation. Or, use acidophilus powder as a douche. Mix $1/_2$ teasp. into douche water.

• **Restore intestinal integrity.** L-glutamine, 2000mg daily, rebuilds healthy intestinal mucosa to prevent candida toxins from leaking into the bloodstream. Glutamine synthesizes N-Acetyl-Glucosamine (NAG), the principal constituent of the mucopolysaccharides involved in maintaining gastrointestinal structural integrity. NAG itself, 1 TB 2 times daily, is a valuable gut protector which promotes the growth of friendly bacteria while blocking Candida yeast.

• **Strengthen your liver** so it can filter candida toxins from your blood. Add B-complex 100mg to your daily program.

• **All candida sufferers have exhausted adrenals.** That's why they feel so tired. Herbs like licorice rt. and sarsaparilla can recharge adrenal health. Crystal Star ADRN™ extract, 15 drops under the tongue 2x daily, or ADRENOTONIC by Herbs, Etc.

• **Get plenty of rest!** Too much stress and too little rest are Candida relapse triggers. Daily R & R is critical for long-term recovery.

Note: It can take up to 6 months to rebuild your health from a candida infection. Some people feel better right away. Others experience a short "healing crisis" (usually a sign that toxic yeasts are being cleared from the body), characterized by headaches, skin rashes and poor digestion. (Yeasts are living organisms, part of your body. Killing them off can be traumatic.) The rewards of renewed vitality and health are well worth it.

Candida Yeast Cleansing Diet (a four to six week diet plan)

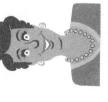

The food recommendations for the initial diet are critical for reducing candida yeast proliferation to normal levels. To overcome a candida infection, your diet must simultaneously nourish your body while starving candida of the foods that support its growth.

—**Do not eat the following foods for the first month to 6 weeks:** Sugar or sweeteners of any kind, gluten bread and yeasted baked goods, dairy products (except plain kefir or kefir cheese, yogurt or yogurt cheese), smoked, dried, pickled or cured foods, mushrooms (except anti-fungal shiitakes), nuts or nut butters (except almonds or almond butter), fruits, fruit juices, dried or candied fruits, coffee, black tea, carbonated drinks (phosphoric acid binds up calcium and magnesium), alcohol or foods containing vinegar. Avoid antibiotics, steroid and cortico-steroid drugs, and tobacco. This is a long, restrictive list, but for the first critical weeks, when energy-sapping yeasts must be deprived of nutrients and killed off, it is the only way.

—**Acceptable foods during the first stage:** Fresh and steamed veggies (especially onions, garlic, ginger, cabbage, and broccoli), raw cultured sauerkraut, poultry, seafoods and sea greens, olive oil, eggs, mayonnaise, brown rice, amaranth, buckwheat, barley, millet, miso soup and tofu, vegetable pastas, plain or vanilla yogurt, rice cakes-crackers, some citrus fruit and herb teas. Have a green drink, green tea and miso soup every day. This is a short list, but diet restriction is the most important way to stop candida yeast overgrowth. Note: Drink 8-10 glasses of bottled water each day of your cleanse (can include herbal teas). Water lubricates and flushes wastes, toxins and dead yeast cells from the body.

—**On rising:** take 2 tsp. cranberry concentrate, with 1 tsp. cider vinegar and 1 tsp. maple syrup in water; or a fiber cleanser like AloeLife FIBERMATE or Crystal Star FIBER & HERBS CLEANSE™; or a cup of Crystal Star GREEN TEA CLEANSER™, or Gaia Herbs 2 week CANDIDA SUPREME VITAL CLEANSE.

—**Breakfast:** a veggie omelette with broccoli; or scrambled eggs with onion, shiitake mushrooms and peppers; or brown rice with onions and carrots; or oatmeal with 1 TB Bragg's LIQUID AMINOS; or oatmeal sweetened with stevia and sauteed veggies.

—**Mid-morning:** have a vegetable drink (page 569) with Monas CHLORELLA or Omega Nutrition VITALITY SUPERGREEN or Crystal Star SYSTEMS STRENGTH™; or a cup of miso soup with sea greens; and a cup of echinacea or chamomile tea.

—**Lunch:** have a fresh green salad with lemon/coconut, olive or flax oil dressing and seafood, chicken or turkey; or a vegetable or miso soup with sea greens; or steamed veggies with brown rice.

—**Mid-afternoon:** have potato corn chowder with crackers; or some raw veggies dipped in lemon/coconut, olive, or flax oil dressing; or mineral water and hard boiled egg with sea vegetable seasoning.

—**Dinner:** have broiled fish or chicken with raw sauerkraut or green beans; or steamed vegetables or baked potato sprinkled with sea greens and Bragg's LIQUID AMINOS; or a vegetable stir fry with brown rice, sea veggies and miso soup.

—**Before Bed:** chamomile tea, Red Star nutritional yeast in water, or miso soup with sea greens.

Recipes to help a candida cleansing diet: •DETOXIFICATION FOODS; •HEALING DRINKS; •SOUPS, LIQUID SALADS; •ENZYME-RICH FOODS; •SALADS, HOT and COLD; •MINERAL-RICH •LIGHT MACROBIOTIC EATING.

After your candida cleanse..... keep candida yeast under control

The candida healing-rebuilding process usually takes from 3-6 months for the excess yeasts to be eliminated and friendly flora re-established. Strong immune response, a vital liver and robust colonies of friendly intestinal bacteria are critical to lasting control. The changes in diet, habits and lifestyle are often radical. But most people with candidiasis infection are feeling so bad anyway, that treating the yeasts and the knowledge that they are getting better, pulls them through the hard times. Give yourself all the time you need, at least up to 6 months. Be as gentle with your body as you can. Multiple therapies all at once can be self-defeating, psychologically upsetting, and traumatic on your system. Just stick to it and go at your own pace.

I have been working successfully with candidiasis since 1984 and have found repeatedly that a too-rigid diet does not work over the long term, because the sufferer cannot stick to it (except in a very restricted, isolated environment), and the body becomes imbalanced in other ways. In fact, the disease itself, and the immune response to it, are changing as well. The new candida cleansing program here has been modified to meet changing needs and to take advantage of an ever-widening network of information.

Watchwords to live by for the next six months:

1: **Eat plenty of beta-carotene-rich foods,** and iodine and potassium-rich foods. They are the most effective food nutrients against candida. My favorite food for these nutrients is sea vegetables - all kinds, in soups, on rice or a healthy pizza, or in a salad.

2: **Use raw sauerkraut in your diet.** It is a superfood for conquering candida. Dr. Elson M. Haas, M.D., director of the Preventive Medical Center of Marin, CA., Gary Ross, M.D. of Health & Medical Clinic of San Francisco, CA, nutritional authority Donna Gates, and many other candida experts report amazing accounts of candida sufferers who report substantial improvement in their condition after eating cultured vegetables (raw sauerkraut). Use Rejuvenative Foods RAW SAUERKRAUT or VEGI-DELITE, or make the cultured vegetables yourself. For an effective recipe, call BODY ECOLOGY 360-384-1238; E-mail bodyeco@aol.com; www.bodyecology.net.

3: **Eat alkalizing foods**... about 80% alkaline-forming foods and 20% acid-forming foods. Alkalizing foods: fresh, steamed, baked or grilled vegetables, sea greens, brown rice, millet, quinoa, and amaranth, herbs and herb teas, sprouts and seeds (except sesame seeds), lemons, limes, unsweetened cranberries, cultured foods (like raw cultured veggies, yogurt, kefir, apple cider vinegar), and almonds. Acid-forming foods to avoid: animal foods like beef, poultry, eggs, fish and shellfish, buckwheat, and unrefined oils. Note: Nutritional yeast does not cause or aggravate candida albicans yeast overgrowth. It is one of the best immune-enhancing foods available.

4: **Eat three to four small meals a day.** Be careful not to overeat or you will divert your body's energy from cleansing to digestion.

5: **Restricting all sugar in your permanent diet is essential**... this means: fruits (except those listed above), all sugary foods or sweeteners (Equal, NutraSweet, etc.), soft drinks, wheat flour foods, beans, tofu, nuts and nut butters, all alcoholic beverages, commercial vinegars or condiments. If you crave sweets, use the herb Stevia in your tea.

6: **Watch your food-combinations.** Excess yeasts will not disappear if you are combining foods that aren't compatible. Instead, they'll ferment, produce sugars and alcohol, and feed the yeast. People with candidiasis have weak digestion, so good food combining is even more important. (See page 398 for a Food Combining Chart.)

Candida 3-Month Healing Diet

Diet change is the most effective way to rebuild strength and immunity from candida overgrowth. Clinical testing shows that a program with plant enzyme therapy, probiotics, certain herbal extracts and organic minerals is effective in treating candida. The initial cleansing diet here concentrates on releasing dead yeast cells from the body. This phase may require 2-3 months for complete cleansing. It may also be used as the basis for a "rotation diet," in which you slowly add back individual foods during healing that caused an allergic reaction to candida. As you start to see improvement, and symptoms decrease (usually after two months), start to add back some whole grains, fruits, juices, a little white wine, some fresh cheeses, nuts and beans. Go slowly, add gradually. Test for food sensitivity all along the way until it is gone. Don't forget that sugars and refined foods will allow candida to grow again.

Note: Superfood therapy is critical to success with candida: add often, any time. - Crystal Star ENERGY GREEN™; Unipro PERFECT PROTEIN; Nutricology PROGREENS with EFA's; Futurebiotics VITAL K; Omega Nutrition VITALITY SUPERGREEN; Green Foods GREEN MAGMA.

On rising: take 2 tsp. cranberry concentrate, or 2 tsp. lemon juice in water, or a fiber cleanser like AloeLife FIBERMATE or Crystal Star FIBER & HERBS CLEANSE™, or a cup of Crystal Star GREEN TEA CLEANSER™ if you have gas.

Breakfast: take ALL 1 VITAMIN/MINERAL drink in water; then take 1 or 2 poached or hard boiled eggs on rice cakes with butter or flax oil; or almond butter on rice cakes or wheat free bread; or oatmeal with 1 TB Bragg's LIQUID AMINOS; or amaranth or buckwheat pancakes with a little butter and vanilla; or a vegetable omelette with broccoli; or scrambled eggs with onion, shiitake mushrooms and red pepper; or brown rice with onions and carrots; or oatmeal or cream of buckwheat.

Mid-morning: a vegetable drink (page 569), see note above, or Monas CHLORELLA, or Crystal Star SYSTEMS STRENGTH™; a cup of miso soup with sea greens snipped on top; or a cup of pau d'arco tea, echinacea or chamomile tea, or mineral water.

Lunch: have a green salad with lemon-coconut oil, olive or flax oil dressing, some seafood, chicken or turkey; or a vegetable or miso soup with sea greens snipped on top with butter and cornbread; Rejuvenative Foods VEGI DELITE cultured veggies; or steamed veggies with brown rice; or open face, wheat-free bread, with mayonnaise or butter, veggies, seafood, or turkey.

Mid-afternoon: have some rice crackers, or baked corn chips, with a little kefir cheese or butter; or some raw veggies dipped in lemon-oil dressing or spiced mayonnaise; or a small mineral water and hard boiled or deviled egg with sea greens seasoning.

Dinner: baked, broiled or poached fish or chicken with steamed brown rice or millet with flax oil and veggies; or a tofu and veggie casserole with sea greens; or a baked potato with Bragg's LIQUID AMINOS, or a vegetable stir fry with brown rice, sea greens and a miso or light broth soup; or a vegetarian, chapati crust pizza with snipped sea greens on top; or chicken, tuna or wheat-free pasta salad, with mayonnaise or lemon/oil dressing.

Before bed: have herb tea - chamomile, peppermint, or Crystal Star AFTER MEAL ENZ™ extract drops in water, or miso soup.

Recipes to help your candida healing diet: •SUGAR-FREE SPECIALS; •HEALING DRINKS; •BREAKFAST; •CULTURED HEALING FOODS; •WHEAT-FREE BAKING; •DAIRY-FREE COOKING; •LIGHT MACROBIOTIC EATING.

Herb and Supplement Choices

• *Rotate anti-yeast and anti-fungal products, so that yeast strains don't build up resistance to any one formula.*

Kill the yeasts: Pau d'arco tea, 4 cups daily (also soak nails for nail fungus, or use as a douche for vaginal fungus); Echinacea extract or echinacea-barberry extract (if diarrhea), 15 drops 4x daily; Crystal Star CAND-EX™ caps, 6 daily with CRAN-PLUS™ tea. Add *Black Walnut* extract and *Garlic* 10 capsules daily; *Olive Leaf* extract eats candida - East Park Olive Leaf extract or Nutricology PROLIVE, up to 1500mg daily; Nature's Secret CANDISTROY or Omega Nutrition ECO RENEW. Transformation PUREZYME helps destroy Candida.

Clean out the dead yeasts and parasites: Crystal Star BWL-TONE IBS™ caps; Renew Life PARAGONE.

Detoxify the liver: Crystal Star LIV-ALIVE™ caps; Pure Planet RED MARINE ALGAE PLUS, or 2 TBS snipped sea greens daily; Milk Thistle Seed extract; Planetary TRIPHALA caps.

Enhance adrenal and thyroid activity: Crystal Star SYSTEMS STRENGTH™ drink; Crystal Star ADR-ACTIVE™ caps or Enzymatic Therapy ADRENAL complex; Biotin 1000mcg with Nature's Secret ULTIMATE B tabs, and taurine 500mg.

Fight fungus, inhibit yeast overgrowth with EFA's: Evening Primrose Oil, 1000mg 4 daily; Solaray CAPRYL, or Solgar caprylic acid up to 1200mg; Oregano oil, 1 drop 2x daily in 1 tsp. flax oil; Coconut oil is a rich source of caprylic acid with 50% lauric acid - Omega Nutrition COCONUT OIL.

Probiotics re-establish internal balance: Omega Nutrition ECO RENEW; UAS DDS-PLUS with FOS.

Enzyme therapy for allergies: Bromelain 1500mg daily; Transformation PUREZYME; Glutamine to increase IgA levels.

Bodywork and Lifestyle Techniques

Use applied kinesiology to test for food and product sensitivities - a significant concern for candida sufferers.

Avoid antibiotics, birth control pills and steroids unless absolutely necessary.

Enema: Take an enema the night before or the morning of your cleanse. Flushing the colon is one of the best ways to jump start a candida cleanse because it immediately begins the release of dead yeast cells and toxins from the body.

Irrigate: Have at least one colonic during your cleanse for best results.

Healing vitamin D sunlight therapy: Get 15 minutes of early morning sun every day to synthesize vitamin D in the body for immune response and body strength.

Exercise: Take a brisk walk for more body oxygen, and a positive mind and outlook. They are essential to overcoming candida body stress. Try a good hearty laugh every day.

Rest: Candida infection often means interrupted sleep patterns. Adequate rest is primary for the body to overcome debilitating, yeast-induced fatigue.

Flower remedies work extremely well for candida sufferers: Natural Labs Deva Flower CLEANSING REMEDY or FEAR-FULNESS (dread is a primary emotion described by candida and chronic fatigue syndrome victims); Nelson Bach RESCUE REMEDY (for stress).

Microcurrent therapy: Patents have been awarded documenting that microcurrents neutralize pathogens, fungi, virus, bacteria, and parasites. Call Sota Instruments for information on this subject - 800-224-0242.

Can't find a recommended product? Call the 800 number listed in Product Resources for the store nearest you and for more info.

Healing Hashimoto's

Hashimoto's is an autoimmune disorder where the immune system suddenly attacks healthy tissue. The thyroid bears the brunt of this disease. Hashimoto's is the most frequent cause of hypothyroidism (low thyroid), and the most common cause of enlarged thyroid (goiter) in America. Iodine depletion from X-rays or low dose radiation (like mammograms) may be a prime factor in development of the disorder. Hashimoto's is related to disorders like diabetes, adrenal exhaustion, Graves' disease and vitiligo. At its worst, Hashimoto's can completely destroy the thyroid gland. Most prevalent in menopausal women (usually with high stress lives), almost one in ten women over the age of 65 have early-stage hypothyroidism clearly linked to Hashimoto's! I myself have seen numerous instances of Hashimoto's in the Southern California entertainment industry in both men and women. In fact, for a long time, Hashimoto's was being defined as a high-stress, deadline-driven disease because it so often occurred in people with high pressure media jobs.

The disease is on the rise as environmental chemicals add their effects to thyroid health and balance. New cases come from war-torn areas like Southeast Asia. Surprising numbers have been recorded in young women (between 16 and 35) in the Middle East since the Gulf War's pollution. Experts speculate that Eastern Europe will soon show thyroid health problems from the Bosnia-Kosovo-Chechneya conflicts where military chemicals damage air, water and food supplies.

Do you think you might have Hashimoto's?

While Hashimoto's itself is generally painless, an unbalanced thyroid invariably causes over-production of estrogen and its attendant problems for women (like painful fibroids, sore breasts, endometriosis and excess bleeding during and between periods).

   —Are you always depressed and tired for no reason? Have you lost your enthusiasm for life?
   —Do you have unexplained weight gain?
   —Are you overly sensitive to cold?
   —Do you have chronic constipation?
   —Is your skin and hair unusually dry? Do you have thin falling hair? Are your nails unusually brittle?

Hashimoto's hypothyroidism can be easily determined by a medical blood test. But the conventional medical treatment is a lifelong prescription of synthetic thyroid hormone. For many women especially, the drug of choice, Synthroid is linked to severe headaches, insomnia, bone loss and rapid heart contractions. Natural treatments for Hashimoto's focus on rebalancing glandular health, reducing symptoms and normalizing immune response. Shifting the emphasis away from drugs toward natural therapies can greatly raise your own healing capacities.

If you're under treatment for Hashimoto's, consult your physician. A glandular product may be an effective alternative to hormone replacement drugs like Synthroid: Nutricology's TG100 Organic Glandulars. (800-545-9960) Note: In some states, you'll need a prescription from a licensed health practitioner for this type of glandular compound. Note: Do not take iron supplements along with thyroid hormone medication.

Hashimoto's Healing Diet

A fresh foods, immune-boosting diet full of fruits and vegetables is the mainstay of protection and treatment for this disease. Its focus is on rebuilding immune strength to promote normal metabolism and defense against recurrence. If you already have Hashimoto's, avoid "goitrogen" foods that prevent your body's use of iodine, like cabbage, turnips, peanuts, mustard, pine nuts, millet, tempeh and tofu. (Cooking these foods inactivates the goitrogens.) Avoid saturated fats, sugars, white flour and red meats.

Watchwords:

1—Take a veggie drink (pg. 569) or a potassium drink (pg. 568), or a green drink like Crystal Star SYSTEMS STRENGTH™ drink, Green Kamut JUST BARLEY, Omega Nutrition VITALITY SUPER GREENS or Transitions EASY GREENS drink several times weekly.

2—Avoid table salt, but eat plenty of iodine-rich foods: sea greens (2 TBS daily over rice, soup or a salad), sea foods, fish, mushrooms, garlic, onions and watercress.

3—Eat vitamin A-rich foods: yellow vegetables, eggs, carrots, dark greens.

4—Watch your water. Cancer of the thyroid has been linked to highly fluoridated water.

—**On rising:** take 2 TBS cranberry concentrate in a glass of water; or ALL 1 VITAMIN/MINERAL drink, or Nature's Plus SPIRUTEIN.

—**Breakfast:** have grapefruit, pineapple, papaya or other fresh fruit; or yogurt with fresh fruit on top; or poached, baked or scrambled eggs with cottage cheese, and whole grain toast or muffins with a little butter; or oatmeal with a little vanilla and butter or Bragg's LIQUID AMINOS; or whole grain pancakes or granola with apple juice, and yogurt or kefir with fresh fruit.

—**Mid-morning:** have a green drink (page 569) or Monas CHLORELLA drink with 1 teasp. Bragg's LIQUID AMINOS; or a small bottle of mineral water with a piece of fresh fruit; or an herb tea, like Crystal Star HIGH ENERGY™ or FEEL GREAT TEA™.

—**Lunch:** have a green salad with Italian or non-dairy light dressing; and a veggie sandwich on whole grain bread; or a light Asian ramen noodle soup and stir-fried vegetables; or a baked potato with a little butter, and a green salad; or seafood and vegetable pasta with a light dressing and a green salad; or a whole grain chapati or burrito with a bean or veggie filling.

—**Mid-afternoon:** have an herb tea such as Crystal Star RELAX™ TEA; or fresh carrot juice; and a hard boiled or deviled egg with sesame salt, a non-dairy dip, and baked chips; or a cup of miso or other light soup with sea greens snipped on top.

—**Dinner:** have baked or grilled, fish, chicken or turkey, with steamed veggies and rice; or a spinach pasta and veggie casserole; or an oriental stir-fry with miso soup and sea greens; or a light Italian vegetable meal with whole grain or vegetable pasta, and a light vegetable soup; or a light egg dish with white wine and yogurt sauce in place of dairy, and a green salad.

—**Before bed:** have a cup of relaxing herb tea, such as chamomile, or Crystal Star GOOD NIGHT™ TEA; or a teasp. of Red Star nutritional yeast in a cup hot water, for relaxation and B vitamins.

Recipes to help your Hashimoto's diet: •**BLENDING EAST and WEST FOODS;** •**HEALING DRINKS;** •**SOUPS, LIQUID SALADS;** •**ENZYME-RICH FOODS;** •**SALADS;** •**FISH and SEAFOODS;** •**LIGHT MACROBIOTICS.**

Herb and Supplement Choices

• **Raw glandular therapy helps dramatically:** Nutricology TG-100 capsules (highly recommended); Nutri-PAK thyroxin-free double strength thyroid; Premier Labs RAW THYROID complex; Enzymatic Therapy THYROID/TYROSINE COMPLEX; or Tyrosine 500mg with Lysine 500mg 2x daily.

• **Herbal iodine reduces goiter symptoms and balances thyroid activity without side effects:** Add sea greens first - kelp, dulse and nori, rich in natural iodine, 2 TBS daily; or New Chapter OCEAN HERBS; Crystal Star IODINE SOURCE™ extract or IODINE/POTASSIUM™ caps; Nature's Path TRACE-MIN-LYTE. Add 2 cups of burdock tea daily to flush the liver, and EVENING PRIMROSE OIL, 1000mg 4 daily, for EFAs.

• **Boost your adrenals:** Adrenal health and thyroid balance go hand in hand in Hashimoto's. Add sea greens. (See above.) Crystal Star ADRN-ACTIVE™ (almost immediate energy).

• **Treat constipation:** Herbal bowel cleansers like aloe vera, slippery elm and marshmallow rt. don't create dependency; Crystal Star BWL-TONE I.B.S.™, or Rainbow Light EVERYDAY FIBER SYSTEM; Vitamin C with bioflavonoids 3000mg daily.

• **Hashimoto's can accelerate atherosclerosis.** Boost circulation and repair nerves: *Hawthorn* and *Ginkgo Biloba* extracts 3x daily; CoQ$_{10}$ 100mg daily; *Gotu kola* extract caps, 6 daily; *Siberian Ginseng* extract 2x daily; *Cayenne* caps 3 daily.

• **For dry skin:** Herbal Answers HERBAL ALOE FORCE GEL

• **For thyroid-related hair loss:** Feed your hair - sea greens for minerals and EFA's, 2 TBS daily, or Nature's Path TRACE-MIN-LYTE, or Crystal Star IODINE-POTASSIUM caps; B-vitamins 150mg daily for 2 months or molasses 2 TBS daily; cysteine 2000mg daily; *Ginkgo Biloba* extract 120mg daily.

Bodywork and Lifestyle Techniques

• The drug *levothyroxine*, frequently given for hypothyroidism can cause significant bone loss. Ask your doctor. Avoid antihistamines and sulfa drugs.

• **Take a brisk half hour walk daily;** exercise increases metabolism and stimulates circulation.

• **Sun bathe in the morning.** Sea bathe and wade whenever possible.

• **Avoid fluorescent lights and fluoride toothpaste.** They deplete vitamin A in the body. If you work under fluorescents, take Emulsified A 25,000IU 3x daily, or beta carotene 100,000IU daily, with vitamin E 400IU daily.

• **For goiter:** Apply BLACK WALNUT extract as a throat paint, and take $\frac{1}{2}$ dropperful 2x daily; or apply calendula compresses twice a day for a month.

• **Thyroid acupressure point:** Press hollow at base of the throat to stimulate thyroid, 3x for 10 seconds each.

Can't find a recommended product? Call the 800 number listed in Product Resources for the store nearest you and for more info.

Healing Fibromyalgia

Fibromyalgia is an arthritic muscle disease that has taken over the lives of more than 10 million midlife American women. Our parents and grandparents called it rheumatism. But, fibromyalgia has the added problem of exhaustive fatigue and 70% of fibromyalgia sufferers share symptoms with Chronic Fatigue Syndrome (CFS), TMJ, and rheumatoid arthritis, such as pain all over the body with tender spots that hurt when pressed. There is considerable depression that often involves deep-seated resentment, and chronic headaches with nerve and hormone imbalances that impair deep sleep. A stress-related immune disorder, the central cause seems to be a low level of serotonin in the brain and reduced growth hormone. Regular exposure to chemical contaminants, a high-stress lifestyle, and deficiencies in key nutrients, like magnesium, manganese, vitamin B-1 and antioxidants are also consistently a problem for Fibromyalgia sufferers. Like other immune breakdown illness, science can't pinpoint an exact cause of fibromyalgia, so they label it untreatable, largely because NSAIDS drugs do not help. However, FM may be vastly helped by natural therapies.

Do you think you might have fibromyalgia? Here are the signs:

1) musculoskeletal pain in at least three "tender" points on the body lasting three months or more
2) persistent, diffuse musculo-skeletal pain that is generally worse when you wake up
3) persistent, exhausting fatigue and weakness; being overweight and a smoker compounds these symptoms
4) irritable bowel syndrome, often with chronic diarrhea; stomach and digestive problems like leaky gut
5) chronic headaches or migraines, often accompanied by mental confusion
6) unexplained anxiety or depression, usually with nightly interrupted sleep
7) hypoglycemia, or unexplained allergies, often with heart palpitations or shortness of breath as reactions
8) paresthesias (prickling or burning sensation on the skin).

Traditional medicine focuses on using non-steroidal anti-inflammatory drugs like aspirin, ibuprofen (Advil/Motrin) or naproxen sodium (Aleve) to relieve aches and pains. Americans take over 85 million aspirin alone every single day, much of it for this type of long term pain. Continued use, however, of these types of pain-killers can actually worsen symptoms, cause intestinal permeability (leaky gut syndrome) and increase food sensitivities, which then depresses the immune system even further! Natural treatment for fibromyalgia is all about supernutrition, normalizing body systems, reducing pain, and re-establishing normal sleep patterns.

1: **A diet for HYPOGLYCEMIA (page 408) is a good place to start.** Keep your diet at least 50% fresh foods during intensive healing time. A largely vegetarian diet is beneficial on blood toxins and fibrinogen that affect coagulation. Add cruciferous veggies like broccoli for 3-indole carbinole to reduce pain. Reduce processed foods, sugars, and saturated fats. Avoid red meats and caffeine. Write down the foods you eat and how you feel after you eat them. Cut out for a week foods that seem to aggravate symptoms to see if symptoms improve. If they do, eliminate them. Dairy foods, caffeine, wheat, oats, chocolate and canola oil are common suspects.

2: **Green foods rich in chlorophyll and magnesium are essential.** Chlorophyll molecular structure is nearly identical to human hemoglobin, carrying magnesium in its center instead of iron. Eating chlorophyll plants is like giving yourself a little "transfusion." Have a green drink every day. Green Kamut BEST OF GREENS, or Crystal Star ENERGY GREEN are good choices.

3: **Increase ATP (energy) production in the muscle cells to reduce pain.** A primary marker for fibromyalgia is a magnesium deficiency in the cells, so a magnesium/malic acid combination is often successful. Malic acid, in foods like apples, improves ATP synthesis. A recent study shows that a magnesium/malic acid combo relieves fibromyalgia pain in only 48 hours. The same study showed that after 4 to 8 weeks, muscle swelling and tenderness lessened significantly. Ethical Nutrients MALIC/MAGNESIUM.

4: **Herbal analgesics accelerate pain relief without causing liver toxicity,** gastrointestinal problems or stomach bleeding like aspirin or NSAIDS. Ginger is one of the best. It modulates prostaglandins to control pain and inflammation safely. Add 2 tsp. ginger to a recipe for a therapeutic dose. Biochemics PAIN RELEAF is a topical formula that improves circulation, reduces inflammation and temporarily numbs aches.

5: **Relieve Irritable Bowel Syndrome symptoms with gentle herbs.** Include a cup of peppermint tea with your meals whenever possible. As a natural anti-gas and anti-spasmodic, peppermint is a specific for I.B.S. Both American and European studies repeatedly confirm its success.

6: **Lower your homocysteine levels:**
— 4 garlic capsules (1200mg a day) to maintain aortic elasticity.
— B_6, 50mg and folic acid 800mg to help break down homocysteine.
— red wine, 1 glass with dinner.

7: **Balance serotonin production.** Low levels of serotonin may be one of the primary causes of pain and disrupted sleep. (Just getting a good night's sleep is often enough to completely turn this disease around.) **Two suggestions:** —Massage therapy is a boon for fibromyalgia because it is a natural pain killer that boosts serotonin. In a study of 30 women with fibromyalgia, massage therapy provided the best results over many other therapies! —St. John's wort modulates serotonin production in the brain for better sleep. It also plays a role in melatonin secretion - Nature's sleep aid. A whole herb combination is superior to standardized St. John's wort products, linked to side effects like GI distress, fatigue and photosensitivity. A St. John's wort combination can also relieve depression related to fibromyalgia. Try Crystal Star's DEPRESS-EX™ CAPS.

8: **Exercise is a key.** Low impact aerobics (especially swimming and stationary bicycling) is one of the most effective fibromyalgia treatments. Start slow and stick with it. Light walking for 5 minutes every day, even if it's just around your house, can accelerate recovery.

9: **SAMe** (*S-Adenosyl-L-methionine*), a derivative of the amino acid methionine, is a promising fibromyalgia therapy. Forty-seven patients receiving 200mg intra-muscularly of SAMe once a day, and 400 to 800 mg twice a day, depression, anxiety and tenderness all reduced significantly.

Bodywork and Lifestyle Techniques

• Those with fibromyalgia are generally not physically fit. Build up a slow, low-impact aerobic exercise program - 20 minutes a day for body oxygen and muscle tone.

• Add light weight bearing exercise for 10 minutes a day to start.

—**Relaxation techniques are crucial:**

• Choose from meditation, guided imagery, yoga, biofeedback, and progressive muscle relaxation - all of which have had success with fibromyalgia in developing a positive mind/body stance to work with the disease.

• Regular monthly massage therapy treatments have had notable success.

• Local, gentle heat applications are effective, especially with a gentle massage.

Herb and Supplement Choices

• **Reduce inflammation, manage pain:** Allergy Research BIOGEN GH or BIOGEN PRO; MSM caps 800mg daily or Futurebiotics MSM; Crystal Star PRO-EST BALANCE™ roll-on; Quercetin 1000mg and bromelain 1500mg daily; Solaray TUR-MERIC (curcumin). Apply Biochemics PAIN RELEAF lotion; Transitions PRO-GEST wild yam cream; Wakunaga GLU-COSAMINE SOOTHING CREAM cream.

• **Balance brain chemistry and nerve transmission:** Ginkgo Biloba improves memory and circulation; Crystal Star RELAX CAPS™, 6 daily as needed; Gotu kola extract or Solaray CENTELLA ASIATICA caps; Crystal Star ADRN-ACTIVE™ capsules for adrenal deficiency.

• **Improve musculo-skeletal system:** Acetyl-L-Carnitine 1000mg daily; Glucosamine-chondroitin combination, a cartilage nutrient-1500/1200mg 6 daily; Crystal Star AR-EASE™ caps, joint rebuilder and collagen tonic; very relieving; Burdock tea 2 cups daily as a blood cleanser for the musculo-skeletal system. Take with Crystal Star FEM SUPPORT™ extract and una da gato caps for best results.

• **Enhance your natural energy sources:** Crystal Star MEN-TAL INNER ENERGY™ with kava kava and ginseng; Country Life sublingual B-12, 2500mcg.

• **Natural antidepressants raise serotonin levels:** SAMe (S-adenosyl methionine) 800mg daily boosts serotonin-dopamine levels; St. John's wort, 300mg daily; Enzymatic Therapy KAVA-TONE for headaches. Rosemary tea, a memory booster.

Can't find a recommended product? Call the 800 number listed in Product Resources for the store nearest you and for more info.

Conquering Chronic Fatigue Syndrome

Chronic Fatigue Syndrome (CFS) is sometimes referred to as a condition without a cause. In reality, the opposite is true. There are a wealth of causative factors. Most researchers accept that a wide group of viruses are involved. Epstein-Barr virus (EBV), herpes simplex viruses (genital and oral), and cytomegalovirus (CMV) are clearly implicated. Candida albicans yeast and parasite infestations are highly suspect. CFS's association with hypoglycemia is well-known. Incredibly, new research shows that the polio virus, considered conquered, may be resurfacing 30 years after childhood vaccinations against it, as Post-Polio Syndrome, now seen as Chronic Fatigue. Environmental contaminants contribute by lowering immune response and allowing CFS a path to develop through exhausted adrenal glands. As immunity drops lower, almost anything can be the final trigger for CFS. Onset is abrupt in 90% of cases.

Chronic Fatigue Immune Dysfunction Syndrome (CFIDS) has been known since the 1800s. CFS, as it's known today, is most prevalent in western industrialized countries where a 40, even 60 hour work week is the norm for one or more wage earners in a household, along with raising children. The problem is getting worse, affecting close to 2 million people in America today. Over 85% of CFS victims are women between 30 and 50, who are outgoing, productive, independent, active overachievers. It seems the overworked, overstressed "superwomen" of the 90s are paying the price of their hectic lifestyles in terms of health. No conventional medical treatment or drug on the market today can help fatigue syndromes; most hinder immune response and recovery. The only long term success I have ever seen with CFS was produced with a good lifestyle program, not a pill.

Do you have Chronic Fatigue Syndrome?

Fatigue syndromes are quite difficult to diagnose and treat. The outward symptoms mimic a wide variety of degenerative diseases - mononucleosis, HIV infection, candidiasis, cytomegalovirus, M.S., lupus, Lyme disease and fibromyalgia. There are many AIDS-like reactions, but CFS does not kill, is not sexually transmitted as once thought, and tends to go into remission. Get tested for viral titers that measure your body's reaction to the virus, or elevated levels of EBV anti-bodies so that your treatment will be correct.

Here's what to look for:

—**Early symptoms:** persistent, debilitating fatigue that is not helped by bed rest, and that is severe enough to reduce average daily activity below 50% percent of normal for at least 6 months. The person experiences classic flu or mononucleosis symptoms - chronic low grade fever, throat infections, muscle weakness, lethargy, digestive disturbance, and sore lymph nodes in the armpit and neck.

—**Second symptoms:** ringing in the ears, exhaustion, chronic depression and self-doubt, moodiness and irritability, fogginess, disorientation and muddled thinking, continued low grade infection and fever, worsening allergies, diarrhea, sharp muscle aches.

—**Third symptoms:** extreme exhaustion, paranoia, herpes infections, aching ears and eyes, night sweats, blackouts, almost constant infections, numbness in the limbs, weight loss and loss of appetite, MS-like nerve disorder with heart palpitations and vertigo.

Knowledge is part of the cure for CFS. Watchwords to recognize:

1: **CFS develops from retro-viruses that attack a weakened immune system.** It is prolonged by: candida or mononucleosis; food allergies; long emotional stress (or low levels of cortisol, a stress response immune hormone); chemical pollutants; smoking; long use of antibiotic or steroid drugs; a low nutrition diet. Have a test to rule out candida yeast, mononucleosis, or herpes before you start a healing program.

2: **Chronic Fatigue Syndrome takes longer to overcome than Candida or Herpes.** The symptoms are similar, but the viral activity is more virulent and debilitating to the immune system; entrenchment in the adrenal glands, the liver and circulatory system is deep-seated. It takes two to four weeks to notice consistent improvement, six months or longer to feel normal. However, most people do respond to natural therapies in three to six months. Many achieve near normal functioning in two years.

3: **Mind and attitude play a critical role in immune strength and energy levels for overcoming CFS.** Don't get so wound up in the strictness of your program that it further depresses you and takes over your life. The people who learn to manage mental, emotional and physical stress in their lives recover fastest. Laughter is still the best medicine.

4: **High homocysteine levels are a risk factor for CFS.** Lower your homocysteine levels naturally: – 4 garlic capsules (1200mg a day) to maintain aortic elasticity; – B_6 50mg and folic 800mg to help break down homocysteine; – red wine, 1 glass with dinner.

5: **Severe chemical sensitivities are part of CFS for 67% of victims after exposure to air pollution or chemical smoke fumes.** Try to avoid these elements. Take a sauna once a week if possible to boost toxin elimination and speed healing.

6: **Chronic Fatigue is linked to low blood pressure.** If you think you have CFS, check your blood pressure first. Your systolic blood pressure should be below 120 and your diastolic blood pressure should be below 80 to be at optimal levels. If your blood pressure drops to 90/60 or below, you may feel light-headed and should consult a health professional.

7: **Herbal adaptogens restore energy and fight stress reactions.** Brazilian Rainforest herb suma and Siberian ginseng are used successfully by herbalists. Crystal Star GINSENG SIX™ SUPER TEA, and Rainbow Light ADAPTOGEM caps are good choices.

8: **Essential fatty acids are a key to controlling inflammation and allergies.** Evening primrose oil, about 1000mg 4 times daily, has been found to improve symptoms for 85% of CFS patients.

9: **If you've had mononucleosis, CFS can reactivate the Epstein Barr Virus.** Get a simple clinic test for EBV. Then, use vitamin C up to 10,000mg a day or to bowel tolerance as a natural anti-infective. Add 2,000mg of L-lysine daily to reduce EBV viral count.

10: **Consider NADH** (*nicotinamide adenine dinucleotide*). Studies show NADH, a naturally occurring coenzyme, 10mg to 15mg daily, alleviates the major symptoms of Chronic Fatigue, especially with long-term supplementation. Available in health food stores.

11: **Consider Alpha Lipoic Acid, a superb free radical scavenger.** Free radical damage is profound in CFS. Alpha lipoic acid also has the ability to detoxify and strengthen the liver, always impaired in Chronic Fatigue. Jarrow Formulas ALPHA LIPOIC ACID 100mg, or LIPOIC ACID by Source Naturals.

Chronic Fatigue diet protocol is effective for other opportunistic diseases: *HIV infection, Lupus, M.S., Candidiasis, Herpes, Rheumatic Fever, Meningitis, Mononucleosis, Venereal Warts (HPV), Hepatitis, Toxic Shock Syndrome, Lyme Disease, Parasite Infestation, Eczema and Psoriasis.*

Chronic Fatigue Healing Diet

A high resistance, immune-strengthening diet is primary to success over fatigue syndromes. I don't recommend a liquid fast since it is often too harsh for an already weakened system. The initial diet should, however, be as pure as possible, in order to be as cleansing as possible. For several months at least, the diet should be vegetarian, low in dairy and gluten foods, and saturated-fat free. This means eliminating meats, dairy foods except yogurt, fried and fatty foods, with no yeasted breads. Avoid alcoholic drinks, nicotine, refined sugars, artificial sweeteners like aspartame (Nutrasweet), and caffeine. These substances exacerbate CFS symptoms the most. Drink lots of fresh liquids, and clear the bowels daily.

The ultra purity of this diet controls the multiple food sensitivities of CFS. Keep the diet at least 50% fresh foods during intensive healing time. Include defense foods often: cruciferous vegetables; antibody forming foods: onions and garlic; oxygenating foods: wheat germ; high mineral, B-complex foods: sea greens, brown rice; high fiber foods: prunes and bran; cultured foods: yogurt and miso; protein foods: sea foods and whole grains. All produce should be fresh and organically grown for best results.

Keep new cell development strong with protein. Take a protein drink every morning: Solgar WHEY TO GO (lactose-free); Crystal Star SYSTEMS STRENGTH™ (also combats hypothyroidism), and GREEN TEA CLEANSER™ to detox; Nutricology PRO-GREENS with EFA's, or Pines MIGHTY GREENS with EFA's; YS ROYAL JELLY blend with ginseng, pollen and propolis (add to hot water and take as a tea).

—**On rising:** take 2 TBS. cranberry concentrate in 8-oz. water with $^1/_2$ teasp. ascorbate vitamin C crystals, or use a green tea blood cleansing formula, like Crystal Star GREEN TEA CLEANSER™ with $^1/_2$ teasp. acidophilus powder.

—**Breakfast:** have a glass of fresh carrot juice, with 1 TB. Bragg's LIQUID AMINOS; and whole grain muffins or rice cakes with kefir cheese or yogurt cheese; or a protein drink (see above) with fresh fruit and $^1/_2$ teasp. acidophilus powder.

—**Mid-morning:** take a potassium drink (pg. 568) with 1 TB. Bragg's LIQUID AMINOS, and $^1/_2$ teasp. ascorbate vitamin C crystals; and another fresh carrot juice, or pau d' arco tea with $^1/_2$ teasp. acidophilus powder.

—**Lunch:** have a green leafy salad with lemon-flax oil dressing; add sprouts, tofu, avocado, nuts and seeds; or have an open-face sandwich on rice cakes or a chapati, with yogurt cheese and fresh veggies; or have a cup of miso soup with brown rice and sea greens snipped on top; or have some steamed vegetables and a cup of pau d'arco tea with $^1/_2$ teasp. acidophilus powder.

—**Mid-afternoon:** have a carrot juice with 1 TB Bragg's LIQUID AMINOS; and a green drink, or Monas CHLORELLA, Green Foods GREEN MAGMA or Crystal Star GREEN ENERGY GREEN™ drink.

—**Dinner:** have a baked potato with Bragg's LIQUID AMINOS or lemon/oil dressing and a fresh salad, and black bean or lentil soup; or spinach or artichoke pasta with steamed vegetables and a lemon-flax oil dressing; or a Chinese steam/stir-fry with shiitake mushrooms, vegetables and brown rice. Sprinkle $^1/_2$ teasp. acidophilus powder over any cooked food at this meal.

—**Before Bed:** take 8-oz. of aloe vera juice with $^1/_2$ tsp. ascorbate vitamin C; and a papaya juice with $^1/_2$ tsp. acidophilus powder.

Recipes to help a candida cleansing diet: • DETOXIFICATION FOODS; • HEALING DRINKS; • SOUPS, LIQUID SALADS; • ENZYME-RICH FOODS; • SALADS, HOT and COLD; • MINERAL-RICH • LIGHT MACROBIOTIC EATING.

Herb and Supplement Choices

•**Fight the viral infection:** *St. John's wort* (also an antidepressant); Crystal Star ANTI-VI™ tea or extract; Nutricology PROLIVE (olive leaf extract tabs); Garlic capsules 8 daily; Nutribiotic GRAPEFRUIT SEED EXTRACT capsules. Vitamin C with bioflavonoids, ¹/₄ teasp. every half hour to bowel tolerance - to flush the tissues and act as an anti-viral agent, for 10 days. Then reduce to 3 - 5000mg daily.

•**Take non-depleting energizers:** MICROHYDRIN (Healthy House); Carnitine 2000mg daily; Country Life sublingual B-12, 2500mcg; Ethical Nutrients MALIC-MAGNESIUM caps; Imperial Elixir SIBERIAN GINSENG; Crystal Star ADRN-ACTIVE™ caps or extract, with BODY REBUILDER™ 4 daily. Kal NADA 10mg each morning; CoQ-10 60 mg 4 daily.

•**Enzyme therapy:** Transformation DIGESTZYME with meals, PUREZYME between meals; Nature's Plus Bromelain 1500mg daily.

•**Relieve muscle pain; boost healing blood supply:** Lysine 500mg 4x daily; Magnesium 1000mg daily; Chamomile tea, 2 cups daily; Hawthorn extract 2x daily.

•**Balance your body chemistry:** Suma extract, Ginseng-Reishi mushroom extract, Siberian ginseng extract, or •Rainbow Light ADAPTO-GEM. Crystal Star PRO-EST BALANCE™ roll-on, with maitake mushroom caps for 3 months. UAS DDS-PLUS with FOS.

•**Detoxify and repair your liver:** Milk thistle seed extract; Crystal Star LIV-ALIVE™ caps; Biotec CELL GUARD, 6 daily; B-complex 100mg daily with extra biotin 1000mcg.

•**Strengthen the nervous system:** SAMe to boost serotonin, dopamine and phos. serine levels, 800mg daily.; Ginkgo Biloba extract as needed; Evening Primrose oil 4000mg daily.

Bodywork and Lifestyle Techniques

Note: High doses of aspirin, NSAIDS and cortisone for pain can hamper your body's ability to keep bone strength and adrenal health.

•**CFS symptoms are greatly reduced by aerobic exercise.** Even light stretching, tai chi, or short walks are noticeably effective when they are done regularly every day. Take a daily deepbreathing walk for tissue oxygen. Walk for a half hour to stimulate lymphatic system and cerebral circulation.

•**Early morning sunlight** on your body every day for Vit.D.

•**Apply Earth's Bounty O₂-SPRAY** onto soles of the feet for body oxygen. Alternate use, one week on and one week off. Too much reactivates symptoms. A little is great; a lot is not.

•**Relax.** An optimistic mental attitude and frame of mind play a major role in releasing body stress, a big factor in lowered immunity. Remember that immune stimulation itself has an anti-viral effect.

•**Stretching exercises and massage will cleanse the lymph system** and enhance oxygenation. Use hot and cold alternating hydrotherapy to stimulate circulation.

•**Take a wheat grass enema**, once a week, to help detoxification.

•**Avoid tobacco in all forms.** Nicotine destroys immunity.

•**Overheating therapy helps control retro-viruses.** See page 462 for at-home technique.

•**Microcurrent therapy:** Patents have been awarded documenting that microcurrents neutralize pathogens, fungi, virus, bacteria, and parasites. Call Sota Instruments for information on this subject - 800-224-0242.

Can't find a recommended product? Call the 800 number listed in Product Resources for the store nearest you and for more info.

Overcoming Colon and Bowel Problems

Most diseases we endure today have their roots in poor drainage. The key to modern health is continually removing toxic wastes and pollutants from our bodies. It starts with back-up and fermentation in the colon, like a walking pressure cooker, and ends with the body actually re-absorbing unreleased waste material, which settles in weak cells unable to "clean house." Continuing accumulation of this poisonous build-up results in disease.

A fiber-rich diet is the age-old key to preventing most of these problems. Daily fresh vegetables and whole grains virtually guarantee a fully active elimination system, good digestion, low cholesterol and balanced blood sugar. Even a gentle, gradual change from a low fiber, low residue diet helps almost immediately, and it's better than a drastic program for relieving pain and inflammation in the colon. In fact, a slow, but complete switch to a high fiber diet over several months gives your body much better therapy than just adding a fiber supplement or a few fiber foods to your regular diet.

Do you have signs of colon and bowel problems? Take the following COLON PROTECTION TEST

1: **Bowel movements should be regular daily, and almost effortless.**
2: **The stool should be almost odorless (signalling increased transit time in the bowel with no fermentation).**
3: **There should be very little gas or flatulence.**
4: **The stool should float rather than sink.**

Is the state of your colon putting you at risk for colon cancer?

People with chronic constipation or diarrhea are in a high risk category for colon cancer. Colon cancer is the second most common cancer for both men and women in the U.S.. U.S. colon cancer rates are 500% greater than the rest of the world! Over 175,000 Americans will be diagnosed this year. Over 60,000 people will die of colon cancer... even with all the advanced techniques of modern medicine.

—**Overweight men are at the highest risk.** An astonishing number of men eat a low fiber diet (even with all the media attention) and that's the biggest culprit. Fiber is the transport system of the digestive tract, moving food wastes out of the body before they have a chance to form potentially cancer-causing chemicals.

—**A high fat diet is the second highest risk factor.** Fatty meats are the primary culprits. The saturated fats and dense protein from red meats are thought to be involved in 40 to 60% of colon cancer cases Meat is hard to digest, too, so more of it reaches the large intestine, where it can be harmful. Red meat animals are those more likely to have man-made hormone injections now linked colon cancer. Most red meat is barbecued today, a process that generates carcinogenic hydrocarbons on the meat surfaces.

You'll notice improvement in your waste elimination problems fairly quickly after diet improvement. There is no instant, easy route. It takes from 3 to 6 months to rebuild bowel and colon elasticity with good systole-diastole action. An herbal colon health formula can help in this effort for normalization.

If you use over-the-counter antacids or take frequent rounds of antibiotics, they maybe doing you more harm than good. Antacids neutralize stomach HCl needed for digestion and food assimilation, and inhibit production of friendly digestive bacteria. In addition, over use of laxatives to correct poor elimination irritates bowel membranes, and may almost bring normal systole-diastole activity to a halt. A vegetable fiber diet is both prevention and cure. I also recommend taking an acidophilus complex supplement, like Nutricology SYMBIOTICS with FOS, about $1/_4$ teasp. in water 3x daily, with 100mg B-COMPLEX daily. Long use of antibiotics or antacids kills friendly bacteria in the digestive tract, and aggravates elimination problems.

Experts tell us that 95% of all disease is linked to constipation and colon toxicity from three basic areas:

1) Non-food chemicals in our food and pollutants in the environment, ranging from relatively harmless to dangerous. A clean, strong system can metabolize and excrete many of these, but when we're constipated, they are stored as unusable substances. As more and different chemicals enter the body they tend to interact with those that are already there, forming mutant, second generation chemicals far more harmful than the originals. Evidence in recent years shows that most bowel cancer is caused by environmental agents taken in through diet and air pollution.

2) Over-accumulated body wastes and metabolic by-products that are not excreted properly. Unreleased wastes can also become a breeding ground for parasite infestation. A nationwide survey reveals that one in every six people studied has one or more parasites living somewhere in their bodies! An astounding figure.

3) Slow elimination time, allowing waste materials to ferment, become rancid, and then recirculate through the body tissues as toxic substances, usually resulting in sluggish organ and glandular functions, poor digestion and assimilation, lowered immunity, faulty circulation and tissue degeneration.

The body can tolerate a certain level of contamination. But when that individual level is passed, and immune defenses are low, toxic overload causes illness. The programs in this chapter include specifics for restoration diets for both bowel and bladder areas, with watchwords to keep in mind so that problems don't return and the solution becomes long term.

The diets in this section can solve faulty waste elimination problems: *Chronic Constipation or Diarrhea, Irritable Bowel Syndrome, Colitis or Spastic Colon, Crohn's Disease, Diverticulitis, Gas, Bloating and Flatulence, Bad Breath and Body Odor, Hemorrhoids, Varicose Veins, Low Energy, and Intestinal Parasites.*

Diet to Rebuild Colon and Bowel Health

The colon and bowel are the depository for all waste material after food nutrients are extracted. Unprocessed food decays and forms gases as well as 2nd, even 3rd generation toxins, and the colon becomes a breeding ground for putrefactive bacteria, viruses, parasites, yeasts and more. Most naturopaths believe that this old, infected material in bowel pockets (diverticula), often reabsorbs into the body, causing up to 90% of all disease. Ideally, one should eliminate after each meal, but experts say the average American is 50,000 bowel movements short over a lifetime because our bowels are so sluggish. Bowel transit time should be about 12 hours. Healthy intestines are your body's second immune system. Take in plenty of fiber and liquids, exercise regularly and have a regular daily time for elimination. If you've had years of chronic constipation, start with the short 3-day colon cleansing juice diet (pg.153).

Watchwords: 1: Fiber foods, like prunes are the diet key - most experts recommend 40-45 grams daily: fiber isn't digested; it simply moves through your system, helping other foods move along with it. 2: Follow a low fat, largely vegetarian diet, with plenty of intestinal brooms - fruits, whole grains, greens, veggies and cultured foods like yogurt. 3: Avoid high fat, sugary, fried foods and dairy foods; they don't allow your body to get rid of waste easily. 4: Drink 6-8 glasses of healthy liquids every day; avoid cow's milk.

—**The night before your restoration diet,** make an easy fiber drink: mix equal parts of flax seed, pumpkin seed and oat bran in water. Let sit overnight. Take 2 TBS in the morning in juice. Or soak a mix of dried prunes, figs and raisins and blackstrap molasses.

—**On rising:** take a glass of lemon juice and water, or a glass of aloe vera juice or Herbal Answers HERBAL ALOE FORCE juice with herbs, with 1/4 teasp. acidophilus added; or Crystal Star CHO-LO FIBER TONE™ capsules or drink in apple or orange juice.
—**Breakfast:** take 2 TBS of your dried fruit-molasses mix with yogurt or apple juice; add 2 teasp. nutritional yeast or Lewis Labs FIBER YEAST to oatmeal or granola, and top with yogurt or apple juice; or have a bowl of mixed fresh fruits with yogurt.
—**Mid-morning:** take a fresh carrot juice or veggie drink (page 569). Monas CHLORELLA, Nutricology PRO GREENS with flax, or Crystal Star ENERGY GREEN™ drink; or green tea or Crystal Star GREEN TEA CLEANSER™ to alkalize the system.
—**Lunch:** have a fresh green salad with lemon/olive oil dressing, or yogurt cheese or kefir cheese; or steamed veggies and a baked potato with yogurt cheese or kefir cheese; or a fresh fruit salad with a little yogurt or raw cottage cheese topping.
—**Mid-afternoon:** have another fresh carrot juice, or Green Kamut Corp. GREEN KAMUT; and-or green tea or slippery elm tea; and-or some raw crunchy veggies with a vegetable or kefir cheese dip, or soy spread.
—**Dinner:** have a large dinner salad with black bean or lentil soup; or an oriental stir fry and miso soup with sea greens snipped on top; or a baked vegetable casserole with a yogurt cheese sauce; or a spinach pasta with a light lemon or yogurt sauce.
—**Before bed:** have apple or papaya juice; or a glass of aloe vera juice or Crystal Star BIOFLAV, FIBER & C SUPPORT™ drink.

Recipes to restore colon health: •**BREAKFAST and BRUNCH;** •**DAIRY-FREE COOKING;** •**SOUPS, LIQUID SALADS;** •**ENZYME-RICH FOODS;** •**SALADS;** •**MINERAL-RICH FOODS;** •**LOW FAT FOODS;** •**HIGH FIBER FOODS.**

Herb and Supplement Choices

• **Cleanse old wastes:** Crystal Star FIBER & HERBS CLEANSE™ capsules 6 daily (1 to 3 months, complete cleanse); Nature's Secret A.M./P.M. ULTIMATE CLEANSE; Earth's Bounty OXY-CLEANSE removes old hardened wastes.

—**For a quick occasional cleanse:** take 3000 to 5000mg vitamin C with bioflavonoids over a two hour period; or Crystal Star LAXA-TEA™ to flush wastes gently over a 24-hour period; or Zand QUICK CLEANSE.

• **Prevent constipation:** Omega-3 flax seed caps; magnesium 400mg daily; (Think twice about drugstore antibiotics, antacids or milk of magnesia; they kill friendly intestinal flora.)

—**Probiotics prevent constipation, overcome antibiotic residues:** Jarrow Corp. JARRO-DOPHILUS + FOS; UAS DDS-PLUS with FOS; Transformation PLANTA-DOPHILUS (also for liver function); Prevail INNER ECOLOGY.

• **Normalize digestive functions:** Solaray TETRA CLEANSE or Nature's Way 5 SYSTEM CLEANSE; Fennel-ginger caps 4 daily; Garlic caps, 4 daily; Turmeric or goldenseal-myrrh extract drops in water enhance bile flow.

• **For a healthy, odor-free stool:** Planetary Formulas TRIPHALA; Apple pectin tabs; Milk thistle seed, or dandelion extract enhances bile output and softens stool.

• **Natural laxatives and regulators:** Bee pollen 2 tsp. daily; Senna leaf/pods (sparingly, a little goes a long way); una da gato caps 6 daily; Cascara caps increase peristalsis.

• **Enzyme therapy re-establishes acid-alkaline balance:** Prevail FIBER-ZYME 2x daily; Papaya enzymes 1000mg daily, to digest milk proteins and sugars; Peppermint or ginger tea provide plant enzymes that specifically balance digestion.

Bodywork and Lifestyle Techniques

• **Consider a catnip or dilute liquid chlorophyll enema once a week to keep cleansing going.** (See page 571 for instructions.) Note: Enemas may be given to children. Use small amounts according to size and age. Allow water to enter very slowly; let them to expel when they wish.

• **Or take a colonic irrigation to start your program.** A grapefruit seed extract colonic is extremely effective; a wheat grass retention enema is effective if there is colon toxicity along with constipation. (Dilute to 15 to 20 drops per gallon of water.)

• **Take a brisk walk daily** to encourage free-flowing elimination.

• **Get early morning sunlight** on the body every day possible for purifying vitamin A and vitamin D.

• **Apply warm ginger compresses** to lower spine and stomach to stimulate systol/diastol activity.

• **Be sure all food is well chewed.** Eat smaller meals more frequently rather than large meals to allow the body to process easily during healing.

Can't find a recommended product? Call the 800 number listed in Product Resources for the store nearest you and for more info.

Diet to Heal Irritable Bowel

A chronically inflamed, painful colon is often a result of food allergies (65%), usually a gluten reaction to wheat, cheese, corn, eggs, or other food sensitivity. Lactose intolerance symptoms mimic those of IBS and colitis. Fast foods (full of chemicals), fried foods (full of fat), refined foods (low in fiber) and sugars aggravate irritable bowel. Most victims are women between 20 and 40 with stressful jobs or lifestyles. Many also have bouts of candida yeast infection. Colon membranes become irritated, and the body forms pouchy pockets in reaction. In severe cases (ulcerative colitis), ulcerous lesions line the sides of the colon. Natural therapies are effective and reduce the need for drugs. Many sufferers see dramatic results. Diet changes are a must. Healing herbs and supplements will not work without diet changes. If there is appendicitis-like sharp pain, seek medical help immediately.

Do you think you might have irritable bowel?

—Have you noticed unexplained weakness, lethargy and fatigue? Are you anemic?
—Do you have abdominal cramps, distention and pain (relieved by bowel movements), especially within an hour after eating?
—Do you have recurrent constipation, usually alternating with bloody diarrhea? Do you have evident mucous in your stool?
—Do you have rectal hemorrhoids, fistulas or anal fissures; urgency to defecate; dehydration and mineral loss?
—Have you lost weight lately without trying? Is your abdomen always distended even though you are thin?
—Are you a heavy smoker or caffeine user?
—Have you been under a great deal of emotional stress? Are you usually depressed and anxious?
—Have you recently taken one or more courses of antibiotics?
—Is there a history of irritable bowel in your family?

—**During the acute stage of irritable bowel pain:** Go on a mono diet for 2 days with apples and apple juice.

—Then eat a low fat diet with plenty of fiber, but low roughage. Foods should be lightly cooked, never fried, with few salts.
—Include fresh fruits, fruit fiber from prunes, apples and raisins, green salads with plenty of alfalfa sprouts for vitamin K, and a light olive oil and lemon dressing, whole grain cereals like oatmeal or brown rice (not wheat), and steamed veggies.
—Have a glass of mixed vegetable juice daily for the first two weeks. Have fresh carrot juice at least 3x a week. Keep your body well-hydrated - 6 to 8 glasses of water a day.
—Eat cultured foods, such as yogurt and kefir and Rejuvenative Foods VEGI DELITE for friendly intestinal flora.
—Eat smaller, frequent meals. No large meals.
—Clean up your diet: Avoid coffee and caffeine foods. Eliminate nuts, seeds, dairy and citrus while healing. Cut back on saturated fat as much as possible. Eliminate refined sugars, sorbitol and wheat foods (the most irritating) of all kinds. Spicy foods are an irritant.

After your mono diet...

—**On rising:** take 2 fresh squeezed lemons, 1 TB maple syrup in 8-oz. of water; or a glass of aloe vera juice; or apple juice.

—**Breakfast:** have a fruit fiber mix of prunes, raisins and apples. Top with a little yogurt, vanilla kefir or apple juice; or apple-alfalfa sprout juice for vitamin K.

—**Mid-morning:** an IBS healing juice: 4 handfuls greens: 1 spinach, 1 parsley, 1 kale, and 1 parsley, 2 large tomatoes, $1/4$ head green cabbage, 4 carrots w/ tops, 1 garlic clove and 2 stalks celery w/ leaves, a 4-oz. tub fresh alfalfa sprouts and sprigs of fresh mint. or a green drink, like Monas CHLORELLA, Wakunaga KYO-GREEN with EFA's, or Crystal Star ENERGY GREEN™drink.

—**Lunch:** have a simple green salad with a special GINGER-FLAXSEED DRESSING for 2 cups: blend 1 cucumber chopped, $1/2$ cup sunflower seeds, 1 TB flax seeds, 1 TB fresh grated ginger, 1 teasp. sesame oil, and $1\ 1/2$ cups water; have a veggie juice like PERSONAL V-8 (page 569). Or take Crystal Star CLEANSING & PURIFYING™ tea with 2 Transformation DIGESTZYME caps.

—**Mid-afternoon:** have a carrot juice; or an herb tea like nettles, green tea, an apple juice, or apple/alfalfa sprout juice. Or have a superfood green drink, like Crystal Star ENERGY GREEN™ with1 tsp. nutritional yeast and 1 tsp. wheat germ added

—**Dinner:** have steamed brown rice and mixed steamed vegetables. Sprinkle with snipped, dry sea greens (like dulse or kelp). Use 1 TB flax or olive oil, and 1 TB Bragg's LIQUID AMINOS. Or make a high luster skin broth: In $2\ 1/2$ cups water, cook 2 cups chopped fresh mixed vegetables, add 1 tsp. miso and 2 TBS chopped dried sea greens. Or have some Rejuvenative Foods VEGI DELITE for friendly intestinal flora.

—**Before Bed:** have Crystal Star CHOL-LO FIBER TONE™ drink, or AloeLife FIBER MATE drink at bedtime for 2 weeks; or another aloe juice drink; or papaya or apple juice; or Red Star nutritional yeast broth for B vitamins; or a gentle cleansing booster like Crystal Star BWL TONE I.B.S.™ caps to soothe irritation while stimulating the body to eliminate wastes.

For the next 6 days:
Have 2 to 3 glasses of any blend of mixed vegetable juices throughout the day. Don't eat any solid food during the day. Have steamed brown rice and mixed vegetables for an early dinner each evening. Drink at least 6 to 8 glasses of pure bottled or mineral water throughout the day for best results.

Recipes to restore bowel tone: • BREAKFAST and BRUNCH; • DAIRY-FREE COOKING; • SOUPS, LIQUID SALADS; • ENZYME-RICH FOODS; • HEALING DRINKS; • MINERAL-RICH FOODS; • LOW FAT FOODS; • HIGH FIBER FOODS.

Herb and Supplement Choices

• **Relieve the pain and inflammation:** Take una da gato (cat's claw) extract, 3 capsules or 3 droppers daily -usual results in 5 days); peppermint oil or Now PEPEPERMINT oil is a specific for colitis and IBS, 2 capsules 3x daily, or 5 drops in tea. I like Crystal Star GREEN TEA CLEANSER™ 2 cups daily with up to 5 drops peppermint oil added, 2x daily. Glutamine 500mg 4x daily; Planetary Formulas TRIPHALA caps or Crystal Star BWL-TONE IBS™ (results within 2 to 3 days). Curcumin caps twice daily; High Omega-3 flax oil 3 caps daily.

• **For painful spasms:** Crystal Star RELAX CAPS™, ANTI-SPZ caps or CRAMP BARK COMPLEX™ extract. Apply warm ginger compresses to spine and stomach.

• **Neutralize the allergen:** Crystal Sar BITTERS & LEMON CLEANSE™ drops, or Milk Thistle Seed drops in water each morning. Alta Health CANGEST powder (for wheat allergies);

• **Soothe the intestines:** Take chamomile tea 4 cups daily; slippery elm or pau d' arco tea as needed; take an electrolyte replacement drink if there is diarrhea.

• **Enzyme therapy restores the entire digestive system:** Bromelain 1500mg daily; American Health papaya enzyme chewables; Biotec BIO-GESTIN; pancreatin 1400mg before meals; Enzymatic Therapy chewable DGL tabs before meals, PEPPERMINT PLUS (enteric-coated peppermint oil) between meals and GUGGUL-PLUS each morning. Natren TRINITY powder in water to rebalance bowel flora.

• **Immune system support is crucial:** Allergy Research Group NAG 500mg or Source Naturals Glucosamine sulfate 500mg for mucous membrane health. Royal Jelly with ginseng 2 tsp. daily. Sun Wellness Chlorella powder in water.

Bodywork and Lifestyle Techniques

Watchwords:

• Do not take aspirin. Use an herbal analgesic, or non-aspirin pain killer.

• Avoid antacids. They often do more harm than good by neutralizing body HCl.

• Consciously practice relaxation techniques like meditation to reduce stress.

Bodywork:

• Effective gentle enemas rid the colon of fermenting wastes and relieve pain:

–Peppermint tea
–White oak bark
–Slippery elm
–Chamomile
–Lobelia

• Reduce stress: Biofeedback is especially helpful for IBS.

• Acupressure helps: Stroke abdomen up, across and down.

Can't find a recommended product? Call the 800 number listed in Product Resources for the store nearest you and for more info.

Urinary Tract Infection Healing Diet

Recurrent bladder infections are common in women; less common in men (infection for them is largely tied to prostate problems). Bladder infections are the most frequent reason a woman seeks medical attention; pain can be all-consuming during the acute stage. Over 75% of American women have at least one urinary tract infection in a ten year period, almost 30% have one once a year. Staph and strep infections, and diabetes may also affect the kidneys, making the problem more serious - an alarming number of cases result in kidney failure. Note: The active chemical in many spermicidal creams and foams, nonoxynol-9, causes recurring cystitis and yeast infections. Some oral contraceptives are also implicated. Treatment should begin at the very first sign of infection. Consult a holistic clinic if there is no improvement within 5 days.

Do you fear you have a urinary tract infection? One or more signs should alert you if you have pain.

—Do you have frequent, urgent, burning, painful urination, especially at night?
—Is your urine strong, turbid, foul-smelling, cloudy or bloody?
—Do you have lower back pain and pain below the navel? (pain above the waist may be a **kidney infection or kidney stones**)
—Do you have frequent chills and fever as the body tries to throw off infection?
—Do you frequently use spermicidal creams or foams?
—Have you had a recent staph, strep or chlamydia infection that was treated by antibiotics?

Watchwords to prevent and avoid urinary tract infections:

1—**Changing body pH is important.** Eat a yeast-free diet, with no baked breads during healing. **Purify the urinary tract** with watermelon seed tea or a carrot-beet-cucumber juice every other day to reduce infection.

2—**Flush the bladder:** Most UTI's are not a problem of bacteria getting into the bladder but of bacteria getting out. Dilute cranberry juice (unsweetened), 6 to 8 glasses daily (cranberries contain substantial D-Mannose against E. coli infection). **Increase urine flow:** Drink 10 glasses of distilled water, diluted, unsweetened fruit juices and herbal teas daily to keep acid wastes flushed

3—**Avoid acid-forming foods:** caffeine, tomatoes, cooked spinach, chocolate. Avoid sugary foods, carbonated drinks, fried, salty and fatty foods, pasteurized dairy foods. Reduce meat protein. **Add alkalizing foods:** celery, watermelon, ume plum balls, blueberries, green drinks, potassium broth, garlic and onions.

4—**Superfoods that help a bladder infection:** Green Foods GREEN MAGMA; Sun Wellness CHLORELLA 2 pkts. daily; Crystal Star BIOFLAV. FIBER & C SUPPORT™ with cranberry; Crystal Star ENERGY GREEN™; Transitions EASY GREENS; Rainbow HAWAIIAN SPIRULINA; Futurebiotics VITAL K drink daily; Aloe Falls ALOE JUICE with ginger.

Diet to Heal a Bladder Infection

Be sure to drink 6 to 8 glasses of bottled water every day to flush toxins and release acid wastes. Don't take iron supplements during healing. Avoid caffeine, soft drinks, salt, pasteurized dairy products, and citrus juices during this diet.

—**During acute stage:** take 2 TBS cider vinegar and honey in water each a.m., yogurt at noon, a glass of white wine at night.

Then for 1 or 2 days:

—**On rising:** take a glass of lemon juice and water, with 1 teasp. acidophilus liquid; or 3 teasp. cranberry concentrate in a small glass of water with $^1/_4$ teasp. ascorbate C crystals; or 2 TBS. cider vinegar in a glass of water with 1 teasp. honey.

—**Breakfast:** have a glass of watermelon juice, or another glass of cranberry juice with $^1/_4$ teasp. vitamin C crystals; and/or a glass of organic papaya or apple juice with $^1/_4$ teasp. high potency acidophilus complex powder.

—**Mid-morning:** take a cup of watermelon seed tea. (Grind seeds, steep in hot water 30 minutes, add 1 teasp. honey); or a potassium drink (page 568), with 2 teasp. Bragg's LIQUID AMINOS; or a cup of Crystal Star BLDR-K™ TEA.

—**Lunch:** have a green drink (see page 569), or Sun Wellness CHLORELLA, or Green Foods GREEN MAGMA granules in water; or a glass of carrot juice, or carrot/celery juice; or carrot-beet-cucumber juice, every other day.

—**Mid-afternoon:** a healing tea, like parsley-oatstraw-plantain tea, or cornsilk tea; or Crystal Star BLDR-K™ tea; or watermelon seed tea.

—**Dinner:** have another carrot juice, with 1 teasp. liquid chlorophyll or spirulina added; or another cranberry juice with $^1/_4$ teasp. ascorbate vitamin C crystals with bioflavs added; or Crystal Star BIOFLAV. FIBER & C SUPPORT™ drink.

—**Before Bed:** take a glass of papaya or apple juice with $^1/_4$ teasp. high potency acidophilus complex powder.

After pain subsides and healing begins, add the following foods to your daily diet to complete your healing regimen:

—**Breakfast:** add some fresh tropical fruits, like papaya, mango, or bananas to the above diet.

—**Mid-morning:** have a green drink like Sun Wellness CHLORELLA, Green Foods GREEN MAGMA, or Crystal Star ENERGY GREEN™, or a glass of apple juice, or dandelion or parsley tea.

—**Lunch:** add a green salad with lots of cucumbers, spinach, watercress and celery, with lemon/oil or cottage cheese dressing; or a Chinese vegetable salad with bok choy, daikon, pea pods, bean sprouts, with a cup of miso noodle soup with sea greens.

—**Mid-afternoon:** add celery and carrot sticks with kefir or yogurt cheese; or fresh apples and pears with kefir or yogurt dip.

—**Dinner:** add brown rice with tofu and steamed veggies; or steamed asparagus with miso soup and sea greens; or baked or broiled salmon with rice and a spinach salad; a glass of white wine is fine at dinner for alkalizing and relaxation.

—**Before Bed:** have an apple or papaya-mango juice; or miso soup with sea greens; or nutritional yeast broth in hot water.

Recipes to restore bladder health: •DETOXIFICATION FOODS; •DAIRY-FREE COOKING; •SOUPS, LIQUID SALADS; •ENZYME-RICH FOODS; •HEALING DRINKS; •MINERAL-RICH FOODS; •LOW FAT FOODS; •SALADS.

Herb and Supplement Choices

•**Control infection and bacterial adhesion:** Crystal Star BLDR-K COMFORT™ caps, 2 every 3 hours at the first hint of a bladder infection, and/or BLDR-K™ tea (with two ANTI-BIO™ capsules each time if problem is severe). D-Mannose by Biotech Pharmacal, Ark., inhibits E. coli infection (powder- 1 tsp. in water every 3 hours); or take cranberry caps every 3 hours. Nutribiotic GRAPEFRUIT EXTRACT caps 2 daily, and a glass of water with 1 tsp. baking soda in it. Homeopathic cantharis can sometimes stop a UTI immediately.

—If infections develop regularly after intercourse, rinse the vagina with goldenseal-echinacea tea.

•**Curb pain and inflammation:** Goldenseal-echinacea extract; or Futurebiotics VITAL K and uva ursi caps for 14 days to disinfect. On the tenth day, begin Solaray CRAN-ACTIN caps or Natural Balance CRAN-MAX caps, 2 daily; Herbal Magic URINARY TEA, or uva ursi tea daily for 10 days, then cat's claw extract for 10 days for chronic infections.

•**Reduce painful spasms:** to a sitz bath, add 3 drops tea tree oil, 2 drops bergamot oil, 2 drops juniper oil, 2 drops thyme oil, 1 drop eucalyptus oil. Sit in it twice daily for $1/2$ hour. Or massage your abdomen with a blend of 1-oz. almond oil, 3 drops sandalwood oil, 2 drops cedarwood oil, 2 drops cypress oil, 1 drop lavender, 1 drop frankincense oil.

•**Re-establish vaginal flora to reduce recurrence:** use a lactobacillus suppository, or 1 TB acidophilus powder in warm water as a douche for 4 days after treating a UTI with antibiotics; take JARRO-DOPHILUS 6 daily with garlic caps 6 daily; take ascorbate vitamin C 1000mg and Lysine 1000mg every 2 to 3 hours.

Bodywork and Lifestyle Techniques

•**Acupuncture can sometimes relieve pain almost immediately.** Biofeedback and acupuncture have also been successful for incontinence in both women and men, regardless of cause.

•**Apply wet heat,** or hot comfrey compresses across lower back and kidneys or take hot sitz baths to relieve pain and ease urination.

•**For accompanying hemorrhage,** take 1 oz. marshmallow rt., steep in 1 pt. hot milk. Take every $1/2$ hr. to staunch bleeding.

•**Take a mild catnip or chlorophyll enema** to clear acid wastes.

•**Lifestyle Watchwords:**
—Dyes in colored toilet paper may contribute to bladder infections.
—Do not use a diaphragm if you are prone to bladder infections.

388

Can't find a recommended product? Call the 800 number listed in Product Resources for the store nearest you and for more info.

Conquering Digestive Disorders

Most digestive disorders are long standing, deeply ingrained from inherited eating habits and early lifestyle. Low enzyme activity is the origin of almost every digestive problem because enzymes are critical to proper metabolism. Poor metabolism is at the root of health problems from obesity to arthritis, even to some kinds of cancer. Food allergies and sensitivities are also increasing in America as more chemicals are added to our food and soil, and as more foods are refined and genetically altered. Low enzymes mean you have little protection from food allergens.

High fat foods with chemical additives cause the worst digestive problems. Too much meat, especially red meat which stays in the stomach too long, and too little fiber which favors constipation, are not far behind. Low stomach HCL and bile reduces digestion of acids and proteins, resulting in an over-acid system and fermentation. Many meals in today's busy lifestyles are hurried and eaten under stress, leading to poor digestion. But since life isn't going to slow down, a conscious effort must be made to break the vicious digestive circle. It is never easy to change daily habits. Keep remembering how much better you will feel.

Find a way to relax before you eat. Breathe deep. Do some mild stretches. Listen to easy music. Lighten up your meals. Simplify complex meals. Eat less concentrated foods. Take two capsules of acidophilus before each meal to build up your friendly bacteria.

5 Easy Steps to Less Indigestion, Heartburn and Gas

1: Take ENZYMES. America is an enzyme deficient nation. We eat on the run, under stress, out of boxes or cans. Many of the foods we eat are so processed they are completely devoid of nutrients. More importantly, they lack enzymes! Enzymes are the spark plugs for every body function. We are each born with a limited supply of enzymes which become depleted with age. But enzymes can be easily brought into your body through fresh foods. If your food is cooked, microwaved, or processed above 118° Fahrenheit, its enzymes are destroyed. If the foods you eat don't have enough enzymes for digestion, the body has to pull from reserves in your liver or pancreas, weakening enzyme-dependent processes like detoxification or hormone secretion. Without enough enzymes for digestion, bacteria feed off the undigested food in your GI tract, a process that generates gas, bloating, heartburn and constipation. In almost every case, when someone with digestive disorders adds more plant enzymes either through fresh foods or enzyme supplements, digestive problems dramatically lessen. People carrying extra weight from body congestion often drop up to 10 lbs. People who are constipated become more regular. People with food allergies are often able to overcome them. Amylase, the plant enzyme which digests starches, renders gluten-rich grains like wheat and rye harmless to people with gluten enteropathy, a severe intestinal malabsorption syndrome caused by an allergy to gluten grains. (See pages 30-31 **About Enzymes** for more.) Have a green salad every day! And consider DIGESTZYME by Transformation, especially good for women, or POWER-PLUS FOOD ENZYMES by Herbal Products and Development, especially good for men.

2: Take PROBIOTICS. Meaning "for life", probiotics are friendly bacteria, like Lactobacillus acidophilus and Bifidobacteria bifidum, that inhabit your digestive tract and maintain the inner ecology critical to digestion. They keep out pathogens like viruses, yeasts and harmful microorganisms by competing with them for space in the gastrointestinal tract. Probiotics are a powerful preventive against digestive problems like diarrhea, constipation, more serious problems like inflammatory bowel disease, even colon cancer. University of Delaware research finds that bifidobacteria can actually remove cancer cells or the enzymes which lead to their formation!

Your natural probiotics are depleted by: chemicals in your food or environment (like chlorine in drinking water), a stressful lifestyle, excessive alcohol, smoking and some prescription drugs. Over-using antibiotics, is the biggest offender in probiotic depletion. (In France, Japan and India, doctors routinely recommend acidophilus when they prescribe antibiotics.) Probiotics keep your digestion smooth. Eat cultured foods rich in these organisms, like yogurt, kefir or raw sauerkraut. Consider high quality probiotic supplements like Ethical Nutrients INTESTINAL CARE or UAS Labs DDS-PLUS with FOS.

3: Begin good **FOOD COMBINING.** Sometimes, it's not what you eat that's making you sick, it's the way you eat it. Different foods need different enzymes to digest properly. Your intelligent body activates the proper enzyme when it detects a certain food in your mouth. (That's why digestion actually begins in your mouth.) When you eat foods that need widely different enzymes for digestion, the food tends to stay too long in your stomach waiting for digestion. It starts to ferment instead, leading to gas, constipation or diarrhea - clear signs that food is not being assimilated well. Proper food combining can make a lot of difference to your digestion.

Most experts think human digestion evolved very early, when our species ate almost all fresh or dried foods. Foods we ate together fell naturally into certain harvest times and seasons, and we developed the capacity to digest them at the same time. Today we eat any type of food we want when our taste-buds want it. Enzymes which digest one type of food but are incompatible with another type eaten in the same meal, get either blocked or confused, and we get the non-compatible food signs of gas and bloating.

Yet our digestive systems adapt somewhat to our eating habits. Unless your digestion is seriously compromised, you probably don't need to follow all the food combining rules. Sometimes we let these things control our lives and lose the pleasure of eating.

I try to follow just two principles: 1: I eat fruits alone and on an empty stomach in the morning. 2: I don't eat fruits and vegetables together. Check out page 398 in this chapter for a Good Food Combining Diet, and a Good Food Combining Chart.

4: Eat more **FIBER.** Why is fiber so good for us? Fiber from whole grains, fruits and vegetables lowers harmful LDL cholesterol levels linked to heart disease. It speeds weight loss by suppressing the appetite and reducing colon congestion. It improves glucose tolerance for people with diabetes. It provides protection against breast and colon cancer development, diverticulitis and irritable bowel. Fiber also keeps the digestive system running smoothly by decreasing the transit time of food in the intestines.

But, most people don't get enough fiber from their diets. Today's statistics tell us that most Americans need to double their fiber intake to get the 30 to 35 grams a day recommended for digestive health. Six half-cup servings of whole grains, cereal or legumes and 4 servings of fresh fruits and vegetables each day give you the fiber you need. Fiber supplements are good as an addition, not a substitute. Try Nature's Secret ULTIMATE FIBER, or All One TOTALLY FIBER COMPLEX.

5: Eat more **ALKALINE FOODS.** The typical American diet relies on too many acid-forming foods. They're the primary cause of GERD

(Gastro-Esophageal Reflux Disorder), the most common cause of heartburn for 40 million Americans. Our bodies by design are slightly alkaline, with a pH of 7.4. When our systems become too acidic, alkaline minerals like sodium, calcium, potassium and magnesium are pulled from reserves to restore alkaline pH. But disrupting mineral balance becomes dangerous. Even small mineral deficiencies are linked to severe depression, osteoporosis and premature aging. Acidity is also implicated in chronic fatigue syndrome, arthritis, cancer, allergies and fungal infections. Bring more alkaline foods into your diet to ease indigestion and heartburn.

—**Acid-forming foods to limit:** refined sugars, white flour, alcohol, sodas, coffee and caffeine foods, red meat, fried, fatty foods.
—**Alkaline-forming foods to increase:** mineral water, land/sea vegetables, sea salt, herbal teas, miso, brown rice, honey, fruits.

Have you become a victim of antacids?

15 million Americans have heartburn daily. Americans spend $1.7 billion on indigestion remedies each year! But antacids are designed to provide temporary relief. Evidence is piling up that excessive use of over-the-counter antacids may wreak havoc on digestive health. They may even become a health problem themselves because they radically change your digestive chemistry.

Do any of these problems pertain to you?

1) The tolerance effect: The more you use antacids, the more you need them. Antacids neutralize stomach HCl (hydrochloric acid), needed for digestion, or they block it, confuse the body and disrupt its normal processes. If you take a lot of antacids, your body overcompensates, producing excess stomach acid.

2) Antacids disrupt your pH balance: Optimum pH is between 7.35 and 7.45. If you take lots of antacids, your GI tract fluctuates between over alkaline and over acid, leading to problems like diarrhea or constipation, gallbladder disorders and hiatal hernia. A friend thought his heartburn symptoms would improve if he doubled his acid blocker dosage. He ended up in the bathroom all night, passing completely undigested food. Disrupting body pH alters your bowel ecology, too, potentially causing dramatic overgrowth of harmful microorganisms…. like candida yeasts.

3) Pernicious ingredients: Many antacids contain aluminum which causes constipation and bone pain. Others overdose you on magnesium causing diarrhea. Some contain both aluminum and magnesium, and you may get alternating constipation and diarrhea. Antacids full of sodium may cause water retention. Most are laden with chemical coloring agents that can cause allergic reactions in some people or lead to "mood changes" and "mental alterations" if taken regularly. And that's the way many people take them.

4) Some drugs interact with antacids: People on drug therapy for HIV know antacids decrease their HIV drug absorption by up to 23%. Oral contraceptives like "the pill" may lose their effectiveness if taken with antacids. People using NSAIDS drugs for arthritis along with antacids suffer $2^1/_2$ times more serious gastrointestinal complications than those taking a placebo! Antacids not only block drug absorption, they also block your food absorption of nutrients, especially B_{12}, necessary for virtually all immune responses.

5) Some antacids build up and impede body processes: I know a woman who was hospitalized three times for kidney stones. Her physician advised her to stop taking her antacids because the unabsorbed calcium in them was causing her kidney stones.

Diets to Overcome Food Allergies and Sensitivities

Allergies, intolerances and sensitivities to foods or food additives are the fastest growing form of allergic reactions in the U.S. today, as people are more exposed to chemically altered foods. Food intolerances are often confused with food allergies.

A **food allergy** is an antibody reaction — an immune system response to a food your body views as a pathogen. Food allergies may be hereditary; a child is twice as likely to develop food allergies if one parent has them, four times as likely if both parents have them. In addition, when too much fat, and lack of stomach HCl hamper digestion of proteins and acids, these two powerful elements enter the bloodstream undigested. The immune system responds with prostaglandins and histamines; food allergy symptoms result.

A **food intolerance** is an enzyme deficiency to digest a certain food. For example, people with a lactose intolerance experience the bloating, cramping and diarrhea of an allergy reaction, but the symptoms are really due to a deficiency of the enzyme lactase, which helps digest milk sugar. The fastest growing group of foods causing intolerances are food additives — sulfites, nitrates, colorants, preservatives, water pollutants, and heavy metals found in contaminated seafood.

Food sensitivities are similar to allergy reactions, but differ in that no antigen-specific antibodies are present. Common food sensitivities include those to wheat, dairy foods, fruit, sugar, yeast, mushrooms, eggs, corn and greens. These foods may be healthy in themselves, but they are often heavily sprayed or treated; in the case of animal products, also injected with antibiotics and hormones. A food sensitivity is usually not a permanent allergy response.

Is your body showing signs that you have a food allergy?

- Are you unable to eat normal amounts of a food? Are you nauseated after eating?
- Do you get cyclical headaches with mental fuzziness after eating? Is your child irritable, flushed and hyperactive after eating?
- Do you get heart palpitations, with sweating, rashes or puffiness around the eyes after eating?
- Does your abdomen become excessively swollen after eating with heartburn or stomach cramps?
- Have you gained significant weight even though your diet hasn't changed?
- Do you have Crohn's disease, hypothyroidism or hypoglycemia?

If you answer yes to most of these questions, you may have an allergy, intolerance or sensitivity to certain foods or food additives, another kind of Type 2 allergy. Regardless of the food, the reaction symptoms are similar. Inflammation occurs from histamine release into tissue mast cells, walling off the affected body area until immune agents can restore health. But this process takes time. If the body is re-exposed before health is renewed, inflammation and symptoms, especially mucous congestion, become chronic.

In addition to food allergies, the diets in this chapter improve associated problems: *Chronic Gastric Pain, Hiatal Hernia, Gallbladder Disease and Gallstones, Stomach Ulcers, Chronic Gas and Bloating, Crohn's Disease, Colitis and Irritable Bowel Syndrome, Diverticulitis, Bad Breath and Body Odor, Heartburn, Chronic Constipation or Diarrhea.*

A Three-Day Food Allergy Cleansing Diet

Diet change and supplementation with herbs are the best and quickest means of overcoming food intolerances, and restoring digestive tract and immune system integrity. A food elimination-rotation diet can help you identify suspected allergen foods, especially if you are overweight, have candida, sluggish thyroid or hypoglycemia. However, it generally takes quite a bit of time to find the offending foods. To make it easier, eliminate common food allergens first - like wheat, dairy foods, chocolate, eggs, sugar, corn, yeast and sprayed foods. Tune into your personal diet history and try to eat ONLY the foods you least suspect of causing symptoms during the elimination phase of the diet. Safer food choices: rice milk, goat's milk, almond milk, flat breads, quick breads, brown rice, millet, buckwheat, amaranth, quinoa, date sugar, maple syrup, almond butter, sesame butter, egg replacer made from flax or arrowroot.

Coca's pulse test can help you detect food allergens (see page 570).
New blood tests available over-the-counter can also identify food allergies.

The short cleanse below is designed to rid your body of food allergens. It may also be used as the basis of a food elimination diet to determine specific allergens. (To determine personal sensitivities, suspected foods should be introduced in small amounts, one at a time.) Note: You may also follow this elimination diet with the ALLERGY CONTROL DIET next page.

—**On rising:** take 2 fresh lemons squeezed in a glass of water with 1 packet of Monas CHLORELLA granules.
—**Breakfast:** take a glass of cranberry-apple or papaya juice; and some citrus or non-sweet fruits such as pineapple or kiwi.
—**Mid-morning:** a green drink (page 569), or Green Kamut Corp. JUST BARLEY, or Crystal Star ENERGY GREEN DRINK™, and some fresh vegetable snacks with a little sesame salt.
—**Lunch:** a glass of pineapple/coconut juice for protein; or a fresh carrot juice, with a green salad and lemon-olive oil dressing.
—**Mid-afternoon:** take a cup of alkalizing herb tea, such as catnip, alfalfa-mint, or peppermint tea.
—**Dinner:** have another small green salad with lemon-olive oil dressing; or a glass of apple-alfalfa sprout juice.
—**Before bed:** have a relaxing tea, such as chamomile or scullcap tea; or a glass of pineapple/papaya juice, or apple juice.

Notes:
—Drink 6 glasses of water daily to flush allergens through your system.
—Take 2 TBS apple cider vinegar with honey at each meal if desired to acidify saliva.
—Be sure, for these three days, that you eat only organically grown, fresh foods - no pre-prepared foods, that might have fillers, additives or hidden sugars or chemicals.

Recipes that can help your allergen cleansing diet: •DETOXIFICATION and CLEANSING FOODS; •HEALING DRINKS; •SOUPS - LIQUID SALADS; •DAIRY-FREE RECIPES.

Diet to Overcome Food Allergies and Sensitivities

This diet stage should be used for 30 days or more to rebalance, alkalize and energize. It is dairy and gluten free, and does not include other common allergens, like corn, yeast, soy foods, mushrooms, eggs, refined sweeteners, or sea foods (like shellfish) currently at risk of contamination. It is rich in minerals and enzyme-producing foods, and uses good food combining techniques for optimal absorption. Be sure you're omitting any foods containing sulfites, nitrates, nightshade plant derivatives (like tobacco and Motrin), colorants, preservatives and additives.
See THE ART OF FOOD EXCHANGES on page 136 for foods you can use in place of those that are causing digestive problems.

—**On rising:** take a glass of lemon juice with 1 teasp. maple syrup; or cranberry juice with a little honey and ginger; or add New Chapter GINGER WONDER syrup to any drink to help block inflammation.

—**Breakfast:** take a supplement drink like All One MULTIPLE VITAMIN and MINERAL drink, or a green superfood & protein drink, like Ethical Nutrients FUNCTIONAL GREENS in apple juice, or Crystal Star BIOFLAVONOID, FIBER & C SUPPORT™ drink to guard against leaky-gut; or some oatmeal or wheat-free grain cereal with apple juice or yogurt, and 1 TB maple syrup.

—**Mid-morning:** have a green drink (page 569), or Monas CHLORELLA, or Green Foods GREEN MAGMA; or a glass of fresh carrot juice; and a cup of light noodle soup with sea greens snipped on top and perhaps some cubes of almond cheese.

—**Lunch:** have a green salad with a light dressing, and a cup of vegetable or onion soup; or some steamed vegetables and a baked potato with yogurt or kefir cheese topping; or a fruit salad with cottage cheese.

—**Mid-afternoon:** have a glass of apple juice, or an alkalizing herb tea, such as a hibiscus cooler, comfrey leaf, or alfalfa/mint tea.

—**Dinner:** have a Chinese stir-fry with greens, rice noodles, and a sweet and sour sauce; or a baked or broiled fish like salmon or sea bass with brown rice and peas; or a dinner salad with nut and seed toppings and a yogurt dressing; or a baked vegetable casserole with a cup of black bean or lentil soup; or roast turkey slices from free-run organic turkeys, with a salad and baked potato with almond or rice cheese on top. A little white wine (a cultured food) is fine before meals.

—**Before bed:** have a glass of apple, pineapple or papaya juice; or a cup of miso soup with sea greens.

Notes:
• An insidious effect of food allergy is weight gain. Eliminate wheat from your diet to stop allergy-related weight gain.
• Eat plenty of plant foods - fresh vegetables, fruits, fruit and veggie juices, sea greens, whole grains, nuts, seeds and beans.
• Add ½ teasp. spirulina or chlorella granules to any juice or drink throughout the day to neutralize allergens and aid elimination.
• Don't forget cultured foods for digestive flora; use unsaturated vegetable oils. Drink bottled water if possible.
• Eat smaller meals. Chew food very well.

Recipes that can help your allergen cleansing diet: •MINERAL- RICH RECIPES; •ENZYME-RICH RECIPES; •CULTURED HEALING FOODS; •DAIRY FREE RECIPES; •WHEAT FREE RECIPES; •HEALTHY CONDIMENTS/SEASONS.

Herb and Supplement Choices

Take only hypoallergenic supplements; free of corn, wheat, yeast, soy, egg, milk and sugar derivatives, with no fillers or additives.

•**Cleanse the G.I. tract:** Crystal Star BITTERS & LEMON CLEANSE™; or green tea; or aloe vera juice each morning.

•**Produce antihistamines:** Crystal Star ANTI-HST™ or ALRG™ caps; CoQ-10 60mg 3x daily.

•**Reduce allergic reactions:** CC Pollen ALLER BEE-GONE, MSM 400-1000mg 2x daily; Crystal Star GINSENG-REISHI extract; Omega-3 flax oil with meals for essential fatty acids (EFA's). For bloating, $\frac{1}{2}$ tsp. baking soda in water.

—**For gluten intolerance:** (See also Diet for Candida Albicans page 365) Crystal Star CAND-EX™ caps especially if unexplained weight gain; Bio-Allers FOOD ALLERGY GRAIN.

—**For lactose intolerance:** Lactaid drops or tablets; Country Life DAIRY-ZYME; Prevail DAIRY ENZYMES.

•**Add a digestive & proteolytic enzyme formula:** Use a full spectrum digestive enzyme like Herbal Products POWER PLUS ENZYMES, and a protease formula like Transformation PUREZYME. Quercetin 500mg daily between meals with bromelain 500mg 3x daily for antioxidant activity plus enzymes.

•**Add probiotics:** Acidophilus before meals; aloe vera juice with 2 tsp. bee pollen granules after meals for best enzyme activity. For a sour stomach: lime juice and a pinch ginger.

•**Herbal enzymes boost immunity - normalize digestion:** Milk thistle seed extract; Dandelion root-nettles tea; Echinacea-goldenseal root caps; •Gaia SWEETISH BITTERS or add a dropperful of Crystal Star PRE-MEAL ENZ™ EXTRACT to water and take before meals; or a dropperful of AFTER MEAL ENZ™ EXTRACT to water after meals.

Bodywork and Lifestyle Techniques

Note: Food allergies are common in children; many result from feeding babies meats and commercial dairy foods before 10-12 months. Babies do not have the right enzymes to digest these foods. Feed mother's milk, rice milk or goat's milk for 10 months to avoid food allergies.

•**Diagnose:** Use Coca's Pulse Test or muscle testing to identify allergens. (See page 570, and pages 466-467) Both skin-prick and RAST tests used by many allergists often misdiagnose food allergies unless a rotation-reintroduction diet is also used.

•**Enema:** Consider a garlic-catnip enema to cleanse the digestive tract and balance colon pH.

•**Avoid caffeine, aspirin, and cortisone drugs.** Each of these can damage the stomach and intestinal walls, and cause gastritis and ulcers.

• **No smoking before meals.** Nicotine magnifies allergies almost more than any other substance.

• **No fluids with meals** - especially no sodas or carbonated drinks. Phosphoric acid binds up many digestive enzymes.

•**Eat relaxed.** Tension and stress reduce the body's ability to deal with allergens.

Can't find a recommended product? Call the 800 number listed in Product Resources for the store nearest you and for more info.

About Good Food Combining

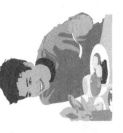

Keep it simple. The human digestive system works best when the number of different foods in a meal is small - about four or five. Each category of foods —fruits, starches, proteins, sweets, etc. requires different acid/alkaline mediums, different enzymes and different digestion times. Eating foods together that have drastically different digestive needs often results in poor assimilation. The body simply passes foods through with no digestion, or holds them back to wait for the proper enzyme medium. Sometimes the unassimilated food decomposes in the digestive tract and then ferments, producing gas along with resulting heartburn or elimination problems.

People have known about good digestion and good food combining for centuries. In simpler times, when we ate with the harvests and seasons, food combinations almost fell into place by themselves. Things that were available at the same time were eaten at the same time.... and so our digestive systems adapted. Today, we can have literally any food, any time, from any where, at any season. Food combinations come from all over the globe. We eat summer, winter, spring and autumn foods in any combo or all together.

America's "melting pot" of ethnic foods, fast foods and pre-prepared foods is one of the worst for good food combining or easy digestion. Most of us start off "not right" each morning because we eat citrus juice, coffee and bread or grain together. We continue through the day drinking milk with meals, eating fruits with meats, veggies and grains. At the end of the day we have a heavy, concentrated starch and protein meal that discourages enzyme activity. A lot of food is only partially digested, or not digested at all, left in the stomach, fermenting and causing gas. Undigested or poorly digested food is a primary cause of the epidemic food intolerances and sensitivities we experience today.

It can get very confusing. Yet, food combining is only one factor in healthy eating. It doesn't guarantee good digestion. Overeating, eating under stress or fatigue, eating before strenuous exercise, or during strong emotional experiences also reduces digestive capacity. Caffeine and alcohol retard digestion considerably. Fever and inflammatory illness may partially suspend digestion to conserve energy. As your diet incorporates more fresh, unprocessed foods, good food combining naturally becomes part of good eating habits. I have included a simple chart on the basics of good food combining. (See page 398.)

<u>Here's the bottom line:</u>

1) Small amounts of poor combinations don't seem to cause problems, and sometimes really enhance taste and enjoyment, such as a handful of raisins in a cake, or a whole grain cereal with a little apple juice or yogurt.

2) Fruits of all kinds are better eaten fresh, by themselves, in the first half of the day.

Enzyme-Rich, Good Food Combining Diet

Ease your new diet into your life. This diet improves faulty food combining gently and moderately by avoiding red meats, caffeine, sugary, fatty and fried foods. It keeps your system alkaline by avoiding dairy products (except cultured dairy foods, like yogurt, cottage cheese, and kefir that offer "friendly flora"). It's full of enzyme-rich foods like fresh vegetables and fruits (like papaya and pineapple) to keep digestion strong.

You can use this diet for a lifetime. It is varied, yet observes good food combinations for easiest digestion. It features simple, lightly cooked high mineral dishes. It emphasizes high fiber to give you a feeling of fullness with very little calorie expenditure. It maintains proper acid/alkaline balance, and stimulates and increases your own enzyme production.

Note: Most commercial antacids neutralize stomach acid, generally making the condition worse, as the stomach produces more acids in an attempt to achieve enzyme rebalance. Experts tell us that Tagamet and Zantac, drugs prescribed regularly for ulcers and gastric problems, can be addictive in the long term. They also inhibit bone formation and proper liver function.

—**On rising:** have grapefruit, papaya, or apple juice; or 2 TBS cider vinegar in water with 1 tsp. maple syrup and 1 tsp. acidophilus; or 10 drops Crystal Star BITTERS & LEMON CLEANSE™ extract in water; or aloe vera juice with 1 tsp. chlorophyll liquid.

—**Breakfast:** have a high fiber, whole grain cereal, or granola with yogurt, apple juice or vanilla rice or almond drink; or fresh fruit with yogurt or kefir; or oatmeal or buckwheat pancakes with a little maple syrup or apple juice, kefir, or miso sauce.

—**Mid-morning:** have some whole grain muffins and a green drink, or a green superfood drink; or carrot juice with 1 teasp. spirulina granules or chlorophyll liquid added, and some whole grain crackers with kefir cheese or a vegetable dip.

—**Lunch:** before eating, have another glass of aloe vera juice with 1 teasp. acidophilus liquid; then have a green veggie salad, and a cup of miso soup with sea greens snipped on top; or a baked potato with yogurt cheese or non dairy topping, and a green salad; or cole slaw with yogurt dressing and cornbread.

Note: Follow any above choice with Crystal Star AFTER MEAL ENZ™ extract for enzyme stimulation.

—**Mid-afternoon:** have some crunchy raw veggies with kefir or yogurt cheese or a veggie dip, and a mineral drink, such as Crystal Star SYSTEMS STRENGTH DRINK™; or a mild herb tea, such as comfrey, slippery elm or peppermint tea.

—**Dinner:** take another lemon and water drink or aloe vera juice with acidophilus liquid before eating: then have some brown rice with tofu and veggies; or an oriental stir-fry with brown rice and miso soup; or grilled fish or seafood dinner with a light vegetable quiche with yogurt-wine sauce; or some millet or bulgar grains with steamed veggies and teriyaki sauce or light yogurt/chive dressing; or a hearty veggie stew with whole grain bread.

Note: A little white wine at dinner can often help digestion.

—**Before bed:** have some pineapple/papaya juice, or apple juice; or make a broth with Red Star nutritional yeast; or alfalfa/mint tea.

Recipes for your enzyme-rich diet: •SALADS-HOT and COLD; •SUGAR-FREE RECIPES; •ENZYME-RICH RECIPES; •CULTURED HEALING FOODS; •DAIRY FREE RECIPES; •HIGH FIBER RECIPES; •HIGH MINERAL RECIPES.

GOOD FOOD COMBINATIONS

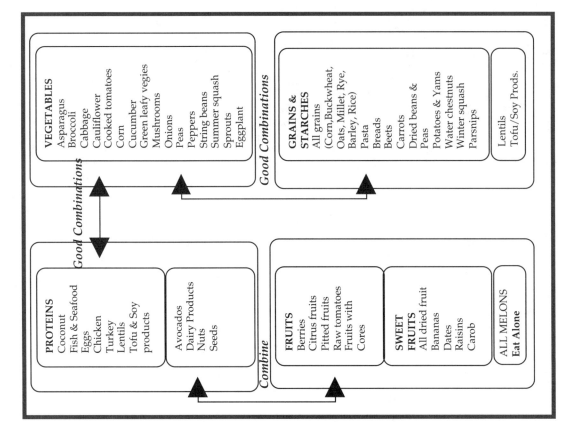

Good Combinations

VEGETABLES
Asparagus
Broccoli
Cabbage
Cauliflower
Cooked tomatoes
Corn
Cucumber
Green leafy vegies
Mushrooms
Onions
Peas
Peppers
String beans
Summer squash
Sprouts
Eggplant

Good Combinations

**GRAINS &
STARCHES**
All grains
(Corn,Buckwheat,
Oats, Millet, Rye,
Barley, Rice)
Pasta
Breads
Beets
Carrots
Dried beans &
Peas
Potatoes & Yams
Water chestnuts
Winter squash
Parsnips

Lentils
Tofu/Soy Prods.

PROTEINS
Coconut
Fish & Seafood
Eggs
Chicken
Turkey
Lentils
Tofu & Soy
products

Avocados
Dairy Products
Nuts
Seeds

Combine

FRUITS
Berries
Citrus fruits
Pitted fruits
Raw tomatoes
Fruits with
Cores

**SWEET
FRUITS**
All dried fruit
Bananas
Dates
Raisins
Carob

ALL MELONS
Eat Alone

Herb and Supplement Choices

• **Add enzymes:** Bromelain 1500mg daily; Transformation DIGESTZYME; American Health PAPAYA CHEWABLES; Crystal Star SYSTEMS STRENGTH™ drink; Pancreatin capsules 1400mg; Herbal Products and Development POWER PLUS ENZYMES; Garlic/parsley caps.

• **Add cultured foods:** like yogurt, kefir, miso and cultured vegetables like Rejuvenative Foods RAW SAUERKRAUT.

• **Add green superfoods:** chlorella, spirulina, or liquid chlorophyll daily.

• **For heartburn:** Crystal Star GINSENG/LICORICE ELIXIR™; L-glutamine therapy 1500mg daily for long-term relief; Prevail ACID EASE or Betaine HCl caps after meals.

• **Relieve gas:** take pinches cinnamon, nutmeg, ginger, cloves in water-drink down. Ginger capsules 2 to 4 as needed; 2 to 4 peppermint oil drops in water (also for irritable bowel).

—**For belching and burping:** AkPharma BEANO drops; Prevail BEAN-VEGI formula; Country Life DIGESTIVE formula.

—**For cramping and diarrhea:** Take activated charcoal tabs - short term; Apple pectin tabs; Crystal Star CRAMP BARK COMBO™ caps.

• **Add probiotics:** UAS Labs DDS-PLUS with FOS; Ethical Nutrients INTESTINAL CARE; Premier Labs MULTI-DOPHILUS caps or Nature's Path FLORA-LYTE.

• **Complete digestion with teas:** Mint or alfalfa-mint tea; Catnip-fennel-lemon peel tea; Chamomile tea; Wild yam tea, especially if you have eaten too much refined sugar.

• **Bitters herbs help stop heartburn:** Crystal Star AFTER MEAL ENZ™ extract in water or PRE-MEAL ENZ™ before meals; BITTERS & LEMON CLEANSE™ extract each morning.

Can't find a recommended product? Call the 800 number listed in Product Resources for the store nearest you and for more info.

Dealing with Blood Sugar Blues Naturally

It's the bittersweet truth: Even after decades of warnings about their dangers we are a nation addicted to sugar and artificial sweeteners like aspartame. Some of us to the point of body destruction! The average American eats more than 150 pounds of refined sugar every year —up from one-half pound of sugar a year in the 1800's. Sugar has become an entire food group, counting for an astounding 20% of total daily calories for adult Americans. The news is even worse for U.S. kids, who eat enough sugar to account for half of their daily calories! The problem is so out of control that 46 health advocacy groups signed a letter to the U.S. government Dec. 31, 1998, urging it to commission more funds for studies on sugar before the problem gets worse.

Are you confused about sugar? We need sugar, in the form of glucose or blood sugar, to live. But, our bodies get enough glucose from eating complex carbohydrates like vegetables, whole grains and legumes. We don't need to get it from simple carbohydrates like sugar or corn syrup. Refined sugar first appeared as a "military drug" during the War of 1812 as a light, quick energy source for armies. It's a revealing sugar fact that when sugar was used by Napoleon's army, he lost his first battle! Sugar existed only as a medicinal until the end of the last century, when it entered into regular food supply. What we know as sugar today is actually a heavily refined substance that qualifies more as a drug than a food! Just two teaspoons of refined sugar is enough to throw off your body chemistry.

A high sugar intake heavily stresses your pancreas, causing abnormal insulin production, and inviting health problems like diabetes and hypoglycemia. A sugar heavy diet suppresses immune response because refined sugar destroys the ability of white blood cells to kill germs for up to 5 hours after consumption! Sugar also disrupts hormonal health, and feeds candida yeast and some cancers.

Too much sugar invariably leads to nutritional deficiencies, because sugar robs the body of B vitamins, minerals like magnesium and zinc, and trace minerals like copper and chromium. Your heart, kidneys and liver all suffer as the result of too much sugar. Eating too much sugar accelerates the aging process of your cells! High sugar consumption is directly related to obesity, coronary thrombosis and periodontal disease. Hyperactivity and Attention Deficit Disorder (ADD) are aggravated by sugar. Sugar even affects energy and mood. Most of us know that our energy drops after a sugar binge, but did you know that too much sugar can cause depression? A University of Alabama study finds people in major depression benefit from eliminating refined sugar from their diet.

Hidden sugars like "high fructose corn syrup," in almost all commercial sodas and juices today, are no good for health either. Studies from Israel reveal that rats fed a high fructose diet age faster because changes in their collagen result in premature skin wrinkling and sagging. Studies also show that sodas sweetened with high fructose corn syrup cause mineral losses of phosphorous and calcium, which may contribute to osteoporosis. Sugar-free artificial sweeteners, which many people think are healthier than sugar, are actually toxic chemicals — not foods you should include in your regular diet. Every time I see someone use an artificial aspartame sweetener like Equal, I cringe. New studies are pouring in on how these poisons are setting up an environment for ravaging illnesses like lupus, multiple sclerosis and Alzheimer's disease that are rising in America.

The leader of today's artificial sweeteners is aspartame, a substance that has received more complaints about adverse reactions than any other food ingredient in FDA history. Aspartame's major brand names, NutraSweet and Equal, have taken the place of saccharin in pre-prepared foods and drinks, and that means we get a lot of it. Some people have immediate, serious reactions from aspartame – extreme dizziness, headaches, throat swelling, allergic reactions and retina deterioration are just a few documented side effects. The American College of Physicians says aspartame is causing a plague of neurological diseases in the U.S.. Pregnant and lactating women, toddlers or allergy-prone children, and those with PKU, should avoid aspartame products.

Scientists at the World Environmental Conference recently presented information on aspartame's terrible side effects: If aspartame's temperature exceeds 86° F, the wood alcohol in it converts to formaldehyde, the same substance used to embalm the dead. Formaldehyde causes methanol toxicity in the body. Over time, methanol toxicity is deadly, mimicking the symptoms of multiple sclerosis, fibromyalgia and lupus (diseases common for diet soda drinkers). The conference study found that cases of M.S. and lupus are actually misdiagnosed "aspartame disease." Eliminating aspartame can cause a complete remission of symptoms for some people.

Aspartame can wreck your eyesight and memory. Formaldehyde builds in the retina from aspartame causing blurred or tunnel vision, visual disturbances like bright flashes or black spots, and may even cause retinal detachment. Aspartame also alters delicate brain chemistry, aggravating Parkinson's disease and increasing Alzheimer's risk. Without the other balancing amino acids found in protein, aspartame's ingredients, aspartic acid and phenylalanine, deteriorate brain cells, leading to memory loss, especially significant for the elderly who consume chemically sweetened beverages at record levels.

Gulf War Syndrome is believed to be directly related aspartame poisoning! Guess what sat for weeks at a time in the blistering desert heat for our troops in Desert Storm? Diet sodas sweetened with aspartame. By the time, our soldiers drank them, aspartame's chemical structure was so altered by the heat, the soldiers got sick almost immediately.

Epileptic, grand mal seizures are a side effect of aspartame. At high altitudes, this effect is magnified, sometimes causing sudden memory loss, visual problems and epileptic seizures. Reports in the magazines Flying Safety and Navy Physiology recount several instances where pilots who had Equal in their coffee went into epileptic convulsions! Aspartame contains 10% methanol which can cause oxygen deprivation. At high altitudes, this effect is magnified, sometimes causing sudden memory loss, visual problems and epileptic seizures. Reports in the magazines Flying Safety and Navy Physiology recount several instances where pilots who had Equal in their coffee went into epileptic convulsions!

Brain tumors rates have increased 10% since aspartame was added to our food supply. The new statistics add validation to the studies done in the 70's with lab animals who were fed aspartame, then showed an unusually high number of brain tumors.

Finally, the very people for whom artificial sweeteners are developed are its biggest victims. Aspartame is dangerous for people with blood sugar problems like diabetes and hypoglycemia. Aspartame, 200 times sweeter than sugar, keeps blood sugar levels out of control by disrupting the way your body uses insulin. Diabetes and hypoglycemia may progress and worsen. Some diabetic patients have even lapsed into comas and died after switching to aspartame sweeteners. Eyes diagnosed with diabetic retinopathy are often victims of aspartame toxicity instead. Neurological damage, memory loss and confusion, and dramatic changes in appetite and weight are frequently a problem for diabetic and hypoglycemic patients hooked on this chemical.

If you use aspartame foods regularly (read labels carefully), problems are one of our countries biggest health threats. There patent recently expired, we'll be seeing even more aspartame drink), molasses, rice syrup and fruit juice concentrates may even for people with blood sugar problems. (See below.)

or eat lots of sugary foods you should know that blood sugar are already 5,000 products containing aspartame. (Since the in foods.) Healthier sweeteners like honey, amazake (sweet rice be a better choice. The herb, stevia, is a healthy sweetening choice.

Do you have the blood sugar blues? There are body signs to watch for. Taking your blood sugar when you get up in the morning can give you some helpful clues. For a non-diabetic, blood sugar should be below 150 in the morning before eating and below 150 two hours after a meal. For a diabetic, blood sugar should be between 80-120 in the morning before a meal and less than 180 two hours after a meal. If your blood sugar gets higher than 230 or lower than 70, you should consult with your physician about treatment for possible diabetes or hypoglycemia. Regular hypoglycemic blood sugar swings may be a sign that you're at risk for adult onset diabetes. Home blood glucose monitoring kits such as Lifescan /Johnson & Johnson ONE TOUCH PROFILE are reliable.

Have you heard about Stevia? Why does our FDA keep trying to railroad it off store shelves? Here's the story in a nutshell.

Stevia is a natural sweetener, safe even for diabetics. Yet it's been an herb under fire from the U.S. FDA. I remember well when stevia was literally ripped off health food store shelves, its makers dragged to jail, their offices ransacked and computers confiscated. Stevia rebaudiana or "sweet herb," native to Paraguay, is an herb with a turbulent story. Not because it is unsafe or has rampant side effects, but because it is big competition for the billion dollar U. S. commercial sweetener market, especially Nutra-Sweet.

Stevia has a centuries' long history of safe use as a natural, herbal sweetener. In South America, it's been used since the 16th century to sweeten foods and as a key ingredient in medicinal teas. Stevia has been grown in England since WW II as an inexpensive sugar substitute. The Japanese widely embraced stevia as a natural sweetener. Stevia now holds 47% of the Japanese sweetener marketplace and has been enjoyed for over 25 years as a regular part of their diet. U.S. distribution began in the late seventies, as Americans demanded healthier alternatives to refined sugar and chemical sweeteners. Stevia immediately became a formidable rival to saccharin and aspartame sweeteners in the U.S. marketplace, widely used throughout the 80's. It wasn't long before the backlash began. The FDA admits it received trade complaints (not safety complaints) from sweetener companies about stevia in the early 80's.

In 1991, the FDA put an import ban on all stevia products to stop any "unapproved" use of the herb in the U.S., saying stevia was a food additive and should not be declared safe unless proven safe by U.S. (not foreign) research. Yet stevia, in its whole, unadulterated form, is a food, NOT a food additive, that meets the GRAS (generally recognized as safe) food criteria. Extensive modern research and experience with stevia in Japan and Brazil has proved stevia to be safe and non-toxic.

The truth: stevia was literally run out of the marketplace by a money driven conspiracy of manufacturers of other sweeteners like Nutrasweet (aspartame) and saccharin to maintain control of the U.S. market. Stevia is still the target of FDA attack. In 1997, the FDA prepared a document with 19 "unresolved concerns" on stevia's safety. According to the FDA, certain studies indicated that stevia might contribute to hypoglycemia. Researcher, Mauro Alvarez Ph.D. , **whose work was cited in the document**, vehemently disagrees with the FDA conclusions.

In a direct quote, Alvarez said, "The only possible way to report that the stevia results showed detrimental effects is to take the information out of context...If this is the case, then the FDA scientists are incompetent or have as their objective, keeping the plant away from American consumers by attributing to it safety issues that don't exist." (Ironically, the FDA has received more complaints on side effects of aspartame (Nutrasweet) than any other substance in the agency's history! Yet FDA continues to give aspartame thumbs up for safety!)

As of this writing (2001) the pressure from the FDA is intense. No educational materials on stevia can make any claims of stevia as a natural sweetening agent. In 1998, the FDA demanded a Texas-based stevia company to burn all its stevia books. Burning books!? I spoke with Robert McCaleb, president of the Herb Research Foundation about stevia safety: "The Herb Research Foundation has reviewed the literature on the safety of stevia and concludes unequivocally that stevia is safe for use in food and should be allowed as a food by the FDA. I strongly disagree with the FDA's tactics of destroying literature."

Can Americans ever enjoy the benefits of this "good for you" sweetener?

Stevia is a low calorie, non toxic sweetener even for people with blood sugar problems like diabetes and hypoglycemia for whom refined sugar and chemical sweeteners can be poison. Today, in South America, stevia is recommended to diabetic and hypoglycemic patients as a healthy sweetener and blood sugar regulator. Health experts say that stevia may soon be regarded as one of the most "good for you" sweeteners on earth!

Unlike sugar, stevia does not cause tooth cavities. Instead, stevia is a potent herbal antibiotic, actually helping prevent tooth decay and gum disease. Regular stevia users report fewer colds and flu. Other studies find stevia lowers high blood pressure. (Stevia does not seem to affect normal blood pressure indicating that your body uses it as a balancer, instead of a drug.) Stevia can even be used as a weight management aid because it contains no calories, while significantly increasing glucose tolerance and inhibiting glucose absorption. People whose weight loss problems stem from a craving for sweets report that it decreases their desire for sugary foods. Many users report that stevia tea reduces desire for tobacco and alcoholic beverages. A facial mask of water-based stevia extract (full of AHA's) effectively smoothes out skin wrinkles while healing skin blemishes, including acne. A drop of the extract may be applied directly on a blemish outbreak for fast results, sometimes within 24 hours.

Can Americans get and use stevia today?

Strangely, the FDA allows the same stevia that it condemns as a food to be sold as a dietary supplement. Even though it is not labeled a sweetener, once you buy it, you can use it any way you like. It has a slight licorice flavor that most people find pleasant. But, remember... stevia is 200 times sweeter than sugar. Just one teaspoon of dried leaves is sweeter than 1 full cup of sugar! A tiny pinch of dried leaves is all you need to sweeten a drink or cooking liquid. Liquid extracts and powders are recommended for cooking and as tabletop sweeteners. The powdered extract should be mixed with water and used by the drop according to directions. Body Ecology SWEET 'N BETTER (liquid concentrate) @ 800-511-2660 and Now STEVIA EXTRACT (powder) @ 800-999-8069 –both quality stevia products.

The diets in this section help sugar-related problems: *Epilepsy, Hyperactivity, Diabetic Retinopathy, Mood and Personality Swings, Schizophrenia, Cataracts and Glaucoma, Drug and Alcohol Addiction, Adrenal Exhaustion, Male Impotence, Unexplained Weight Gain, Gingivitis.*

Controlling Diabetes Naturally

Diabetes is on the rise in America... and it's almost always a result of our western "civilized" diet. Type 1 diabetes, a juvenile condition, is more severe and almost entirely dependent on insulin to sustain life. Type 2, adult-onset, non-insulin dependent diabetes, affects about 85% of diabetics, striking one in 20 Americans. With its complications, it is the third leading cause of death in the U. S.. It's a chronic degenerative disease in which disturbances in normal insulin mechanisms impair the body's ability to use carbohydrates. Type 2 diabetics produce insulin, the hormone that helps convert food into energy, but it isn't used properly (insulin resistance), so glucose builds up in the bloodstream, depriving cells of nutrients. The pancreas produces little or no insulin, so diabetic blood sugar levels fluctuate dramatically between too low and too high. The end result is extreme fatigue, lost job productivity and serious health complications. Diet improvement is absolutely necessary to overcoming diabetes.

Do you think you or your child might have diabetes? Here are the signs.

Type II - Adult-Onset Diabetes
–Are you always thirsty? Do you urinate too often?
–Do cuts and bruises heal slowly?
–Have you lost weight but weren't on a diet?
–Are you constantly tired? or drowsy?
–Do you get frequent infections?
–Do you get leg cramps, or prickling in your fingers or toes?
–Have you experienced episodes of impotence?
–Is your vision blurry from time to time?

Juvenile Diabetes
–Is your child unusually thirsty?
–Does he or she urinate too often?
–Is your child extremely hungry?
–Is your child unusually irritable?
–Is he or she unusually tired? or drowsy?
–Has your child lost weight lately?

Both types common today - juvenile onset diabetes (type 1) and adult onset diabetes (type 2) are serious. Preliminary studies suggest juvenile diabetes is linked to cow's milk consumption in infants. Research from the journal, Diabetes Care in 1994, showed that infants fed a cow's milk formula in the first three months of life have a much higher risk of developing juvenile-onset diabetes.

Adult onset diabetes is clearly a "civilization" disease caused by our common Western diet – long-term overload of refined carbohydrates (white bread and pastries) too many sugar-laced foods, and low fiber. Obesity, lack of exercise, a family history of diabetes, and being African American also increase your risk for adult onset diabetes. High blood sugar usually indicates high triglycerides, too.

Sixteen million Americans have adult onset diabetes today. Experts think up to 8 million more have the disease but don't know it! Heart disease, high blood pressure, retinopathy (loss of vision), nerve damage, obesity, kidney malfunction, accelerated aging (from arteriosclerosis), food allergies and circulatory problems all face diabetics with much more ferocity than non-diabetics. Diabetics are 250 times more likely to suffer a stroke! Women with diabetes run a much greater risk of heart attack than either diabetic men or non-diabetic women.

Diabetes Control Diet

Diabetic proneness is often hereditary, and is usually brought on by dietary habits that include too many sugary foods and refined carbohydrates. Pancreatic activity is damaged, the body loses the ability to produce enough insulin, and high blood sugar results. As less and less insulin is produced, simple sugars, which require large amounts of insulin for metabolism, accumulate in the body and are stored as fat. The following diet, in addition to reducing insulin requirements and balancing blood sugar, has the nice "side effect" of healthy weight loss.

This diet supplies slow-burning, complex carbohydrate fuels that do not need much insulin for metabolism. Meals are small, largely vegetarian, and low in fats of all kinds. Proteins come from soy foods and whole grains that are rich in lecithin and chromium. Fifty percent of the diet is based in fresh or simply cooked vegetables for low calories and high digestibility. Avoid caffeine and caffeine foods, hard liquor, food coloring and sodas. Even "diet" sodas have phenylalanine that can affect blood sugar levels.

—**On rising:** take the juice of two lemons in a glass of water with 2 teasp. Monas CHLORELLA granules.

—**Breakfast:** have aloe vera juice, or ALL ONE VITAMIN-MINERAL drink mix in apple juice or water to regulate and balance sugar curve; or make a mix of 2 TBS <u>each</u>: nutritional yeast, toasted wheat germ, lecithin granules and rice or oat bran. Sprinkle some on your choice of breakfast foods, or mix into yogurt with fresh fruit and grated almonds on top; or have 1) poached egg on whole grain toast; 2) granola with apple juice or vanilla soy milk; 3) buckwheat pancakes with apple juice or molasses.

—**Mid-morning:** have a green drink like Crystal Star ENERGY GREEN™ or Green Foods GREEN MAGMA; and whole grain crackers or muffins with a soy spread or kefir cheese; and a sugar balancing herb tea, such as licorice, dandelion, or pau d'arco tea.

—**Lunch:** have a green salad, with celery, sprouts, green pepper, marinated tofu, and mushroom soup; or baked tofu, tofu burgers or turkey with steamed veggies and rice or cornbread; or a baked potato with yogurt or kefir cheese, or soy cheese and some miso soup with sea greens; or a whole grain sandwich, with avocado, low fat or soy cheese, a low fat spread and watercress.

—**Mid-afternoon:** have a glass of carrot juice; and/or fruit juice sweetened cookies with a bottle of mineral water or herb tea; or watercress-cucumber sandwiches with a kefir cheese sandwich spread; or a hard boiled egg with sesame salt, or a veggie dip.

—**Dinner:** Keep it light - have baked or broiled seafood with brown rice and peas; or a Chinese stir-fry with rice, veggies and miso soup; or Spanish beans and rice with onions and peppers; or a light Italian polenta with a hearty vegetable soup, or whole grain or veggie pasta salad; or a mushroom quiche with whole grain crust and yogurt/wine sauce, and a green salad. A little white wine is fine with dinner for relaxation and has surprisingly high chromium content. Beware anything more than moderate alcohol, it can cause blood sugar to soar.

—**Before bed:** take a heaping teasp. Crystal Star CHOL-LO FIBER TONE™ mix in apple juice; or Red Star nutritional yeast or miso, 1 teasp. in warm water.

Recipes for a diabetes control diet: •BREAKFAST and BRUNCH; •PROTEIN without MEAT; •SUGAR-FREE FOODS; •ENZYME FOODS; •SALADS, HOT and COLD; •MINERAL- RICH FOODS; •SANDWICHES; •HIGH FIBER FOODS.

Bodywork and Lifestyle Techniques

• **Don't smoke.** Nicotine increases the desire for sugar and sugary foods. Don't stop or reduce insulin without monitoring by your physician.

• **Use all sweeteners sparingly,** on special occasions for longevity and better health.

• **Walking is good exercise for diabetics** to increase metabolic processes and reduce need for insulin.

• **Alternate hot and cold hydrotherapy** to stimulate circulation. See pg. 463.

• **A regular deep therapy massage** is effective in regulating sugar use through the body.

• **Avoid phenylalanine.** No Nutra-Sweet or Aspartame products. (Check labels on colas, diet drinks, etc.) They may trigger diabetes.

• **If you're overweight, loose the excess.** Poor bio-chemistry often results from being overweight. A fiber weight loss drink, like Crystal Star CHOL-LO FIBER TONE™ or AloeLife FIBER-MATE are effective.

Herb and Supplement Choices

• **Stabilize blood sugar:** Crystal Star SUGAR STRATEGY HIGH™ capsules to encourage insulin balance; GTF Chromium or chromium picolinate 100mcg 2x daily; Siberian ginseng extract or Grifron MAITAKE MUSHROOM caps to stabilize blood sugar. Crystal Star GINSENG-LICORICE ELIXIR™ or dandelion-licorice tea; vitamin E 800IU daily; fenugreek seed, bitter melon or rosemary tea balance blood sugar. Neem and turmeric powders ($^1/_4$ tsp. each in 1 tsp. honey before a meal).

• **Lower blood sugar levels:** Alpha Lipoic acid 600mg daily lowers glucose levels up to 30%; Crystal Star GINSENG 6 SUPER TEA™ or Bilberry extract; or Olive Leaf extract; high dose biotin - 3000mcg daily; Vitamin C 3000mg daily with magnesium 400mg daily combats insulin resistance.

• **Normalize pancreas activity and insulin function:** Take gymnema sylvestre extract before meals to help repair damage; Ester C 3000mg daily increases insulin tolerance, normalizes pancreatic activity. Glutamine 1000mg with carnitine 1000mg; Nutricology PRO-LIVE olive leaf extract as directed; DHEA 25mg daily increases cell sensitivity to insulin. *Burdock, Pau d'arco or Astragalus* tea, 2 cups daily for 3 months; raw pancreas glandular or Premier VANADIUM 25mcg daily.

• **Prevent nerve damage with EFA's:** Evening Primrose Oil capsules 1000mg daily, Omega-3 flax or fish oil (for DHA) 3000mg daily.

• **Raise antioxidants:** Pycnogenol or grape seed PCO's 200mg daily.

• **Boost energy:** Crystal Star ADR-ACTIVE™ caps for cortex support with BODY REBUILDER™ for stable energy. Spirulina tablets 6 daily to elevate mood.

Can't find a recommended product? Call the 800 number listed in Product Resources for the store nearest you and for more info.

Hypoglycemia Control Plan

Hypoglycemia and diabetes stem from the same causes. Hypoglycemia is caused by sugary food overload, but a hypoglycemic's body reacts to the sugar in the opposite way. The pancreas produces too much insulin rather than too little. The blood sugar swings are just as wild, though. In fact, regular hypoglycemic episodes can be a marker that your body is on the pathway to diabetes. If your adrenals are exhausted (they sit atop your kidneys and they hurt when pressed if they're exhausted), if you diet excessively, or if you abuse drugs or alcohol, you're on a road to hypoglycemia.

There are two types of hypoglycemia: 1) Endogenous hypoglycemia, related to a serious medical condition such as liver disease, is the most serious and requires immediate medical supervision; 2) Reactive hypoglycemia, which happens a few hours after a meal, is the type we're talking about in this section. Reactive hypoglycemia occurs when the excess insulin secreted by the pancreas lowers blood sugar to the point of body disruption. This form of hypoglycemia is an internal body condition, not a disease. It is less severe than endogenous hypoglycemia, but symptoms become apparent swiftly. Your decision making and thinking abilities are affected first, because your brain requires 50% of all blood glucose as an energy source to think clearly.

Do you think you have low blood sugar? Here are signs to watch for:

The importance of correct diagnosis and treatment of sugar instabilities is essential. The human body possesses a complex set of checks and balances to maintain blood glucose concentrations within a narrow range. Blood sugar control is influenced by the pituitary, thyroid and adrenal glands, as well as the pancreas, liver, kidneys and even the skeletal muscles. Hypoglycemia symptoms are often mistaken for other problems. Low blood sugar is the biological equivalent of a race car running on empty. It is not so much a disease as a symptom of other disorders. Some of the symptoms can be improved right away by eating something, but this does not address the cause.

—memory lapses and mental dullness
—mood swings, especially aggressive behavior
—depression and anxiety
—insomnia
—blurry vision that goes to frequent headaches or migraines
—periodic ravenous hunger, especially cravings for sweets
—shakiness, racing heartbeat resulting in temporary incoordination
—severe PMS

If you have any of these symptoms regularly for two weeks or more, you should consult with a physician to determine whether you have hypoglycemia. Hypothyroidism or chronic stress can mimic hypoglycemia symptoms. A blood test is a quick way to determine whether hypoglycemia is causing your symptoms. Home blood glucose monitoring kits are also available from your pharmacist.

Hypoglycemia in children is widely indicated as a cause of both hyperactivity and learning disorders. Chronic negativism, mood swings, aggressive behavior, and obstinate resentment to all discipline are reasons for at least taking the self-test below, as well as a Glucose Tolerance Test from a physician. I find that for children, the condition can only be managed by a diet from which all forms of concentrated sugars have been removed, including fruit juices.

Natural therapies can help you reduce blood sugar swings.

Natural therapies for hypoglycemia are much the same as those for diabetes because the conditions are so closely related and their underlying causes are similar. Like diabetes, hypoglycemia responds quickly to natural therapies. The rewards of a commitment to a diet change are well worth it.

1: **Avoid refined carbohydrates** like pastas and white bread, and sugary foods which cause blood sugar to rise rapidly. Your pancreas will over-produce insulin to clean up the excess blood glucose, which then may cause your blood sugar levels to drop, prompting the hypoglycemic reaction.

2: **A low glycemic diet is a good answer for dealing with hypoglycemia.** See the next page for a hypoglycemia control diet.

3: **Avoid "trigger" foods like alcohol, cheese, vinegar, condiments like ketchup and mayonnaise, and salad dressing.** Hypoglycemics get a double whammy if they have food allergies, because the pancreas often over-secretes insulin in response to an allergen food in addition to its sugar response. Drinking alcohol on an empty stomach is especially dangerous!

4: **Keep a sugar-free, high protein drink on hand for acute reactions,** for immediate relief and returned well-being. Try Crystal Star's SYSTEMS STRENGTH™ drink mix, (excellent results) or Nutricology's PRO-GREENS with EFA's.

5: **Boost brain power.** Eat plenty of brainy foods like soy lecithin, wheat germ and nutritional yeast to increase neurotransmitter activity and improve memory.

6: **Supercharge your adrenals for long-term recovery.** When blood glucose is low, the adrenals compensate by secreting extra adrenaline which brings sugar levels back up. Eventually, the adrenals become exhausted by repeated attempts to normalize your blood sugar. Consider vitamin C with bioflavonoids 1-3000mg daily to revitalize the adrenal glands. Crystal Star GINSENG/LICORICE ELIXIR extract also provides adrenal support and helps stabilize blood sugar levels.

7: **Take plant enzymes with meals to enhance sugar absorption.** Herbal Products and Development POWER-PLUS ENZYMES and Transformation DIGESTZYME are high potency digestive enzyme formulas.

8: **Hypothyroidism is regularly involved with hypoglycemia.** Iodine and potassium rich sea greens like dulse, wakame and sea palm can reactivate the thyroid and increase body energy.

9: **Gentle whole herbs fight stress reactions linked to hypoglycemia.** Consider kava kava, passionflowers and scullcap.

10: **Normalize blood sugar swings with herbs and nutrients.** Crystal Star's SUGAR STRATEGY LOW™ is designed to balance blood sugar levels and encourage a feeling of well-being; or Gaia Herbs DEVIL'S CLUB SUPREME. (Devil's Claw herb can improve carbohydrate and sugar metabolism.)

Diet for Hypoglycemia Control

The key factors in hypoglycemia are stress and poor diet... both a result of too much sugar and refined carbohydrates, like pastries and desserts. These foods quickly raise glucose levels, causing the pancreas to over-compensate and produce too much insulin, which then lowers body glucose levels too far and too fast. The diet on this page supplies your body with fiber, complex carbohydrates and proteins - slow even-burning fuel that prevents sudden sugar elevations and drops. Eat small frequent meals, with plenty of fresh foods to keep sugar levels in balance. I recommend a diet like this for 2 to 3 months until blood sugar levels are regularly stable.

Diet watchwords: 1) Eat potassium-rich foods: oranges, broccoli, bananas, and tomatoes. 2) Eat chromium-rich foods: nutritional yeast, mushrooms, whole wheat, seafood and sea greens, beans and peas. 3) Eat high quality vegetable protein at every meal.

—**On rising:** take a "hypoglycemia cocktail:" 1 teasp. each in apple or orange juice to control morning sugar drop: glycine powder, powdered milk, protein powder, and nutritional yeast; or a protein/amino drink, such as Monas CHLORELLA, Wakunaga KYO-GREEN with EFA's, or Crystal Star SYSTEMS STRENGTH™.

—**Breakfast:** the most important meal of the day for hypoglycemia - include $1/3$ of daily nutrients; have oatmeal with yogurt and fresh fruit; or poached or baked eggs on whole grain toast with butter or kefir cheese; or whole grain cereal or pancakes with apple juice, soy milk, fruit, yogurt, nuts or fruit sauce; or tofu scrambled "eggs" with bran muffins, whole grain toast and butter; or my favorite: brown rice with tofu and tamari sauce and steamed veggies for breakfast.

—**Mid-morning:** have a veggie drink (page 569), Green Foods GREEN MAGMA with 1 teasp. Bragg's LIQUID AMINOS, or Crystal Star ENERGY GREEN™ drink as a liver nutrient; or a sugar balancing herb tea, such as licorice, dandelion, or Crystal Star SUGAR STRAT-EGY LOW™ tea; and some crisp, crunchy vegetables with kefir or yogurt cheese;

—**Lunch:** have a fresh salad, with cottage cheese or soy cheese, nuts, noodle or seed toppings, and lemon oil dressing; or a high protein sandwich on whole grain bread, with avocados and low-fat cheese; or a bean or lentil soup with tofu or shrimp salad or sandwich; or a seafood and whole grain pasta salad; or a vegetarian pizza on a chapati crust with low fat cheese.

—**Mid-afternoon:** have a hard boiled egg with sesame salt, and whole grain crackers with yogurt dip; or a licorice herb tea, such as Crystal Star GINSENG/LICORICE ELIXIR™ drops in water; another green drink, such as Vibrant Health GREEN VIBRANCE with spirulina; or yogurt with fruit, nuts and seeds.

—**Dinner:** have some steamed veggies with tofu, or baked or broiled fish and brown rice; or an Oriental stir fry with seafood and vegetables; or a vegetable Italian pasta dish with verde sauce and hearty soup (add green beans for pancreatic support); or a Spanish beans and rice dish, or paella with seafood and rice; or a veggie quiche and a small mushroom and spinach salad.

—**Before bed:** have a cup of Red Star nutritional yeast or miso broth; or papaya juice with a little yogurt.

Recipes to control hypoglycemia: •**BREAKFAST and BRUNCH;** •**PROTEIN without MEAT;** •**SUGAR-FREE FOODS;** •**SANDWICHES;** •**ENZYME-RICH FOODS;** •**HEALING DRINKS;** •**MINERAL-RICH FOODS;** •**HIGH FIBER FOODS.**

Herb and Supplement Choices

• **Help your body rebalance sugar levels:** Crystal Star SUGAR STRATEGY LOW ™ capsules and tea; Crystal Star GINSENG 6 SUPER TEA™ helps remove sugar from the blood; Crystal Star CHOL-LO FIBER TONE™ or other fiber cleanse morning and evening to absorb excess carbohydrates and balance sugar curve. Vitamin C 3000mg with bioflavonoids or Ethical Nutrients SU-PER FLAVONOID C. (Take vitamin C immediately during an attack).

—**Adrenal tonics help handle stress:** Crystal Star ADRN-ACTIVE™ caps or ADRN™ extract nourishes exhausted adrenals; Beehive Botanical or Y.S. ROYAL JELLY with ginseng caps; Gotu kola caps, 2 daily; Country Life GLYCEMIC FACTORS and MOOD FACTORS capsules; Transformation ULTRA-ZYME to support adrenals; *Evening Primrose Oil* caps 2000mg; B Complex 100mg 2x daily with extra PABA 100mg, and pantothenic acid 500mg.

• **Stabilize blood sugar swings:** Glutamine 500mg daily; Crystal Star GINSENG-LICORICE ELIXIR™ drops as needed; 1 teasp. each: spirulina granules and bee pollen granules in a fruit juice, or Rainbow Light HAWAIIAN SPIRULINA, between meals. Take aloe vera juice concentrate before meals (add pinches of cinnamon, ginger and nutmeg to help control cravings).

• **Enzyme therapy for glucose homeostasis:** CoQ-10 60mg 3x daily for 3-6 weeks; Pancreatin 1200mg with meals; Prevail GLU-COSE FORMULA; Alta Health CANGEST before meals, especially if candida yeast is also a problem.

• **Chromium may be critical:** GTF Chromium 200mcg; Solaray CHROMIACIN; Chromium picolinate 200mcg daily; Premier Labs VANADIUM, 25mcg.

Bodywork and Lifestyle Techniques

—**Lifestyle changes for hypoglycemia pay off handsomely for total health, too.**

• Eat 6 to 8 mini-meals throughout the day to keep blood sugar levels up. Large meals throw sugar balance way off, especially at night.

• Eat relaxed, never under stress.

• Relaxation techniques that are successful for hypoglycemia include regular massage therapy treatments.

—**Bodywork:**

• Get some exercise everyday to work off unmetabolized acid wastes.

• Some oral contraceptives can cause glucose intolerance and poor sugar metabolism. Ask your doctor.

Can't find a recommended product? Call the 800 number listed in Product Resources for the store nearest you and for more info.

Infections: Fighting the New Supergerms

Supergerms like E. coli, salmonella, antibiotic-resistant pneumonia and staph infections are a real danger in the U.S. today, largely caused by the over-use of antibiotics! In the last fifteen years, infectious diseases jumped from the fifth leading cause of death to the third leading cause in the U.S.. At least 30 new diseases from supergerms have emerged in the last 20 years. Many experts believe hundreds more are on the way, especially new drug-resistant strains migrating around the world as infected people travel or move.

Strains of drug-resistant tuberculosis and pneumonia are targeting people with compromised immune systems. Staph infections, once easily treated by penicillin, are now 95% resistant to conventional treatment! Virulent staph organisms are resistant to the most powerful new antibiotics. Supergerms in our foods are leaping on the U.S. radar with E. coli contaminated beef and other foods.

What's causing the supergerm epidemic?
—substandard conditions in the agriculture industry.
—exposure to infected animals and contaminated foods.
—lowered immune response from pollution, chemical toxins and poor diet.
—over-use of antibiotics is one of the biggest offenders. There's now a global effort to fight the problem of antibiotic overloading!

Has antibiotic therapy backfired?
The antibiotics that came into being during World War II saved many lives. But we've made ampicillin and tetracycline practically useless today. Antibiotics are such powerful drugs that they can't be taken casually or indiscriminately the way we take them now. For example, thousands of antibiotics are prescribed to treat the viruses that cause colds and flu. But using antibiotics to get rid of a virus or an allergy-related condition like chronic bronchitis, is ineffective. Worse, it also reduces that antibiotic's ability to treat any future bacterial infections. The more antibiotics you take, the more an infection strain will try to find another way to survive and attack! And there's a new problem. Some people, understandably, in an effort to limit their antibiotic intake, stop taking an antibiotic before the prescription is completed. But, if you don't take the full course of antibiotics, you give germs that haven't been destroyed an opportunity to mutate against the drug.

Even if you don't take antibiotics regularly, you may not be immune. Low dose antibiotics come into your body through commercial meats, dairy foods and produce without you even knowing it. About 40% of the antibiotics produced in the U.S. each year are fed to cattle, pigs and chickens. An astounding 300,000 pounds of antibiotics was sprayed on apples and pears in 1998 to prevent a blight! Many household cleaning supplies contain antibiotics to keep your home "germ-free," but when those antibiotics saturate your home, otherwise harmless germs can transform into something more dangerous. Triclosan, a widely used antibacterial household chemical, causes certain bacteria to mutate into new strains resistant to treatment.

Don't get me wrong. There are times when antibiotic therapy is necessary to arrest death or stabilize a life-threatening infection. But I feel short term or emergency use makes the most sense.

What can you do to fight supergerms?

1: Use antibiotics only when needed and use as directed. Ask your physician if a prescribed antibiotic is really right for your type of infection. 2: For basic household cleaning, stick with environmentally sound cleaners free of antibiotics. 3: Buy organic meats and dairy foods to avoid antibiotic overload. I find myself eating more foods from the sea because they are free of hormone and antibiotic injections. Free range turkeys have a more natural diet than commercial animals and their meat is free of antibiotics, too.

Do natural remedies hold real answers to fighting supergerms?

Herbs are at their best stimulating immune response and working with the body's natural safeguards. Since herbs are really foods, you don't get many interactions the way you might when you combine two different drugs. Certain plant remedies are a good choice for supergerm protection. Many can even help knock out supergerms if you're already sick.

IMMUNE BOOSTERS: Herbal immune boosters strengthen the body against supergerm infection.

—**Echinacea:** Echinacea increases your body's levels of the antiviral substance interferon, and prompts the thymus, bone marrow and spleen to produce more immune cells for disease protection. Echinacea increases phagocytosis, the process by which pathogens are engulfed by immune system "eater" cells.

—**Astragalus:** Astragalus boosts natural killer activity and enhances interferon production for protection against harmful bacteria and viruses. It is particularly beneficial for respiratory illnesses because it can promote the regeneration of bronchi cells.

Note: Echinacea and astragalus work well in combination for deep immune system activation. Look for formulas with both herbs for the best results.

HERBAL LYMPH FLUSHERS: Herbal lymphatic system flushers render disease-causing wastes innocuous.

—**Echinacea:** Echinacea extract is one of the best lymph cleansers to keep the body disease free and to build body defenses.

—**Seaweed baths:** A seaweed bath once a week during high risk seasons stimulates lymphatic drainage to rid your body of disease-causing toxins. The electromagnetic action of seaweed releases excess fluids from congested cells and dissolves fatty waste and toxins through the skin, replacing them with immune boosting minerals. An added perk of bathing in sea greens? You'll keep off excess weight and cellulite. A sluggish lymphatic system is directly related to cellulite formation.

—**Bitters herbs:** Your liver produces most of your body's lymph, the lymphatic fluid rich in lymphocytes, special white blood cells which form the overall defense of the body. Herbal bitters like turmeric, cardamom and lemon peel recharge the liver and lymphatic system, and boost immune response against supergerm infection.

ORGANISM KILLERS: Plants may be the best tool to wipe out supergerms...

—**Olive leaf extract:** Olive leaf extract kills 56 different pathogens. Park Research, of Henderson, Nevada finds that it may remedy as many as 120 illnesses. Serious infections like herpes, tuberculosis and pneumonia respond to olive leaf. Olive leaf extract is an ideal preventive for persons traveling to third world countries where supergerm infections and diarrheal illnesses are common.

—**Tea tree oil:** Tea tree oil kills antibiotic-resistant staph infection, even at low concentrations of .5%. Tea tree can attack both growing and dormant bacteria, something most antibiotic drugs can't do. Add 1-3 drops of tea tree oil to an infuser and breath deeply to fight off most respiratory infections. Pure tea tree oil is potent. Do not take internally unless under the guidance of a health professional experienced in appropriate use of essential oils. Diluted mouthwashes, lozenges, drops, etc. are okay used as directed.

—**Garlic:** Nature's antibiotic, garlic is effective against severe infections like dysentery and H. pylori (responsible for most stomach ulcers), including antibiotic-resistant strains. It is an amazing immune booster. In one study, immune cell activity increased 140% in people who ate 2 bulbs in 2 days' span and an amazing 156% in people who took 1800 mg of an aged garlic product.

—**Oregano oil:** Oregano has over fifty compounds with anti-infective action. It inhibits candida yeast, bacteria, viruses and parasites. Oregano especially inhibits bacteria on foods; cooking with oregano may help prevent food borne illness. Oregano oil products should contain about 65% carvacrol and 5% thymol. Oregano oil is powerful. Use only as directed.

—**Probiotics:** Acidophilus can suppress even virulent strains of E. Coli, staph, candida and salmonella in the intestinal tract.

Choose the right remedy for your infection:

Staph infection:

–Use anti-infectives like GRAPEFRUIT SEED EXTRACT, TEA TREE OIL, UNA DA GATO and PROTEASE ENZYMES.

–Use QUERCETIN, BROMELAIN and TURMERIC EXTRACT to take down inflammation.

–Use VITAMIN C with BIOFLAVONOIDS to flush infection wastes.

Bacterial infection:

–Use OREGANO OIL, OLIVE LEAF EXTRACT, AGED GARLIC EXTRACT, ECHINACEA EXTRACT, or an herbal antibiotic formula with herbs like echinacea, goldenseal, capsicum, myrrh and propolis to destroy the active microbes.

–Use PROPOLIS, PROBIOTICS like acidophilus and lactobacillus, GARLIC or ASTRAGALUS EXTRACT to boost immunity.

–Use QUERCETIN, BROMELAIN and TURMERIC EXTRACT to take down inflammation.

–Use VITAMIN C with BIOFLAVONOIDS, or an herbal formula with herbs like cornsilk, juniper, uva ursi, dandelion, ginger, marshmallow, goldenseal root, and parsley to flush infection wastes.

Viral infection:

–Use OLIVE LEAF EXTRACT, GARLIC, or an herbal anti-viral formula with lomatium, St. John's wort and usnea.

–Use MAITAKE MUSHROOM D-FRACTION or an herbal formula with goldenseal, astragalus, myrrh, maitake, reishi, echinacea and propolis to boost immune response.

Some say herbal antibiotics may be our only hope. New medical antibiotics being developed to address the supergerm problem aren't scheduled to hit the market until the year 2002!

Healing Colds, Sore Throat and Sinus Infections

Respiratory illnesses of all kinds are more than common in our society today. Americans catch about 66 million colds a year. During high risk seasons, over one-third of the U.S. population has had a cold or flu within the last 2 weeks. Your body is giving you a "cell phone call" when you get a cold. A cold is often part of your natural detox mechanism; it's your body way of relieving itself of wastes, toxins and bacterial overgrowth that have built up to a point where your immune response can't overcome them. Your body opens up and drains its channels of elimination, through coughing, sneezing, diarrhea, etc. A cold can be a friendly enemy - your wonderful, immune system working to rebuild a stronger, cleaner system. To get over a cold, work with your body, not against it. Natural remedies are effective in speeding recovery and reducing discomfort for the vast majority of respiratory diseases.

Do You Have a Cold or the Flu?

Colds and flu are separate upper respiratory infections, triggered by over 200 hundred different rhino-viruses. (Outdoor environment, drafts, wetness, temperature changes, etc. do not cause either of these illnesses.) The flu is more serious, because it can spread to the lungs, and cause bronchitis or pneumonia. Nose, eyes and mouth are usually the sites of invasion from cold viruses. The most likely target for the flu virus is the respiratory tract. Viruses don't breathe, digest food or eliminate, but they replicate themselves with a vengeance. The following symptom chart can help identify your problem and allow you to deal with it better.

A cold profile looks like this:
—Slow onset. No prostration. Body aches - largely due to the release of interferon (an immune stimulator).
—Rarely accompanied by fever and headache.
—Sore throat, sinus congestion, listlessness, runny nose and sneezing.
—Mild fatigue and weakness as a result of body cleansing.
—Mild to moderate chest discomfort, usually with a hacking cough.
—Sore or burning throat common.

A flu profile looks like this:
—Swift and severe onset. Early and prominent prostration with flushed, hot, moist skin.
—Usually accompanied by high (102°-104°) fever, headache and sore eyes.
—Chills, depression and body aches.
—Extreme fatigue, sometimes lasting 2-3 weeks.
—Acute chest discomfort, with severe hacking cough.
—Sore throat occasionally.

For 92 million Americans (1 in 3), a chronic sinus infection is a daily energy drain. When the thin, air-filled chambers of the sinuses become obstructed, mucous and infected pus collect in the sinus pockets causing pain and swelling. Chronic sinusitis, which according to new research may be a fungal infection, also results in nasal polyps and scar tissue. Suppressive over-the-counter sinus medications can both trigger a sinus infection by not allowing draining of infective material, and aggravate a sinus infection by driving it deeper into sinus cavities. Natural healing methods revolve around relieving the cause of the clogging and inflammation.

Do you have a sore throat due to a cold, or a more serious strep throat?

—Strep throat onset is rapid; *onset of a sore throat that comes before a cold is slow.*
—Strep throat is very sore; *the throat is not so sore if it's part of a cold.*
—Strep throat is accompanied by a fever and aches; *if your sore throat is part of a cold, there's only mild achiness.*
—Strep throat is accompanied by swollen lymph nodes; *in a sore throat that's part of a cold, lymph nodes aren't sore.*
—Antibiotics work for strep throat; *they don't usually work for a cold.*
—Strep throat is hoarse, from inflamed vocal chords; *sore throat due to a cold has a raspy, breathy voice (sometimes laryngitis).*
—Strep throat usually has complications, like pneumonia or ear infections; *a sore throat with a cold is accompanied by sinusitis.*

Drugs and over-the-counter medicines only relieve the symptoms of infection. They do not cure it, and in my experience, often make the situation worse by depressing immunity, drying up needed mucous elimination, and keeping the virus or harmful bacteria inside the body. I find most drug store remedies halt the body cleansing-balancing process, and generally make the cold last longer. Antibiotics are not effective against virally caused infections, and aspirin can enhance the reproduction of viral germs. Unfortunately, whatever temporary relief aspirin might afford, it may make it easier for viruses to multiply and spread.

Do you have chronic colds?
An ounce of prevention is worth a pound of cure. Keep your immune system strong.
1) A daily walk revs up immune response, puts cleansing oxygen into your lungs, and keeps your mood positive. It works wonders!
2) Take vitamin C 1000mg every hour, in powder form with juice, throughout the day. Take zinc lozenges as needed.
3) Smoking or alcohol suppress immunity. Refined foods, sugar, and dairy foods increase production of thick mucous.
4) Nutrient absorption is less efficient during a cold. A vegetarian diet is much easier on your digestion during a cold.
5) Drink plenty of liquids; 6-8 glasses daily of fruit and vegetable juices, herb teas and water to flush toxins out of your system.
6) Keep warm. Don't worry about a fever unless it is prolonged or very high.
7) Take a hot bath or sauna. Lots of toxins release though the skin. Increase room humidity so mucous membranes remain active.
8) Go to bed early, and get plenty of sleep. Most regeneration of cells occurs between midnight and 4 a.m.

Healing diets for respiratory infections, colds and flu, etc. also help: *Asthma, Seasonal Allergies, Pleurisy, Adrenal Exhaustion, Tuberculosis, Emphysema and other Smoking Diseases, Chronic Cough, Ear Infections, Cystic Fibrosis, Sinusitis, Tonsillitis, Taste and Smell Loss.*

Cleansing Diet for Colds, Sinus Infection, Sore Throat

Avoid refined flours, sugar and pasteurized dairy foods. They increase production of thick mucous. When the acute stage has passed, eat light meals, including plenty of fresh and steamed vegetables, fresh fruits and juices, and cultured foods for friendly intestinal flora. Light meals with rich plant nutrients are the easiest to assimilate.

Start with a 24-hour mucous elimination diet. You'll get better results from your cold remedy diet if you allow your body to rid itself first of toxins and mucous accumulations before attempting to change your eating habits. Green drinks and vegetable broths promote mucous elimination.

Before you begin: make up garlic syrup: soak a chopped garlic bulb in 1 pt. honey and water overnight; take a teasp. every hour during your 24-hour cleanse. Take grapefruit or cranberry juice throughout the day, or Crystal Star GREEN TEA CLEANSER™ to combat infection.

—**On rising:** take a glass of lemon juice, honey and water with a pinch cayenne pepper each morning to thin mucous secretions.

—**Breakfast:** take a potassium drink (page 568), or aloe vera juice, or Barleans BARLEANS GREENS. Take Crystal Star BIOFLAV., FIBER & C SUPPORT™ drink for nasal congestion; and take 3 garlic capsules and $1/2$ teasp. vitamin C or Ester C powder in water.

—**Mid-morning:** have a fresh carrot juice; or dilute pineapple juice, or a pineapple/papaya juice, or cranberry/apple juice; and/or a cup of comfrey/fenugreek tea, green tea or Crystal Star X-PECT™ TEA.

—**Lunch:** have a hot vegetable, miso or onion broth, or Crystal Star SYSTEMS STRENGTH™. Take Crystal Star BIOFLAV., FIBER & C SUPPORT™ drink for nasal congestion; and take 3 garlic capsules and $1/2$ teasp. vitamin C or Ester C powder in water.

—**Mid-afternoon:** take another green drink like Monas CHLORELLA, or SYSTEMS STRENGTH™. Dissolve low zinc lozenges under the tongue, or Crystal Star ZINC SOURCE™ drops in water as a nasal rinse for sinusitis or on back of the tongue to kill pathogenic throat bacteria. Or use New Chapter GINGER WONDER syrup as a gargle.

—**Dinner:** have a potassium drink, or miso soup with sea greens; or a glass of carrot juice. Take Crystal Star BIOFLAV., FIBER & C SUPPORT™ drink for nasal congestion; and take 3 garlic capsules and $1/2$ teasp. vitamin C or Ester C powder in water.

—**Before bed:** take a hot lemon and honey drink; or hot apple or cranberry juice; green tea; or garlic/miso soup each night

Watchwords:

—Go to bed early. Most regeneration of cells occurs between midnight and 4 a.m.

—Take a hot sauna or a hot bath. Many toxins will pass out through the skin.

—Use Crystal Star BIOFLAV., FIBER & C SUPPORT™ drink if you also have sinusitis. It clears congestion in 15 to 20 minutes.

—Then follow the diet on the next page for 3 to 5 days. It's loaded with vitamin C, and can produce symptomatic relief from many respiratory problems in under 48 hours.

Healing Diet for Colds, Sinus Infection, Sore Throat

After your congestion cleanse, eat only fresh foods for the rest of the week to cleanse encrusted mucous deposits. Have plenty of leafy greens. Eat plenty of plain yogurt. Drink 8 glasses of healthy liquids, fruit and vegetable juices, broths, herb teas (especially green tea and peppermint tea), and water to relieve congestion and other symptoms. (1 to 2 teasp. Bragg's LIQUID AMINOS may be added to any broth or juice.)

Eat light meals - fresh and steamed vegetables, fresh fruits and juices, and cultured foods like Rejuvenative Foods VEGI-DELITE for friendly intestinal flora. Boost immunity with glutathione foods: avocado, asparagus, watermelon, oranges, peaches, and green superfoods like chlorella and barley grass. Add plenty of garlic, onions and mustard. Avoid the pasteurized dairy products, starches and refined foods that are the breeding ground for congestion. All respiratory infections benefit from a non-clogging diet.

Note: **Effective gargles for sore throat:** 1) lemon juice and brandy; 2) black tea; 3) liquid chlorophyll in water with pinches of cayenne; 4) lemon juice and sea salt in water; 5) cider vinegar and honey in water every hour until relief.

—**On rising:** take a glass of cranberry, apple or aloe vera juice; or a glass of lemon juice in hot water with 1 teasp. honey.
—**Breakfast:** take green tea, or a cup of Crystal Star GREEN TEA CLEANSER™, or Crystal Star SYSTEMS STRENGTH™ drink, Monas CHLORELLA or Green Foods GREEN MAGMA to regenerate immune response; and take 3 garlic capsules, or garlic/ginger tea, and ¹⁄₂ teasp. ascorbate vitamin C or Ester C powder in water.
—**Mid-morning:** Balance your intestinal structure with Solgar WHEY TO GO protein drink; or have a fresh carrot juice; or a glass of cranberry/apple juice; or a cup of miso soup with sea greens snipped on top; or CC Pollen DYNAMIC TRIO drink, or Crystal Star ENERGY GREEN drink.
—**Lunch:** Have a green leafy salad with lemon/oil dressing to give your bowels a good sweeping; and/or a hot vegetable, miso or onion broth, or Rejuvenative Foods VEGI DELITE cultured veggies; or steamed veggies with brown rice. Take Crystal Star BIOFLAV., FIBER & C SUPPORT™ drink for nasal congestion; take 3 garlic capsules and ¹⁄₂ teasp. vitamin C powder in water.
—**Mid-afternoon:** have a cleansing herb tea, such as alfalfa/mint or Crystal Star X-PECT™ TEA; or another green drink such as Wakunaga KYO-GREEN, or Crystal Star ENERGY GREEN™.
—**Dinner:** have a hot veggie broth, or miso soup with sea greens; or a tofu and veggie casserole with sea greens; or a baked potato with Bragg's LIQUID AMINOS, or a vegetable stir fry with brown rice, sea greens and miso soup. Take Crystal Star BIOFLAV., FIBER & C SUPPORT™ drink for nasal congestion; and 3 garlic capsules and ¹⁄₂ teasp. vitamin C powder in water.
—**Before bed:** take another hot water, lemon and honey drink; or hot apple or cranberry juice; or Red Star Nutritional Yeast or miso broth.

Recipes to help a cold or sinus infection: •DETOXIFICATION FOODS; •HEALING DRINKS; •SOUPS, LIQUID SALADS; •ENZYME-RICH FOODS; •SALADS, HOT and COLD; •MINERAL-RICH •LIGHT MACROBIOTIC EATING.

Herb and Supplement Choices

• **During initial stage:** Vitamin C crystals, $1/4$ teasp. every half hour to bowel tolerance to flush and neutralize toxins; COLLOIDAL SILVER drops every 3 hours.

• **During acute phase:** Crystal Star FIRST AID CAPS™ every hour during acute stages to promote sweating and eliminate toxins (a preventive in initial stage); Zand HERBAL LOZENGES, Crystal Star ZINC SOURCE™ throat spray or Beehive Botanical PROPOLIS THROAT SPRAY every 2 hours.

• **Relieve infection:** Crystal Star ANTI-BIO™ caps to flush lymph glands; Enzymatic Therapy ESBERITOX chewables. **Throat coats:** Crystal Star COFEX™ TEA, or elderberry-mint-yarrow tea; apply hot ginger compresses to chest.

• **A great "cold" cocktail:** To a glass of aloe vera juice: add $1/4$ teasp. vitamin C crystals, 2 tsp. Nature's Way SAMBUCOL elderberry syrup, $1/2$ teasp. turmeric powder (or open a curcumin capsule), 1 capsule echinacea, $1/2$ tsp. propolis extract.

• **Congestion cleansers:** Cayenne-ginger caps; Echinacea-goldenseal caps; Crystal Star X-PECT™ tea; Zand DECONGEST extract; Boiron OSCILLOCOCCINUM; Nutribiotic GRAPEFRUIT SEED extract spray, or gargle.

• **For strep throat:** Crystal Star ANTI-BIO™ extract every hour, or ANTI-VI™, or Usnea extract or Crystal Star BIO-VI™ extract; Nutribiotic GRAPEFRUIT SEED extract in water; glutamine 1000mg 2x daily; Zinc lozenges to kill throat bacteria; or Crystal Star ZINC SOURCE™ drops (apply directly on throat); take vitamin C 5000mg daily, and Lysine 1000mg; Colloidal silver drops for a week, or Nature's Path SILVER-LYTE liquid; Planetary OLD INDIAN COUGH SYRUP.

• **For sinusitis:** Nutribiotic NASAL SPRAY & EAR DROPS.

Bodywork and Lifestyle Techniques

• **Regular exercise encourages immune response.** Even just a short walk every day, puts cleansing oxygen into the lungs, restoring vitamin D in the body, and fresh air into the brain.

• **Take a hot 20 minute bath or sauna at the onset** of a cold, flu or any respiratory problem to stimulate the body's defenses and increase elimination of toxins through the skin.

• **Stimulate easier breathing by massaging** and gently scratching the lung meridian from the top of the shoulder to the end of the thumb to clear chest mucous. Massage therapy opens up blocked body meridians.

• **Essential oils:** Assist your lung cleanse by using oregano, tea tree, and eucalyptus oils (singly or in combination). Put a total of 15 drops essential oils in 1-oz of a carrier oil (such as jojoba) and rub on the chest. Inhalant: 6 drops of essential oils added to one quart hot water - inhale the steam:

–Eucalyptus opens sinus passages.

–Wintergreen relieves nasal congestion.

–Mint or chamomile relieve headaches.

–Tea tree oil combats infection.

–Oregano oil combats lung infection, thins mucous.

• **A catnip enema** to cleanse infection from strep throat.

• **For chronic sinusitis** - Acupuncture is effective.

–**Acupressure points:** 1: Massage under big toes for 1 minute. 2: Squeeze ends of each finger and thumb hard for 20 seconds. 3: Press thumb and index finger gently on the top of your nose on either side for 5 seconds. Repeat 3 times.

• **Sinusitis:** Nasal salt irrigation clears breathing: add $1/2$ tsp. sea salt to 1 cup warm water. Fill a dropper with liquid, tilt your head and fill each nostril; then blow your nose.

Can't find a recommended product? Call the 800 number listed in Product Resources for the store nearest you and for more info.

Healing Flu, Bronchitis and Pneumonia

Like a cold, the flu is an upper respiratory infection caused by a rhino-virus. Unlike a cold, flu infections are more severe, longer-lasting and highly contagious. Some twenty thousand people die each year from flu. Some people become incapacitated for weeks at a time. Flu treatment works best in stages for complete recovery. The ACUTE, infective stage (aches, chills, prostration, fever, sore throat, etc.), usually lasts for 2 to 4 days. The RECUPERATION, healing stage, (replenishes the body's natural resistance), should be followed for 1 to 2 weeks. The IMMUNE SUPPORT stage should be followed for 2 to 3 weeks, especially in high risk seasons. Recovery from flu is often slow with a good deal of weakness. Flu shots can affect immune response. Beware. Colds and flu are different. It's important to know what ails you before you can treat it. See page 413 for the differences.

Chronic bronchitis is an infectious inflammation of the bronchi. Experts see it as a direct result of prolonged exposure to irritants like cigarette smoke and environmental chemicals. The typical victim is forty or older, with lowered immunity from stress, fatigue or smoking. Viral bronchitis affecting women, is very hard to treat, lasts from 3 weeks to 5 months, and does not go away on its own. Chronic bronchitis can be incapacitating and lead to serious lung disease. Acute bronchitis is generally self-limiting, like a bad chest cold, with eventual complete healing.

Pneumonias and pleurisy are inflammatory lung diseases. Bacterial pneumonia is caused by staph, strep or pneumo-bacilli; it responds to antibiotics, both medical and herbal. Viral pneumonia is an acute systemic disease caused by virulent viruses which does not respond to antibiotics. Herbal antivirals have shown some success. Pleurisy, an inflammation of the pleura membrane surrounding the lungs, often accompanies pneumonia. Pneumonias drastically weaken the immune system. It can take 3 months to recover strength and up to 2 years to be able to resist a cold without falling victim to another bout of pneumonia.

Do you have Flu, Bronchitis, or Pneumonia? Here are some ways to tell: see page 413 for flu symptoms.
—<u>Acute Bronchitis:</u> deep chest cold; slight fever; headache, nausea, lung and body aches; hacking, mucous-producing cough.
—<u>Chronic Bronchitis:</u> bronchial tissue inflamed; mucous thick and profuse; difficult breathing from clogged airways; repeated attacks of acute bronchitis; chest congestion; mucousy cough and wheezing for 3 months; fatigue, weakness and weight loss.
—<u>Pneumonia:</u> inflamed lungs and chest pain; aggravated flu and cold symptoms, worsening after 5 days; swollen lymph glands; difficult breathing; heavy coughing and expectoration; back and body aches; chills and high fever; sore throat; inability to "get over it"; fluid in lymph and lungs; great fatigue which remains for six to eight weeks even after recovery.

Flu, bronchitis and pneumonia can be serious diseases. Do not risk your health if you have major difficulty breathing. Short term heroic medicine may be necessary. Newer broad spectrum drugs can sometimes give your body a "breather" from the infection trauma and are less harmful to normal body functions than most primary antibiotics. Ask your physician.

Healing Diet for Flu, Bronchitis and Pneumonia

1: Get rid of the infected, thick mucous with the cleansing diet below for 1 to 3 days. Then follow a vegetarian, light "green" diet, high in vegetable proteins, low in meat, dairy foods and animal fats, for 3 weeks to allow lungs to heal easily. Avoid sugars, dairy foods, starchy and fatty foods during healing to reduce congestion (these foods allow a place for the virus to live).

2: Take cleansing broths, hot tonics, high vitamin C juices, vegetable juices (page 569) and green drinks (pg. 569). Avoid alcohol.

3: Take flax seed tea each night during acute stages to cleanse the colon (where infected mucous builds up).

4: During the recuperation stage: Have a salad every day, cultured foods: Rejuvenative Foods VEGI DELITE, yogurt and kefir, for friendly flora replacement, and steamed vegetables with brown rice for strength.

5: Avoid alcohol and tobacco - immune suppressors. Avoid caffeine foods - inhibit iron and zinc absorption.

6: As an emergency measure for sinusitis, take fresh grated horseradish root in a spoon with lemon juice. Hang over a sink immediately to expel large quantities of mucous.

7: If you just can't seem to "get over it:" make up 1 gallon of Crystal Star CLEANSING & PURIFYING™ tea, and take 5 to 6 cups daily with 15 FIBER & HERBS CLEANSE™ capsules daily until the virus is removed.

The night before you begin.....

—Take your choice of gentle herbal laxatives. Make a traditional onion-honey syrup: Put 5 to 6 chopped onions and $1/_2$ cup honey in a pot and cook over very low heat for two hours. Strain and take 1 TB every two hours for the next 3 days.

The next day....

—**On rising:** Take a hot lemon and maple syrup drink with water each morning, or a cup of green tea, or an aloe vera juice to rebalance body chemistry; or fresh carrot juice, or potassium drink (pg. 568), or Crystal Star SYSTEMS STRENGTH™ drink.

—**Breakfast:** have grapefruit juice with 1 TB of a green superfood, like Transitions EASY GREENS or Wakunaga KYO-GREEN; or pineapple juice as a natural expectorant - add 1 TB of a green superfood like Monas CHLORELLA for detox support.

—**Mid-morning:** take a carrot juice or mixed fresh vegetable juice such as Personal Best V-8 (page 569).

—**Lunch:** have a Potassium Juice (page 568), Green Foods GREEN MAGMA or Crystal Star ENERGY GREEN.

—**Mid-afternoon:** have a mucous cleansing tea like Crystal Star X-PECT™ tea or mullein tea with New Chapter GINGER WONDER SYRUP.

—**Dinner:** have a warm Potassium drink (page 568), or Nature's Path TRACE-MIN-LYTE for energy and electrolytes. Or try a stomach soothing, rich in zinc, vitamin A, C, potassium and magnesium electrolytes broth: In $2 1/_2$ cups water, cook $1 1/_2$ cups fresh mixed vegetables (carrots, broccoli, dark leafy greens, celery and parsley), with 1 TB. miso. Strain and take broth.

—**Before Bed:** have cranberry or celery juice or a cup of miso soup with Red Star nutritional yeast.

Recipes to help a flu, bronchitis, pneumonia diet: •DETOXIFICATION FOODS; •HEALING DRINKS; •SOUPS, LIQUID SALADS; •ENZYME-RICH FOODS; •SALADS; •MINERAL-RICH FOODS •LIGHT MACROBIOTICS.

Bodywork and Lifestyle Techniques

•**Air pollutants** are probably responsible for more chronic bronchitis than any other one cause. Avoid smoking, second hand smoke and smog-plagued areas.

•**Take a hot sauna;** follow with a brisk rubdown, and chest-back percussion with a cupped hand to loosen mucous.

•**Apply:**

—alternating hot and cold witch hazel compresses to the chest. Use eucalyptus oil in a vaporizer.

—a hot cayenne/ginger poultice: Mix powders - $\frac{1}{2}$ teasp. cayenne, 1 TB lobelia, 3 TBS slippery elm, 2 TBS ginger and enough water to make a paste. Leave on chest 1 hour.

—a mustard plaster to chest to stimulate lungs and draw out poisons: Mix 1 TB mustard powder, 1 egg, 3 TBS flour and water to make a paste. Leave on until skin turns pink.

—tea tree oil on the chest, or apply Earth's Bounty O₂ OXY-SPRAY on the chest.

•**Do deep breathing exercises daily,** morning and before bed to clear lungs especially during recovery. Breathe in, pushing abdomen out, then from chest to completely fill upper and lower lungs.

•**Avoid inhaling cold air.** Cover mouth and nose with a scarf so that infectious pathogens are not sucked into the lungs.

•**Get plenty of rest.** Get a complete massage therapy treatment to cleanse remaining pockets of toxins, and clear body meridians. Plus it makes you feel so good again!

•**Overheating therapy helps deactivate viruses:** See page 571 for "How To Take An Overheating Bath" in your home. Or take an oxygen bath. Use 1 to 2 cups 3% H_2O_2 to a tub of water. Soak 20 minutes.

Herb and Supplement Choices

•**Acute flu stage:** Vitamin C crystals: $\frac{1}{4}$ teasp. every half hour to bowel tolerance to flush out infection. Crystal Star FIRST AID CAPS™ to raise body temperature and reduce virus replication; Nutribiotic GRAPEFRUIT SEED extract drops; or Olive leaf extract capsules 2 to 6 daily.

•**Flu infection fighters:** Crystal Star ANTI-VI™ extract 4x daily, or ANTI-BIO™ caps every 2 hours until improvement; Nature's Path Silver-Lyte ionized silver; Oregano oil capsules, 3x daily; MICROHYDRIN, from Healthy House; Boneset tea (or homeopathic Eupatorium Perfoliatum) or Nature's Way SAMBUCOL elderberry syrup, inhibits flu virus.

•**Speed up recovery time:** Glutamine 1000mg 3x daily; astragalus or reishi mushroom extract 4x daily; Nutricology GERMANIUM 150mg; Calendula tea 4 cups daily.

•**Restore immune response:** Nutricology NAC a powerful immune booster, 1000mg daily, or Nutricology LACTOFERRIN with colostrum; Panax ginseng or astragalus to boost lymphocytes and interferon; Monas CHLORELLA;OPC's from white pine or grapeseed, 100mg 3x daily; CoQ-10, 60mg 3x daily; Source Naturals OPTI-ZINC 30mg daily.

•**Bronchitis, for inflammation and infection:** Oregano oil as directed. Crystal Star BRNX™ extract with ANTI-BIO™ caps 6x daily; usnea extract or Crystal Star BIO-VI™ extract for direct effect. Reishi mushroom extract, or Crystal Star GINSENG-REISHI extract, for T-cell defense. Flora VEGE-SIL or Crystal Star SILICA SOURCE™ for bio-available silica.

•**Expectorants relieve irritating mucous:** Lobelia extract drops in water as needed; apply cayenne-ginger compresses to chest. NAC (N-acetyl-cysteine), or Nutricology NAC 2 daily.

Can't find a recommended product? Call the 800 number listed in Product Resources for the store nearest you and for more info.

Controlling Your Weight

The latest statistics are shocking. **One out of every two Americans is overweight.** This doesn't count kids who are rapidly becoming an overweight generation. Right now, two-thirds of Americans are trying to lose weight. Amazingly, of those, only 20% are actually reducing their calories or exercising. Next to smoking, obesity is the second leading preventable cause of death in the United States, contributing to an excess of 300,000 deaths each year. The natural recommendations presented on this page can be used successfully for a wide variety of men and women struggling with their weight. Notes: Yo-yo dieting increases the risk of gallstones. For the best results, start slowly on your weight loss program and stick with it. The four keys to an effective weight control diet: low fat, high fiber, regular exercise, lots of water.

The Six Most Common Weight Loss Blockers

There are almost as many different weight loss problems as common and developed comprehensive programs to address you make the decision to be a thin person, identify your most be more than one. When results in the primary area begin to Take additional supplements after the first program is well

there are people who have them. I've identified six of the most them. Each of the six plans has years of success behind it. Once prominent weight control problem, especially if there seems to pay off, secondary problems are often overcome in the process. underway if lingering problem spots exist.

1: Lazy Metabolism and Thyroid Imbalance. If you've experienced weight gain after 40 or after menopause, thyroid malfunction and lowered metabolism may be to blame. Huge new studies reveal that as many as 1 in 10 women over 65 have the early stages of hypothyroidism!

The signs: 1) General weakness and fatigue, especially in the morning; 2) Digestive disturbances like heartburn, unusual bad breath or body odor; 3) Unexplained depression and anxiety; 4) Breast fibroids; 5) Hair loss, especially in women.

Recommendations: To boost metabolism and support your thyroid, add seaweeds like kelp, dulse and nori, rich in natural iodine, to your daily diet. Sea greens are also available in capsules or extracts, like New Chapter OCEAN HERBS and Crystal Star's IODINE POTASSIUM™ caps. Add thermogenic spices like cinnamon, cayenne, mustard and ginger to speed up your fat burning process. Try dipping raw veggies in mustard throughout the day. One teasp. of mustard can increase metabolism 25% for up to 3 hours!

Note: if you have the slightest tendency to wheat or gluten allergies (you'll bloat when you eat them), avoid breads and pastries.

2: Sugar Craving and Blood Sugar Imbalances. Dieters who cut their fat intake to almost zero often try to make up for the missing fats by adding more sugar for better taste. But, sugary foods are usually empty calories... the downfall of dieters. And they raise insulin levels too much – your body's signal to make fat, no good for weight loss.

The signs: 1) Moodiness, being easily frustrated with a tendency towards crying spells; 2) Great fatigue (especially after sugar binges); 3) Having a wired feeling that is only relieved by eating sweets.

Recommendations: Increase your intake of healthy essential fatty acids (EFA's) from sources like seafood, sea greens, spinach or flax seed oil to reduce the cravings. Take EVENING PRIMROSE OIL, an easy-to-use EFA source, 3000mg daily. Eat more fiber. You'll have less cravings for sugar. High fiber foods improve the control of glucose metabolism and help promote weight loss and regularity. Target excess sugar in the blood with herbs for weight loss. Crystal Star GINSENG-LICORICE ELIXIR™ or Herbal Magic HYPOGLY-HERBAL. Take a dry sauna every day possible for 15 minutes. Raising your body temperature with dry heat really helps balance sugar levels and accelerate weight loss.

3: Overeating Fat and Calories. Overeating and eating too much fat are big reasons why it's so hard for Americans, particularly men, to lose weight. Men are often encouraged to dip into second, even third helpings as a sign of manliness or approval for the cook. Men also tend to overeat when they're under stress, tired, or on-the-run.... circumstances under which many American men eat today. Our lifestyles don't help. 45% of every food dollar is spent on eating out, and restaurant portions are bigger than ever as consumers demand more food for their money.

The signs: 1) Binging on junk foods, especially fatty, sugary foods, about every ten days; 2) Eating all your calories at one meal and then trying to eat nothing for the rest of the day when you're dieting (most people can't do it); 3) Having second and third helpings at a meal but still feeling hungry.

Recommendations: Control your portions so you don't overeat. Reduce fats to no more than 20% of your food intake. (Don't replace fats with fat substitutes like Olestra.) An herbal appetite suppressant with St. John's wort can curb cravings for fatty foods. Hypericin, one of St. John's wort's constituents, makes the user feel full, much the same way the drug fenfluramine does, but without the hazards of heart valve damage. Try Crystal Star APPE-TITE™ caps with St. John's Wort, Nature's Secret THINSOLUTION or Natural Balance SEROTHIN.

4: Liver Malfunction and Cellulite Formation. Your liver is responsible for fat metabolism. Liver malfunction is also directly related to sugar metabolism. Add to that the fact that most of us have a liver that's overloaded with toxic build-up today and you have three reasons why liver health is related to weight problems. A poorly functioning liver is almost always involved in cellulite formation, too. Women are hardest hit by cellulite because their skin fibers are thinner than a man's. Fatty wastes become lodged beneath the skin's surface more easily in a woman when the liver or lymphatic system is sluggish.

The signs: 1) Extreme, unrelenting fatigue; unusual depression and sadness; 2) Unexplained, pudgy weight gain; 3) Heartburn and constipation that worsen after fatty meals; 4) Food and chemical sensitivities; 5) Bulging, dimply, skin on hips, buttocks, thighs and knees (women); torso and stomach (men).

Recommendations: A two-week course of herbal bitters can regenerate the liver by increasing bile production. Try Crystal Star BITTERS & LEMON™ extract, or Gaia Herbs SWEETISH BITTERS ELIXIR. Detox your liver with Monas CHLORELLA. Add B complex, like Nature's Secret ULTIMATE B to assist liver detoxification and fat metabolism. Cellulite Tip: Seaweed body wraps are especially good because they also squeeze cellulitic waste back into the working areas of the body so it can be eliminated. Check out your nearest day spa for a good program.

5: Poor Circulation and Low Energy. A lifestyle with little exercise slows down circulation, metabolism and elimination, factors which impede successful weight loss. For some dieters, initial weight loss is rapid, but then a plateau is reached and further weight loss becomes difficult. Restricted food intake slows down metabolism, and affects circulation.

The signs: 1) Hands, feet, face and ears become cold regularly; 2) Poor memory; 3) Ringing in the ears.

Recommendations: For circulation stimulation: Futurebiotics CIRCUPLEX or Rosemary Gladstar's BUTCHER'S BROOM caps, or add CoQ-10, 100mg daily. Mineral electrolytes, like Nature's Path TRACE-LYTE turn body energy circuits back on. Dry brush your skin before showers to speed up circulation.

6: Poor Elimination. An astounding 30 million Americans have chronic constipation.... and it can be a major factor in weight control. If your colon is sluggish, your body hangs on to toxins and wastes that would normally be removed through elimination channels. This build-up of waste materials in your blood and bowel slows down all systems and your weight loss program.

The signs: 1) frequent bad breath, body odor and coated tongue; 2) infrequent bowel movements.

Recommendations: Try an easy fiber drink. Take 2 TBS of aloe vera juice concentrate in juice each morning. Add 2 capsules of an herbal formula like Crystal Star FIBER & HERBS CLEANSE™, or Herbal Magic COL-LIV HERBAL. Use massage therapy on your lower back (near the kidneys) to relieve colon congestion. If you get backaches when you're constipated, your transverse colon is probably blocked up by impacted wastes. Sometimes a little light massage work can help to break up the congestion and release the accumulated materials.

Note: Changing diet composition is the key. The importance of cutting back on saturated fat cannot be overstated. Saturated fats are hard for the liver to metabolize. Focus on healthy fats from seafood, sea greens, nuts and seeds which curb cravings by initiating a satiety response.

Watchwords:

—**Fat isn't all bad.** It's your body's chief energy source. Most overweight people have too high blood sugar and too low fat levels. This causes constant hunger; the delicate balance between fat storage and fat utilization is upset; and your ability to use fat for energy decreases. Eating fast, fried, or junk foods aggravates this imbalance. You wind up with empty calories and more cravings. Fat becomes non-moving energy; fat cells become fat storage depots. But don't replace fats with fat substitutes like Olestra. Fake fats fool your tastebuds, not your stomach. In one study, people who replaced 20% of their fat with fake fats were still hungry at the end of the day and they ate twice as much food as normal! Fake fats are nutrition thieves. Eating a one ounce portion of olestra potato chips on a daily basis reduces blood carotene levels by 50%!

—**Water can get you over diet plateaus.** Dehydration slows resting metabolic rate (RMR) and can cause waste products like ketones to build up in tissues. Drink juices or green tea in the morning to wash out waste products.

—**A little caffeine after a meal raises thermogenesis** (calorie burning) and boosts metabolic rate. Use fat burning spices like ginger, cinnamon, garlic, mustard and cayenne.

—**High fiber fruits and veggies are a key to successful body toning.** Have an apple every day!

Herb and Supplement Choices

• **Stimulate BAT thermogenesis:** Evening Primrose oil 3000mg daily; Carnitine 3000mg daily; Crystal Star THERMO-CITRIN® GINSENG™ caps; Source Naturals DIET PHEN; Natural Balance ULTRA DIET PEP; Nature's Secret ULTIMATE WEIGHT LOSS; Diamond Herpanacine DIAMOND TRIM.

—**Deficiencies can lead to food binges:** B-complex with extra B-6 200mg (boosts serotonin and metabolizes carbohydrates); lack of minerals leads to sugar craving: Crystal Star MINERAL SPECTRUM™ or ZINC SOURCE™ caps.

• **Control food cravings:** Crystal Star APPE-TITE™ caps with St. John's Wort; Nature's Secret THIN SOLUTION; 5-HTP as directed; chromium picolinate (400mcg); L-glutamine 2000mg, spirulina and bee pollen for sugar cravings; Natural Balance SEROTHIN caps with 5-HTP.

• **Natural fat blockers:** Health from the Sun CLA (conjugated linoleic acid) up to 2000mg daily; fat digesting enzymes, like Prevail FAT ENZYME; garcinia cambogia in formulas like Now's CITRI-MAX or Natrol CITRI-MAX PLUS; Pyruvate aids in transforming blood sugar into energy, 5 grams daily; Twin Lab PYRU-VATE FUEL; Chitosan reduces absorption of fats; Natural Balance FAT MAGNET. *Note: Gastrointestinal problems may result from excessive use of pyruvate or chitosan.*

• **Good fats help burn bad fats:** Barleans OMEGA-3 FLAX OIL or Omega Nutrition ESSENTIAL BALANCE help overcome binging; Co-enzyme A Technology BODY IMAGE; Richardson Labs CHROMA-SLIM - a lipotropic-carnitine formula.

• **Boost metabolism:** Enzymatic Therapy THYROID/TYROSINE caps; for compulsive eating, tyrosine 1000mg with zinc 30mg daily. Enzymatic Therapy 7-KETO NATURAL LEAN.

Bodywork and Lifestyle Techniques

• **Daily exercise is the key to permanent, painless weight control.** Exercise releases fat from the cells. (Exercising early in the day can raise metabolism as much as 25%! Exercising before breakfast is best because the body dips into its fat stores for quick energy.)

—Even if eating habits are just slightly changed, you can still lose weight with a brisk hour's walk, or 15 minutes of aerobic exercise.

—One pound of fat represents 3500 calories. A 3 mile walk burns up 250 calories. In about 2 weeks, you'll lose a pound of real extra fat. That's 3 pounds a month and 30 pounds a year without changing your diet. It's easy to see how cutting down even moderately on fatty, sugary foods in combination with exercise can still provide the look and body tone you want.

• **Exercise promotes an afterburn effect,** raising metabolic rate from 1.00 to 1.05-1.15 per minute up to 24 hours afterwards. Calories are used up at an even faster rate after exercise.

• **Weight training exercise increases lean muscle mass,** replacing fat-marbled muscle tissue with lean muscle. Muscle tissue burns calories; the greater the amount of muscle tissue you have, the more calories you can burn. This is very important as aging decreases muscle mass. Exercise before a meal raises blood sugar levels and thus decreases appetite, often for several hours afterward.

• **Deep breathing exercises increase metabolic rate.** See pg. 472 of this book.

Can't find a recommended product? Call the 800 number listed in Product Resources for the store nearest you and for more info.

Intense Fat and Sugar Cleanse

Is your body showing signs that it needs a fat and sugar cleanse?

—Is cellulite collecting on your hips, thighs or tummy? Cellulite is a mixture of fat, water and wastes trapped beneath the skin.

—Are your upper arms slightly flabby or your waistline noticeably thicker? Have your wrists and ankles thickened?

—Does your face look jowly or puffy?

If your diet problem is eating too much fat and sugars, try my light detox from fats and sugars for 1 to 3 days. It makes you feel terrific and it's so easy. Sugary foods and highly processed foods like fast foods, are so devoid of digestive enzymes that they collect as excess fat. Further, if you are congested, your body tries to dump its metabolic wastes to get them out of the way — one of the places that receives metabolic wastes is excess fat. Start the night before with a green leafy salad to give your intestines a good sweeping. Dry brush your skin all over for five minutes before you go to bed to open your pores for the night's cleansing eliminations.

—**Upon rising:** have a cup of green tea to cut through and eliminate fatty wastes. For maximum results, add drops of ginseng extract to control sugar cravings, or licorice extract for maximum sugar stabilizing.

—**Breakfast:** have a Fat Melt Down Juice: juice 2 apples, 2 pears, 1 slice of fresh ginger to help reduce fat from places where it is stored in cellulite. The ginger stimulates better blood circulation.

—**Mid-morning:** have a superfood drink once a day. Green superfoods help cleanse your body of fatty build-up.

—**Lunch:** enjoy a mixed vegetable juice, like Knudsen's VERY VEGGIE. Even regular V-8 juice works just fine.

—**Mid-afternoon:** Take a glass of papaya-pineapple juice, or Crystal Star LEAN & CLEAN™ SUPER TEA or a cup of green tea to enhance enzyme production. Enzymes are a dieters best friend!

—**Dinner:** Have some miso soup with snipped sea greens. Seaweeds add minerals and improve sluggish metabolism. Add spices like cinnamon, cayenne, mustard and ginger to speed up the fat burning process.

—**Before bed:** have a cup of apple juice, licorice or peppermint tea to rebalance and restore normal body pH.

Watchwords:

• **Focus on reducing fats and sugars in your diet.** Add more fiber to get rid of excess sugar, especially from whole grains, legumes like peas, and vegetables. High fiber foods improve glucose metabolism, help promote weight loss and reduce cravings for sugar.

• **Take a 15 minute dry sauna several days a week for a month.** Raising your body temperature with dry heat really helps balance sugar levels. When I worked at a European spa, we used this technique for weight loss and blood sugar problems with great results!

• **Expert dieters drink 8 glasses of water a day.** Water naturally suppresses appetite and helps maintain a high metabolic rate. In fact, water is the most important catalyst for increased fat burning. It enhances the liver's ability to detox and metabolize so it can process more fats. Don't worry about fluid retention; high water intake decreases bloating, because it flushes out sodium and toxins.

Herb and Supplement Choices

• **Deep liver cleanser:** The liver is your body's chemical plant for fat metabolism. Weight gain and energy loss are often the result of a liver which has become enlarged through overwork, alcohol exhaustion or congestion. Crystal Star CEL-LEAN™ caps or Herbasway LIVER ENHANCER tea.

• **Essential fatty acids:** Without essential fatty acids (EFA's), poor fat metabolism is certain. Unhealthy excess fluid retention is also controlled by EFA's. EFA deficiency increases appetite and promotes obesity.

—**EFAs to consider:**

   Flax Oil -1 or 2 TBS. over a salad.

   Evening Primrose Oil - 1000mg daily.

   CLA - an Omega-6 fatty acid with fat-burning properties, 1800mg daily.

• **Capillary strengthening:** you must tighten capillary walls in order to keep extra fat and cellulite from returning. Bioflavonoids are important: Ethical Nutrients SUPER FLAVONOID C; Crystal Star BIOFLAV. FIBER & C SUPPORT™ drink or CEL-LEAN™ tea.

• **Appetite suppressant help:** Crystal Star APPE-TIGHT™ is a mild, subtle herbal formula that helps you from overeating; Nature's Secret THIN-SOLUTION; Gaia Herbs DIET SLIM; Source Naturals DIET-PHEN.

• **Enzyme support:** Transformation Enzyme BALANCE-ZYME PLUS for weight loss.

• **Electrolytes dramatically boost energy levels:** Arise & Shine ALKALIZER; Nature's Path TRACE-LYTE LIQUID MINERALS.

Bodywork and Lifestyle Techniques

• **Enema:** Take an enema the first day of your excess fat cleanse to help release toxins out of the body.

• **Exercise:** Exercise promotes an "afterburn" effect, raising metabolic rates for up to 24 hours afterwards. Exercise before a meal raises blood sugar levels and decreases appetite, often for several hours after the exercise. Good exercise for women with the little tummy bulge that appears at menopause? Do hard tummy sucks to the count of 100 each morning. It works!

• **Dry brushing:** Fatty wastes can get trapped beneath the skin's surface easily (especially in women) when the liver or lymphatic systems are sluggish. Use a natural bristle brush - brush vigorously in a rotary motion and massage every part of your body in this order: feet and legs, hands and arms, back and abdomen, chest and neck. Five to fifteen minutes is the average time.

• **Massage:** Have a massage therapy treatment at the end of your cleanse to move excess fluid wastes and unattached fats into elimination systems, and to stimulate skin circulation.

• **Bathe away excess fats:** Crystal Star HOT SEAWEED BATH; or a sea salt bath: add 1 cup Dead Sea salts, 1 cup Epsom salts, $1/2$ cup regular sea salt and $1/4$ baking soda to a tub; swish in 3 drops lavender oil, 2 geranium drops oil, 2 drops sandalwood oil and 1 drop neroli oil.

Can't find a recommended product? Call the 800 number listed in Product Resources for the store nearest you and for more info.

Weight Control After 40

There's no doubt about it. Weight loss gets more difficult after 40. The latest figures show that body fat typically doubles between the ages of 20 and 50. Everybody goes through a change of life, and those middle years affect our body shapes, too....for both men and women. One of the worst problems America's fitness oriented population faces in their 40's and 50's is a disconcerting body thickening and a slow, steady rise in weight. It seems to happen with everybody, even people who have always been slim, who have a good diet, and who regularly exercise.

For women, a major calorie-burning process grinds to a halt after menopause. A woman's menstrual cycle consumes extra calories. Some experts say that the metabolic rise in the last two weeks of year. Those calories really start to add up when menstrua- the menstrual cycle accounts for 15,000-20,000 calories per tion ceases! While a woman needs to work a little harder to lose that extra fat later in life, once her body adjusts to its new hormone levels, weight gain stabilizes, becomes man- ageable, and, in many cases, falls back to premenopausal levels. Lower testosterone levels in andropausal men can mean a decrease in muscle mass and increase in fat storage. But, most men, by cutting back on fat and adding more fiber to their diets can lose the middle-age spread. I've been working for several years to develop natural weight control techniques for people trying to maintain slimness and tone after their metabolism changes. For weight loss after 40, begin with two starting points: 1) Improve body chemistry at the gland and hormone level; 2) Re-establish better, long-lasting metabolic rates.

1:   LOVE YOUR LIVER. The liver is your body's chemical plant responsible for fat metabolism. It is intricately involved with hormone functions, so it is the prime target to optimize for weight loss after 40. Weight gain and energy loss signal a liver that has enlarged through overwork, alcohol exhaustion and congestion. A good thermogenesis (calorie-burning) herbal formula with ginseng works extremely well. I have used • Crystal Star's THERMO-GINSENG™ extract for many years with success. • Herbs, Etc. GINSENG SEVEN SOURCE is a good choice; or add liver tonics: fresh vegetable juices, dandelion greens, milk thistle seed extract (accelerates liver regeneration by a factor of four); • Enzymatic Therapy SUPER MILK THISTLE COMPLEX with artichoke; • Herbs Etc. LIVER TONIC; or a liver tonic tea: 4-oz hawthorn berries, 2-oz. red sage, and 1-oz. cardamom seeds. Steep 24 hours in 2 qts. water. Add honey. Take 2 cups daily.

2:   CONSCIOUSLY EAT LESS. As metabolism slows, you don't need to fuel it up as much, because your body doesn't use up nutrients like it once did. If you eat like you did in your 20's and 30's, your body will store too much, mostly as fat. New research shows that moderate food intake may extend lifespan by as much as ten years!

• **Make sure you are eating a low fat diet.** Even with all the fat-conscious foods on the market today, Americans still consume one-third of their calories as fat. Your fat intake should be about 20% for weight control, 15% or less for weight loss. But remember: no-fat is not good for weight loss, either. Your body goes into a survival mode if you eliminate all fat, shedding its highly active lean muscle tissue to reduce your body's need for food. When lean muscle tissue decreases, fat burning slows or stops.

• **Control your food portions.** Portion control is a cornerstone of weight control. Even if your diet is healthy and reasonably low in fat, there's no way you can eat all you want of anything. Eat smaller meals every 2 to 3 hours to keep your appetite hole from gnawing, and to keep metabolic rate high. Small meals virtually prevent carbohydrates and proteins from being converted to fat.

• **Control hunger with safe herbal appetite suppressants.** Serotonin is the brain chemical linked to mood and appetite. Serotonin balancers like St. John's wort, 5-HTP, and evening primrose oil help stabilize mood and reduce food cravings. Herbal weight loss compounds can address almost every individual problem of weight control. Superfood herbs like barley grass, spirulina, sea greens and alfalfa can be a key to controlling appetite. Take a green drink with these low-calorie foods in mid-afternoon to rapidly decrease a craving for high-calorie foods. Crystal Star's ENERGY GREEN™ drink can raise both metabolic rate and activity levels.

• **Control your cravings.** The herb gymnema sylvestre can help control sugar cravings. Gymnema binds with sugar receptors in the mouth, causing sugary foods to lose their appealing sweet flavor, an effect that can last for up to 2 hours. Seven different clinical studies show garcinia cambogia or HCA (hydroxycitric acid) reduces food intake an amazing 46% when taken orally. Gaia Herbs combines gymnema and HCA in their product •DIET SLIM.

3: RAISE YOUR METABOLISM. A higher metabolic rate means you burn more fat, lose weight easier, and maintain your ideal body weight more comfortably.

• **Don't skip meals, especially breakfast.** Breakfast is the worst meal to skip if you want to raise metabolism. It sends a temporary fasting signal to the brain that food is going to be scarce. So stress hormones increase, and the body begins shedding lean muscle tissue in order to decrease its need for food. By the time you eat again, your pancreas is so sensitized to a lack of food, that it sharply increases blood insulin levels, your body's signal to make fat. Eating early in the day, when your metabolism is at its best, and hours of activity ahead in which to burn fats is the best for weight loss. Reduce both sugars and fats - they slow metabolism. Fats have twice the calories, gram for gram, as protein and complex carbohydrates. They also use only 2% of their calories before the fat storage process begins. Protein and carbohydrates burn almost 25% of their calories before storing them as fat. Limit alcohol consumption, even wine, to two glasses or less a day. With seven calories per gram, alcohol sugars shift metabolism in favor of fat depositing; too much alcohol burdens the liver and stimulates the appetite.

• **Eat fat-burning foods.** Foods that raise metabolism are fresh fruits and vegetables (full of enzymes), whole grains and legumes. Eat fruits for breakfast or between meals. If you eat them with or after meals, the fructose is likely to be converted to fat by the liver. Sea greens work especially well for women to recharge metabolism and balance thyroid activity. Sea greens are also a rich source of fat-soluble vitamins like D, and K which help balance estrogen, and DHEA. Two tablespoons a day are a therapeutic dose. Add them chopped and dried to any salad, soup, rice dish or omelet. Or, add 6 pieces of sushi daily to your diet.

• **Re-activate your fat-burning systems with herbs.** Herbal adaptogens like panax and Siberian ginsengs, suma, gotu kola, and licorice root normalize body homeostasis; ginkgo biloba and hawthorn boost circulation; bee pollen, alfalfa, and phytohormone-containing herbs like sarsaparilla and black cohosh support the liver; spices and sea greens like cayenne, ginger, kelp and spirulina help the thyroid govern metabolism. Crystal Star FEEL GREAT™ caps are a whole body tonic to enhance fat burning and well-being.

• **Amino acids boost metabolism and keep lean muscle.** —L-Phenylalanine (LPA), suppresses appetite, boosts energy and reduces food craving. (Avoid phenylalanine if you take anti-depressants, have high blood pressure, or are pregnant.) —L-Tyrosine is a thyroid precursor and reduces appetite. —L-Carnitine suppresses appetite, accelerates fat metabolism and helps control sugar levels. —Ornithine (1000mg daily) helps boost metabolism and curb appetite. Amino acid metabolic products for weight maintenance include MYOPLEX LITE by EAS, and AMINO BALANCE by Anabol Naturals.

• **Drink plenty of water.** Drink at least six 8-oz servings of water daily, even if you're not thirsty. Water naturally suppresses appetite, helps maintain a high metabolic rate, promotes good digestion and regular bowel movements, and actually reduces fat deposits. Water may be the most important catalyst for fat burning, because it increases the liver's detoxification and fat metabolism activity. Don't worry about fluid retention. High water intake actually decreases bloating, because it flushes out sodium and toxins. Low water intake causes **more** fat deposits. Expert dieters drink eight glasses of water a day. They know each pound of fat burned releases 22 ounces of water which must be flushed away along with the metabolic by-products of fat breakdown.

4: EXERCISE FOR SURE. Getting regular exercise is a standard we should all strive for. The newest studies find that regular exercise extends life-span and cuts the risk for heart attack in half! But, recent statistics from the National Institutes of Health find that 58% of adult Americans get no or little exercise. Daily exercise is the key to permanent, painless weight control. No diet will work without exercise; with it, almost every diet will. Exercise before a meal raises blood sugar levels, increases metabolism and decreases appetite. Even if you just slightly change your eating habits, you can still lose weight with a brisk hour's walk. Calories continue to be burned at a greater pace for several hours after you have exercised! In addition, exercise improves your mood and emotional health through endorphin release in the brain. Exercise also transports oxygen and nutrients through the body, and helps eliminate carbon dioxide and toxins from the tissues. Exercise not only helps you look better, it helps you feel better.

• <u>Get moderate doses of sunlight.</u> The sun receives a lot of criticism today, but sunlight in moderation boosts metabolism and digestion. Sunlight can produce metabolic effects in the body similar to that of physical training. Eat outdoors when you can.

Thermogenesis is Critical to Weight Loss after 40.

Thermogenesis is about fat burning. About 75% of the calories you eat work to keep you alive and support your resting metabolic rate. The rest are stored as white fat, or burned up by brown adipose tissue, (BAT), your fat-burning factory. Brown fat is the body's chief regulator of thermogenesis, so the more active your brown fat is, the easier it is to maintain a desirable weight. Dieters who rely solely on restricting their calorie intake usually end up disappointed, because extreme calorie restriction lowers the rate of thermogenesis. Your body actually burns less fat than it did before you started dieting. People who yo-yo on and off low calorie diets have even more problems. When a yo-yo dieter begins to increase calorie intake after dieting, their metabolic rate does not return to pre-diet levels, so they store more calories as fat than they did before they started!

Middle-aged spread means too little thermogenesis after eating, but the amounts of heat (calorie burning) vary widely. Lean people experience a 40% increase in heat production after a meal. Overweight people may have only an increase of 10%. Obesity occurs primarily when brown fat isn't working properly, only a little thermogenesis takes place, and the body deals with the excess calories by storing them as fat. During our mid-life years, starting in our early 40's, a genetic timer shuts down the thermogenic mechanism. Turning this timer back on is the secret to re-activating thermogenesis and a more youthful metabolism. Here's how brown fat works to stimulate thermogenesis: A protein, called uncoupling protein, breaks down, or uncouples, the train of biochemical events that the cells use to turn calories into energy. Brown fat cells continue to convert calories into heat as long as they are stimulated, and as long as there is white fat for them to work on. Brown fat activity is also self-perpetuating, because it energizes more uncoupling proteins, produces more brown fat cells, and results in substantially more excess calories being burned off as heat through thermogenesis.

Research into the genetic basis of obesity shows that some people are not born with enough brown fat. People who eat lightly but still can't lose weight, gain more weight in middle age because the little brown fat they did have is reduced even further. Thermogenesis research demonstrates that it is possible to reverse this aberration. Thermogenic herbs have been successful at reactivating brown fat in middle age. They can increase calorie burning without additional diet changes or exercise, although these things offer additional benefits. 1) Thermogenic herbs increase blood flow to lean muscle tissue, so it works faster and longer. 2) Thermogenic herbs suppress appetite. You eat less with less effort. 3) The longer you take thermogenic herb formulas, the more effective they tend to become, because they help your body produce enough thermogenic activity to make a difference.

Weight control tips just for women over 40:

1— **Eat only when you're hungry.** Eating when you're stressed or depressed is a sure way to overeat. Listen for real physical hunger before you start to eat. Sometimes, what we think are hunger pangs, are really thirst pangs. Drink lots of water when you first feel hunger, then wait 10 or 15 minutes before you decide to start eating. Then, serve yourself a portion that is only as big as your clenched fist. Take small bites, and eat slowly. Remember, it takes 10 to 15 minutes for the stomach to signal the brain that it is full. So, if you just keep eating, you will overeat.

2— **Recharge your metabolism.** Sea greens help recharge metabolism and help balance thyroid activity after menopause. Just add two tablespoons, chopped, dried to any salad or soup. Sea greens are available at Oriental markets or any health food store. Or add 6 pieces of sushi (any kind) twice a week to your diet.

3— **Eat more whole foods,** in their natural, unprocessed state, especially nutritious foods, like dense grains (such as brown rice) at lunchtime. They will help carry your body through the day by providing B vitamins and minerals for foundation strength.

4— **Breathe deeply.** It may sound too easy, but breathing processes 70% of the body's wastes. Shallow breathing can slow down metabolism and the body's natural process of detoxification. Breathing deeply from the abdomen will deliver the right amount of oxygen to all your cells, help get rid of fat, increase your energy and boost metabolism. It also helps regulate heart rate, lower blood pressure and oxygenizes your cells to stimulate healing.

5— **Use aromatherapy.** New research shows that the smell of banana, green apple and peppermint can help reduce weight!

6— Do aerobic exercises! Aerobic exercise combined with a low fat, low calorie, fresh foods diet is particularly good for women. No long term weight control plan will work without it. One study found that overweight women who cut their calories and added an aerobic exercise program had significantly less PMS problems, such as mood swings and poor concentration. They also had lower blood levels of monoamine oxidase, an enzyme linked to PMS; and they lost an average of 36 pounds.

7— Take a brisk walks after dinner because it also helps boost liver activity for fat metabolism. (The liver metabolizes fats and dumps a lot of its wastes at night.) It may also help you live longer. A new study in the Journal of the American Medical Association revealed that taking just 6 brisk, half-hour walks a month cuts risk of death up 44% (compared to no doing no exercise).

Can a woman beat cellulite?

Men and women have different kinds of body fat. Women have a gynoid pattern of fat distribution that generally accumulates over the hips and buttocks. Men have an android pattern of fat that resides mainly in the abdominal region. It is much harder for women to lose fat in their problem areas than men. After menopause, women tend to have more fat and less lean muscle tissue than women who are still menstruating.

Eighty-six percent of American women over the age of 25 have cellulite deposits on the hips and thighs. Cellulite is actually a combination of fat, water and trapped wastes beneath the skin that the body isn't able to eliminate through normal channels. Fatty wastes get trapped beneath the skin's surface when the liver or lymphatic systems are sluggish. Cellulite is mainly a women's problem, because women's skin fibers are thinner, more delicate than men's. Cellulite is tough to get rid of. It often doesn't go away even after regular exercise. (Men aren't totally immune to cellulite - they get it on their "love handles.") Liposuction for cellulite is a billion dollar business, the most often performed surgery. But surgery is not your only option.

Do you have cellulite? When you squeeze your fatty areas, the skin ripples like a orange peel or has the texture of cottage cheese. If it is smooth, it is regular white fat.

Do thigh creams work for cellulite? Some of them do! Both men and women benefit from using natural smoothing creams which help reduce the look of cellulite by stimulating circulation to that area for better elimination of wastes. Massage and knead them into problem areas twice daily to help break up and release cellulite deposits. Try Crystal Star's THERMO CEL-LEAN™ TONING GEl.

Cellulite control relies on liver health:

1: Drink green tea to optimize your liver's ability to digest excess fats, 2 cups a day in the morning and early afternoon. Green tea can change the metabolic pattern of the liver by changing the ratio of two metabolic enzymes, *cytochrome P450* and *glucuronyltransferase*, to help the body excrete toxic compounds and fatty wastes. Moreover, green tea has been found to protect against cancers of the lungs, skin, liver, pancreas, and stomach, protect the heart, lower cholesterol and regulate blood sugar and insulin levels. Green tea is also a gentle cleanser which leaves you feeling refreshed and invigorated. Tea, anybody? Take green tea in the morning for the most benefits throughout the day.

2: Take Milk Thistle Seed extract for long term liver support, 10 to 15 drops under the tongue for 1 to 3 months, to gently cleanse the liver and improve its function. More than 300 studies show that silymarin, one of milk thistle's constituents, can prevent toxins from even entering the liver and can actually increase the liver's ability to generate new, healthy cells.

3: Take B vitamins. B-vitamin deficiencies cause problems with the metabolism of fats and carbohydrates. For some people, this one change in nutrition makes all the difference to their ability to lose cellulite.

4: Use dry skin brushing. Drink 8 glasses of water daily to help dump congested wastes. Then dry brush cellulite away. The best time for a dry brush massage is upon arising in the morning and again before going to bed at night. Take a shower or rubdown with a sponge or wet towel to wash away dead skin particles loosened by the brushing. (Or, go for a swim.) Use a natural bristle brush - not synthetic. Start with the soles of the feet - brush vigorously making rotary motions and massage every part of your body in this order: feet and legs, hands and arms, back and abdomen, chest and neck. Five to fifteen minutes is the average time.

Dry skin brushing:
  –Effectively removes the dead layers of skin and other impurities, and keeps pores open.
  –Stimulates hormone and oil producing glands.
  –Has a powerful rejuvenating influence on the nervous system by stimulating nerve endings in the skin.
  –Revitalizes and rejuvenates the skin, and helps to tone and tighten the skin.

Weight control tips for men over 40:

1— Control your portions. Don't overeat. It's a big problem for men. Overeating is a problem for American men, who are encouraged to dig in to second and even third helpings as a sign of manliness, or approval for the cook. Overeating happens when you eat lots of highly processed, chemical-laced foods, and junk food snacks that don't have much nutrition to help you feel full. Overeating happens when you eat under stress or on-the-run....the very circumstances under which many men in America eat. Drink plenty of water to naturally suppress appetite and maintain a high metabolic rate.

2—Take enzymes with meals to help prevent gas, heartburn and indigestion naturally. Enzymes work in my experience, far better than antacids. They speed up digestion and keep the entire digestive tract free of waste build-up. The best enzymes come from fresh plant foods. Cooking largely destroys them. So have a fresh salad at least once a day for weight control. And if you can't make them, take them. I regularly recommend Nature's Secret REZYME to men with success.

3—Eat more whole foods, in their natural, unprocessed state. I especially recommend eating more fruits in the morning to men because they offer a blood sugar-raising glycogen energy punch, and are easily digested and assimilated.

432

4—Exercise is one of the main pillars of weight control for men.... even more than women. Exercising just 25 to 30 minutes a day will help you lose about 20 pounds a year, improve your energy and stamina, recharge your cardiovascular health and increase your life span!

5—Metabolism is the key to weight management. Metabolism, the process by which you burn calories, slows down once you get past forty, but you can reactivate it. In men, metabolism is most affected by calorie-burning lean muscle mass. The more muscle you have, the better your metabolism rate. In one study, men who did intense strength training exercises raised their metabolism for 15 hours after their workout! Incorporate weight bearing exercise into your program for faster metabolism. But be reasonable about it. Many weight bearing exercise injuries are the result of overzealous people who tried to lift too much weight, lifted the wrong way or simply lifted for too long. Start slow and stick with it.

6—Certain spices work well for men to increase the thermogenesis (calorie-burning) process. Spices like cinnamon, cayenne, mustard and ginger can speed up a man's fat burning process. Try dipping raw veggies in mustard throughout the day. One teasp. of mustard can increase metabolism 25% for up to 3 hours! The amino acid arginine 1000mg daily is also a useful tool for men trying to reactivate metabolism, because of its support for increasing lean muscle mass.

7—Men have android fat patterns that tend to be distributed in the abdomen area. In other words, guys get potbellies! There are two types of fat, subcutaneous and visceral. A man with a hard potbelly has more visceral fat, or fat that lies between the muscles and organs. Soft bellies, in contrast, are largely comprised of subcutaneous fat just beneath the skin, and harder to get rid of. Men have more visceral fat than women..... one reason why they seem to be able shake extra pounds easier than women. However, hard bellies, formed from visceral fat, are linked to cardiovascular diseases and intestinal problems. Reducing fat and exercising regularly is an effective solution that often works quickly for men.

8—Keep your liver healthy! The poor health of your liver may be causing that potbelly. The liver is the major fat metabolizing organ of the body! Did you know that a man who is thin everywhere else but has a protruding stomach often has an enlarged liver? Keeping it healthy is essential to body balancing and weight management for men.

Signs and symptoms that your liver needs some TLC:
  –great tiredness
  –unexplained weight gain
  –poor digestion
  –depression, melancholy
  –food and chemical sensitivities

Recipes for an adult's weight loss diet: •DETOX / CLEANSING; •DAIRY-FREE; •FISH / SEAFOOD; •ENZYME-RICH FOODS; •SUGAR-FREE SWEETS; •LOW FAT / VERY LOW FAT; •SALADS; •BLENDING EAST and WEST.

Weight Control for Kids

Today's children are becoming an overweight generation. America's adults may be paying more attention to their diets, but statistics show that U.S. kids are the fattest they've ever been. An estimated 14% of children over the age of 6 are obese. Until the 1960's, weight control wasn't much of a problem for kids. But the fifties ushered in the fast food era - refined, chemicalized foods that changed people's metabolism and cell structure. As the fifties kids became parents, they passed on immune defense depletions and digestion problems to their kids who are now the parents of the overweight, undernourished kids of today. Obesity rates for young children jumped 54% between 1960 and 1981, and 30% for teenagers. They jumped another 50% between 1981 and 1998.

It's only the beginning. T.V. food advertising especially targets kids who are eating an ever widening array of chemical-laced, genetically altered foods, and junky foods with too much fat, salt, sugar and calories. Some kids eat out of a box most of the time!

U.S. schools have dropped the ball for children's health. A 10-year study by the President's Council on Physical Fitness showed two very disconcerting facts in the last decade: 1) 85% of the children and teenagers tested failed basic fitness tests; 2) as many as 90% of American children already have at least one risk factor for a degenerating disease. The telecommunications age has brought kids computers, T.V.'s, and video games - and a lot less active playtime. (Today's kids get less exercise and outdoor play than any previous generation.) P.E. classes in U.S. schools, most sports and many extra-curricular activities have been dropped, and our kids are paying the price. Most kids attend only 1 or 2 physical education classes a week. Forty percent of boys ages 6-12 can't touch their toes; American girls actually run slower today than they did 10 years ago. P.E. teachers have been reassigned to other classes in a full 75% of U.S. schools.

Today's kids watch up to 24 hours of TV a week. By the time U.S. kids reach their senior high school year, they've spent over 3 years of their lives watching TV. Even more alarming, heart disease is now traceable to early childhood. U.S. doctors are discovering that many American teens (even some 3 year olds) already have fatty deposits on their coronary arteries. Today's kids rely on junk foods. Children are rewarded with food for good behavior or denied food for punishment from an early age. As they grow older, kids tend to continue that cycle by rewarding themselves with salty, sugary, fatty snacks, soft drinks, and nitrate-loaded lunch meats before parents even come home from work.

Overweight children face early diseases, low self-esteem, depression and rejection by peers. Getting weight problems under control at an early age is the best choice for later health. As an obese child grows older, he or she doubles the likelihood of adult obesity. But, crash diets are not the solution for kids (or adults). Changing the focus to health, to having a fit body instead of a thin body can make all the difference in a weight management program. Kids need mineral-rich building foods, fiber-rich energy foods, and protein-rich growth foods.

I recommend a light detox to start a good weight control program for an overweight child, who usually has "toxic overload" from too many chemical-laced foods. A gentle detox normalizes body chemistry. Avoid all highly processed, junky foods, red meats and dairy foods, except yogurt during this detox.

1 to 3-Day Junk Food Detox for Kids

—**On rising:** give citrus juice with 1 teaspoon of acidophilus liquid, or a glass of lemon juice and water with honey or maple syrup.
—**Breakfast:** offer fresh fruits, such as apples, pineapple, papaya or oranges. Add vanilla yogurt, rice milk, almond milk or soymilk.
—**Mid-morning:** give fresh carrot juice. Add $^1/_4$ teasp. ascorbate vitamin C or Ester C crystals to neutralize body toxins.
—**Lunch:** give fresh raw crunchy veggies with a yogurt dip; or a fresh veggie salad with lemon/oil or yogurt dressing.
—**Mid-afternoon:** offer a refreshing herb tea, such as licorice or peppermint tea with honey.
—**Dinner:** give a fresh salad, with avocados, carrots, kiwi, romaine and other high vitamin A foods; and a cup of miso soup.
—**Before bed:** offer a relaxing herb tea, like chamomile tea, or Crystal Star GOOD NIGHT™ tea. Add $^1/_4$ teasp. vitamin C or Ester C crystals; or a cup of MISO broth for strength.

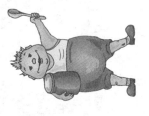

Light-Right Diet for Kids

After the light detox above, begin a healthy diet. **Breakfast is a key to weight loss for kids.** A high fiber breakfast cuts a child's calorie intake by up to 200 calories a day and holds a child's energy and hunger til lunchtime. Add plenty of fresh enzyme-rich foods. Many of today's diets don't work because they rely on microwaved foods - a process that kills the enzymes. Enzyme dead foods create a nutritional gap for our kids (some experts say we would die if all we ate was microwaved foods). For children, this also means weight gain and constipation, a major problem for kids that eat a lot of dairy foods like milk, cheese and ice cream. 20% of Caucasian children and 80% of black children don't produce lactase, the enzyme necessary to digest milk.

Snacks, lunch foods and meals can be satisfying and delicious without adding significant amounts of sugar, fat or salt. In fact, young children need two or three snacks daily to have a nutritious diet, because their stomachs don't hold all they need in just three meals. Kids need mineral-rich building foods, fiber-rich energy foods, and protein-rich growth foods.

Changing the type of food eaten without restricting the amount can result in easy, spontaneous weight loss. Plenty of fresh fruit, un-buttered spicy popcorn, and sandwich fixings are good defenses against junk foods. The following diet serves as an easy weight control guideline for kids. It has passed many tests on both overweight and "couch potato" kids for foods that they will eat.

Two enzyme-rich juice recipes that even the pickiest of kids will ask for again and again.
1: GREEN DRINK FOR KIDS: Make it in a juicer. Make it easy. Use any fresh veggies that your child likes most. Include green leafy vegetables like spinach, sunflower greens and lettuces. I find that kids like baby veggies. Consider baby bok choy, baby carrots and sprouts. Don't forget sweet tasting veggies like cucumbers, celery and tomatoes.

2: ENERGIZING FRUIT SMOOTHIE: Use fresh fruit, not canned or frozen. Blend 1 banana and 1 orange with apple juice. Add half a papaya or one-quarter of a fresh pineapple.

Note: If you don't have a juicer, give your child a plant enzyme supplement to keep his metabolism going strong, like Prevail's CHILDREN'S DIGESTION FORMULA or Transformation's DIGESTZYME, both quality products I've worked with.

—**On rising:** give a vitamin/mineral drink like ALL ONE MULTIPLE VITAMINS & MINERALS or Nature's Plus SPIRUTEIN (lots of flavors), or 1 teaspoon liquid multi-vitamin in juice (such as Floradix CHILDREN'S MULTI-VITAMIN/MINERAL).

—**Breakfast:** have a whole grain cereal with apple juice or a little yogurt and fresh fruit; if more is desired, whole grain toast or muffins, with a little butter, kefir cheese or nut butter; add eggs, scrambled or baked (no fried eggs); or have some hot oatmeal or kashi cereal with maple syrup, and yogurt if desired.

—**Mid-morning:** snacks can be whole grain crackers with kefir cheese or low-fat cheese or dip, and a sugarless juice or sparkling fruit mineral water; or some fresh fruit, such as apples with yogurt or kefir cheese; or dried fruit, or fruit leather; or fresh crunchy veggies, like celery, with peanut butter; or a no-sugar dried fruit, nut and seed candy bar (you can easily make one) or a dried fruit and nut trail mix, stirred into yogurt.

—**Lunch:** have a fresh veggie, turkey, chicken or shrimp salad sandwich on whole grain bread, with low-fat or soy cheese and mayonnaise. Add whole grain or corn chips with a low-fat veggie or cheese dip; or a hearty bean soup with whole grain toast or crackers, and crunchy veggies with garbanzo spread; or a baked potato with a butter, kefir cheese, or soy cheese, and a green salad with light dressing; or a vegetarian pizza on a chapati or pita crust; or whole grain spaghetti or pasta with a light sauce and Parmesan cheese; or a Mexican bean and veggie, or rice or whole wheat burrito with a light natural no-sugar salsa.

—**Mid-afternoon:** have a sparkling juice and a dried fruit candy bar, or fruit juice-sweetened cookies; or some fresh fruit or fruit juice, or an amazake drink with whole grain muffins; or a hard boiled egg, and some whole grain chips with a veggie or low-fat cheese dip; or some whole grain toast and peanut butter or other nut butter.

—**Dinner:** have a light pizza on a whole grain, chapati or egg crust, with veggies, shrimp, and soy or low-fat mozzarella cheese topping; or whole grain or egg pasta with vegetables and a light tomato and cheese sauce; or a baked Mexican quesadilla with soy or low-fat cheese and some steamed vegetables or a salad; or a stir-fry with crunchy noodles, brown rice, baked egg rolls and a light soup; or some roast turkey with corn bread dressing and a salad; or a tuna casserole with rice, peas and water chestnuts, and toasted chapatis with a little butter.

—**Before bed:** a glass of apple juice or vanilla soy milk or flavored kefir. A snack of unbuttered, spicy, savory popcorn is good and nutritious anytime.

Recipes for a child's weight loss diet: •**BREAKFAST - BRUNCH;** •**DAIRY-FREE;** •**SANDWICHES;** •**ENZYME-RICH FOODS;** •**SUGAR-FREE SWEETS;** •**MINERAL-RICH RECIPES;** •**HIGH PROTEIN** without **MEAT;** •**HIGH FIBER.**

Sports Nutrition and Healing Diets

Optimizing your Exercise and Sports Performance

The latest statistics are shocking! We may all know exercise is critical to good health, that exercise speeds results in weight loss and strengthens our hearts, but new National Institute of Health studies reveal that as many as 58% of adult Americans get no or little exercise. A sedentary lifestyle has the same effect on heart disease risk as smoking a pack of cigarettes a day! Regular exercise is also a significant part of a healing program. It strengthens your whole body — muscles, nerves, blood, glands, lungs, heart, brain, mind and mood. It increases your metabolic rate, muscle mass, oxygen uptake, circulation, and boosts the enzymes that help your body burn fat. Exercise is the key to stress control, low cholesterol and a sharper memory. It also stimulates antibody production, enhances immune response, and reduces fatigue. Exercise is the best mood elevator of all! By releasing pain-relieving endorphins, exercise reduces anxiety, relieves depression and extends your lifespan.

Exercise is integral to good nutrition. Most of us notice that when we're exercising we're not hungry. We're thirsty after a workout as our bodies call for water and electrolyte replacement, but not hungry. One of the reasons rapid results are achieved in a body streamlining program is this phenomenon. Muscles become toned, heart and lungs become stronger, and fats are lost, but the body doesn't call for calorie replacement right away. Its own glycogens lift blood sugar levels for a feeling of well being. **Exercise becomes a nutrient in itself.**

Exercise optimizes metabolism, especially brown fat activity. Brown fat is highly active metabolically, very different from yellow fat (the kind you see deposited around your body). Brown fat is bound to your skeleton and is filled with tiny, brown-colored, mitochondria and cytochromes, chemical powerhouses that produce energy in your cells. Brown fat is thermogenically responsive. When you take in excess calories, your body compensates in part by producing more heat to burn them off instead of storing them as yellow fat. Brown fat activity explains why some people can overeat and stay slim while other people gain weight easily. Brown fat becomes less active and less thermogenically responsive as we age. Instead of calories being burned off, they get stored as yellow fat. Keep your brown fat activated to control your weight as you age. Brown fat activity goes down if your diet is poor and you don't get regular exercise. Not exercising causes lean muscle tissue to break down, leaving you flabby, with less energy, and ultimately, with even less brown fat activity to burn calories.

Exercise is as available as your front door. A daily, thirty minute walk, breathing deeply, for even a mile a day ($\frac{1}{2}$ mile out, $\frac{1}{2}$ mile back) makes a big difference to brown fat activity. Exhaling deeply releases metabolic waste along with CO_2; inhaling deeply floods your body with fresh oxygen. A walk cleans your circulatory system, and improves muscle tone. It reduces heart attack risk, especially in women. Think of sunlight on your body as heliotherapy adding natural vitamin D for skin and bone health.

If you don't exercise, you'll not only lose muscle, you'll lose about 1% of your bone mass every year… it can begin as early as age 35. There is an exercise program for you no matter what age you are or what shape you're in. You don't need to overdo it to reap the rewards. Two studies in the Journal of the American Medical Association show moderate exercise is as beneficial for the cardiovascular system and overall fitness as high intensity workouts. My 87-year old father is a cancer survivor who goes to exercise classes several times a week… he looks and feels great.

Pick an exercise that you enjoy and stick to it! Dancing is one of the best aerobic exercises I know. Legs and lungs both show rapid improvement, not to mention the fun you have. Any kind of dancing is a good workout, and the breathlessness you feel afterward is the best sign of aerobic benefits. Swimming works all parts of your body at once. Noticeable upper arm and thigh definition improvement comes quickly with regular swimming. Just fifteen to twenty steady laps, two or three times a week, and a more streamlined body is yours. (I use water weights when I swim to maximize my exercise.) Cycling gets you somewhere while you exercise. Walking, jogging or cycling all increase both muscle and bone mass. High energy exercise classes are available, everyday, everywhere at low prices.

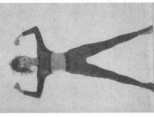

If your schedule is so busy that you hardly have time to breathe, let alone exercise, but still want the benefits of bodywork, there is an all-in-one aerobic exercise. It has gotten resounding enthusiasm and response rates for aerobic activity and muscle tone - all in one minute. The exercise sounds very easy, but is actually very difficult, and that is why it works so well. You will be breathless before you know it.

Simply lie flat on your back on a rug or carpet. Rise to a full standing position any way you can, and lie down flat on your back again. That's the whole exercise. Stand and lie down, stand and lie down – for one minute. Typical repetitions for most people with average body tone are six to ten times in 60 seconds. The record time for an athlete in top competitive condition is 20-24 times in a minute. Repeat only as many times as you feel comfortable and work up gradually. It is worth a try because it exercises muscles, lung capacity and circulatory system so well... but don't overdo it.

Whatever exercise program you choose for yourself, make rest a part of it. Work out harder one day, go easy the next; or exercise for several days and take two days off. It's better for body balance, and will increase your energy levels when you exercise the next time. After a regular program is started, exercising four days a week will increase fitness level; exercising three days a week maintains fitness level; exercising two days a week will decrease a high fitness level. But any amount of exercise is better than nothing at all.

Choose those that work for you conveniently and easily. Vigorous physical exercise is the most efficient way to burn yellow fat, but every series of stretches and exercises you do tones, elasticizes, shapes and contours your skin, connective tissue and muscles.

Eating for Energy and Performance

Body building is 85% nutrition.

Nutrition is the most important factor for exercise or sports performance, at any level. Long-term, optimal nutrition is the basis for high performance. Protein or carbo-loading before an event can't make up for nutrient short-falls. No anabolic supplement of any kind can give you athletic excellence if you have an inferior diet. Good nutrition helps eliminate fluctuating energy levels, abnormal fatigue, and susceptibility to injury or illness. When you eat junk foods, you pay the penalty of poor performance.

Analyzing a high performance diet: Sixty to seventy-five percent should be in clean-burning complex carbohydrates - from whole grains, pasta, vegetables, rice, beans and fruits. They improve performance, promote muscle fuel storage, and absorb easily without excess fats that slow down weight loss and sap energy.

Twenty to twenty-five percent should be in protein from whole grains, nuts, beans, low fat dairy foods, soy foods, yogurt, kefir, eggs, some poultry, fish, and seafood. Vegetable protein is best for mineral absorption and bone density. Strength and muscle mass decline if you get too little protein. But eating too much protein, especially from red meats (as is in the highly popular "Zone" and "Zone clone" diets) hampers performance. Excess amino acids from too much protein cause toxic ammonia to form in the body. Too much protein overloads your kidneys (you'll feel lower back pain) as your body struggles to eliminate waste from inefficient metabolism. (See "Protein in a Healing Diet" on pg 40 of this book for more.)

Ten to fifteen percent of an athletic diet should be in energy-producing fats necessary for glycogen storage. The best fats for athletes are mono-or polyunsaturated oils, a little butter, eggs, nuts and seeds, low fat cheeses, avocados and whole grain snacks.

Other diet fuel should be liquid nutrients: fruit juices for natural sugars, mineral waters and electrolyte replacement drinks for potassium, magnesium and sodium, and "superfoods." Superfoods are highly concentrated, bio-available nutrients that can give an athlete the edge in strength and stamina. Green superfood blends contain concentrates of spirulina, alfalfa, chlorella, barley grass, blue-green algae and wheat grass. Bee pollen and royal jelly are rich in essential nutritional elements. Aged garlic has valuable properties for the athlete, providing potent antioxidants for free radical protection.

Drink plenty of water. Without ample fluids, waste and impurities don't get filtered or released, and the liver doesn't metabolize stored fats for energy. Six to eight glasses of water a day are a must, even if you don't feel thirsty.

Here's why. A few fluid facts for athletes:

• Two-thirds of your body water is inside your cells (intracellular fluid); the remaining one-third is outside cells (extracellular fluid); only a small portion is in blood plasma.

• Dehydration during prolonged exercise causes a drop in blood volume, increases stress on the heart by forcing it to pump harder. Water's most important function? For athletes it's regulating body temperature via sweating (you need water to sweat).

• A body water loss of 4% to 6% reduces muscle endurance and muscle strength. A loss of more than 6% of body weight through sweating causes severe heat cramps, heat exhaustion, heat stroke, coma, and in some cases of long distance runners without water, even death.

• Potassium, magnesium, iron, and other minerals are also lost in sweat. Drink at least 16-oz. of water two hours before exercise to prepare for exercise-related water-mineral loss.

A diet to improve sports performance also enhances other body needs: *Faster Healing of Wounds-Injuries, Endurance and Stamina, Chronic Constipation, Muscle Tone, Glands, Hormone Balance, Stimulates Metabolism, Overcomes Fatigue, Prevents Osteoporosis.*

Note: See pages 446 and 448 for a FOOD EXCHANGE LIST and a FOOD AMOUNTS CHART by diet so you can adjust individual needs.

Sports Enthusiast's Diet

This diet is for the naturally athletic person who works out for fitness and muscle tone 3 or 4 times a week, but not for competition. It is low in fats, emphasizes complex carbohydrates for smooth muscle use, has moderate protein, and may be used successfully as part of a weight control plan. Complex carbohydrates also produce glycogen for the body, resulting in quicker energy. The diet is designed to quickly build up body nutrients and strength with energizing, "refueling" meals. Drink 6 to 8 glasses of bottled water daily for a clean, hydrated, and well-regulated system.

—**On rising:** take 1 teasp. molasses, 2 teasp. bee pollen granules, and 1 teasp. spirulina in apple, or pineapple juice; or 1 TB All ONE VITAMIN/MINERAL drink mix in juice or water.

—**Breakfast:** take a high protein drink, such as Nature's Plus SPIRUTEIN; or make a protein drink with soy protein powder, 1 egg, 2 teasp. nutritional yeast, 1 teasp. spirulina powder, 2 teasp. toasted wheat germ and 1 teasp. sesame seeds; or see the suggestions on page 445 for good protein energy drinks; then have some muesli or whole grain granola, such as coconut/almond granola, with yogurt and fresh fruit, apple juice or soy milk topping; or hot oatmeal with maple syrup, or whole grain (buckwheat) pancakes with maple syrup; or a poached egg on a whole grain English muffin, with a little butter and Bragg's LIQUID AMINOS;

—**Mid-morning:** take a high potency enzyme/mineral drink such as Crystal Star SYSTEMS STRENGTH DRINK™, or Amazake rice drink; or Crystal Star RAINFOREST ENERGY TEA™ with fresh fruit; or miso soup with sea vegetables snipped on top; or a green drink or vegetable juice, or Sun Wellness CHLORELLA.

—**Lunch:** have a baked potato, with butter and 1 teasp. Bragg's LIQUID AMINOS; and/or a spinach or other green leafy salad; or a vegetable frittata or low-fat veggie pizza; or a seafood salad, spinach or veggie pasta salad (hot or cold), with whole grain muffins; or a roast turkey sandwich on whole grain bread with greens and mayonnaise; or tofu or steamed veggies with brown rice and tamari; or some low-fat cheeses or cottage cheese with fresh fruit; or a high protein salad or sandwich with avocados and sprouts.

—**Mid-afternoon:** have some low-fat yogurt with nuts, seeds, or fresh fruit; or a hard boiled or deviled egg with sesame salt for dipping, and a bottle of mineral water; or a cup of Crystal Star FEEL GREAT TEA™ with some whole grain crackers and a low-fat dip; or some dried or fresh fruit with kefir cheese for dipping.

—**Dinner:** have a low-fat Italian meal with whole grain or vegetable pasta, a soup and antipasto; or bulgar, brown rice, or other whole grain pasta/vegetable casserole; or baked, broiled or grilled fish or seafood with a salad and whole grain bread; or a roast or baked poultry entree with brown rice or other whole grain, and a small salad; or a dinner omelet or quiche, with a green leafy salad; or a hearty vegetable soup or stew with rye or pumpernickel bread.

Note: A little wine with dinner is fine for better digestion, raising HDLs, and relaxation.

—**Before bed:** a cup of Red Star nutritional yeast broth for B vitamins and relaxation; or pineapple-coconut juice or organic apple juice.

Recipes to help your sports enthusiast diet: •COMPLEX CARBS for ENERGY; •BREAKFAST and BRUNCH; •HIGH PROTEIN without MEAT; •SALADS; •ENZYME-RICH; •MINERAL-RICH; •SANDWICHES; •HIGH FIBER RECIPES.

Herb and Supplement Choices

•**Superfoods for strength and faster recovery:** Nutricology PROGREENS; Pines MIGHTY GREENS; Nature's Secret ULTI-MATE GREEN; Crystal Star ENERGY GREEN drink mix.

•**Protein-Amino Drinks:** muscle building and endurance: Twin Lab AMINO FUEL; Unipro PERFECT PROTEIN; PureForm WHEY PROTEIN; Bee pollen full spectrum aminos.

•**Sports Drinks/Electrolyte Replacements:** Use after exercise to replace minerals. Anabol Naturals CARBO SURGE; Nature's Path TRACE-LYTE liquid electrolytes; Knudsens RE-CHARGE; Twin Lab ULTRA FUEL; Unipro ENDURA.

•**Stimulants:** quick energy. Natural Balance RIBOSE RIBO-MAX to replenish ATP energy; Crystal Star ACTIVE PHYSICAL ENERGY™ or HIGH PERFORMANCE™ caps.

•**Fat Burners:** Metabolize fats, enhance muscle growth. Nature's Path SLIM-LYTE 1200; Anabol Naturals GH RELEASERS - metabolic fat burner; Pinnacle ALPHADOPA GROWTH POPPERS.

•**Sports Bars:** Power Foods POWER BARS; Unipro BURN BAR; EAS® MYOPLEX LITE™.

•**Recovery Acceleration:** Proteolytic Enzymes break down scar tissue build-up and shortens recovery time. Bromelain-Papain 1500mg - for muscle and ligament repair and strength. Natural Balance RIBOSE RIBO-MAX to replenish ATP energy.

•**Free Form Amino Acids:** activators to increase strength. Anabol Naturals GH RELEASERS to burn fats for energy; Anabol Naturals AMINO BALANCE - 23 crystalline free-form aminos; Carnitine,1000mg to strengthen heart; Glutamine, 1000mg growth hormone release; Anabol Naturals AMINO NITRO MAX, BCAAs for ATP energy conversion; Unipro BCAA 1000.

Bodywork and Lifestyle Techniques

•**Weight training.** It's good for everybody, no matter what your sport, age or fitness goals. Women do not get a bulky physique from lifting weights. They have low levels of testosterone, which influences their muscle development. *Note: Vitamin E prevents muscle damage from weight training.*

•**Recuperate.** Muscles don't grow during exercise. They grow during rest periods. Alternate muscle workouts with rest days. Exercise different muscle sets on different days.

•**Breathe deep.** Lung capacity is a prime training factor. Muscles and tissues must have enough oxygen for stamina. Breathe in during exertion, out as you relax for the next rep. Vigorous exhaling is as important as inhaling for an athlete, to expel all carbon dioxide and increase lung capacity.

•**Stretch out.** Muscle extensions before and after a workout keep cramps down and muscles loose. Get morning sunlight on the body every day possible for optimal absorption.

•**No pain does not mean no gain.** Your exercise doesn't have to hurt to be good for you. Take your pulse during a workout to determine if it is demanding enough to strengthen your heart, but not too demanding. Place the first two fingers on your carotid artery just below the jaw line. Use a watch to count the number of beats for six seconds while you are moving, then add a zero to that number. This gives your heartbeats per minute. A heart rate between 70 and 85% of your age-range maximum is an ideal workout zone. Examples: 30 to 35 years - 133 to 157 beats per minute: 35 to 40 years - 130 to 153 beats per minute; 40 to 45 years - 126 to 149 beats per minute.

Note: A resting heart rate for a fit adult is 65 to 80 beats per minute.

Can't find a recommended product? Call the 800 number listed in Product Resources for the store nearest you and for more info.

Do You Really Need Steroids For High Performance?

As standards of excellence rise in sports competition, steroid use, legal and illegal is increasing. Steroids lead to wholesale destruction of gland tissue, stunted growth from bone closure, male testicle shrinkage, low sperm counts (noticeable after only a few months), male breast enlargement, weakened connective tissue, jaundice, poor circulation, and hostile personality behavior and facial changes.

<u>ANDRO</u> (*androstenedione*) a superhormone steroid, rates high popularity today. ANDRO, a by-product of DHEA is synthesized from the seeds of the Scotch Pine tree. Studies show ANDRO increases the body's testosterone supply up to three times the normal level. However, ANDRO should be used cautiously, and under the supervision of a health professional. It can boost testosterone levels too much and too fast, causing aggressive behavior and acne. ANDRO may actually convert into estrogen in the body, leading to breast growth or water retention in men. And, the conversion of androstenedione to estrogen accelerates aging in both men and women! Don't use ANDRO if you have any hormone-related problems like cancers of the breast, prostate or testes. People with acne, liver disorders, BPH, dysmenorrhea or Cushing's adrenal syndrome should avoid ANDRO.

<u>Creatine</u>, a steroid-like supplement, is a booming $100 million business. It's found in large amounts in the muscles, formed when the amino acids arginine, methionine and glycine combine in the body. Food sources are meats and fish. Creatine helps provide ATP energy for muscles and is especially useful for the rapid, explosive movements required in competition. Rod Fleming, a registered physical therapist, says, "Dehydration is consistently a problem for people using creatine. I have personally seen unusual muscle tears (pectoral) in people taking creatine. I advise against it." If you choose to try creatine, take it only as directed and drink plenty of fluids. (Don't mix it with fruit juice; creatine can react with fruit juice and transform into creatinine, a metabolic waste product.)

<u>Ribose</u> is a simple sugar our cells use to convert nutrients into ATP. As a supplement with some advantages over ANDRO and creatine, ribose increases energy stores in the heart and muscle cells, especially useful for people with cardiac insufficiency (diminished blood flow to the heart) and athletes who want to increase muscle endurance and decrease recovery time. Natural Balance RIBOSE RIBOMAX, a maintenance doses equal 3 to 5 grams per day.

<u>Can herbal steroids do the strength enhancement job?</u> There are no magic bullets for energy or endurance in sports, but plant-derived steroids called phytosterols do have growth activity similar to that of free form amino acids and anabolic steroids. Amino acids can act as steroid alternatives to help build the body to competitive levels without chemical steroid consequences. They also help release growth hormone, detox ammonia, promote fast recuperation, increase stamina, and support peak performance.

<u>The most well-known of these herbs are:</u> Tribulus Terrestris, an ancient treatment for low libido and impotence, increases stamina. Damiana, a mild aphrodisiac and nerve stimulant. Sarsaparilla (Smilax), coaxes the body to produce more testosterone and cortisone. Saw Palmetto, increases blood flow to the sexual organs; balances testosterone. Siberian and Panax Ginsengs, for over-all body balance and energy. Yohimbe, a testosterone precursor for body building, and potent aphrodisiac for both men and women.

High Performance Training Diet

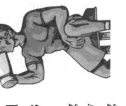

Athletics are about body/energy efficiency. This diet focuses on energy for competitive sports. Sports tests show that adjusting the diet before competition can increase endurance 200% or more – well worth consideration.

This training diet is high in complex carbohydrates for maximum fuel use for muscles. It has plenty of amino acid precursors to enhance the body's own growth hormone production; it is vitamin and mineral rich for solid building blocks. The old watchword of great protein increase for performance has changed as athletes realize the undesirable effects too much protein can cause; especially excess uric acid and its burden on the kidneys and liver. Muscle mass is not increased by excess protein.

Athletes' nutrition needs are considerably greater than those of the average person. They need concentrated nutrition for long range energy reserves. Normal RDAs are far too low for high performance or competition needs. Body composition, not body weight, is the important consideration. Both diets in this chapter are useful for a serious athlete. Competitive training and a training diet alone cannot insure success. Rest time and building energy reserves are necessary to tune the body for maximum efficiency.

When not in competition or pre-event training, extra high nutrient amounts are not needed, and can be hard for the body to handle. A reduced density diet is better for maintaining tone. Some supplement guidelines are given in this diet, since how and when supplements are taken during training is as important as which ones are taken. Additional suggestions are listed in the supplement and herb section following the diet.

—**On rising:** take a nutrient supplement, such as ALL ONE VITAMIN/MINERAL drink in pineapple/coconut juice; or vanilla soy milk with 2 teasp. bee pollen and 1 teasp. barley green or spirulina granules; or Crystal Star SYSTEMS STRENGTH™ high mineral drink mix in water.

   If this is a rest day, now is a good time to take the nutritional supplements: B-complex 150mg; A high potency multi vitamin such as Weider MEGABOLIC PAK or PureForm LIQUID VITAMIN; Vitamin C 1000 to 2000mg. with bioflavonoids and rutin,or ESTER-C with minerals and electrolytes; Nature's Path CAL-LYTE or HEMA-LYTE iron, electrolytes; Bromelain 1500mg. for muscle/ligament repair; MSM caps help to rebuild and protect joints from injuries.

—**Breakfast:** take more liquid nutrition, in a high-powered protein drink, such as Twin Lab AMINO FUEL or Max Muscle SUPERPRO for off days, Twin Lab CREATINE FUEL PLUS or Champion PRO-SCORE 100 for workout days; or make your own drink from soy protein powder, an egg, 2 tsp. Red Star yeast, 2 tsp. toasted wheat germ, 1 tsp. spirulina, and 1 tsp. sesame seed; then, have some muesli or whole grain granola with yogurt and fresh fruit, or soy or rice milk topping; or hot oatmeal with maple syrup, or whole grain pancakes with maple syrup or honey; or a poached egg on a whole grain English muffin, with a little butter and Bragg's LIQUID AMINOS; or hot brown rice; or an omelet with veggie filling, or tofu "scrambled eggs" with vegetables.

   If this is a training day, take amino acid, herbal or protein supplements now and 25 minutes before your workout: Chromium picolinate 250-500mcg to increase muscle mass and reduce body fat; CoQ-10, 100mg, or DMG (Di-Methylglycine) to boost oxygen delivery; Unipro TRIBULUS SYNERGY for testosterone support; Crystal Star HIGH PERFORMANCE™ for stamina; an anabolic natural steroid, Radiant Life SUMAX (like dianabol without the side effects), Natural Balance RIBO-MAX, Champion MUSCLE NITRO (BCAAs to increase endurance, and ATP build-up).

443

—**Mid-morning:** have an Amazake rice drink; or carrot juice with 1 teasp. Bragg's LIQUID AMINOS; or Monas CHLORELLA or Crystal Star ENERGY GREEN™, or a natural energy bar, like Power Foods POWER BARS or EAS® MYOPLEX DELUXE with 8-oz. water; or a dried fruit or nut snack mix; or yogurt with fresh fruit or nuts; or Alacer HIGH K COLA mineral drink after a workout.

—**Lunch:** whole grain or veggie pasta; hot with veggies and a light sauce, cold with greens or seafood and a light dressing; or a pita or burrito filled with veggies or seafood; or a whole grain bread sandwich with turkey, cheese, avocado and sprouts; or a baked potato with butter and 1 teasp. Bragg's LIQUID AMINOS, and a green salad; or a tofu, brown rice and veggie frittata/casserole; or some cheeses or cottage cheese with fresh fruit and whole grain muffins or bread; or a seafood, chicken or other high protein salad and whole grain bread.

—**Mid-afternoon:** Amazake rice drink, or yogurt with fresh fruit; or a bean dip, kefir cheese, soy cheese or low-fat cheese with whole grain crackers, or raw veggies; or a hard boiled egg with sesame salt dip, some whole grain crackers, and an energizing herb tea, such as Crystal Star HIGH ENERGY TEA™ or RAINFOREST ENERGY TEA™, or Siberian ginseng tea; or fruit juice sweetened cookies or granola bars; or a high energy sports bar like Power Foods POWER BARS or EAS® MYOPLEX DELUXE with mineral water.

—**Dinner:** Whole grain or veggie pasta Italian style with a light sauce and whole grain bread; or a hearty soup or stew with a green salad and whole grain bread; or a brown rice or other whole grain and vegetable casserole; or whole grain and bean Mexican meal (easy on the salsas, fats and sweeteners; no fried food); or baked, grilled or broiled poultry or seafood with soup and a green salad; or a vegetarian pizza with chapati or flour tortilla crust, or an egg pizza with vegetable toppings; or a vegetable quiche with whole grain crust and low fat cheeses.

   Note: Have a little red or white wine with dinner for relaxation, minerals and polyphenols.

—**At bedtime:** 1 teasp. Red Star yeast broth in a cup of hot water for relaxation and B-complex vitamins.

For both training and off days, this is a good time to take the following supplements: B-complex 150mg; high potency potassium-magnesium-bromelain combo to relieve muscle fatigue and lactic acid build-up; or a cal-mag-zinc combo to prevent muscle cramping and maintain bone integrity; Anabol Naturals GH RELEASERS to burn fat and release natural growth hormone while you sleep.

Recipes to help your sports training diet: •COMPLEX CARBS for ENERGY; •BREAKFAST; •SOUPS; •HIGH PRO-TEIN without MEAT; •SALADS; •ENZYME-RICH; •SANDWICHES; •MINERAL-RICH; •HIGH FIBER RECIPES.

Herb and Supplement Choices

• **High Protein Drinks:** Unipro MYO SYSTEM XL and PERFECT PROTEIN drink; Twin Lab AMINO FUEL liquid and CREATINE FUEL PLUS; PureForm WHEY PROTEIN.

• **Antioxidants:** CoQ-10 100mg daily; Source Naturals DMG 100mg; Nature's Path HEMA-LYTE w. electrolytes; Nutricology GERMANIUM 150mg.

• **Amino Acids:** Arginine-ornithine-lysine to metabolize fats, carnitine to strengthen muscles, Anabol Naturals AMINO BALANCE, AMINO NITRO MAX; Unipro AMINO 1000; Champion MUSCLE-NITRO for ATP energy conversion.

• **Non-steroidal Anabolics:** Radiant Life SUMAX 5, shown to be as effective as the illegal synthetic steroid, dianabol without the side effects. Highly recommended. Natural Balance RIBOSE RIBO-MAX to replenish ATP energy.

• **Testosterone to increase muscle hardness:** Unipro TRIBULUS SYNERGY; Country Life LIQUID FARMACY SUPER STRENGTH YOHIMBE (use with caution); Crystal Star ACTIVE PHYSICAL ENERGY™ with panax ginseng; raw orchic extract, 6 to 10x strength; Futurebiotics MALE POWER.

• **Fat Burners:** Anabol Naturals GH RELEASERS - metabolic fat burner; Unipro TRI-METABOLIC; Bricker Labs CUT-UP PLUS; MAXIMAL BURNER - with HCA.

• **Vitamins and Minerals:** Weider MEGABOLIC PAK; Unipro TRI-METABOLIC; PureForm LIQUID VITAMIN.

• **Recovery Acceleration:** EAS® BETAGEN™, Champion CORTISTAT-PS to reduce cortisol levels and REVENGE sports drink to reduce lactic acid; Alacer MIRACLE WATER for electrolytes; Unipro GLUTAGEN, Now MSM caps to rebuild joints.

Bodywork and Lifestyle Techniques

• **Supplement your major sport with other fitness activities** such as bicycling, jogging/walking, swimming or aerobics. This will balance muscle use, and keep heart and lungs strong.

• **Recuperation time is essential for optimum growth.** Muscles grow during rest periods. Alternate muscle workouts and training days with rest days, or exercise different muscle sets on different days, resting each set in between.

• **Deep breathing and lung capacity are training keys.** Muscles must have oxygen for endurance and stamina. Breathe in during exertion, out as you relax for the next rep. Vigorous exhaling is as important as inhaling for the athlete, to expel all carbon dioxide and increase lung capacity.

• **How much fat are you burning?**
—Check your heart rate to see how many fat calories you're burning during your workout. If your heart rate is 70% of the maximum, you are burning 20% fat of your total calories per hour of exercise time. If your heart rate is 45% of maximum, you are burning 40% fat of the total calories per hour/exercise time. More fat is burned in low intensity activities because you can take in extra oxygen needed to burn it - more than twice as much as carbohydrates per fat gram.

—**Calorie burning choices:** —Aerobic dancing- 300-700 calories per hour; —Calisthenics- 360 calories per hour; —Cross Country Skiing- 350-1,400 calories per hour; —Cycling- 200-850 calories per hour; —Running- 400-1,300 calories per hour; —Stretching- 60-120 calories per hour; —Swimming- 380-850 calories per hour; —Walking- 240-430 calories per hour; —Water Aerobics- 180-880 calories per hour; —Weight training- 260-480.

Can't find a recommended product? Call the 800 number listed in Product Resources for the store nearest you and for more info.

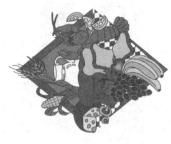

Food Exchanges

Any food in a category may be exchanged one-for-one with any other food in the same category. Portion amounts are given for a man weighing 170 pounds, and a woman weighing 130 pounds.

See diet amounts on page 448.

Grains, Breads and Cereals: One serving is approximately one cup of cooked grains.

—brown rice, millet, barley, bulgur, kashi, couscous, corn, oats, or whole grain pasta;

—or one cup of dry cereals, such as bran flakes, Oatios, or Grapenuts;

—or three slices of wholegrain bread; or three six-inch corn tortillas; or two chapatis or whole wheat pita breads;

—or twelve small wholegrain crackers; or two rice cakes.

Vegetables:

Group A: One serving is as much as you want.

—Chinese greens and peas, raw spinach and carrots, celery, cucumbers, endive, sea greens, watercress, radishes, green onions.

Group B: One serving is 2 cups cabbage or alfalfa sprouts;

—or 1 ¹⁄₂ cups cooked bell peppers or mushrooms;

—or one cup cooked asparagus, cauliflower, chard, sauerkraut, eggplant, zucchini or summer squash;

—or ³⁄₄ cup cooked broccoli, green beans; onions or mung bean sprouts; or ¹⁄₂ cup vegetable juice cocktail.

Group C: One serving is approximately 1 ¹⁄₂ cups cooked carrots;

—or one cup cooked beets, potatoes, or leeks; or one cup fresh carrot or vegetable juice;

—or ¹⁄₂ cup cooked peas, corn, artichokes, winter squash or yams.

Fruits: One serving is approximately one apple, nectarine, mango, pineapple, peach, pear or orange;

—4 apricots, medjool dates or figs; or half a honeydew or cantaloupe;

—4 cups small watermelon chunks;

—or 20 to 24 cherries or grapes; or one and a half cups strawberries or other berries.

Dairy: One serving is approximately one cup of whole milk, buttermilk or full fat yogurt, for 3mg of fat;

—or one cup of low-fat milk or yogurt, for 2gm. of fat;

—or one cup of skim milk or non-fat yogurt, for less than 1gm. of fat;

—or one ounce of low fat hard cheese, such as swiss or cheddar;

—or 2 ounces low-fat yogurt cheese, kefir cheese or soy cheese for 2gm of fat

—or 6 TBS of non-fat dry milk or soy milk powder for less than 1gm of fat.

Poultry, Fish and Seafood: One serving is approximately 4-oz. of white fish skinned, for 3gm of fat;

—or four ounces of chicken or turkey, white meat, no skin for 4gm of fat;

—or one cup of tuna or salmon, water packed for 3gm of fat;

—or one cup of shrimp, scallops, oysters, clams or crab for 3 to 4gm of fat.

Note: I recommend avoiding red meats – beef, veal, lamb, pork, sausage, ham, and bacon. They are high in saturated fats and cholesterol, and unsound as a use of planetary resources. Many are routinely injected with hormones and antibiotics.

High Protein Meat and Dairy Substitutes: One serving is approximately four ounces of tofu (one block);

—or $^1/_2$ cup low fat or dry cottage cheese; or $^1/_3$ cup ricotta, parmesan or mozzarella;

—or one egg; or $^1/_2$ cup cooked beans or brown rice.

Fats and Oils: One serving is approximately one teaspoon of butter, margarine or shortening for 5gm of fat;

—or one tablespoon of salad dressing or mayonnaise for 5gm. of fat;

—or 2 teaspoons of polyunsaturated or monounsaturated vegetable oil for 5gm. of fat.

The following foods are high in fat: amounts are equivalent to 1 fat serving on the diet chart. Use sparingly.

—2 tablespoons of light cream, half and half, or sour cream; 1 tablespoon of heavy cream;

—$^1/_6$ slice of avocado; $^1/_4$ cup of sunflower, sesame, or pumpkin seeds;

—12 almonds, cashews or peanuts; 20 pistachios or Spanish peanuts; 4 walnut or pecan halves; 2 macadamia nuts.

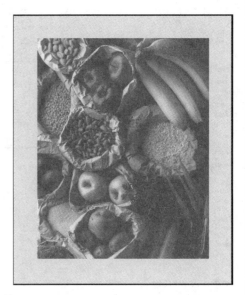

Food Amounts Chart by Diet

Sports Enthusiast Daily Diet For Men

Calories 2800
Protein 17%
Carbos 70%
Fat 13%

Whole Grains
6 servings

Group A Vegetables
all you want

Group B Vegetables
6 servings

Group C Vegetables
6 servings

Fruits
5 servings

Dairy Foods
3 servings

Seafood/Poultry
2 servings

Fats
5 servings

Sports Enthusiast Daily Diet For Women

Calories 2000
Protein 17%
Carbos 70%
Fat 13%

Whole Grains
4 servings

Group A Vegetables
all you want

Group B Vegetables
4 servings

Group C Vegetables
3 servings

Fruits
3 servings

Dairy Foods
2 servings

Seafood/Poultry
1 serving

Fats
3 servings

High Performance Daily Diet For Men

Calories 2800
Protein 17%
Carbos 70%
Fat 13%

Whole Grains
6 servings

Group A Vegetables
all you want

Group B Vegetables
7 servings

Group C Vegetables
8 servings

Fruits
6 servings

Dairy Foods
4 servings

Seafood/Poultry
5 servings

Fats
6 servings

High Performance Daily Diet For Women

Calories 2800
Protein 17%
Carbos 70%
Fat 13%

Whole Grains
6 servings

Group A Vegetables
all you want

Group B Vegetables
6 servings

Group C Vegetables
5 servings

Fruits
4 servings

Dairy Foods
3 servings

Seafood/Poultry
3 servings

Fats
3 servings

Scale servings up or down to fit your individual weight and type of active diet.

Healing Diets for Kids

Healthy children develop powerful immune systems in infancy. Unless unusually or chronically ill, a child often needs only the subtle body-strengthening forces that nutritious foods, herbs or homeopathic remedies supply, rather than the highly focused medications of allopathic medicine which can have such drastic side effects on a small body.

Still, the undeniable ecological, social and diet deterioration in America during the last fifty years has had a marked effect on children's health. We see evidence of it in every aspect of their lives — declining educational performance, learning disabilities, mental disorders, obesity, drug and alcohol abuse, hypoglycemia, allergies, chronic illness, delinquency and violent behavior; they're all evidence of declining immunity and poor health.

You can get a lot of help from the kids themselves in a natural health boosting program. Kids don't want to be sick; they aren't stupid; they don't like going to the doctor any more than you do. They often recognize that natural foods and therapies are good for them. Children are naturally immune to disease. A nutritious diet and natural health enhancer like herbs help keep them that way.

A Good Diet Heals and Prevents Childhood Diseases

Diet is your most important weapon in safeguarding your child's immunity defenses against disease. Pathogenic organisms and viruses are everywhere. But they aren't the major factor in causing disease if the body environment is healthy. Well-nourished children are usually strong enough to deal with infection successfully. They either don't catch the "bugs" that are going around, they contract only a mild case, or they develop healthy, short-duration reactions, and get the problem over with quickly. This difference in resistance and immune response is the key to understanding children's diseases.

A wholesome diet can easily restore a child's natural vitality. Even children who have eaten a junk food diet for years quickly respond to a diet of fresh fruits, vegetables, whole grains, and less dairy and sugar. I have noted substantial improvement in as little as a month's time. A child's hair and skin takes on new luster — they fill out if they are too skinny, and lose weight if they are fat. They sleep more soundly. Their attention spans markedly improve, and many learning and behavior problems lessen or disappear.

Keep it simple. Let kids help prepare their own food. Let kids help prepare their own food, even though they might get in the way and you feel like it's more trouble than it's worth. You'll be giving them a better understanding of good food (they're also more likely to eat the things they have a hand in making). Keep only good nutritious foods in the house. Children may be exposed to junk foods and poor foods at school or friend's houses, but you can build a good, natural foundation diet at home. For the time that they are at home, they should be able to choose only from nutritious choices.

Kids have extraordinarily sensitive taste buds. Everything they eat is very vivid and important to them. The diet programs I offer in this section have lots of variety, so they can experiment and find out where their own preferences lie. There are plenty of snacks, sandwiches, fresh fruits, and sweet veggies like carrots — all foods children naturally like.

Should your child have vaccinations?

Do you know why you get most childhood diseases only once? It's because the memory T-cells of your immune system work like a natural vaccination. They actually remember the first time a disease attacked during childhood, and prepare a defense against further infections of it with the antibodies that were formed **the FIRST time it entered the body.** Current immunization theory tries to work on this principle, but your memory T-cells don't always recognize a man-made vaccination pathogen.

There has been an overwhelming emphasis placed on the need for vaccinations at an early age for children and pets in our society. Wide-ranging vaccinations are one of the biggest dilemmas facing immunologists today. Medical scientists are finding something unexpected when the children who received broad spectrum vaccinations in the nineteen-sixties and seventies grew into adulthood. While the children may have avoided the childhood disease they were vaccinated against, an above average number contract the diseases as adults instead (for example chicken pox and new strains of measles), as well as other stronger diseases that a healthy adult should be able to fend off (like chronic flu infections). Many speculate what naturopaths have known for years.... that when a child is not allowed to go through childhood diseases, the memory T-cells never build up immune defenses against them. I believe we're trying to fool Mother Nature when it's much smarter to work with her plan for immune defense.

I believe too many questions about vaccinations remain unanswered. How necessary are they? What do they do in our bodies? How do they affect our immune systems? Our understanding of how the immune system works is far from complete, especially about how the immune system responds to vaccines in the long term, or how after vaccination, the immune system interacts with variables such as environmental or chemical agents.

The immune system is highly complex, the most delicately balanced system in the body. Vaccines are designed to create antibodies for the diseases they "protect" against. Yet, as we've just seen, antibodies aren't really necessary for your body to defend or protect against disease.

What about chicken pox, the most controversial of the childhood immunizations? Chicken pox is much more serious in adults than in children. The protective effect of the chicken pox vaccine may wear off later in life. Many experts today admit that the only real immunity from chicken pox comes from having it once, **not vaccination.**

I predict that we're going to find out this same truth about many childhood vaccinations. As a naturopath, I feel that mild childhood diseases like chicken pox are really gifts in disguise to strengthen a child's immunity against future illness. Remember: Kids don't want to be sick; they aren't stupid; and they often recognize natural foods and therapies that are good for them. Children are naturally immune to disease. A nutritious diet can help keep them that way.

The diets in this chapter are effective for several childhood problems: *Acute Bronchitis, Chest Congestion, Chronic Constipation, Indigestion, Gas and Flatulence, Diarrhea, Chicken Pox, Jaundice, Mumps, Measles, Whooping Cough, Thrush and Fungal Infections, Low Immunity, Allergies and Food Sensitivities, Hyperactive Behavior, Colds, Flu and Sore Throat, Parasites and Worms, Chronic Earaches.*

Purification Diet for Children

A healing diet for common childhood diseases, including measles, mumps, chicken pox, strep throat and whooping cough, is simple and basic. It's a therapy that starts with a short liquid elimination fast, followed by a fresh foods diet in the acute stages. When the crisis has passed, and the child is on the mend with a clean system, begin an optimal nutrition diet, like the one on the following pages, to prevent further problems, and boost energy.

Use this 1 to 3-day diet for initial or acute symptoms when a liquid detox is not desired. A fresh foods diet serves cleansing activity while the light solid foods start to rebuild strength. Dairy products, except for yogurt should be avoided.

Watchwords:

1: **Start the child on cleansing liquids** as soon as the disease is diagnosed to clean out harmful bacteria and infection. Give fruit juices such as apple, pineapple, grape, cranberry and citrus juices, or give Crystal Star FIRST AID TEA FOR KIDS™. The juice of two lemons in a glass of water with a little honey may be taken once or twice a day to flush the kidneys and normalize body chemistry.

2: **Alternate fresh fruit juices during the day** with fresh carrot juice, potassium or veggie drink (pages 568,569), bottled water, and clear soups. Encourage the child to drink as many healthy cleansing liquids as she or he wants. Light smoothies are favorites with kids. Avoid dairy products.

3: **Offer herb teas throughout the cleanse.** Children respond to herb teas quickly, and they like them more than you might think. Make them about half adult strength. Add a little honey or maple syrup if the herbs are bitter.

4: **I recommend acidophilus culture compounds** to get a child over the hump of a childhood disease. They restore friendly bacteria in the G.I. tract, especially if the child has taken a course of antibiotics. Acidophilus makes a big difference in both recovery time and immune response. Bifidobacteria provides better protection for infants and children than regular acidophilus strains. Nutrition Now RHINO ACIDOPHILUS (a great-tasting, chewable tablet with 4 strains of beneficial bacteria plus Vitamin C for children ages 4 and older), Solaray BABY LIFE, or Ethical Nutrients INTESTINAL CARE powder work well for children. Use about $^1/_4$ teasp. at a time in a glass of water or juice three to four times daily.

—**On rising:** Give citrus juice with $^1/_4$ teasp. acidophilus powder; or 2 TBS lemon juice in water with maple syrup.

—**Breakfast:** Offer a choice of favorite fresh fruits. Top with vanilla yogurt, Rice Dream or soy milk if desired.

—**Mid-morning:** Give a vegetable or potassium drink (page 568) or fresh carrot juice. Add $^1/_4$ teasp. ascorbate vitamin C or Ester C crystals with bioflavonoids.

—**Lunch:** Give fresh raw crunchy veggies with a yogurt dip; or a fresh veggie salad with yogurt dressing.

—**Mid-afternoon:** Offer a refreshing herb tea, such as licorice or peppermint tea; or Crystal Star FIRST AID TEA FOR KIDS™ to keep the stomach settled and calm tension; or another vegetable drink with $^1/_4$ teasp. vitamin C added.

—**Dinner:** Give a fresh salad, with avocados, carrots, kiwi, romaine and other high vitamin A foods; and/or a cup of miso soup or other clear broth soup with Chinese noodles if desired.

—**Before bed:** Offer a relaxing herb tea, like chamomile or scullcap tea, or Crystal Star GOOD NIGHT TEA™ or a cup of miso broth for strength and B vitamins. Snip 1 teasp. dry sea greens on top if desired.

451

Optimal Nutrition for Children

We live in the most affluent country in the world, yet many of our children's basic nutritional needs are not met. Even American Pediatrics magazine says only a tiny 1% of American kids meet the USDA requirements for all five food groups. Only 36% eat 2 to 4 servings of vegetables a day; even less eat the recommended 5 vegetable servings a day. Instead fats and sugars supply an astounding 40% of American children's daily nutrients! Because much of our agricultural soils are depleted, and most of our foods are sprayed or gassed, many micronutrients like vitamins and minerals are no longer sufficiently present in our foods. The most common childhood nutrient deficiencies are calcium, iron, B-1, and vitamins A, B-complex and C. Offer organic foods to your child whenever possible. An Environmental Health Perspectives study shows children regularly exposed to pesticides have serious problems, like low stamina, underdeveloped hand-eye coordination, and poor attention span and recall. Make sure you graphically show your child what junk and synthetic foods are. Because of TV advertising and peer pressure, kids often really don't know what wholesome food is, and think they are eating the right way. Your presence as a loving parental authority is a powerful influence. Gather your family together for a meal at least once a day to establish good eating habits for your kids.

Use superfoods for kids! Superfoods are concentrated nutrients widely popular with adults today (check out the many superfoods listings in this book). They're just as good in healthy diet programs for kids. Mix them in or sprinkle them on other foods to increase the nutritional content of any meal. Superfood supplements put some great nutrients into fussy eaters. Crystal Star SYSTEMS STRENGTH™ drink mix is a potent vegetarian blend of sea greens, herbs, and foods like miso, soy protein, nutritional yeast and brown rice. Add it to soups, sauces, even salad dressings. Green Foods BERRY BARLEY ESSENCE has a natural raspberry-strawberry taste kids like. Kids also like bee pollen, a highly bio-active superfood often called "nature's complete nutrition," because it is so full of balanced vitamins, minerals, proteins, EFA's, enzymes, and essential amino acids. Its sweet flavor works well sprinkled on cereals or in smoothies.

Diet tips to help keep your child healthier and happier:

It's a lot easier said than done to change old dietary patterns to healthier eating.... for anybody, but especially for kids. A good way to start is to find something delicious to replace whatever is being taken away.

For example:
—**If you want your kid to eat more fruits and vegetables,** start with food forms that children go for, like dried fruit snacks, and smoothies for fruits. Sandwiches, tacos, burritos and pitas easily hold vegetables. Most kids like soup with vegetables. Let them add sauces or flavors they like.
—**To encourage your child to drink more water instead of carbonated sodas** or sweetened drinks, keep plenty of natural fruit juices and flavored mineral water around the house.
—**To reduce the amount of sugar your child eats,** buy sugar-free snacks. Replace sugar-filled cereals with granola or oatmeal with healthy toppings. Offer dried fruit. Almost every kid likes raisins. Or try CC Pollen Co. BUZZ BARS.

452

—**If you want more whole grains in your child's diet,** start by keeping only whole grains in the house. Kids love bagels and pastas, which come in a wide variety of whole grain options. Brown basmati rice is much tastier than white rice if your kid is a "rice kid." Stuffing is a big favorite. Popcorn is a healthy snack. Season it with tamari or a seasoning blend instead of gobs of butter and salt.

—**To add healthy cultured foods to your child's diet,** keep an assortment of yogurt flavors with fruit for snacks in the fridge. Offer delicious kefir cheese for snack spreads instead of sour cream.

—**To reduce the amount of meat and dairy protein your child is eating,** keep tasty plant protein available. Kids like tofu and grain burgers, especially with their favorite trimmings. Most kids like beans — look for healthy chili blends. Stock peanut butter, nuts and seeds, like almonds, sunflower seeds and pumpkin seeds for snacks. Use them as toppings for soup, salad crunchies, smoothies and desserts. (Seeds and nuts give kids unsaturated oils and EFA's.) Eggs are a good protein choice for kids.... one of Nature's perfect foods that's gotten a bad rap. Most kids like deviled eggs, and eggs are great in honey custards, another kid favorite.

—**If you want to add more seafood to a child's diet,** start with favorites like shrimp, tuna fish or salmon.

This sample diet for optimal health for your child has been kid-tested for taste.

—**On rising:** offer a protein drink like ALL 1 VITAMIN-MINERAL, especially if the child's energy or school performance is poor; or if the child always seems to be ill; or 1 teasp. liquid multi-vitamin in juice, like Floradix CHILDREN'S MULTI-VITAMIN/MINERAL.

—**Breakfast:** have granola with apple juice or yogurt and fresh fruit; or whole grain toast or muffins, with butter, kefir cheese or nut butter; add eggs, scrambled or baked (no fried eggs); or have hot oatmeal or puffed kashi cereal with maple syrup or yogurt.

—**Mid-morning:** whole grain crackers with kefir cheese or dip, and fruit juice; or fresh or dried fruit, or fruit leathers with yogurt or kefir cheese; or crunchy veggies with peanut butter or a nut spread; or a sugar-free candy bar, or trail mix, stirred into yogurt.

—**Lunch:** have a veggie, turkey, chicken or shrimp sandwich on whole grain bread, with low fat cheese. Add corn chips with a low fat dip; or bean soup with whole grain toast, and a small salad or crunchy veggies with garbanzo spread; or a vegetarian pizza on a chapati crust; or spaghetti or pasta with parmesan cheese sauce; or a Mexican bean and veggie, or rice burrito with fresh salsa.

—**Mid-afternoon:** have a sparkling juice and a dried fruit candy bar; or fresh fruit or fruit juice, or a kefir drink; or a hard boiled egg and some whole grain chips with a veggie or low fat cheese dip; or some whole grain toast and peanut butter or other nut butter.

—**Dinner:** have a veggie pizza on a chapati or egg crust, with veggies, shrimp, and low fat cheese topping; or whole grain or egg pasta with vegetables and a light tomato/cheese sauce; or a baked Mexican quesadilla with low fat cheese and some steamed veggies or a salad; or roast turkey with cornbread dressing and a salad; or a tuna casserole with rice, peas and water chestnuts.

—**Before bed:** a glass of apple juice or a little soy milk, Rice Dream or flavored kefir.

Recipes for a kid's nutrition diet: • DETOX FOODS; • HEALING DRINKS; • SOUPS, LIQUID SALADS; • ENZYME-RICH FOODS; • BREAKFAST; • MINERAL-RICH; • SANDWICHES; • HIGH PROTEIN COOKING; • HIGH FIBER.

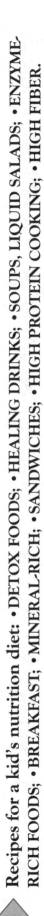

Herb and Supplement Choices

• **Acidophilus, liquid or powder:** give in juice 2 to 3x daily for good digestion and assimilation. Nature's Path FLORA-LYTE, or Solaray BABY LIFE are excellent for children. Nutrition Now RHINO ACIDOPHILUS (chewable tablets for children ages 4 and older). Add vitamin A & D in drops if desired.

• **Vitamin C, or Ester C:** for powder form with bioflavonoids: give in juice, $\frac{1}{4}$ teasp. at a time 2x daily. For chewable wafers, use 100mg, 250mg, or 500mg potency according to age and weight of the child.

• **A sugar-free multi-vitamin and mineral supplement:** in either liquid or chewable tablet form. Some good choices are from Floradix, Prevail, Solaray and Mezotrace. A vitamin/mineral drink, such as 1 teasp. Floradix CHILDREN'S MULTIVITAMIN liquid in juice, Prevail CHILDREN'S MULTI-VITAMIN & MINERALS caps, or Nutrition Now RHINO CHEWY VITES. Continue to give them until the child is symptom free.

• **Continue cleansing, purifying herbal teas:** especially Crystal Star FIRST AID TEA FOR KIDS™. Clear your child's chest congestion with herbal steam inhalations. Use eucalyptus or tea tree oil, or Crystal Star RSPR TEA™ in a vaporizer help to keep lungs mucous free and improve oxygen uptake.

• **Use a mild herbal laxative:** like Nature's Secret ULTIMATE FIBER, in half dosage for regularity.

• **Use garlic oil:** drops or open garlic capsules into juice for natural antibiotic activity; or give Crystal Star ANTI-BIO™ caps or extract in half dosage or Wakunaga KYOLIC liquid in juice.

• **Boost immunity:** open Colostrum caps and sprinkle into baby or children's food - FIRSTFOOD COLOSTRUM (Healthy House).

Bodywork and Lifestyle Techniques

• **Continue with herbal baths, washes and compresses to cleanse toxins coming out through the skin.** Oatmeal baths help neutralize rashes coming out on the skin. Herbal baths help induce cleansing perspiration, too, but the child should be watched closely all during the bath to make sure he or she is not getting too hot. Make up a big pot of calendula or comfrey tea for the bath water. Rub the child's body with calendula or tea tree oil, or Tiger Balm to loosen congestion after the bath.

• **Give a soothing massage** before bed.

• **Get some early morning sunlight** on the body every day possible .

• **Give a gentle enema** at least once during the detox cleanse to clear the child's colon of impacted wastes that hinder the body's effort to rid itself of diseased bacteria. A catnip tea enema is effective and safe for children.

• **Apply hot ginger-cayenne compresses** to affected or sore areas to stimulate circulation and defense response, to rid the body more quickly of infection. Alternate hot compresses with cold, plain water compresses.

—Dab on with cotton balls, a water infusion of goldenseal, myrrh, yellow dock, black walnut, and yarrow, or Crystal Star ANTI-BIO™ phyto-therapy gel to help heal sores and scabs.

• **Exercise for kids is a primary nutrient for body and mind.** US Public Health studies show a third of American children are unfit! Exercise is a key to health, growth and energy. Don't let your kid be a couch potato, or a computer junkie. Encourage outdoor activity, and make sure your child is taking P. E. classes in school.

Can't find a recommended product? Call the 800 number listed in Product Resources for the store nearest you and for more info.

454

Overcoming Attention Deficit Disorders

Hyperactive behavior and Attention Deficit Disorder are serious problems affecting up to 10% of today's kids. Hyperactivity may be the expression of either hypoglycemia or food allergies or both. Attention Deficit Disorder is slow learning caused by any or all of the learning disorders. Autism is almost a "mind-blind" condition, characterized by withdrawn behavior, lack of emotion and speech, extreme sensitivity to sound and touch. Autistic children have a brain malfunction that creates a barrier between them and the rest of the world. Autism almost certainly has allergy, parasite, yeast infection or fungal links. Some researchers blame heavy metal poisoning (especially lead), that allows excess ammonia waste to build up in a child's brain. Children at greatest risk are male, with a family history of diabetes or alcoholism. Nutrition improvement and stress-calming herbs are the cornerstones of successful treatment in overcoming hyperactivity disorders.

Does your child have an attention deficit disorder?

—Does your child exhibit dramatic mood swings and extreme personality changes?
—Does your child exhibit compulsive-aggressive, destructive behavior? Is your child extremely impatient and defiant?
—Is your child unable to follow directions? or instructions?
—Does your child have an unusually short attention span? Is he or she unable to sit still?
—Does your child have poor motor coordination, a speech impediment or dyslexia?
—Is your child an extremely slow learner? Is he or she unable to reason or think rationally?
—Is he or she abnormally accident prone? Is there evidence of self-mutilation?
—Is your child a chronic liar?
—Does your child have chronic thirst?
—Does your child have a chronic cold symptoms like sneezing or coughing?

Is your child on Ritalin?

The latest research shows an astounding 2.5 million American school children take the narcotic stimulant Ritalin to treat Attention Deficit Disorder. While Ritalin seems to help some kids concentrate, it can also cause elevations in blood pressure, heart rate and respiration, suppress normal appetite and stunt normal growth. Insomnia, facial tics, liver damage and depression are all reported by Ritalin users. Moreover, as an amphetamine-like substance, Ritalin has a high potential for misuse, can cause addiction and may need to be taken your entire life. The latest government research shows 80% of kids taking Ritalin will need to continue taking it into their adolescence; 50% will need to take it as adults! In spite of its drawbacks, the popularity of this drug has become incredible. Some schools reach for it the moment a child get "rowdy." I believe instead of administering more drugs with powerful side effects to our school children, we need to look for natural solutions that support their health so they can learn unimpeded.

Attention Deficit Disorder Healing Diet

Researchers are slowly learning more about what causes this extremely disturbing disorder. Some kids admit they "are feeling crazy" at times when they exhibit ADD behavior. (Certainly their parents and teachers are!) Dietary causes are identified as the first place to look by most experts. Mineral and EFA deficiencies from too many refined, junk foods are always present. (Prescription drugs that block EFA conversion in the brain are culprits, too.) Food allergies to corn, wheat and additives are more than likely. Hypoglycemia, normally an unusual syndrome for a child, is usual.

Clearly, diet improvement is the key to changing ADD behavior. Results are almost immediately evident, generally within 1 to 3 weeks. When behavior normalizes, maintain the improved diet to prevent reversion.

<u>Watchwords:</u>

1: Food sensitivities play a major part in attention disorders. Reduce sugar intake. Make sure any sugary foods allowed are part of a well-balanced meal. Reduce carbonated drinks (excess phosphorus). Eliminate red meats (nitrates).

2: The ongoing diet should be high in vegetable proteins and whole grains, with plenty of fresh fruits and vegetables, and no junk or fast foods. Use organically grown foods when possible. Have a green salad every day.

3: Use applied kinesiology to determine allergens, or test foods like milk, wheat, corn, chocolate, and citrus with an elimination diet to see if they're involved.

4: Include calming tryptophan-rich foods like turkey, tuna, wheat germ, yogurt and eggs. Take a cup of miso soup before bed.

5: Add EFA-rich foods: sea greens, spinach and other leafy greens, soy foods, fish and seafoods.

6: Read food labels carefully. Avoid all food products with preservatives, BHT, MSG, BHA, additives and colors.

7: Superfoods help. Smoothies with green superfoods like Pines MIGHTY GREENS SUPERFOOD BLEND or Vibrant Health GREEN VIBRANCE, Lewis Labs high phosphatide lecithin and-or Red Star NUTRITIONAL YEAST.

8: See the STRESS REDUCTION diet on page 359 for a step-by-step program you can use.

Recipes that can help an ADD diet: •MINERAL-RICH RECIPES; •HEALING DRINKS; •PROTEIN without MEAT; •ENZYME-RICH FOODS; •SUGAR-FREE DISHES; •FISH and SEAFOODS; •SANDWICHES; •DAIRY FREE FOODS.

Herb and Supplement Choices

• **Improve behavior problems:** DMAE, 100 to 500mg daily in divided doses; Crystal Star RELAX CAPS™; Herbs Etc. KIDALIN, Source Naturals FOCUS CHILD; Planetary Formulas CALM CHILD drops as needed. Homeopathic *Camomilla* (very young kids). NADH 2.5mg daily. Rosemary tea.

• **Calming herbs:** Crystal Star CALCIUM SOURCE™ extract in water is a rapid calmative. Crystal Star VALERIAN-WILD LETTUCE extract or Catnip tea for extra calming; gotu kola or hawthorn drops for nerve stress or Taurine 500mg daily.

• **Enhance neurotransmitters - brain serotonin:** Stress B-Complex with extra pantothenic acid 100mg and B$_6$ 100mg; Gotu kola, kava kava or St. John's wort extract drops in water; Ginkgo biloba drops (older kids) 60mg daily also helps inner ear balance; GABA, 100mg; or Phos. Serine 100mg daily.

• **Add electrolyte minerals:** Nature's Path TRACE-LYTE minerals; Add magnesium 400mg and Premier Lithium .5mg. An iron deficiency often results in a learning disability.

• **Minimize allergic reactions:** Chromium 150mcg 3x daily with Vanadium 150mg to regulate blood sugar metabolism.

• **Correct prostaglandin imbalance with EFA's:** Omega Nutrition ESSENTIAL BALANCE Jr.; Black currant or borage oil, Evening Primrose oil, 500mg; Omega-3 flax oil; or NEUROMINS DHA 200mg 2x daily.

• **Homeopathic remedies help ADD:** Hylands CALMS and CALMS FORTE; Nature's Way RESTLESS CHILD.

• **Autism therapy:** Magnesium 400mg, B-complex with extra B$_6$ 100mg (Natren HEALTHY TRINITY for B vitamin synthesis); Black walnut, an anti-fungal medicine. Ask a practitioner for dosage; Vitamin C with bioflavs, up to 2000mg.

Bodywork and Lifestyle Techniques

• Avoid aspirin and amphetamines of all kinds if your child has any of these disorders.

• Prescriptions for Ritalin, Cylertor, and Atarax, short-term sedative drugs for hyperactive disorders, often make the condition worse. Some researchers say Ritalin is almost identical to cocaine! Side effects include nervousness, insomnia, unhealthy weight loss, stunted growth, stomach aches, skin rashes, headaches and hallucinations. Avoid them if you can. Try diet improvement first.

—Bodywork:

• Massage therapy, acupressure and biofeedback have shown some success.

• Take warm baking soda and sea salt baths.

• Use aromatherapy oils such as lavender.

Can't find a recommended product? Call the 800 number listed in Product Resources for the store nearest you and for more info.

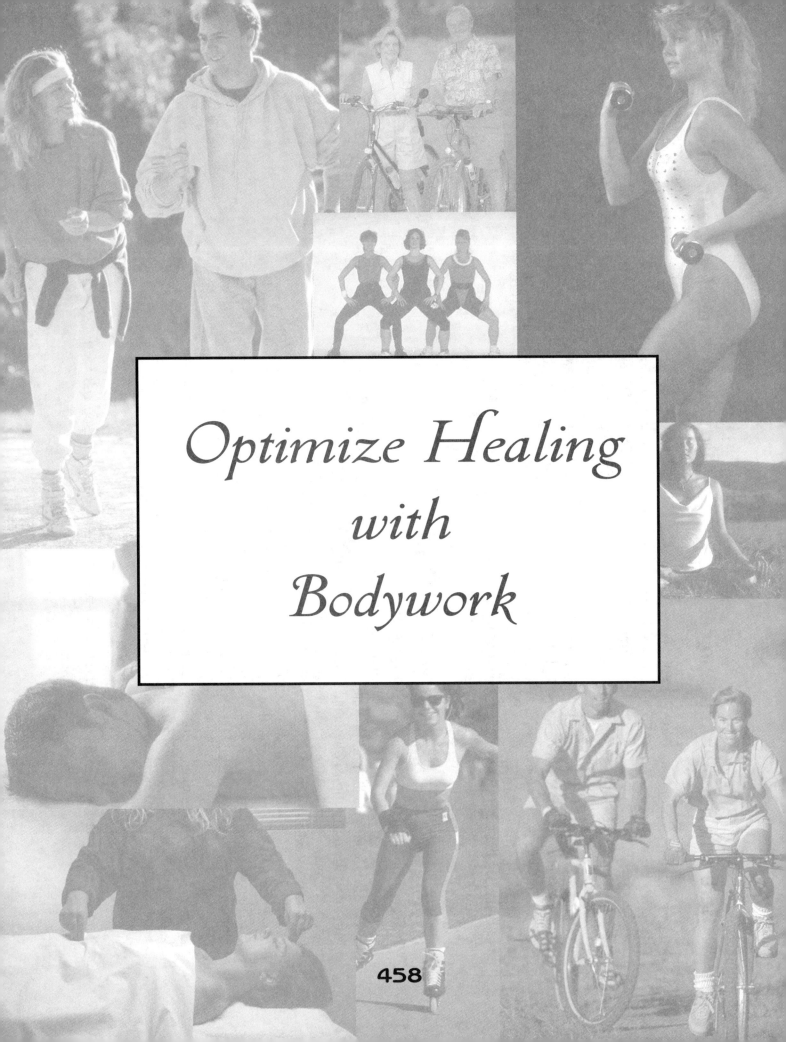

Optimize Healing with Bodywork

Bodywork Techniques Optimize Nutrition

Your body is meant to move. This book focuses on using food and diet as primary tools for healing, but bodywork is the ignition spark that starts the healing process. Body activity moves much more than just your muscles. It uses your skin and lungs for example, as organs of ingestion. Techniques like therapeutic bathing, massage and deep breathing exercises can often bring nutrients into your body more rapidly and more completely than your digestive system. A relaxation process like Zen meditation is a therapeutic technique that connects your mind and body to your healing needs.

Exercise has significant influence on healing

—Exercise speeds up removal Sweating helps expel toxins largest organ of elimination. Tests for example, they excrete poten- heavy metals and pesticide PCBs

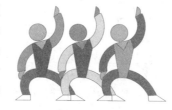

of toxins through perspiration. through the skin, your body's show that when athletes sweat, tial cancer causing elements, like from their bodies.

—Exercise stimulates removal of toxins through deep breathing. Low impact aerobics and stretching build a stronger diaphragm and elasticize your lungs.

—Exercise stimulates metabolism, especially before you eat, to aid in weight loss. Calories are burned at a greater pace for several hours after you exercise.

—Exercise stimulates circulation, lowering blood pressure and preventing heart disease by increasing blood flow. New heart endurance tests show exercise strengthens your circulatory system right down to your capillaries.... even forming new ones!

—Exercise stimulates the lymphatic system. Blood is pumped through your body by your heart, but lymph fluid depends solely on exercise for cleansing circulation.

—Exercise reduces stress by increasing body oxygen levels. It improves your mood while you tone. Endorphins, the body's "feel good" hormones, release into the brain during exercise, explaining the "high" people often experience after exercise.

—Exercise prevents disease. Disease often results from an underactive body. Almost any kind of exercise transports oxygen and nutrients to your cells while it carries away toxins and wastes to your elimination organs.

A moderate exercise program that raises your heart rate for 20 to 30 minutes offers the most benefits for nutrient use.

Water therapy helps you heal in almost every way.

Therapeutic baths are an ancient healing technique

A therapeutic bath is easy, stress-free "medicine." Holistic healing clinics and spas are famous all over the world for their therapeutic baths. They use mineral clays, aromatherapy oils, seaweeds and enzyme-rich herbs to draw toxins out of the body through the skin, and to put healing nutrients into the body through the skin.

For cleansing nutrition, I recommend a therapeutic bath at least once a week to remove toxins coming out on the skin. In essence, you soak in an herbal tea, where the skin takes in the healing nutrients instead of the mouth and digestive system.

Procedure is important for taking an effective healing bath. Before a therapeutic bath, dry brush your body all over for 5 minutes with a natural bristle, dry skin brush to remove toxins from the skin and open pores for nutrients.

Then take the bath in one of the following two methods:
1: Draw very hot bath water. Put herbs, seaweeds, or mineral crystals into a large teaball or muslin bath bag. Add mineral salts directly to the water. Steep until water cools and is aromatic. Rub the body with the solids in the muslin bag during the bath.
OR
2: Make a strong tea infusion in a large teapot, strain and add to hot bath water. Soak as long as possible to give the body time to absorb the healing properties.

—After a bath, use a mineral salt rub, like Crystal Star LEMON BODY GLOW™, a traditional spa "finishing" technique to make your skin feel healthy for hours.

Thalassotherapy uses the sea for healthful bathing

Thalassotherapy is an ageless, health-restorative technique. Thalassa is the ancient Greek word for sea. The Greeks indeed used the sea for their well-being. I myself have seen 2500 year-old healing sites on the Greek islands of Rhodes and Corfu, and the ancient Greek healing center at Pergamum in what is now Turkey. Even judging by the therapeutic centers still known to us, much of the population of the ancient Greek and Roman world soaked in sea water "hot tubs" and heated seaweed baths, drank and inhaled sea water for health, got sea water massages, had seaweed facials and body wraps, and used sea water pools for hydrotherapy and detoxification.

Today, we are learning once again about the ability of the sea to reduce tension and de-stress our bodies, detoxify the skin and improve circulation, relieve allergies, sinus and chest congestion, and ease arthritis symptoms.

Seaweed baths are Nature's perfect body/psyche balancer. Remember how good you feel after an ocean walk? Seaweeds purify and balance the ocean — they can do the same for your body. A hot seaweed bath is like a sauna, only better, because the sea greens balance body chemistry instead of dehydrating it. The electromagnetic action of the seaweed releases body congestion, and dissolves fatty wastes through the skin, replacing them with depleted minerals, like potassium and iodine. Iodine boosts thyroid activity, so nutrients get used before they become fat deposits. Vitamin K in seaweeds boosts adrenal activity, so a seaweed bath helps maintain hormone balance for a more youthful body. A seaweed bath even once a month stimulates lymphatic drainage and fat burning to keep off excess weight, reduce cellulite and rid your body of toxins.

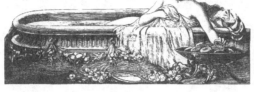

Here is how to take a hot seaweed bath:

If you live near the ocean, gather kelp and seaweeds from the water, (not the shoreline) in buckets or trash cans; carry them home to your tub. Or buy dried seaweeds from your health food store. Crystal Star Herbs packages dried seaweeds, gathered from pristine waters around the San Juan islands, in a made-to-order HOT SEAWEED BATH™.

Place your chosen seaweeds in a tub and run very hot water over them, filling the tub to the point that you will be covered when you recline. The leaves (either dried or fresh) turn a beautiful bright green. The water turns rich brown as the plants release their minerals. Add an aromatherapy oil if desired, to help hold the heat in and boost your detox program. Let the bath cool enough to get in. As you soak, the gel from the seaweed will transfer onto your skin. This coating increases perspiration to release system toxins, and replaces them with minerals by osmosis. Rub your skin with the seaweed during the bath to stimulate circulation, smooth the body, and remove wastes coming out on the skin surface. When the sea greens have done their work, the gel coating dissolves and floats off the skin, and the seaweeds shrivel - a sign that the bath is over.

The release of the gel coating is a natural timekeeper for the bath. Forty-five minutes is usually long enough to balance body pH, encourage liver action and fat metabolism. Skin tone, color, and circulatory improvement are almost immediately noticeable. After the bath, take a capsule of cayenne and ginger to assimilate the seaweed minerals.

No time for a bath? Seaweed facials are great skin tonics

The ancient Greeks said that Aphrodite, the goddess of love, rising out of the foaming sea, owed her supple skin, shiny hair, and sparkling eyes to the plants of the sea. Human body makeup is a lot like that of the ocean, so taking in things from the sea helps replace nutrients we may have lost. Sea plants especially contain minerals that stress and pollution deplete from your skin. Sea plant cell structure allows your skin to easily absorb those minerals.

A seaweed facial stimulates lymphatic drainage and dilates capillaries for better tone. Sea plant mineral salts help your skin hold moisture. When your skin retains moisture it plumps up, smoothing out fine lines and wrinkles. Some sea plants contain elements similar to collagen that make the skin more supple and elastic, and add amazing luster. Most people report better skin texture after a seaweed treatment.

Seaweed wraps are restorative body conditioners.

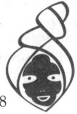

Top European and American spas use thalassotherapy seaweed wraps to rapidly cleanse the body of toxins, and to elasticize and tone the skin. The sea herb and mineral solution easily enters the millions of skin pores to break down and shrink unwanted fatty cells, and cellulite deposits stored in fluids between cells. Wraps are most successful when used along with a short detox program that includes 8 glasses of water a day to flush out the loosened fats and wastes.

I have seen astounding benefits from thalassotherapy wraps during my work with sea herbs in European spas. The results were so amazing I formulated two gel wraps you can use at home.

Here's how: Mix 10 drops <u>each</u> of the herbal extracts for each wrap in aloe vera gel; slather onto your torso, upper arms and thighs to the knee. Have a partner wind plastic wrap several times around your thighs, upper arms and torso to just <u>under</u> the breasts. Lie down on towels, cover yourself with towels or a cotton blanket, turn on soft music and relax for an hour.

1) **Tightening and toning wrap** to improve muscle, vein and skin tone:
   Herbal extracts of Kelp, Cranesbill, White Oak Bark, Marshmallow, Angelica, Rosemary, Lemon Balm and Hawthorn.
2) **Thermogenesis wrap** to enhance metabolism, boost circulation and reduce puffiness:
   Herbal extracts of Bladderwrack or Kelp, Alfalfa, Ginger Root, Dandelion Root, Spearmint, Capsicum and Cinnamon.

Sauna therapy creates a healing, cleansing sweat

An ancient Scandinavian healing technique, today sauna therapy is used all over the world by alternative physicians and clinics to help people release environmental toxins like pesticides and heavy metals. Profuse sweating dramatically increases the detoxifying capacity of the skin.

When body temperature rises enough to cause a sweat, vital organ and gland activity increase, and the skin becomes a "third kidney" to eliminate body wastes through perspiration. A 30 to 40 minute sauna sweat speeds up metabolism, and inhibits the replication of pathogenic organisms. Immune response accelerates. For optimum skin cleansing and restoration, take a sauna once or twice a week. Finish each sauna with a cool shower and a brisk rubdown to remove toxins that are eliminated by the skin.

<u>**The healing benefits of a dry sauna:**</u>
—A sauna creates a fever that inhibits replication of harmful bacteria and viruses.
—A sauna increases leukocytes in the blood to strengthen the immune system.
—A sauna provides a therapeutic sweat that flushes out toxins and heavy metals.
—A sauna accelerates cardiovascular activity and reduces high blood pressure.
—A sauna stimulates vasodilation of peripheral blood vessels to relieve pain and speed healing of sprains, bursitis, arthritis and muscle pain.
—A sauna promotes relaxation and a feeling of well-being.

The benefits of a steam bath are different

Steam baths go back to prehistoric steaming hot springs of our first ancestors. Early man, like primates today in both Japan and Russia, used hot springs to clean and warm themselves, and to remove parasites.

Just as with dry heat saunas, ancient Greeks and Romans used wet steam baths to sweat for health. Hot steam particularly helps respiratory diseases and rheumatic pain. The humid heat of a steam bath is ideal for skin tone and texture.

A steam bath works quicker than a sauna, cleansing the body in about 15 minutes compared to 30 to 40 minutes in a sauna. The powerful detoxification, healing process of hyperthermia does not take place until the body reaches 101-103° F. In a dry heat sauna, your body's cooling mechanism retards hyperthermia by natural evaporation. In a steam bath, evaporation is not possible so there is no loss of body heat. In fact, steam condensation actually becomes the heat transfer mechanism on the body.

Hydrotherapy showers are popular today

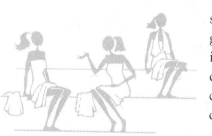

Alternating hot and cold showers open and stimulate the body's vital healing energies. Alternating hydrotherapy is effective for improving circulation and energy levels, relieving throbbing and cramping, toning muscles, and relaxing bowel and bladder tightness. The form of hydrotherapy below is easy and convenient for home use.

—Begin with a comfortably hot shower for three minutes. Follow with a sudden change to cold water for 2 minutes. Repeat this cycle three times, ending with cold. Follow with a full or partial massage, or a brisk towel rub and mild stretching exercises.

Baking soda bath therapy

A simple baking soda bath is a remarkable healing treatment if you suffer from too little sleep, high stress, too much alcohol, caffeine or nicotine, chronic colds or flu, or over-medication. Baking soda balances an over-acid system leaving you refreshed and invigorated, with extra soft skin.

<u>Here's how to take a baking soda bath</u>:
Fill the bath with pleasantly hot water to cover you when you recline. Add 8-oz. baking soda and swirl to dissolve. Soak for 20 to 30 minutes. When you emerge, wrap up in a big thick towel or a blanket and lie down for 15 minutes to help overcome any feelings of weakness or dizziness that might occur from the heat and toxin release. Zia Wesley-Hosford author of Face Value, recommends this rest time for a face mask, since the hot water will have opened up the pores for maximum benefits.

What are ozone pools and oxygen baths?

Ozone (O$_3$), or "activated oxygen," is the fresh, clean scent you smell in the air after a thunderstorm. Amazingly, O$_3$ can also help purify your body. Ozone is the most powerful natural oxidizer – and one of the fastest, safest, detoxifiers known. Professional spas use ozone pools in their treatments to destroy water and airborne viruses, cysts, bacteria and fungi on contact. Ozone pool baths are actually the next generation of oxygen baths; you can use them in your own home healing plan. They noticeably increase energy and tissue oxygen uptake.

<u>Here's how to take a healing oxygen bath:</u>
—Pour about 1 cup of food grade 35% hydrogen peroxide in to a bath. Oxygen baths are stimulating rather than relaxing. Most people notice a significant energy increase within 3 days. Other benefits include body balance and detoxification, reduction of skin cancers, clearing of lung congestion, and arthritis and rheumatism relief.

—Certain herbs used in a bath also supply oxygen through the skin. Rosemary is one of the best and most popular; peppermint and mullein are also effective. Just pack a small muslin bath or tea bag with the herb, drop it into the tub or spa, and soak for 15 to 20 minutes. Use the bag as a scrub during the bath to smooth and tone your skin.

Can you sweat out arthritis?

An arthritis elimination sweating bath can release a surprising amount of toxic material that aggravate your joints. Epsom salts or Dead Sea salts, along with herbs that have diaphoretic action, can play a big part in the success of the bath.

<u>Here's how to take the arthritis bath:</u>
Make a simple tea of elder flowers, peppermint and yarrow. Drink hot just before the bath so you'll sweat. Pour 3 pounds of Epsom salts, or enough Dead Sea salts for 1 bath, into very hot bath water. Rub arthritic joints with a stiff brush in the water for 5 to 10 minutes; stay in the bath for 15 to 25 minutes. On emerging, do not dry yourself. Wrap up immediately in a clean sheet and go straight to bed, covering yourself with several blankets. Protect your mattress with a sheet of plastic. The osmotic pressure of the Epsom salt solution absorbed by the sheet will draw off heavy perspiration. The following morning the sheet will be stained with wastes excreted through your skin - sometimes the color of egg yolk. (This is a strong detox procedure and it happens relatively quickly. Consult a health professional if you have a weak heart or high blood pressure.)

Improvement after an arthritic sweat bath experience is noticeable. Repeat the bath once every two weeks until the sheet is no longer stained, a sign that your body is cleansed. Drink water during the sweat to prevent dehydration and loss of body salts.

A sitz bath puts herbal help where you need it

A sitz bath increases circulation in the pelvic area. Sitz baths help women recover from hemorrhoids and vaginal infections. They help men strengthen the prostate, urinary and anal area. They improve pelvic muscle tone if you suffer from incontinence (a fast-growing group of people in America). The best sitz baths combine herbs with astringent, antiseptic, emollient and hemostatic properties.

<u>Here's how to take a sitz bath:</u>
—For a cold sitz bath, use cold water – about 40° to 85°F. Make a strong, strained tea with a combination of herbs: goldenseal root, marshmallow root, plantain, juniper berry, saw palmetto berry, slippery elm and witch hazel leaf. Add the tea to 3" of water in a tub. Soak in the bath for 5 minutes with enough water to reach your navel, once a day for 5 minutes until healed. Use the strained herbs as a compress on the affected area.

OR

—For a hot sitz bath, add Epsom salts, Breh or Batherapy salts, ginger powder, comfrey or chamomile to the water. Start with water about 100° and increase the heat by letting hot water drip continuously into the tub. The water should cover your hips when seated. Place your feet at the faucet end of the tub so they are soaking in slightly hotter water as the water drips in. Cover your upper body with a towel, and your forehead with a cool, wet cloth. After 30 minutes, rinse off in a quick, cool shower before drying off to stimulate circulation.

Your skin is a key organ for healing

Your body uses your skin to cleanse itself of wastes. Both skin eruptions and perspiration are natural methods by which your body gets rid of harmful substances. You can use this natural process to accelerate your own healing. Herbal compresses and dry skin brushing draw out wastes and release body poisons fast through your skin,

Herbal compresses draw out waste and waste residues, like cysts or abscesses, through the skin and release them into the body's elimination channels. Use alternating hot and cold compresses for best results. Apply the herbs to the hot compress; leave the cold compress plain.

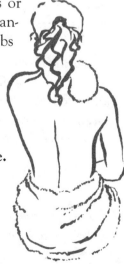

<u>Some effective compresses I use:</u>
—Add 1 teasp. powdered herbs like cayenne, ginger and lobelia to a bowl of very hot water. Soak a washcloth and apply until the cloth cools. Then apply a cloth dipped in ice water until it reaches body temperature. Repeat several times daily.

—Green clay compresses are effective toxin-drawing agents for growths. Apply to gauze, placed on the area, cover and leave all day. Change as you would any dressing when you bathe.

Dry skin brushing helps remove toxins and opens pores for better assimilation of nutrients. Dry skin brushing removes the top layer of old skin, helping to eliminate uric acid crystals and mucous residues. Dry skin brushing also stimulates circulation, cleanses the lymph system and boosts cell renewal. Dry brushing your skin every 24 hours rejuvenates your skin during detoxification. Dry brush before a shower once a week to keep your skin beautiful and keep cellulitic build-up down.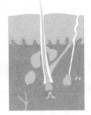

Your technique for skin brushing can make all the difference to its success:
1) Use a natural bristle brush, not synthetic - it scratches skin surface.
2) Do not wet your skin. It stretches the skin and will not have the same effect.
3) All brush strokes should go towards the heart.
4) Especially brush bottoms of your feet, nerve endings here affect the whole body.
5) Use circular, counter-clockwise strokes on the abdomen.
6) Brush lighter strokes over and around the breasts. Do not brush nipples.
7) Dry brushing is best before you bathe in the mornings. Done before bed, it can stimulate too much and may interrupt sleep.
8) Brush the whole body for best results.
9) Wash your brush every few weeks in water and let it dry.

Muscle testing detects energy blocks

Muscle kinesiology is a Traditional Chinese Medicine technique now being enthusiastically rediscovered in America. The word kinesiology means the study of motion, especially how muscles actually move the body. In the natural health field, kinesiology uses principles from Chinese medicine, acupressure and massage to bring the body into balance, and release pain and tension.

Muscle testing is the way most Americans are familiar with applied kinesiology today. Applied kinesiology is based on the premise that muscles, glands, and organs are linked by meridians, or energy pathways throughout the body. Muscle testing is an effective method for detecting and correcting energy movements and imbalances in the body.

Weak muscles indicate an energy flow blockage in one of the body's meridians. Muscle testing reliably identifies weak muscles. A kinesiologist uses stress release techniques to unblock the meridians. The muscles are then retested after visualization, massage techniques and movement exercises; if the muscles have regained strength, the restoration of the energy flow of the meridians is confirmed. Kinesiology does not heal, but rather restores balanced energy flow.

You can use personal muscle testing to determine your own individual response to a food or substance. It's a good technique to use before buying a healing remedy, because it lets you estimate the product's effectiveness for your own body before you buy. You will need a partner for the procedure.

Here's how to use muscle testing:

1: Hold your arm out straight from your side, parallel to the ground. Have a partner place one hand just below your shoulder and one hand on your forearm. Your partner then tries to force your arm down towards your side, while you exert all your strength to hold it level. Unless you are in ill health, you should easily be able to withstand this pressure and keep your arm level.

2: Then, simply hold the item that you desire to test against your diaphragm (under the breastbone) or thyroid (the point where the collarbone comes together below the neck). The item may be in or out of normal packaging, or in its raw state, like a fresh food.

3: Holding the item as above, put your arm out straight from your side as before and have your partner try to press it down again. If the test item is beneficial for you, your arm will retain its strength, and your partner will be unable to force it down. If the item is not beneficial, or would worsen your condition, your arm can be easily pushed down by your partner.

Massage therapy is an amazing healing technique

Massage therapy has been a proven healing technique for thousands of years. Both the ancient Romans and Greeks used massage regularly as a detoxification technique, to promote mucous and fluid drainage from the lungs, and to encourage regular bowel elimination. Modern massage therapy has joined the alternative medicine techniques of chiropractic and reflexology as a viable health discipline. I recommend several massage treatments during a healing program to stimulate the body's immune response and natural restorative powers.

Overwhelming scientific evidence has accumulated over just the last decade to support massage therapy. Here are some of the research findings:

—Massage therapy is especially helpful for pain control, stimulating the production of endorphins, the body's natural pain relievers.
—Massage therapy is an effective cardiovascular treatment, improving blood circulation throughout the circulatory system, and actually helping to prevent heart disease. It is often more helpful than drugs for nerve and gynecological problems like PMS.
—Massage therapy relieves chronic fatigue syndrome, candida albicans, gastrointestinal conditions, epilepsy and psoriasis.
—Massage therapy helps correct poor posture from spinal curvatures or whiplash.
—Massage therapy helps chronic headaches, temporo-mandibular joint syndrome (TMJ), respiratory disorders like bronchial asthma, and emphysema.
—Massage therapy helps break up scar tissue and adhesions.
—Massage therapy effectively reduces inflammation by increasing limbic circulation, especially swelling from fractures, sports injuries or muscle pain after exercise.

<u>**Three types of massage therapy specifically help the body's cleansing process:**</u>
1: Swedish massage uses kneading, stroking, friction, tapping and sometimes body shaking to stimulate and cleanse. These techniques also help cleanse muscle acids, joints, nerves and the endocrine system, by stimulating the body's circulation.

2: Deep tissue massage removes waste in the muscles. Deep tissue therapy uses more direct deep finger pressure across the grain of the muscles to release chronic tension patterns, and stress accumulation. It also boosts circulation to facilitate move-ment of wastes out of muscle tissue. Evidence shows that deep tissue massage can even break up scar tissue and eliminate it.

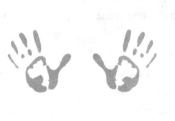

3: Lymphatic drainage massage is a large surface, highly specialized kneading technique, a unique method that uses precise, complex hand movements to encourage the draining of lymph fluids. In comparison, normal massage techniques are much too forceful to allow drain-age in the tissues and may hinder transport. I call the lymphatic system your body's natural antibiotic. Healthy lymph removes body toxins as part of your immune response to disease. Using slow, gentle strokes with a rhythmic pumping action, massage therapy follows the lymph pathways throughout the body to move the flow of lymph and accelerate detoxification.

<u>**Lymphatic massage has four primary effects on your body:**</u>
1: It balances the sympathetic and parasympathetic nervous systems.
2: It activates inhibitory reflexes to decrease or even eliminate pain sensation.
3: It increases lymph flow to clear connective tissue congestion, stimulate capillary blood flow and increase capillary capacity.
4: It boosts immune response by increasing lymph flow and stimulating antibodies.

<u>*Note: Massage is great, but for some health conditions, massage is not a good idea.*</u>
• Don't massage a person with high fever, cancer, tuberculosis or infectious or malignant conditions which might be further spread in the body.
• Don't massage the abdomen of a person with high blood pressure or ulcers.
• Don't massage people with varicose veins, diabetes, or phlebitis.
• Massage no closer than six inches to bruises, cysts, skin breaks or broken bones.
• Massage people with swollen limbs gently, above the swelling, towards the heart.

Hand and foot reflexology is zone therapy

Reflexology, an ancient massage science, believes that all body parts have energy and share information; particularly that each of the body's energy zones are interconnected through the nerve system to specific points on the feet and hands. Reflexology demonstrates that pressure to a particular meridian point brings about better function in all parts of that meridian zone, no matter how remote the point is from the body part in need of healing.

A history of foot massage spans time and place from the Physician's Tomb in Egypt of 2300 B.C. to the Physicians Temple in Nara, Japan of 700 A.D. The ancient Egyptians are believed to have actually developed hand and foot reflexology.

Reflexology is often known as zone therapy and can be used for a measure of self-diagnosis and treatment. Reflexologists look at the feet as a mini-map of the entire body, with the big toes serving as the head, the balls of the feet representing the shoulders, and the narrowing of the foot as the waist area. Ten reflexology zone meridians have been extensively mapped connecting all organs and glands, and culminating in points in the hands and feet. The nervous system is considered an electrical system. Contact can be made through the feet and hands with the electro-mechanical zones in the body to the nerve endings.

The nerve endings are called reflex points. The points on the feet are reflexive, like a knee-jerk reaction. They serve as reflexes for the entire body. Any illness, injury or tension in the body produces tenderness in the corresponding foot zone. The points are manipulated to open blocked energy pathways.

Stress is involved in over 80% of all illness. Reflexology helps the body heal itself by relaxing stress. Its goal is to clear the pathways of energy flow throughout the body, to return body balance, and increase immune response. It does this by stimulating the lymphatic system to eliminate wastes, and the blood to circulate easily to poorly functioning areas. Today, reflexology treatments are used for pain relief, and for faster recovery from injuries or illness without surgery or heavy medication.

Reflexologists rely on an inchworm-like massage motion of the thumb to produce light or deep pressure on each zone, concentrating on the tender spots, which often feel like little grains of salt under the skin.

For your own use, picture your hands and feet as your body's control panels. Get a good reflexology chart — available in health food stores. Then use your fingers or a rounded-end tool to locate the reflex points. Some points take practice to pinpoint. The best rule for knowing when you have reached the right spot is that it is usually very ten-der, denoting crystalline deposits brought about by poor capillary circula-tion of fluids, or congestion in the cor-responding organ. The amount of sore-ness on the foot point normally indicates the size of the crystalline deposit, and the amount of time it has been accumu-lating. For most people, the tenderness is usually accompanied by an immediate feeling of relief in the body organ area as waste deposits break up for removal.

For effective reflexology, press on a reflex point 3 times for 10 seconds each time. Fifteen pounds of applied force on a reflex point is enough to send a surge of energy to remove the obstructive crystals, restore circulation and clear congestion. Use the pressure treatment for twenty to thirty minute sessions at a time, about twice a week. Sessions more often than this will not give nature the chance to use the stimulation or do its necessary repair work. Most people notice frequent and easy bowel movements in the first twenty-four hours after reflexology as the body throws off released wastes.

Reflexology can also be part of a good health maintenance program. You don't have to be sick to appreciate the benefits. Many people simply enjoy the tension release a session gives.

Here are some of the documented health benefits of reflexology therapy:

—**Reduces PMS.** A study published in 1993 in the journal Obstetrics and Gynecology finds women suffering from premenstrual syndrome experience a 40% reduction in symptoms after using reflexology treatments.

—**Improves asthma.** One case study reports a significant improvement in well being and reduction in asthma symptoms after three months of reflexology therapy.

—**Helps balance blood sugar in cases of type 2 diabetes.** Two different studies (one from China; the other from America) reveal reflexology effectively lowers high blood sugar levels in diabetics.

—**Helps restore some movement and sensation for people paralyzed from spinal cord injuries.** Case studies published in the journal Reflexions find some quadriplegic and paraplegic patients respond to reflexology sessions with movement. Other effects noted: some return of bowel and bladder control; induced sweating below the level of the injury; the sensation of bowel rumbling, improved muscle tone; and a decrease in bladder infections.

—**May help dissolve ovarian cysts.** Professional reflexologist Christopher Shirley attests the story of two women scheduled for surgery to remove ovarian cysts who experienced a mysterious disappearance of the cysts (documented by sonograms) after reflexology treatments.

—Medical doctor Julian Whitaker reports that just two weeks of reflexology treatment helped remove a ganglion cyst on his hand.

Polarity therapy is a blend of art and science

Technology graphically shows that the human body consists of electromagnetic patterns. Energy both surrounds the body and courses through it in a continual flow of positive and negative charges. Expressed in ancient times as an aura, this magnetic field makes up our physical, mental, and emotional characteristics, directs body systems and maintains energy balance. A polarity practitioner, popular in holistic spas and detox centers today, accesses the magnetic current to release energy blocks.

Polarity therapy, rooted in Ayurveda, believes that balancing the flow of energy in the body is the underlying foundation of health. Polarity therapy uses diet and exercise for cleansing tissues, increasing energy, improving breath and circulation, and preventing illness. Polarity therapy also treats migraines, low back pain and stress disorders.

Gentle touch induces a relaxed, meditative state to accelerate energy flow throughout the body. There are three types of touch the therapist may use: *rajasic* - gentle and stimulating, *sattvic* - light and balancing, *tamasic* - deep muscle and tissue. The touch may be so light you don't feel anything at all.

Magnet therapy balances negative-positive energy

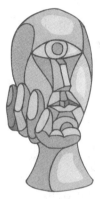

Science has known since the 1950's that a magnetic field is critical to normal body function and coordination. In fact, immune deficiency syndromes like chronic fatigue, and fibromyalgia were first identified as magnetic field deficiency syndromes.

The positive, acid-producing field can create conditions like arthritis, mental confusion, fatigue, pain and insomnia - and encourage fat storage. Culprits producing this field are refined foods, caffeine, nicotine, toxic chemicals in cosmetics and agriculture, auto exhaust, and many prescription drugs.

The negative, alkaline-producing field increases oxygen, encourages deep sleep, reduces inflammation and fluid retention, relieves pain, and promotes mental acuity. A negative field acts like an antibiotic, helping to destroy bacterial, fungal and viral infections because it lowers body acidity.

Does magnet therapy actually work? There seems to be no question that magnets can dramatically influence our health and well being. Russians used magnet therapy during World War II to ease pain, specifically from amputation. At least 50 countries including Germany, Japan and Russia have approved therapeutic magnets for healing. Magnet therapy is being enthusiastically rediscovered in the U.S. by health professionals and health conscious consumers looking for non-invasive, non-toxic solutions to chronic pain. Americans spent $500 million on therapeutic magnets in 1997 alone!

Science is still probing magnet therapy. What we know so far:
Our blood is composed of positively and negatively charged particles. Magnets increase blood flow and therefore more oxygen to areas of the body that need healing.

1: **Magnet therapy balances pH,** establishing an enivironment unfavorable for disease and favorable for healing.
2: **Magnet therapy helps breakdown scar tissue and releases toxins,** accelerating recovery from injury and reducing pain.
3: **Magnet therapy speeds up the movement of calcium to help heal nerve tissue and bones....** and helps eliminate excess calcium in the joints related to arthritis pain.
4: **Magnet therapy stimulates enzyme activity,** vital to healing.
5: **Magnet therapy enlarges blood vessel diameters** and reduces inflammation.
6: **Magnet therapy may offset the effects of free radicals** that contribute to chronic pain and degenerative disease by restoring the body's electrical balance.
7: **Magnet therapy appears to reduce pain by modulating pain receptors** or reducing the activity of brain neurons that cause pain sensations. Magnets may also stimulate the production of endorphins, the body's natural pain killers and mood elevators.

Recently confirmed health benefits from magnet therapy:
—A 1997 study in *Archives of Physical Medicine Rehabilitation* reveals that patients with post-polio pain experience significant, rapid relief when pressure points are exposed to magnets.

—Studies at John Hopkins, Yale and NYU confirm that magnet therapy reduces pain from tendonitis, arthritis and venous ulcers. Other research finds magnet therapy relieves pain from whiplash, head and knee injuries, and menstrual cramps.

—Magnet therapy may be effective for severe depression. An electromagnet, strapped for 5 minutes to the left front portion of the brain, (underactive in depressed people), induces an electric current in the brain and causes brain cells to produce more neurotransmitters that elevate mood. Long term side effects are unknown.

Magnetic sleeping pads, cushions, insoles for shoes, wraps and adhesives, pillow cases, bracelets and necklaces, and massagers are widely available. Use high quality magnets with a gauss strength greater than 400 for best results. If you suffer from chronic pain from arthritis, backaches, migraine headaches, or sports injuries, magnet therapy may be a safe, effective alternative to drugs, medications or invasive treatments. Consider Encore Technology MAGNE-LYFE flexible contour magnets.

Note: Do not use magnets during pregnancy, if you are on insulin, if you have a history of epilepsy or have a pacemaker. Use extreme caution when applying strong magnets on children, particularly on their eyes, brain or heart.

Deep breathing helps you cleanse and heal

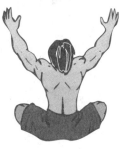

Expand your breathing capacity for better health. Body cleansing and your body's ability to heal are linked to the delivery of oxygen and removal of carbon dioxide. Breathing directly affects lymph circulation. When breathing is restricted, body fluid and wastes from cellular metabolism build up in the lymph. Most of us know that several deep breaths before a hard task clears our mind for the job. But deep breathing does more.... it enhances every body function.

Breathing is controlled by two sets of nerves, the involuntary (autonomic) nervous system, and the voluntary nervous system. Expanding breath capacity improves autonomic nerve functions. Studies show that people suffering from environmental illness have unhealthy, hyperventilating breathing patterns. Hyperventilation contributes to histamine release and altered immune response. Breathing deeply can speed the recovery of environmentally sensitive people.

Good News! **Breathing can even help you burn fat faster!** The special breathing technique below helps you take in more oxygen than normal, which boosts metabolism and prompts your body to burn more stored fat.

　　　1: Inhale quickly through your nose as you pull your mouth into a smile.
　　　2: Pull in your abdomen as you lift your chest upward.
　　　3: Tuck in your pelvis. Squeeze and lift your buttocks.
　　　4: Exhale through your mouth with a blow to force all the air out. Keep your
　　　　　head up, and shoulders back. Keep your rib muscles tight.

Aromatherapy heals through bioelectrical frequency

<u>Did you know that plants have an electrical frequency?</u> Essential plant oils carry a bio-electrical frequency, expressed as hertz. Many of us today understand megahertz rates from our computers and electronic equipment. Plants have a frequency from 0 to 15Hz.; dry herbs have a frequency from 15 to 22Hz.; fresh herbs have a frequency from 20 to 27Hz.; essential plant oils start at 52Hz and go to 320Hz.

<u>Your body has an electrical hertz frequency, too.</u> A healthy body has a frequency between 62 to 78Hz. Disease frequency rates begin at 58Hz. A higher frequency rate destroys an entity of lower frequency. Aromatherapy actually heals through bio-electrical frequency because some high frequency essential oils can create an environment in which disease-causing organisms cannot live. In fact, many aromatherapy oils can affect pathogenic organisms that are resistant to chemical antibiotics. They may turn out to be a good choice for overcoming today's virulent super germs.

Volatile essential oils distilled from plants are the heart of aromatherapy. Seventy-five to one hundred times more concentrated than dried herbs and flowers, aromatherapy oils are potent herbal medicines, able to carry healing nutrients to your body's cells.

<u>Essential oils affect people first through the sense of smell.</u> Information we get through smell is directly relayed to the hypothalamus. Motivation, moods, emotions and creativity all begin in the hypothalamus, so odors affect them immediately. Essential oil molecules work through hormone-like chemicals, so odors can influence hormone levels, metabolism, insulin and stress levels, sex drive, body heat and appetite.

Scents are also intimately intertwined with thought and memory. Studies on brain-waves show that scents like lavender increase alpha brain waves associated with relaxation; scents like jasmine boost beta waves linked to alertness.

<u>Essential oils are not oily.</u> They are non-oily, highly active fluids. You can take them in by inhalation, steams and infusers, or apply topically to the skin. The therapeutic effects of essential oils are due both to their pharmacological properties and to their small molecule size, which allows easy penetration through the skin, the walls of the blood vessels, the lymph system and body tissues — pathways that impact the body's organ, hormonal, nervous and immune systems.

Essential oils assist healing:

• **<u>Their detoxification value is powerful.</u>** When a detoxifying oil is applied, certain toxins like free radicals, heavy metals, fungi, bacteria, viruses and wastes actually attach to the essential oil and are excreted via the skin, kidneys, urine, lungs and bowels. They also cleanse by stimulating sluggish circulation to bring oxygen and nutrients to the tissues, and by accelerating disposal of carbon dioxide and other waste products.

• **<u>They act as blood purifiers and normalizers,</u>** especially against blood stickiness. For example, rose oil helps counteract the toxic blood effects of alcohol. A rose oil and yarrow combination helps normalize a system invaded by pollen and spore allergens.

- **<u>They stimulate immune response,</u>** invigorating white blood cells, and increasing the activity of T-cells, NK-cells, alveolar macrophages and serum antibodies. Studies show all essential oils stimulate phagocytosis, the ability of white blood cells to devour harmful microbes.
- **<u>They improve the immune efficiency of the lymph system,</u>** especially the body's drainage ducts, for better elimination of metabolic residues and toxins. For example, juniper oil enhances the filtration action of the kidneys.
- **<u>The molecules of essential oils have an electromagnetic charge</u>** that influences and balances the charge on our cell magnetic fields, effective for healing.
- **<u>They are natural antioxidants</u>** which destroy free radicals and boost the body's resistance to harmful pathogens of all kinds.
- **<u>Essential oils have antibiotic properties,</u>** but each oil is effective against different pathogens. For example, tests show thyme oil, with the component thymol, is a powerful antibiotic agent against micro-organisms in candida and thrush infections.

Specific oil uses:

- *Eucalyptus, fennel, frankincense, ginger, peppermint and pine*, are expectorants that stimulate the removal of heavy mucous from the lungs and bronchial tubes.
- Citrus oils like *lemon, orange or grapefruit* help fluid retention. *Juniper, sandalwood and cypress* release fluid wastes. *Rose oil and rosemary* help normalize body chemistry, particularly against allergens. *Thyme* oil is an anti-fungal; *marjoram* promotes blood flow; *cedarwood* promotes lymph activity. *Vetiver and cypress* stimulate circulation.
- *Lemon, peppermint, rosemary and thyme* enhance immunity.
- *Orange, juniper berry, basil, and cinnamon* boost energy.
- *Grapefruit, lavender, cypress, basil, and juniper berry* improve skin tone.

FYI: The above oils are by Wyndmere Naturals, 153 Ashley Road, Hopkins, MN 55343, 800-207-8538.

Most essential oils are best delivered through the skin in a massage or bath oil. For best results, mix about 15 drops to 4-oz. of a carrier oil like almond, sunflower, jojoba or a favorite massage oil.

Turn your barriers into stepping stones. Nothing is impossible.

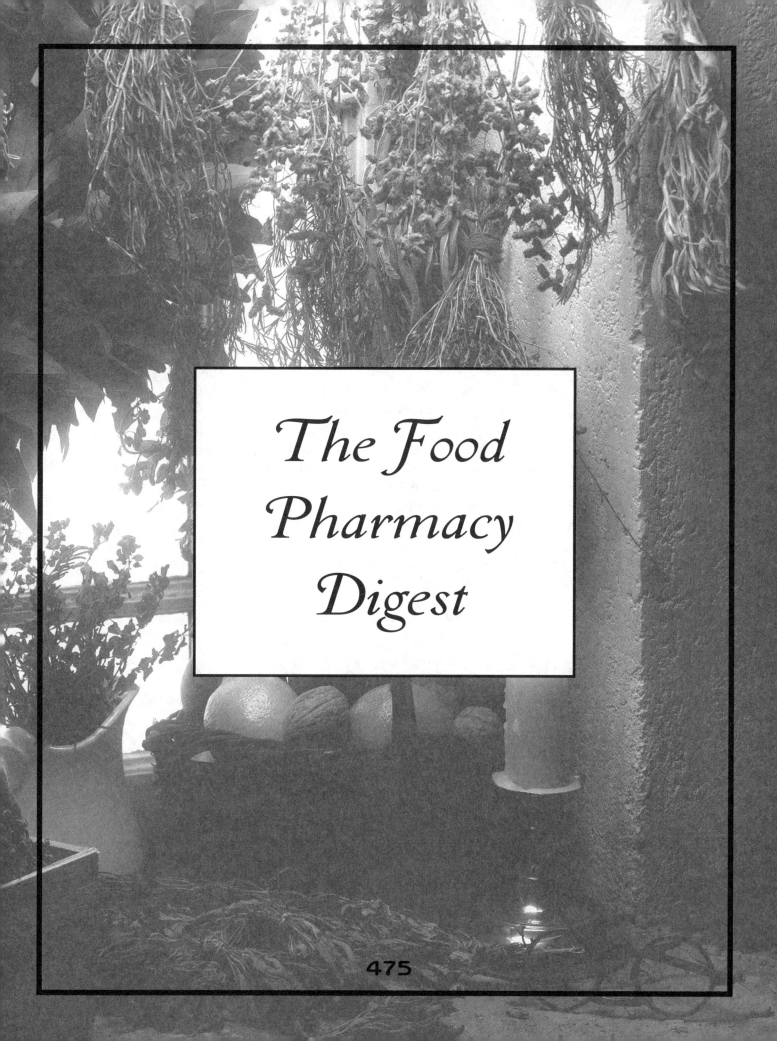

The Food
Pharmacy
Digest

The Food Pharmacy Digest

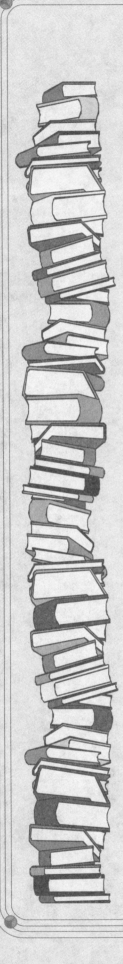

This "quick-look" digest may be the most important section of this book. It's all about getting back to the basics.... because the basics are basics for a reason, like classics are classics for a reason. They stand the tests of time, reliability and value.

Science is validating what natural healers have known for centuries. Food by food; herb by herb, nutrient by nutrient, scientific testing confirms the astounding nutritional profiles of the Earth's plants. Every real, whole food is far more than nourishment, far more than fuel. Every food is medicine, too.

We know herbs are powerful medicine today. We forget that they're also foods. Many have amazing nutritional value.

This section is the "inside story." It's an incredibly complete glossary of the properties and benefits of each food and herb. You'll learn a great deal about what these high nutrition foods can do for your health. Some of the healing foods are unusual; some of the herbs are exotic. Many are also a part of gourmet cooking today.

It's a big list. The Earth is abundant with healing plants, and each plant is incredibly complex. We're just scratching the surface on the research front.

But even if we don't yet know all the valuable elements of each plant, or how the elements all work together, if we eat whole foods and use whole herbs, we'll get all the benefits.

This information can help you build your best healing diet.... customized for your best personal health and well-being.

It's so easy. Here's how to use this section:
1) Check the diet section for your health problem. Note the nutrients you need to help heal it.

2) Then check the food and herb profiles in this section to learn which foods have the nutrients you need.

3) Then look up a recipe that has those foods and add it to your diet.

Need more info on special food nutrients? Check out the Companion Constituent Glossary on page 525.

Section 1 - The Foods

A complete A to Z glossary of foods
with major nutrient values and healing benefits.
Use it to individually tailor your healing program.

ADUKI (azuki) BEANS: very low-fat, easily digested, only 8 to 10 minutes for preparation. Popular in macrobiotic diets. Available in Asian markets and natural food stores.

Nutrient Assets: rich amounts of protein, fiber, potassium, calcium, iron, magnesium, sodium, manganese, vitamin A, beta-carotene, thiamine (B-1), riboflavin (B-2) and niacin (B-3). Beneficial amounts of lignans and fatty acids; rich in protease inhibitors (enzymes that suppress activation of cancer-causing compounds in the intestines).

Health Benefits: provide protein without the fat. A plentiful source of easy-to-digest fiber to keep bowel movements regular and help inhibit diverticular disease, hemorrhoids, and colon or rectal cancer. Aduki bean lignans help reduce breast cancer risk while its fatty acids lower bad LDL cholesterol and blood pressure. Especially beneficial to the kidneys, flushing toxins and releasing wastes through diuretic activity.

ALFALFA SPROUTS: a super low calorie super food — only 10 calories per cup.

Nutrient Assets: no fat or sodium, alfalfa sprouts are an excellent source of vitamin E and phytohormones to protect the heart and enhance sexual function. Vitamin K for blood clotting and plant protein are also widely available.

Health Benefits: a superior detoxification food, alfalfa sprouts have high water content, and a laxative effect to eliminate body toxins. Its high enzymes speed metabolism of heavy, hard-to-digest foods. Diuretic and anti-inflammatory, alfalfa is helpful for PMS bloating and arthritis. Alfalfa is abundant in nitrilosides which break down into chemicals that can selectively destroy cancer cells. For more on alfalfa, see "Nature's Superfoods Help You Heal Faster," pg. 44. *Note: although rare, some people with lupus or rheumatoid arthritis may have sensitivity to alfalfa.*

ALMONDS: easily digested, the most alkalizing of all nuts. For almond oil, see "Fats and Oils," pg 84. There are two kinds of almonds, sweet and bitter. Sweet almonds are a food flavoring; bitter almonds are used as a sedative, topical skin cleanser and in almond oil. Bitter almonds contain *prussic acid* and should not be eaten in large amounts. Both varieties contain high amounts of arginine which may activate the herpes virus in susceptible people.

Nutrient Assets: a high calorie, high fat food rich in minerals (especially potassium and calcium) and vitamin E; contain carbohydrates, protein and magnesium phosphates, ideal for strengthening the body. Almonds contain small amounts of laetrile (B-17), currently being tested as a possible anticancer food (see pg. 538). *Caution: Laetrile can be dangerous in large doses.*

Health Benefits: sweet almonds are a building food, ideal for alleviating heartburn quickly, good for those who have trouble gaining weight. Although almonds have a high fat content, their fat is mainly unsaturated; they may be included in moderate amounts in a diet to lower cholesterol. Bitter almonds can sedate coughs, slightly thin the blood, and are diuretic.

AMARANTH: an incredibly hardy, ancient Aztec grain, now being rediscovered in America. After toasting, popcorn-like amaranth seeds can be added to soups or vegetables or eaten alone.

Nutrient Assets: very high in protein (one cup has 28 grams), making it an exceptional food source for vegetarians. Higher in fiber than wheat, gluten-free corn, rice or soybeans; rich in B-vitamins, calcium, magnesium, iron and the amino acid lysine.

Health Benefits: especially compatible with a diet to control candida albicans yeast. An excellent recovery food, amaranth boosts collagen formation, helps repair damaged tissue and builds muscle protein. Helps alkalize body chemistry to fight the *Herpes Simplex virus*, fever blisters and cold sores. Helps lower high triglycerides, a heart disease risk factor. Amaranth's high lysine content aids calcium absorption; eating it regularly can reduce angina pain.

AMAZAKE: a tasty, rich pudding-like mixture made from fermented sweet brown rice. May be eaten like pudding or other desserts, or as a high protein beverage. Comes in flavors like almond, apricot, cocoa-almond, vanilla pecan, sesame, banana - peanut butter, hazelnut.

Nutrient Assets: amazake is one of the most nutrient-rich drinks known today, high in calcium and whole grain B-vitamins. Amazake is also a good source of magnesium, manganese, potassium, zinc, iron, copper and phosphorus.

Health Benefits: Asian mothers often use nutrient-rich amazake to wean their babies off of breast milk. Amazake can also be used as a power drink after sports or exercise. It is non-dairy making it a good choice for those who are lactose intolerant.

APPLES: a quintessential food for health, apples are low fat, low calorie and an enzyme-rich energy food which help break down and digest other foods. Look for organic, unwaxed apples that aren't treated with fungicides or pesticides.

Nutrient Assets: apples are rich in pectin fiber which binds to and helps eliminate gut toxins, keeping the GI tract healthy and digestion smooth. Apples are a good source of vitamin A carotenes for antioxidant activity, and the flavonoid quercetin.

Health Benefits: fiber-rich apples gently encourage regularity, improve the ability of the intestinal muscles to move waste through, and help lower cholesterol levels. Apples regulate blood sugar against hypoglycemia and diabetes. They keep blood glucose levels up to help you feel full longer during a weight loss diet. Apples reduce your risk for colds and flu. A Michigan State University study shows that 1300 students who ate an apple a day in a 3 year period had less upper respiratory infection and less tension than those who didn't eat apples regularly.

APRICOTS: apricots are sweet fruits related to peach, plum, cherry and almond.

Nutrient Assets: apricots are happy heart foods, with high amounts of magnesium, potassium, pectin, B-vitamins, vitamin C and beta-carotene; low amounts of fat, sodium and cholesterol. Drying apricots concentrates the amounts of nutrients and minerals. Five dried apricots, for example, offer almost 50% of the recommended daily allowance of beta carotene.

Health Benefits: beneficial for blood-related conditions like anemia, acne, toxemia, even tuberculosis. High beta carotene in apricots is especially active against lung, pancreas, larynx and skin cancer. Like almonds, apricot kernels are a source of laetrile (B-17) which should be used with caution. A safe dose for both non-infected and cancer-infected persons may be 10-20 kernels daily. Do not exceed 1 gram daily!

ARROWROOT: powdered cassava plant, used as a thickener for fruit dishes, soups and gravy when a shiny sauce is desired.

Nutrient Assets: contains 20-25% starch, minor proteins and fats. High in calories.

Health Benefits: arrowroot powder helps diaper rash... it's absorbent, soothing, natural, nontoxic; it reduces friction, prevents irritation and helps keep skin dry. It is an easily digested starch. *Note: Sauces thickened with arrowroot become watery if over-cooked or left out too long.*

ARTICHOKES: a thistle that looks like a cabbage, there are three types — the globe artichoke (most common), the Chinese artichoke and the Jerusalem artichoke. Globe artichokes can be steamed, sliced and dipped in a sauce or baked and stuffed. The best ones have brown outer leaves and squeak when you squeeze them.

Nutrient Assets: rich in potassium, calcium, iron, vitamin A, vitamin C and niacin. Low in calories, artichokes are fat-free, but high in natural sodium. Artichokes contain *feylquinic acids* — proven liver protectors. Jerusalem artichokes also contain a carbohydrate called *fructo-oligosaccharides* (FOS) that nourishes friendly bifidobacteria in the digestive tract while reducing harmful bacteria. See "Section Three- The Nutrients," pg. 534 for more information on FOS.

Health Benefits: a powerful liver protector, artichokes increase bile flow and decrease hepatitis risk. Artichokes lower serum cholesterol and blood pressure by increasing cholesterol excretion and decreasing cholesterol synthesis in the liver. Artichokes have compounds similar to caffeine that gently stimulate the brain and nervous system, to offer a pick-me-up sensation.

ARUGULA: a peppery gourmet green. Use fresh with honey-mustard or lemon-pepper dressing; or steam briefly and sprinkle with balsamic vinegar.

Nutrient Assets: a rich source of iron and vitamin C for bone protection and chlorophyll for blood balance. Arugula has vitamin A and 500 carotenoids, of which 10%, including beta-carotene and lutein, are seen as cancer fighting and highly usable.

Health Benefits: a rich source of vitamin A and carotenes, arugula helps prevent stomach, colon, rectum and bladder cancers. Even nicotine-related lung and esophageal cancer may be prevented with a high arugula diet. Arugula's carotenes also make it ideal for the eyes, protecting them from cataracts and macular degeneration, and restoring strength after illnesses like measles, chicken pox, colds, flu, or pneumonia. Helpful for peptic ulcers, hemorrhoids and digestive deficiencies from long-term use of antacids. High iron in arugula is valuable for anemia and restless leg syndrome.

ASPARAGUS: there are three types of asparagus: green, white and, rarely found, purple. The only edible part of the asparagus are the spears which are delicious cooked or raw (canned asparagus has lost most of its nutrients).

Nutrient Assets: low in calories, high in B vitamins, potassium, vitamin A, riboflavin and thiamin, with measurable vitamin C, calcium and iron.

Health Benefits: asparagus is ideal for a healthy heart — it contains no fat, sodium or cholesterol, even assists in lowering blood pressure. Its *asparagine* may be Nature's most effective food diuretic. Its high water content also promotes bowel evacuation. *Aspartic acid* in asparagus neutralizes excess ammonia that causes fatigue. A good source of chlorophyll, asparagus helps build blood and aids liver, skin, ligament and bone conditions.

AVOCADO: considered a fruit, but eaten as a buttery vegetable, <u>avocados only ripen when they're picked</u>. A vegetarian substitute for sour cream, mayonnaise and cheese. Refrigerate to keep them from going rancid.

Nutrient Assets: avocados are cholesterol and sodium-free. They provide high amounts of iron, and are one of the best vegetarian sources of monounsaturated-fat, fiber and protein. Avocados have a high nutrient profile, with minerals like copper, calcium, magnesium, phosphorus, potassium and manganese, and vitamins like A, C and E, and B-vitamins.

Health Benefits: avocados are easily digested and pH balanced to help normalize an over-acid or over-alkaline system. Avocado phytochemicals help fight cancer and heart disease. An abundant source of iron and copper, avocados are useful for blood regeneration, arthritis symptoms and anemia. Monounsaturated-fats in avocados help lower cholesterol. Fat soluble vitamins in avocados make them an "aphrodisiac" food.

BAKING POWDER: a blend of both slow and fast acting leavenings, baking powder substitutes for baker's yeast and allows quick breads like muffins, to rise. I recommend aluminum-free baking powder like Rumford's brand.

Nutrient Assets: baking powder is high in the minerals potassium and sodium, important electrolytes that support heart health, pH balance and energy. It contains chloride, a critical part of the body's electrolytic reactions that allows potassium and sodium to perform their pH balancing functions in the body.

Health Benefits: high potassium in baking powder helps lower blood pressure and also helps people with severe potassium depletion caused by over-use of diuretics, rigorous exercise or severe vomiting. High organic sodium is beneficial for organ, nerve and muscle health.

BANANAS: one of Nature's most nourishing fruits, if it's sprinkled all over with brown freckles it is ready to eat. If the skin doesn't break easily, the banana isn't ripe enough; if the skin feels soggy, it is too starchy.

Nutrient Assets: bananas provide rich fiber and potassium, and high levels of energy giving carbohydrates with no fat! Bananas contain measurable amounts of magnesium, phosphorus, copper and iodine, B-vitamins and C.

Health Benefits: bananas are easily digestible with anti-ulcer and antibacterial activity that inhibits microbes like *bacillus cereus, bacillus coagulans and baccillus sterothenmophilus and clostrodium sporegenes*. Bananas are an athlete's dream fruit, building endurance without weight gain. For weight loss, bananas boost energy and keep you feeling full. For the elderly, bananas prevent constipation caused by a sluggish bowel. Bananas even relieve nausea, especially in kids.

BARLEY: a low gluten grain with a sweet, malty taste. Use it as part of a flour or whole grain mix to lend a chewy texture to cookies and muffins. Barley grass is one of the healing green grasses. See "Nature's Superfoods," pg. 44.

Nutrient Assets: a good source of protein, B vitamins, minerals like calcium, manganese, magnesium, copper, iron, selenium, potassium and protease inhibitors.

Health Benefits: a nutrient-rich, virus-fighting superfood, barley lowers LDL (bad) cholesterol and raises HDL (good) cholesterol through its tocotrienols, which suppress the liver's ability to make bad cholesterol. Balances blood sugar in cases of hypoglycemia and diabetes. Barley is loaded with protease inhibitors that help suppress cancer, especially colon cancer.

BARLEY MALT SYRUP: a mild natural sweetener cooked to a syrup from barley sprouts and water. Only 40% as sweet as sugar and 75% as sweet as honey, barley syrup is a good sweetener for cookies, muffins and quick breads.

Nutrient Assets: barley malt syrup is a complex carbohydrate food (not a simple sugar). Niacin and folic acid are the best represented B-vitamins; magnesium, calcium, iron, phosphorus and potassium are barley's most significant minerals. Barley malt contains large amounts of essential fatty acids. The syrup is a good nutrient source for recovery from illness.

Health Benefits: barley malt's health benefits target the bladder, chest and urogenital areas. It is a digestive tonic, diuretic, mucous cleanser and appetite stimulant. It enters the bloodstream slowly so it doesn't upset blood sugar levels. It helps balance acid-alkaline pH. It may be used as a poultice for burns. Early in this century, barley was used to reduce fevers, prevent gray hair, and alleviate pain and inflammation.

BASMATI RICE: a delicious aromatic whole grain rice, originally from India, but now also grown as a hybrid in Texas. Basmati is better for you than white rice, lighter, easier to digest than brown rice. Available in brown and white varieties, it is aged for at least a year to develop its nutty flavor.

Nutrient Assets: an enzyme and mineral rich energy food; a good source of complex carbohydrates, fiber and a light source of protein. Especially rich in B-vitamins, and minerals like selenium, magnesium, zinc, iron and potassium.

Health Benefits: offers slow calorie burning for sustained energy; an excellent fiber choice for diseases like colon cancer, hemorrhoids or varicose veins, diverticulitis or chronic constipation, gallstones, high cholesterol, high blood pressure and ulcers.

BELGIAN ENDIVE: a white, tangy, tender cone-shaped salad-green, related to chicory. Belgian endive's flavor changes when it is steamed, stewed, broiled or baked, but is delicious both cooked and fresh.

Nutrient Assets: organic sodium, one calorie per leaf, high in protein with minerals like iron, magnesium, potassium and silica, some B-vitamins and vitamin C.

Health Benefits: Belgian endive is considered pain relieving, antispasmodic, expectorant and may be used to help cure insomnia. Because of its silicon content, Belgian endives help renew joints, bones, arteries and connective tissues. As a slight bitter, it improves digestion and stimulates bile flow from the liver.

BELL PEPPER: bell peppers are considered by many nutrition experts to be the perfect pepper, rich in disease-fighting antioxidants. Available in a variety of colors like green, yellow, orange and red, you can eat bell peppers raw in a sandwich or salad, or add them to almost any vegetable dish for more color and spice.

Nutrient Assets: very high in vitamin C and beta carotene (red bell peppers are the highest, containing 20 times the beta carotene and three times the vitamin C of other bell peppers). Also contains some B-complex, calcium, magnesium and potassium.

Health Benefits: an antioxidant food that fights free radical damage to cells and boosts immune response. Its high beta carotene and vitamin C content makes it an excellent choice for heart disease and cancer protection.

BITTER MELON: a wrinkly, cucumber-like Asian vegetable.

Nutrient Assets: a high fiber food with B vitamins and vitamin C, bitter melon contains "compound Q," currently being researched for treatment of AIDS. Bitter melon contains a blood sugar lowering agent called *charantin*, more potent than the diabetic drug *tolbutamide*.

Health Benefits: used in the treatment of diabetes, especially in China and India, to improve glucose tolerance without increasing blood insulin levels. Bitter melon has antibacterial properties against *E. coli.* and helps expel roundworms. Traditionally used in China against asthma, boils, colitis, dysentery, indigestion, earache, eczema and psoriasis, fever, gonorrhea, halitosis (a stomach cleanser), headaches, hepatitis, jaundice (a liver cleanser), hemorrhoids, gout and rheumatism, thrush, tumors and ulcers. *Note: the juice is not recommended for children; remove the seeds - they are slightly toxic.*

BLACK BEANS: a Mexican staple with rice, black beans are an excellent source of protein — especially good as a detoxifying soup. Black beans need overnight soaking and 5 to 8 hours of slow cooking. They are delicious in soups, dips, burritos, burgers and pancakes.

Nutrient Assets: a good source of pectin, fiber and anti-cancerous lignans. High in protease inhibitors, enzymes that counteract activation of cancer-causing compounds.

Health Benefits: black beans are potent healers for the cardiovascular system and work amazingly well to regulate insulin in Type I diabetes. Their fiber helps colon regularity reducing risk for colon cancer. Black beans are kidney strengtheners; they also reduce cholesterol, control blood sugar levels, lower blood pressure, and prevent hemorrhoids and irritable bowel syndrome.

BLUEBERRY: a low calorie sweet berry related to bilberries, huckleberries and cranberries. Blueberries should be plump, dark blue and their soft skin should look as if it's been dipped in powder. Blueberries only last 3 to 7 days after picking and should be refrigerated.

Nutrient Assets: low in calories (81 calories per cup), very high in antioxidant compounds called anthocyanosides, fiber, vitamin C and bioflavonoids.

Health Benefits: a good blood cleanser, laxative and circulatory stimulant, blueberries are especially effective against cataracts and glaucoma, slowing down vision loss and improving the ability of eyes to adjust and focus quickly after exposure to light. Blueberries are loaded with bioflavonoids that fight varicose veins, hemorrhoids and peptic ulcers. Blueberries are anti-bacterial against *E. coli* and urinary tract infections. Dried blueberries are effective for toddler diarrhea (just 2 or 3 dried blueberries are needed). The Journal of Neuroscience shows a diet high in blueberries improves short-term memory and coordination problems.

BOK CHOY: a soft, peppery Asian cabbage, bok choy is sometimes called Chinese chard or Chinese mustard, and has a mild, juicy sweet taste, similar to romaine lettuce. Use bok choy alone, add to soups and salads or use in a delicious stir-fry.

Nutrient Assets: very low in calories (3-oz. has 13 calories) and fat, bok choy is high in potassium (especially cooked), vitamin C and A, with 75% of the RDA for these vitamins. *Dithiolthione* compounds in bok choy fight cancer and boost antioxidant activity.

Health Benefits: an indole-rich green, bok choy speeds up estrogen metabolism, which helps flush excess hormones, making them less available to feed cancer. (May even prevent breast cancer recurrence and metastasis.) Steam or stir-fry bok choy; heavy cooking destroys the indoles, dramatically reducing their therapeutic effects.

BRAN: often called miller's bran or unprocessed bran, the outside shell of the grain, well known these days as a fiber source. Use it as part of a flour mix for texture. Bran from rice or oats is a good wheat alternative.

   Nutrient Assets: extremely high in fiber (5 times the amount of regular whole wheat), and contains B-1 (thiamin), copper and riboflavin.

   Health Benefits: eating bran regularly ensures proper digestion, stimulates bowel nerves and bulks up stool elimination. Bran reduces the risk of constipation-aggravated conditions like diverticular disease, irritable bowel syndrome, hemorrhoids, even varicose veins. Just 2 teasp. of bran 3x daily can reduce diverticular disease symptoms up to 90%! Bran inhibits the reoccurrence of cancerous growths in the colon. It fights breast cancer by lowering cancer-promoting estrogen levels in the blood. Bran fiber decreases levels of estradiol, a cancer promoting hormone. Drink plenty of water with bran to ease digestion at first. *Note: Eat bran in moderation; large amounts of bran can prevent minerals such as copper, iron and zinc from being absorbed by the body.*

   BREWER'S YEAST: (See "Section Three- The Nutrients" on pg. 541.)

   BROCCOLI: every bit of broccoli is edible — stems, buds, leaves, even sprouts. Parboil or steam broccoli heads and stems for best health results — just until it turns bright green and crunchy. The leaves can be cooked just like spinach.

   Nutrient Assets: high calcium, potassium, iron, niacin, folate, vitamin A and C, and fiber. High in *chlorophyll, lutein, sulfarophane and indoles* that possess anticancer properties.

   Health Benefits: antioxidants in broccoli are believed to inhibit the DNA damage that triggers some forms of cancer. Its *indoles and sulforaphane* stimulate the body's natural detoxification systems (phase II enzymes). Two potent broccoli chemical groups, *indoles* and *isothiocyanates*, are credited with its cancer-prevention properties. Broccoli is a good source of beta carotene, also thought to reduce the risk of cancer. Cruciferous vegetables, including broccoli, flush cancer-contributing, excess estrogen from the body. Tests show *sulforaphane*, reduces breast cancer occurrence by up to 60%. Broccoli helps lower both cholesterol and high blood pressure. It is an excellent source of calcium for strong bones. Lutein in broccoli may also protect against colon cancer. For people who don't like broccoli.... three-day-old broccoli sprouts are loaded with cancer fighters (chemoprotective and 20 to 50 times more potent than broccoli itself) and they don't taste like broccoli. You need up to 2 pounds of broccoli in the diet per week to cut the risk of colon cancer in half, *but just one handful of sprouts to do the same job.*

   BROCCOLINI: a hybrid of broccoli and Chinese kale with a mild and sweet taste.

   Nutrient Assets: provides the nutrients found in broccoli and Chinese kale - high levels of vitamins A and C; minerals like calcium, potassium (15%), iron, indoles, sulforaphane, B-vitamins and fiber. Low in calories, broccolini is ideal for weight loss.

   Health Benefits: broccolini's high fiber helps control diabetes by decreasing the need for insulin. (Fiber helps empty the stomach, slowing the absorption of glucose in the intestine.) Like broccoli, broccolini's *indoles* and *sulforaphane* potentiate anticancer activity, and flush excess estrogen from the body to fight hormone-driven diseases like breast cancer. Calcium-rich broccolini helps maintain bone mass against osteoporosis. An antioxidant, broccolini helps prevent free radical damage involved in cancer, arthritis, Alzheimer's, heart disease and aging.

BROWN RICE: a healthier alternative to white rice because the outer shell of bran is still intact. There are many forms of brown rice..... Long grain is dry and fluffy (good for pilafs and stir fries); short grain is soft and sticky (good for molds and shaping). Sweet brown can be used for desserts, wehani for its nutty texture, basmati for aroma, wild rice for chewiness.

Nutrient Assets: full of B vitamins, including B-12, particularly thiamine, biotin and niacin. Rice is one of the few grains that has vitamin E and retains its nutrients even when cooked. Also rich in magnesium, zinc, iron, selenium and potassium.

Health Benefits: lowers blood pressure through its low sodium content. A low calorie (116 per half a cup) food favorable for weight loss. A better tolerated grain than wheat for people with grain allergies. Brown rice nutrients inhibit breast, colon and prostate cancer. May be used to curb diarrhea, even for babies, and prevent kidney stones. For diabetics, brown rice keeps blood insulin and glucose balanced. It calms the nervous system and relieves mental stress. Use brown rice for body cleansing as an effective option to a juice cleanse to improve body definition, weight control and body chemistry. A valuable source of B-vitamins, brown rice clears up skin conditions like psoriasis, helps restore hair loss and supports skin health.

BRUSSELS SPROUTS: the smaller the sprout, the tastier for these cabbages-on-a-stalk. Like all crucifers, cook brussels sprouts to neutralize goitrogens that depress thyroid functions.

Nutrient Assets: a good source of fiber, rich in essential minerals like sulphur, potassium, iron, calcium, magnesium, phosphorus, sodium, zinc, copper and manganese. B-vitamins, vitamin E and vitamin C are also available. Low in fat and calories (only 45 calories per half cup!). Brussels sprouts are packed with anticancer compounds like *chlorophyll, indoles, dithiolthiones, carotenoids and glucosinolates.*

Health Benefits: brussels sprouts greatly reduce the risk of developing stomach, lung, bladder or esophageal cancer and help suppress polyps— precancerous growths in the colon. Brussels sprouts improve enzyme activity in the liver, which in turn, helps the body eliminate one of the most malicious cancer promoters, *aflaxtoxin* —a fungal mold linked to liver cancer. Sulphur in brussels sprouts increases antibiotic and antiviral capabilities against most infectious disease.

BUCKWHEAT: a very hardy grain, growing even in extreme climates. Highly resistant to disease so it is one of the few commercially grown grains that is not contaminated with insecticides. Use the flour in a baking mix for mild taste.

Nutrient Assets: one of the few foods that possesses all eight essential amino acids. Extremely high in lysine, B vitamins and rutin, its minerals include: iron, calcium, magnesium, phosphorus, potassium, sodium and zinc. Buckwheat's rich fiber and silica content help it produce *butyrate*— a short-chain fatty acid.

Health Benefits: a good blood builder and balancer of toxic acid wastes in the body. Buckwheat can be eaten by people allergic to other grains. Especially helpful for those with candida albicans yeast overgrowth because it does not feed the yeasts. Butyrate, produced in roasted buckwheat helps detoxify the intestines and suppresses cancer growth. Rutin in buckwheat helps strengthen capillaries, aids circulation and protects against the effects of radiation — ideal for chemotherapy patients. *Note: Buckwheat is not recommended if you have skin cancers or skin allergies because its astringent action tightens skin and may keep skin cells from cleansing themselves.*

BULGUR: hulled, parboiled cracked wheat, bulgur is best used in a mix of grains, vegetables and legumes. For example, B vitamins in bulgur complement protein in legumes like pinto beans, and high folate vegetables like spinach, asparagus and broccoli.

Nutrient Assets: a high fiber, low calorie food rich in B vitamins and zinc.

Health Benefits: as a member of the wheat family, bulgur helps detoxify the liver. A food for the colon, bulgur's high fiber content stimulates bowel elimination and prevents colon conditions like constipation, irritable bowel syndrome, even development of colon polyps.

CABBAGE: a super nutritious vegetable, cabbage is crispy and has a mildly bitter flavor. Green, red, white and purple varieties are all available. Look for compact, good sized heads with large leaves. Use in soups, stir-frys, steamed, in salads, or raw.

Nutrient Assets: cabbage is high in sulphur, iron, iodine and is a rich source of vitamin C. It's loaded with vitamin E and calcium, and very high in anti-cancer compounds *such as dithiolthiones* and *indoles*. Cabbage juice contains *gefarnate*—an important antiulcer factor.

Health Benefits: antioxidant *dithiolthiones* in cabbage fight cancer, especially cancers of the breast and colon, and also suppress polyp growth. Recent studies show men who eat cabbage at least twice a week reduce their risk of developing cancerous colon polyps by up to 66%! 2 TBS of cooked cabbage daily shows good results against stomach cancer. A powerful intestinal cleanser, cabbage helps prevent harmful bacteria from attaching itself in the stomach and accelerates fecal elimination. A sulphur food, cabbage helps beautify the skin, increase immunity and heal ulcers. A good choice for fibrocystic breast disease because it helps flush excess estrogen from the body. Raw sauerkraut, made from cabbage, cleanses and rejuvenates the digestive tract and boosts the growth of friendly bacteria (acidophilus).

CANNELLINI BEANS: white kidney beans found in Italian markets, cannellini have a rich nutty flavor, and make a tasty addition to minestrone soup and stews.

Nutrient Assets: rich in protein, calcium, phosphorus, potassium and iron. Abundant in manganese, extremely high in fiber and virtually fat free!

Health Benefits: particularly beneficial for persons with joint and bone problems who are often deficient in the trace element manganese. Cannellini beans promote the easy passage of food through the digestive tract. *Lignans* and *protease inhibitors* in cannellini beans offer cancer protection; *Lignans* also regulate blood sugar levels. Other therapeutic benefits: help reduce LDL "bad" cholesterol, lower blood pressure, and prevent hemorrhoids and bowel problems.

CANOLA OIL: from the rapeseed plant, unrefined canola oil has a rich palatable flavor. Use for cooking (not for cooking over 320°F) and in salad dressing.

Nutrient Assets: canola is high in monounsaturated fats, with 10% omega-3 fatty acids, and lower saturated fat than other vegetable oils. Very high (58%) in the fatty acid *oleic acid*.

Health Benefits: a cardiovascular protector that prevents harmful blood clots. Omega-3 fatty acids found in canola oil reduce inflammation and asthma, and maintain healthy skin. Omega-3 fatty acids also inhibit the formation of breast, colon and pancreatic tumors. Oleic acid in canola oil reduces LDL "bad" cholesterol levels without affecting HDL or "good" cholesterol. Use only in moderation. Rape seeds contain *erucic acid*, a compound that may lead to deterioration of the heart, kidneys, adrenals and thyroid. (See "Fats & Oils," page 84)

CAPERS: the flower buds of a Mediterranean shrub, pickled in salt water and vinegar, and used as a condiment in Greek, Italian and Turkish foods. They have a lemon-like taste.

Nutrient Assets: high in sodium, protein, the amino acid tyrosine, and fat. A good choice for vegetarians for high quality protein and fat.

Health Benefits: a brain food which enhances mental clarity. Tyrosine in capers promotes the formation of neurotransmitters that stimulate the brain. Note: high sodium, pickled capers may cause water retention and possibly raise blood pressure.

CAROB POWDER: made from the seed pods of a Mediterranean tree, carob powder is sweet with a chocolate-type flavor. Use in small amounts as a healthy substitute for cocoa.

Nutrient Assets: 45% natural sugars; also contains pectin which aids digestion. Small amounts of fat, low in calories, contains no caffeine.

Health Benefits: offering children sweets made with carob powder instead of refined sugar can help reduce hyperactivity and weight gain, an increasing problem for today's kids directly linked to refined sugar overload.

CARROTS: a sweet root vegetable, carrots can be prepared a variety of ways: sautéed, puréed, boiled, shredded (for salads) or added to soups and casseroles. Choose bulk carrots with rich color that don't seem rubbery.

Nutrient Assets: abundant in beta-carotene (carrot's beta-carotene is not destroyed during cooking, instead cooking enables easier absorption). Also high in calcium, magnesium, phosphorus, potassium, silicon, sodium and vitamin C.

Health Benefits: carrots and carrot juice detoxify all systems in the body. Carrots fight cancer, especially of the stomach, colon, rectum, bladder, and smoking-related esophagus and lungs cancers. A powerful medicinal food for women, an Iowa Women's Health Study shows the more carrots a woman eats, the lower her risk for lung cancer. Research shows women who eat carrots three times a week are half as likely to develop breast cancer. Tests also show that a carrot a day reduces a woman's chance of a stroke by 68%. Carrots are a powerful artery protector, immune booster and infection fighter. Their high beta carotene reduces risk of cataracts, macular degeneration, and angina. Carrots contain essential oils that kill parasites and intestinal pathogens. Carrot soup alleviates constipation, strengthens connective tissue and aids calcium metabolism (see CARROT SOUP recipe, in *Book Two: The Healing Recipes*).

CAULIFLOWER: a member of the cabbage family and relative of broccoli, cauliflower can be served raw in salads, in veggie platters, or lightly steamed.

Nutrient Assets: a low calorie food, high in vitamin C, fiber, potassium, folacin, anticancer *dithiolthiones* and *indoles*, and anti-infective sulphur. Contains protein, calcium, boron, iron, magnesium, phosphorus, zinc, copper, manganese, vitamin A, traces of B-1 through B-9 and vitamin E. Heavy cooking destroys its important nutrients.

Health Benefits: a blood purifying food beneficial for bleeding gums, especially when eaten lightly cooked. Cauliflower improves kidney and bladder health, hypertension and constipation caused by low fiber. Add cauliflower to your anti-cancer, immune boosting diet. Cauliflower helps balance excess estrogen coming from hormone-injected foods or environmental pollutants. *Note: Cauliflower's high sulphur content may cause mild indigestion. Cooking alleviates this problem.*

CELERY: a crunchy, tangy veggie that if stored correctly (0 to 1°C and 98-100° humidity), can be used from 2 weeks up to 2 months after purchase. Enjoy celery raw, in healthy casseroles, and in salads and soups. Select firm bunches with crisp green leaves.

Nutrient Assets: celery has high water content and contains anticancer compounds such as *phthalides* and *polyacetylene*, particularly effective against cigarette smoke. Contains heart protecting quercetin and coumarins. Celery is abundant in minerals like calcium, iron, magnesium, phosphorus, potassium, zinc, copper, manganese.

Health Benefits: a mild diuretic which helps balance body fluids. Celery detoxifies the kidneys and remineralizes the blood. It is an anti-rheumatoid that also lowers blood pressure. Strongly alkaline, eating more celery can help clear up skin problems and aid digestion. As a source of natural calcium and silicon, it can help repair ligaments and bones. *Note: Avoid celery before and after workouts; it may cause an allergic reaction.*

CHAPATIS: Indian flat bread made by kneading together flour, salt, water and canola oil. Use chapatis as a whole grain pizza crust or sandwich "wrap." Chapatis cook quickly (about 2 minutes), but prior to cooking, need to be left in a damp cloth for 30 minutes.

Nutrient Assets: high in B vitamins (with the exception of vitamin B-12), with available vitamin E; omega-3 fatty acids are also present. An excellent source of selenium, chapatis are rich in minerals like calcium, copper, potassium, magnesium, iron, zinc and phosphorus.

Health Benefits: as a rich source of vitamin E, chapatis are a good addition to a healthy heart diet. High selenium content works to protect against free-radical damage and eliminate heavy metals like lead, mercury and aluminum from the body. An easy-to-digest food that helps relieve abdominal gas.

CHEESE: an aged dairy food made from milk curd. Choose low sodium cheeses for better health. You'll never miss the high salt taste. (See pp. 88 for more about healthy cheese choices.)

Nutrient Assets: rich in calcium and protein. Non-fat or low-fat cheeses contain the same nutrients as regular high-fat cheese.

Health Benefits: cheese (especially cheddar cheese) may block cavities due to its calcium phosphate or casein content. High calcium in low fat cheese may also help lower blood pressure. Low-fat, non-fat or rennet-free cheeses can reduce the risk of endometrial cancer and osteoporosis. If you're allergic to cow's milk, choose cheese from goat (chevre) or sheep's milk (feta), less likely to cause reactions. Low-fat cheeses enhance mental clarity.

CHICK PEAS: (also known as garbanzo beans), light brown beans with a crunchy, nutty flavor. Can be made into cakes and puddings, hummus dip, or simply added to salads, casseroles and other tasty dishes. Soak and slow cook for best results.

Nutrient Assets: a high protein food with plenty of vitamin C, calcium, iron, magnesium, phosphorus, potassium, sodium, zinc, copper, manganese, and carotenes for antioxidant activity. A low-fat, high fiber healthy heart food with plenty of anti-cancer protease inhibitors.

Health Benefits: an anti-cancer food which, like all other beans, controls insulin and blood sugar, lowers blood pressure and cholesterol, regulates colon function and prevents constipation. Easy to digest, chick peas also cleanse the arteries and contain choline, an agent that boosts fat metabolism for weight loss.

CHILI PEPPERS: chili peppers are the immature pods of various peppers, such as anaheim, ancho, cayenne, jalapeno, etc., used to add heat and color to Mexican dishes.

Nutrient Assets: low in calories, high in protein, fiber, calcium, iron, magnesium, phosphorus, potassium, sodium, zinc, copper and manganese, chilies contain vitamin A, which promotes resistant to colds, growth and feelings of well being. Chili peppers also contain vitamins B-1 through B-9, which aid in food absorption, mental clarity and nervous system health.

Health Benefits: an important recovery food for colds or flu because they clear excess mucous that harbors infection. A mild stimulant for low energy and a heart protector that lowers cholesterol levels and triglycerides. Chilies clear blood clots, making the circulatory system less vulnerable to arterial blockage and thrombo-embolism (life threatening blood clots). Chilies actually protect the stomach lining, even help limit damage caused by over-use of alcohol and aspirin, or excess fats. Peppers open up sinuses and air passages to relieve asthma. They can be used to speed up metabolism and burn off calories quickly — ideal for weight loss. *Note: Fresh chilies can burn both eyes and skin. Handle them with gloves. Broil them until blistered, then allow them to steam in a paper bag. Run under cold water, slip off skin, and remove seeds and veins before using.*

CILANTRO: fresh coriander leaves are used in Mexican, Chinese and Indian cooking, with a distinct orange-parsley flavor. Dried cilantro has almost no flavor.

Nutrient Assets: low in calories and fat, high in vitamin A, cilantro contains calcium, magnesium, potassium, iron, phosphorus and sodium, B-vitamins and C.

Health Benefits: helps settle the stomach — reduces gas, indigestion, nausea, even vomiting. An anti-inflammatory food for those suffering from arthritis. Purifies the blood and strengthens the cardiovascular system. Cilantro helps retard meat spoilage.

CITRON: a citrus fruit resembling a lemon with thicker skin and bigger size. Citron has a mild lemon-like taste, but is not as sour. The peel is usually desalted and candied. The hard pulp is used to make jelly. Useful in breads, cakes, puddings and candies.

Nutrient Assets: contains protein, calcium, potassium, fiber, iron, phosphorus, beta carotene, B-1, B-2, B-3 and vitamin C. Raw citron has no calories; candied, it has 314 per 100g.

Health Benefits: citron has anticancer capabilities, particularly against pancreatic and stomach cancer. Alleviates seasickness, lung disorders, intestinal problems, and fibromyalgia rheumatic pain. The juice is a purgative that eliminates body toxins. Citron is a traditional remedy for dysentery and can be eaten to overcome halitosis.

COCONUTS: a fruit with a tough, hard shell, soft meat and sweet flavorful juices. For best quality, look for large coconuts; shake and listen for liquid. Coconuts are available dried, desiccated, flaked, shredded or as a cream. More easily digested if eaten with salads and cooked vegetables versus with starchy sugars, including honey.

Nutrient Assets: its saturated fat is primarily medium chain. Its primary fatty acids are *lauric, myristic, palmitic, oleic, caprylic, capric and stearic acids.* Contains organic iodine, calcium, iron, magnesium, phosphorus, potassium, sodium, zinc, copper and manganese. Contains some B vitamins and vitamin C.

Health Benefits: nourishes the thyroid with plentiful natural iodine. Offers easily digested fat for people who have trouble putting on weight.

COCONUT MILK: a bittersweet liquid made from simmering equal parts of shredded fresh coconut and water. Can be used in place of oil, fat and butter. *Note: High in calories and fat, use in moderation. May be used as a good protein source for children.*

    Nutrient Assets: a complete protein food. Has calcium, magnesium, phosphorus, zinc, copper, manganese, B-1, B-3 and vitamin C. Very high in potassium, low in sodium.

    Health Benefits: a rich source of potassium, coconut milk reduces high blood pressure and cardiovascular disease, and may help prevent cancer and strokes. Helps replace body fluids and electrolytes in cases of diarrhea. Coconut protein nourishes the brain. Coconut milk softens and smooths skin, keeping it supple and youthful-looking.

COCONUT OIL: see "oils, vegetable" in this section.

COLLARDS: dark greens related to the cabbage family. Mix into a salad or cook like you would spinach. Use in vegetable dishes, casseroles, soups and stews.

    Nutrient Assets: a high nutrient profile, high in vegetable protein, packed with beta-carotene, calcium, sulphur and lutein. Antioxidant, anti-cancer compounds, dithiolthiones and indoles specifically ward off breast and colon cancer.

    Health Benefits: powerfully anti-cancer and antioxidant, collards are a high sulphur food with antibiotic and antiviral activity. High beta carotene in collards reduces the chance of brain damage during strokes. Collards gently cleanses the liver. *Note: Not recommended for patients with kidney stones; collard oxalates may stress the kidneys.*

CORN: the leading grain grown in the world. For best ripeness, look for cream colored corn with kernels that excrete a milky fluid.

    Nutrient Assets: once blamed for pellagra, a niacin deficiency disease, today experts know corn offers valuable nutrition. A protein and carbohydrate-rich food high in fiber, corn contains minerals like calcium, iron, magnesium, phosphorus and zinc. Also contains vitamins C, beta carotene and B-complex. High in potassium, folic acid, and protease inhibitors.

    Health Benefits: a diuretic and mild brain stimulant, corn helps lower the risk of developing colon, breast and prostate cancers. May reduce menopausal symptoms by mildly boosting estrogen. May prevent dental cavities. Corn strengthens bone and builds muscles. *Note: Corn and corn by-products may aggravate arthritis, chronic fatigue, irritable bowel syndrome and allergy headaches.*

CORNMEAL: a coarsely ground grain used in hot cereals (like porridge), breads, pancakes and muffins. For the most nutrients, choose stone-ground whole-grain corn.

    Nutrient Assets: low in gluten, with fair amounts of protein, fat and fiber. Moderate amounts of iron, calcium, magnesium, phosphorus, potassium, sodium and beta carotene. Commercial "enriched" cornmeal actually contains <u>half</u> the nutrients of whole grain cornmeal.

    Health Benefits: may prevent cancer and lower risk of heart disease and cavities.

COTTAGE CHEESE: a low-fat cultured dairy product. A good substitute for ricotta, cream cheese and processed cheeses full of chemicals. Mix with non-fat or low-fat plain yogurt to add the richness of cream or sour cream to recipes without the fat.

    Nutrient Assets: lactose levels per $1/2$ cup cottage cheese is 0.7-4. Very rich in B-2 (riboflavin); low in fat and sodium; a balanced amount of phosphorus and calcium.

Health Benefits: usually well tolerated by people with slight lactose intolerance. Low in saturated fat for a healthy heart. A good choice for bone health. Boosts immune strength and reduces colds, flu, sinusitis and ear infections. *Note: When over-consumed, all dairy foods can be mucous forming, burdening the respiratory, digestive and immune systems.*

COUSCOUS: precooked semolina, very light, low calorie, and easy and quick to fix. Works well with vegetable casseroles, as a breakfast grain and with legumes, nuts and seeds. Buy whole wheat couscous instead of prepackaged couscous for richer taste and higher nutrition.

Nutrient Assets: a good source of protein, fiber, calcium (for strong bones), magnesium, phosphorus and potassium. Easy to digest; contains lactobacillus which aids digestion of complex carbohydrates.

Health Benefits: helps detox the liver and also supports heart health. A strengthening grain especially good for recovery from illness, stress relief and boosting energy.

CRANBERRY: a tangy, acidic fruit. Look for ones that are plump, firm and a rich red color. Use cranberries to make desserts, jam, jelly, pies, cranberry sauce or relish.

Nutrient Assets: low in calories, an excellent source of fiber, bioflavonoids, vitamin C and potassium. Contains a natural benzoyl peroxide *(vacciniin)* helpful for acne.

Health Benefits: a powerful healing food, cranberries have anti-cancer, anti-infective and immune stimulating qualities. An effective remedy for bladder infections, cranberries actually neutralize harmful *E. coli* bacteria, which cause most bladder infections, before it can spread! A high bioflavonoid food ideal for fighting off colds and flu. *Vacciniin* in cranberries prevents acne-causing bacteria from entering the skin (less breakouts, less severe breakouts). Cranberries reduce risk of gum disease and kidney stones. Also dilate the bronchial tubes — beneficial during an asthma attack.

CREAM OF TARTAR: tartaric acid is derived from fermented grape juice, used as a leavening in baking, and to incorporate air into egg whites. (Substitute $\frac{1}{2}$ tsp. cream of tartar and $\frac{1}{2}$ tsp. baking soda for 1 tsp. baking powder.) Also use to clean copper cookware.

Nutrient Assets: contains calcium, potassium, iron, magnesium, phosphorus, zinc, copper, sodium and manganese.

Health Benefits: help balance the body's pH and maintain the integrity of nerves, and kidney and adrenal glands. A high potassium food for relief of fatigue and muscle weakness.

CUCUMBER: a part of the gourd and squash families, cukes should be firm, shaped like a big pickle. Work well with lemon juice, mayonnaise, sour cream, vinegar and yogurt.

Nutrient Assets: extremely high water content, at least 95%, cucumbers are low calorie with iron, potassium, vitamin A and vitamin C. The rind is very high in vitamin A. The skin is rich in silica and chlorophyll. High in the enzyme erepsin which helps break down protein.

Health Benefits: has laxative and diuretic effects. Helps eliminate harmful substances through the kidneys. Helps dissolve kidney and bladder stones. Can destroy intestinal parasites like tape worms. High minerals in celery balance blood acidity. Celery's high potassium helps regulate blood pressure. Use celery juice to balance out high sugar from beet or carrot juice.

DASHI: a basic healing soup stock and broth used in macrobiotic and Japanese cooking. Make it by simmering a 6" piece of Kombu seaweed with 2 chopped shiitake mushrooms and 2 tsp. tamari in water. Dried bonito (fish flakes) is also regularly added.

Nutrient Assets: high in calcium, iron, potassium, magnesium, iodine, B vitamins, germanium, zinc, bromium, silica, vitamins A, E and C.

Health Benefits: helpful for people suffering from immune compromised diseases and cancer because its mushrooms and seaweed have immune stimulant, anti-cancer activity. Alkalizes and purifies the blood from the effects of a modern diet. Eating dashi regularly increases vitality, improves circulation, and fights colds and flu.

DATE SUGAR: ground up dates. Has half the sweetening power as white sugar, and is much healthier. Use as a sweet topping after removing your dish from the oven.

Nutrient Assets: fair amounts of calcium, phosphorus, boron, potassium and vitamin C with moderate protein, fat, fiber, iron, beta carotene, B-1, B-2 and B-3.

Health Benefits: traditionally used for throat and chest ailments. A gentle fiber source that will not irritate a sensitive bowel (beneficial for people with irritable bowel syndrome). The boron in date sugar strengthens bones — a lack of boron causes brittle bones. Date's boron increases steroid hormones, acting as a gentle natural estrogen therapy for menopausal women. Also an energy booster for sports stamina. Date sugar is linked to lower rates of cancers (particularly pancreatic cancer).

EGGS: one of Nature's perfectly balanced foods. Americans eat as many as 65 billion eggs every year! Try free range eggs for better flavor and broader range of essential fatty acids.

Nutrient Assets: high in amino acids, protein, B vitamins, vitamin A and E, phosphorous and iron; low in saturated fat but contains 213 mg of cholesterol per large egg. The yolk is one of the few foods that provides vitamin D for hormonal health.

Health Benefits: although eggs have been demonized as a culprit in high cholesterol, in reality eggs don't raise cholesterol in people with normal cholesterol levels. The cholesterol content of egg yolks is balanced naturally by the phosphatide content of the whites. A Harvard Nurses' Health Study shows that women who eat an egg a day do not have a higher risk for cardiovascular disease. Eggs are a nutritious choice for teenagers, athletes, the elderly and people who have demanding physical jobs. *Note: eggs cause food allergy symptoms for susceptible people.*

ESSENE BREAD: a sprouted bread of wheat and rye, with no flour, oil, sweetener, salt or leavening.

Nutrient Assets: fairly high in protein and the basic B vitamins; also provides vitamin E and plentiful minerals such as calcium, phosphorus, potassium, magnesium, iron, zinc, selenium and copper.

Health Benefits: a low sodium food — excellent for people trying to maintain healthy blood pressure levels. A building food that promotes energy and stamina, and builds muscles. Can prevent anemia. Helpful for cleaning out clogged arteries, improving hair and nail growth, and bone formation. A gentle laxative. Perfect for people on a restricted allergy diet for food intolerances or candida albicans. A staple food for people on a macrobiotic diet to curb or arrest cancer.

FARINA: finely ground cereal grains known as cream of wheat. Serve with fresh or dried fruits. Add more flavor to farina with spices like cinnamon and nutmeg.

Nutrient Assets: low-fat and low cholesterol. Contains some protein, fiber and B vitamins. Often fortified with iron for blood building.

Health Benefits: a good source of complex carbohydrates for slow calorie burning and sustained energy throughout the day. May not be a good choice for those with blood sugar disorders because it has a high glycemic index.

FAVA BEANS: similar to lima beans. Slow cook for the best results.

Nutrient Assets: contains protein (23%), iron, fiber, vitamin A, vitamin C and potassium. One cup has only 80 calories. Also contain protease inhibitors and L-dopa.

Health Benefits: a good source of protein and fiber that regulates blood sugar for Type I diabetics. Fava beans support the cardiovascular system, lower blood cholesterol and blood pressure. They reduce risk of colon or rectal cancer, diverticular disease, hemorrhoids and chronic constipation. Rich in L-dopa, an amino acid that increases dopamine levels, intimately associated with sex drive in men. A 16-ounce can has almost a therapeutic dose. *Note: some people have a genetic reaction to fava beans. Symptoms: nausea, vomiting, dizziness, anemia after eating.*

FLAX SEEDS: tiny brown seeds from the flax plant used in bread recipes, salads, casseroles, drinks and cereals. I like to add 2 TBS. ground seeds to my favorite smoothie blends. Note: while the seeds have long shelf life, flax seed meal becomes rancid within a few days.

Nutrient Assets: high in protein, omega-3 fatty acids and fiber, flax is the richest source of lignans protective against cancers of the breast and colon.

Health Benefits: helpful for rebuilding nerves and reducing the inflammation of M.S. Use as part of a nutritional program to lower cholesterol, enhance brain activity and promote regularity. High lignans and fiber in flax seed make it a good choice for diabetes prevention.

FLAX SEED OIL: a high omega-3 oil (see "Fats & Oils" page 84.)

Nutrient Assets: flax seed oil, sometimes called linseed oil, is an excellent source of unsaturated fatty acids (EFAs), and is high in calories, protein and fiber. Rich in the minerals potassium, magnesium, calcium, phosphorus and iron, and B vitamins and vitamin E. Contains eight of the essential amino acids and lecithin (for brain health).

Health Benefits: high in omega-3 oils that regulate blood pressure, lower cholesterol and triglyceride levels, and may prolong cancer survival by increasing T-cell levels. A potent detoxifier. Also makes dry brittle hair more lustrous and silky.

FRUCTOSE: a highly refined sweetener that is twice as sweet as white sugar. It is, however, absorbed more slowly into the bloodstream than sugar and does not require insulin for assimilation. (See "Sugars & Sweeteners In A Healing Diet" page 93.)

Nutrient Assets: a low nutrient carbohydrate which provides quick energy for the body.

Health Benefits: reduces fatigue (not caused from lack of sleep), lethargy, pallor, coated tongue, persistent thirstiness and bad breath. Has little effect on blood sugar levels in diabetics and does not tend to cause low blood sugar symptoms in individuals with hypoglycemia. Also prevents cravings for fatty foods — good for weight loss.

GALANGA: a root similar in appearance and taste to ginger root used as a spice for more than a thousand years. In cooking, galanga may be substituted for ginger. Best used in curries and stews. Available in Asian grocery stores.

Nutrient Assets: volatile oil and the acid resin.

Health Benefits: like ginger, galanga is exceptional for reducing nausea and settling an upset stomach. Tones tissues and can reduce fevers. The powder can be used as a snuff for catarrh.

GARBANZO BEANS: (also called chickpeas), meaty, high protein beans. They take a long time to cook, but are excellent in dips and authentic falafels. (For more, see "Protein in a Healing Diet" page 40.) See page 487 of this document.

GHEE: a golden oil that results when white milk solids are removed from melted butter. Also called clarified butter. Considered the best oil in Ayurveda.

Nutrient Assets: high in fat.

Health Benefits: a good food choice in the Ayurvedic tradition for vata body types. A wholesome food included in Rasayana body purification diets.

GOMASHIO: a mixture of sesame seeds and sea salt. Originally only used in Asian cooking, it is a delicious low sodium alternative to table salt, and a good cooking and baking salt.

Nutrient Assets: gomashio is high in minerals and amino acids (the building blocks of protein-important for growth and healing).

Health Benefits: used in macrobiotic diets for hepatitis and illness recovery.

GRAPEFRUITS: a hybrid cross between the pumello and orange.

Nutrient Assets: contain a fair amount of potassium and are very low in sodium. The pulp is very high in vitamin C and a soluble fiber called galacturonic acid. The fresh fruit is high in salicylic acid which helps dissolve inorganic calcium linked to arthritis.

Health Benefits: powerful medicine for the heart, grapefruit's fiber can both lower "bad" (LDL) cholesterol levels and raise "good" (HDL) cholesterol. Grapefruit may even help dissolve plaque already clogging your arteries, possibly reversing atherosclerosis and preventing a heart attack. Counteracts the effects of a high fat diet. Improves the health of the blood by promoting the elimination of old red blood cells from the body. Use the pulp topically to speed wound healing. *Note: Not recommended for children who suffer from epileptic seizures or chronic migraines, as it may aggravate their symptoms. Should not be used in combination with many medications because it can affect their metabolism and cause adverse reactions. Ask your physician.*

HEARTS OF PALM: the edible inner portion of the stem of the cabbage palm tree. Ivory colored with a flavor similar to the artichoke.

Nutrient Assets: low in calories —1 cup has 21 calories. High in vitamin A.

Health Benefits: its vitamin A content helps prevent infectious disease, particularly viral infections such as AIDS. Also aids skin disorders like acne and psoriasis, and may play a role in cancer and cardiovascular disease prevention. Its vitamin A content also boosts immune response, growth and development, strengthens the retina and even improves dry-eye disorder.

HOISIN SAUCE: a thick reddish brown sweet and spicy sauce used in Chinese cuisine. Contains soybeans, garlic, chili peppers and spices.

Nutrient Assets: see soybeans, garlic and chili peppers listings for more information.

Health Benefits: a healthy seasoning choice for people with heart disease because its garlic and chili peppers content can clear the arteries and boost circulation. In addition, may help lower high cholesterol.

HOMINY: white or yellow corn kernels with the hull and germ removed mechanically or by soaking in slaked lime.

Nutrient Assets: high in protein, calcium, iron, magnesium, phosphorus, potassium, sodium, zinc, copper, manganese, vitamin A, B-vitamins and vitamin C. An enzyme-rich food, high in fiber that is easy to digest. Contains protease inhibitors.

Health Benefits: a building food for bone and muscle, and an excellent food for brain and nervous system health. High in protease inhibitors that help protect against colon, breast and prostate cancer. May also lower the risk of heart disease and fight cavities. A good food for menopausal women because it boosts estrogen production.

HONEY: a mixture of sugars formed from bee nectar by the enzyme invertase.

Nutrient Assets: naturally about 38% fructose, 31% glucose, 18% water, 9% other sugars and 2% sucrose.

Health Benefits: a natural sweetener with bioactive, antibiotic and antiseptic properties, honey contains all the vitamins, minerals and enzymes necessary for proper metabolism and digestion of glucose and other sugars. Helps reduce indigestion, respiratory problems and can be used as a gentle antiseptic for the skin. Still, honey is almost twice as sweet as sugar. Avoid it if you have candidiasis or diabetes; use it with great care if you are hypoglycemic.

JICAMA: a beet shaped root vegetable with crisp white flesh. Fresh tasting, it retains its crispiness even when cooked. Add to salads, salsas, stir frys or veggie platters.

Nutrient Assets: contains protein, potassium, iron, calcium and vitamins A, B complex and C. (A three and a half ounce serving of jicama provides about 25% of the recommended daily allowance (RDA) for vitamin C.) Low in calories.

Health Benefits: jicama helps a weight loss diet; it is low in fat, high in fiber and offers the crunch people love. Helps eliminate water retention; good for PMS or hot weather edema.

KALE: a dark green leafy vegetable best known today for its role in protecting against eye diseases like macular degeneration.

Nutrient Assets: high in vitamins C and E, folic acid, beta carotene, lutein and zeaxanthin, calcium, magnesium and essential fatty acids.

Health Benefits: like other dark green leafy vegetables, kale offers a powerhouse of healing for America's nutrient-starved bodies. Tufts University studies say kale is the most antioxidant-rich land vegetable available. Kale is an intestinal sweeper that promotes regularity and helps rid the body of toxins. It's an excellent blood builder for illness recovery and chronic fatigue. Its lutein and zeaxanthine are specific for eye health, reducing risk for macular degeneration in clinical studies. Kale is also a good choice for people with or at risk for cataracts.

KASHI: a delicious 7 grain pilaf mix, available as a puffed cold cereal, or cooked as a grain base for almost any rice or pasta type dish.

Nutrient Assets: an excellent source of protein, complex carbohydrates and fiber.

Health Benefits: a good choice in a diet to help lower cholesterol and manage blood sugar problems like diabetes.

KEFIR: kefir or yogurt as its commonly called is a fermented milk product. It comes plain or fruit-flavored, and may be taken as a liquid or used like yogurt.

Nutrient Assets: contains calcium, protein, vitamin B-3, B-6, folic acid, the enzyme lactase and sometimes *L. acidophilus* (a probiotic). High lactic acid in kefir enhances the absorption of minerals like calcium.

Health Benefits: kefir with *L. acidophilus* stimulates interferon, a natural antiviral that fights off allergic reactions and cancers such as leukemia. Calcium-rich kefir also reduces the risk of endometrial cancer and osteoporosis. Eating kefir for three months during allergy or cold seasons fights hay fever and colds. Kefir helps protect the stomach lining against cigarette smoke and alcohol; a good choice against diarrhea as it boosts the growth of friendly bacteria in the intestines. Helps lower LDL ("bad") cholesterol and raise HDL ("good") cholesterol.

KEFIR CHEESE: a delicious fermented milk product with the consistency of sour cream. I like it better than sour cream for cooking, dips and sauces. *Note: kefir cheese is more perishable than other cheeses.* (See "Cultured Foods" page 57.)

KIWI FRUIT: a tangy, citrusy fruit; the most nutrient-rich of the top 26 fruits consumed in the world today.

Nutrient Assets: low in fat and calories; high in vitamin C, E, chlorophyll, folic acid, inositol, pantothenic acid, fiber, amino acids, potassium (contains more than bananas), and magnesium. Kiwis offer serotonin, plentiful antioxidants, carotenoids (including lutein), flavonoids and phenolics. Contains copper and manganese, both deficient in American diets.

Health Benefits: a nutritional powerhouse that may help prevent heart disease and cancer. Used in TCM to treat breast and stomach cancer. Inhibits animal melanoma cell lines. Its B vitamins and serotonin can help invigorate the brain and manage depression symptoms. High fiber in the fruit detoxifies carcinogens in the intestinal tract before they re-poison the body. High potassium and low sodium in kiwi fruit may even normalize high blood pressure. An anti-aging food that also increases energy.

LECITHIN: a soy derived granular product used as a natural emulsifier for smoothness. It may be substituted for $^1/_3$ of the oil in recipes for a healing diet. A therapeutic food, add 2 teasp. daily to recipes for superior phosphatides, choline, inositol, potassium and linoleic acid.

Nutrient Assets: consists of 15% saturated fat, 11% monounsaturated fat and 45% polyunsaturated fat. Provides choline and inositol, vital for brain and liver health. Just add granules to cereals or yogurts.

Health Benefits: stimulates fat metabolism by the liver and helps the brain convert choline into acetylcholine, necessary for memory, mood and muscle control. May boost adrenals and hormonal health by increasing absorption of vitamins A, D, E and K. Lecithin helps a diet program to lower cholesterol (actually prevents cholesterol from attaching to blood vessel walls and may remove deposits already there). Improves dry skin conditions like psoriasis and reduces brown skin spots. Strengthens the gallbladder. May promote recovery from Multiple Sclerosis by repairing the myelin surrounding damaged MS nerves. May benefit viral infections like herpes and AIDS.

LEMONS, LIMES: used mostly to flavor low calorie dressings, drinks and spreads.

Nutrient Assets: contain high amounts of potassium and vitamin C, bioflavonoids, traces of the B vitamins and minerals, and phytonutrient liminoids (in rinds and seeds).

Health Benefits: tonics for sore throats (especially in hot drinks), soothing for sunburns, effective as cures for hiccups and as remedies for colds and coughs. Stimulate the liver and gall bladder to release toxins and sediment. D-Limonene (a liminoid) in lemons and limes helps dissolve gallstones and has anticancer properties (boosts production of enzymes that deactivate carcinogens). Use the juice externally to wear away warts and corns, destroy harmful bacteria in cuts and infections, and relieve poison ivy. Can be used in shampoos to lighten the hair. A good astringent for oily skin.

MANGOES: A tropical fruit that can be eaten by itself, in salsas and fruit smoothies. Formerly a stranger to U.S. crops, mangoes are now being produced in the U.S. bringing down their cost and increasing their availability.

Nutrient Assets: the best fruit source of cancer-fighting carotenoids including beta carotene. A good source of vitamins C and E, potassium and fiber.

Health Benefits: help promote acid/alkaline balance and strengthen the kidneys. A rich carotenoid fruit to add to your anti-cancer arsenal. A good high fiber choice for cholesterol lowering. Used as a disinfectant for clogged pores and cysts, and for clearing excess heat.

MATZO MEAL: fine crumbs of unleavened bread used as a soup thickener, in Jewish Passover cakes, to thicken soups and as a substitute for flour or bread crumbs.

Nutrient Assets: contains protein, calcium, iron, magnesium, phosphorus, potassium, sodium, zinc, copper, manganese, selenium, B-vitamins and vitamin E. Whole wheat matzo meal contains some barium and vanadium (essential for a healthy heart).

Health Benefits: a high fiber food that prevents constipation. Whole wheat matzo meal promotes liver detoxification. A good source of complex carbohydrates for high energy. Especially beneficial for growing children and underweight people.

MESCLUN: a mix of young, small salad greens that often include arugula, dandelion, frisee, mizuna, oak leaf, mache, radicchio and sorrel.

Nutrient Assets: contains vitamin C, glutathione, and high amounts of iron, calcium and chlorophyll. A rich source of beta carotene, lutein and other carotenoids.

Health Benefits: high calcium in mesclun strengthens bones; high chlorophyll keeps the system flushed, alkaline, and neutralizes toxins linked to degenerative disease. High carotenoids in mesclun are especially useful for cancer protection (particularly stomach, lung, esophagus, colon, rectum and bladder cancers) and to prevent eye diseases like cataracts and macular degeneration. Dandelion greens in mesclun give it blood and lymph cleansing properties.

MILLET: a quick-cooking, balanced amino acid grain.

    Nutrient Assets: a complete protein grain, rich in fiber (about 15%) and silica. Especially high in iron, magnesium, potassium and has a great balance of amino acids.

    Health Benefits: an easy-to-digest, gluten-free food, millet is an excellent choice for those with wheat allergies. An anti-fungal against candida infection. A rich source of fiber and non-meat protein, it is also a good choice for heart disease and cancer protection. Millet warms the body and is a very useful food for those who live in cold climates or who have poor circulation.

MISO: a fermented salty paste made from cooked aged soybeans and grains like wheat, rice or barley. Miso is a tasty base for soups, sauces, dressings, dips, spreads and cooking stock, and is a healthy substitute for salt or soy sauce.

    Nutrient Assets: very high in protein; fairly high in sodium (benefits from soybeans and healing enzymes outweigh the effects of high sodium when used in moderation). Rich in enzymes and phytoestrogens *(genistein)*. Also contains *zybiocolin*, a binding agent. *Note: unpasteurized miso is preferred for a healing diet, since beneficial bacteria and other enzymes, as well as flavor, are still intact. Check in your health food store.*

    Health Benefits: promotes easy digestion and alkalizes the body. Miso's phytoestrogens help counteract cancer-promoting estrogen against breast cancer. May also protect against prostate and stomach cancer. Japanese research shows that a bowl of miso soup daily lowers the risk of stomach cancer by one-third. Miso's *zybiocolin* binds to and eliminates radioactive substances from the body. Also helps neutralize carcinogens from smoking and establishes an immune-enhancing environment.

MOCHI: a chewy, unleavened rice "bread" made from sweet brown rice. Can be used as big croutons in soup, or as a crispy casserole topping. Available today in many flavors like garlic, sesame, plain, cinnamon-raisin, and mugwort.

    Nutrient Assets: high nutrient profile with protein, B-vitamins, including B-12, magnesium, manganese, potassium, iron, zinc, phosphorus, protease inhibitors, copper and calcium.

    Health Benefits: warming and strengthening, good for a recovering body. Mochi works as an antacid, calms the central nervous system, relieves mental stress and strengthens the internal organs. Mochi may even help clear up skin conditions such as acne and psoriasis.

MOLASSES: (blackstrap, unsulphured)- a by-product of the sugar refining process used to sweeten recipes or as a topping on muffins or pancakes.

    Nutrient Assets: plentiful mineral content, particularly high in iron and potassium. The blackstrap variety also contains more calcium ounce for ounce than milk, more iron than eggs, plentiful B vitamins, vitamin E, zinc and is 50% sucrose.

    Health Benefits: 2 TBS daily improve hair growth and color in about 3 months.

MUSHROOMS, WILD (culinary)

    —**Cepe (Porcini):** a rich, meaty mushroom for soups, stews and stuffings.

    Nutrient Assets: contains eight essential amino acids and polysaccharides.

    Health Benefits: anti-tumor properties when given to animals. An immune booster, also used in TCM formulas to relieve muscular pain and leukorrhea.

—**Chanterelle:** golden, trumpet-shaped mushrooms with a light delicate flavor. They are most often used in French and gourmet sauces, or as a special vegetable delicacy.

Nutrient Assets: contains eight essential amino acids and vitamin A.

Health Benefits: a good food choice to strengthen the eyes and prevent night blindness. Benefits dry skin, tones mucous membranes and may boost immunity against respiratory infections. Also has tumor inhibiting properties.

—**Enoki:** tender tiny mushrooms with long slender crunchy stems; delicious barely heated. *Note: do not eat raw regularly - contains a cardiotoxic substance which is sensitive to heat.*

Nutrient Assets: contain phosphorous, iron, fiber, riboflavin and vitamin D.

Health Benefits: anti-cancer in animals tests. May offer protection against liver disease and gastric ulcers. Its lysine is reported to cause increases in weight and stature.

—**Morel:** brown, spongy mushrooms with deep, rich flavor. They go especially well with egg dishes and omelettes, and broiled poultry.

Nutrient Assets: seven amino acids and the sterol *brassicasterol.*

Health Benefits: used in TCM to increase "Qi", reduce mucous congestion and tonify the gastrointestinal tract.

—**Oyster:** fan-shaped pale mushrooms with a delicate flavor like oysters.

Nutrient Assets: contains high protein and minerals, eight essential amino acids, B vitamins and plentiful essential fatty acids.

Health Benefits: used in TCM to strengthen veins and as a mild muscle relaxant. Inhibits cancer in animal tests. Lowers triglycerides, VLDLs (very low density lipoprotein) and total cholesterol. Counteracts toxic effect of excess alcohol on triglyceride levels and liver in animal tests. High iron in the mushroom helps build the blood.

—**Shiitake:** large, dark brown fountain-shaped mushroom with a rich, succulent flavor. An excellent addition to miso broths, brown rice casseroles or Asian recipes. Usually sold dry, just soak in water until soft then remove woody stems and sliver into dressings, soups and salads. Use just a few each time; a little goes a long way.

Nutrient Assets: contains LEM, vitamins, minerals, amino acids, polysaccharides and abundant in nutrients such as potassium, phosphorus, magnesium, calcium, sulphur. Its polysaccharide compounds, lentinan and lentinula have been widely studied for antitumor and immune stimulating properties.

Health Benefits: a tonic mushroom useful for system weakness, general debility and immune defense. At least two different extracts from the mushroom act as immune system stimulators and possess antiviral activities - LEM, an extract from immature shiitake's, and Lentinan, an extract from the mushroom's fruit body. Shiitake mushrooms have very precise activity on immune response: they stimulate the immune system powerhouses, the macrophages and NK (natural killer) cells to act more quickly and aggressively against invading pathogens; they combat existing infections; and they increase antibody production and interferon for greater disease resistance. A compound in shiitake, called eritadenine, lowers serum cholesterol by as much as 45 percent. Also shows healing results against hypertension, cataracts, anemia and immune compromised diseases like Chronic Fatigue, encephalitis, cancer and viral infections like HIV. Shiitake protect the liver, and may even assist the body in making antibodies to Hepatitis B. *Note: In large amounts, may cause diarrhea or skin rash. Consult with your physician if you are taking blood thinners, shiitake has mild anti-clotting properties.*

OATS and OAT BRAN: an excellent fiber grain source to help lower cholesterol and promote regularity. A good addition to any grain or flour mix, but lower in gluten than wheat, so not very effective as a substitute for wheat flour to make cookies or cakes.

Nutrient Assets: low calories, rich carbohydrates for energy, amino acids, B vitamins, vitamin E, and many minerals including calcium, silicon, magnesium and potassium.

Health Benefits: lowers cholesterol and reduces heart disease risk. A good choice to help wean diabetics from insulin therapy. Can be included in small amounts for celiac disease patients who are in remission. Helps promote production of serotonin to elevate mood and reduce depression. A warming food helpful for poor circulation or for those who live in cold areas. Can help boost thyroid activity for hypothyroidism. High silicon strengthens bones and beautifies the skin. Used externally in a poultice, oats can reduce inflammation from eczema, psoriasis or poison oak.

OILS, NATURAL VEGETABLE: these should be unrefined, either cold or expeller pressed, and stored in the refrigerator after opening.

Nutrient Assets: natural oils provide vitamins A, E, lecithin and essential fatty acids. Use olive oil in salads, Italian and Middle Eastern cooking for its superior flavor and poly and mono-unsaturated fat composition. For other uses, use canola oil, or a blend of pressed oils - like a mix of safflower, peanut and soy, with sesame seed oil for flavor. (See "Fats and Oils" page 72.)

—**Avocado Oil:** a rich, sweet oil for salad dressings and grilled greens.

Nutrient Assets: vitamin E, high in monounsaturated fatty acids.

Health Benefits: helps decrease "bad" LDL cholesterol while increasing "good" HDL cholesterol. Protective against heart disease with antioxidant properties to guard against early aging and free radical damage. Used as a moisturizer in many skin care products.

—**Coconut Oil:** one of the most stable oils known, with a shelf life of 18 months. A great cooking oil. At room temperature, coconut oil becomes solid like butter and can be used in place of butter in recipes. (Use $^3/_4$ the amount to obtain the same results).

Nutrient Assets: over 90% saturated fatty acids, 7% oleic acid (MUFA) and 2.5% (PUFA). A rich plant source of anti-infective lauric acid (accounts for 50% of its fatty acid profile). Also contains antifungal *caprylic acid,* and in small amounts, vitamin E.

Health Benefits: medium chain saturates in coconut oil provide energy and do not clog arteries (as was once speculated) like the long chain group do. Used in capsule formulas against candida albicans overgrowth for its caprylic acid. (Don't use if you have ulcerative colitis.) May help reduce viral load in HIV-AIDS. Coconut oil is converted into *monolaurin* in the body which can kill many pathogens like herpes, influenza and pneumonia, and bacteria like *staphylococcus aureus and streptococcus agalactiae.* A good choice for dieters and body builders, coconut oil's medium chain fatty acids stimulate fat metabolism and increase energy. It is also useful for massage, dry skin and hair. *Note: over 40 years ago, diet studies falsely concluded coconut oil raised blood cholesterol. Today, we know that coconut oil has a neutral effect on blood cholesterol.*

—**Corn Oil:** a rich, buttery-flavored oil for baking, sautéing and salad dressings.

Nutrient Assets: high in polyunsaturated fats. Contains some vitamin E.

Health Benefits: used by some manufacturers in capsules as a carrier for vitamins or other supplements. Research shows corn oil frequently contains MSG, a food additive linked to migraines, seizures, even brain degeneration in some studies.

—**Olive Oil:** 1) *Extra Virgin* - from the first pressing, with no additives; highest quality; best flavor and aroma. 2) *Fine Virgin* - good flavor, no additives, but with higher acid content. 3) *Plain Virgin* - slightly off flavor and the highest acidity. 4) *Pure* - from the second pressing, with additives to mellow bitter taste; includes pulp, pit and skin. Include olive oil to add flavor and energy to vegetable sautés, salads and pasta dishes.

Nutrient Assets: high in calories and fatty acids, especially monounsaturated (Omega 9) oleic acid (75%). Also contains vitamin E.

Health Benefits: easy to digest; a nerve tonic; especially helpful for liver and gallbladder problems. A mild laxative, gentle enough for children to use in small quantities. A good choice to help dissolve cholesterol deposits and lower blood pressure. Recent animal studies reveal olive oil may also reduce risk for colon cancer.

—**Palm Kernal Oil:** used mainly in nondairy creamer, candies, dressings and dips.

Nutrient Assets: saturated, with few essential fatty acids.

Health Benefits: avoid in a healing diet; high in saturated fats and low in nutrients.

—**Peanut Oil:** okay for stir-frying at high temperatures to seal in juices and nutrients.

Nutrient Assets: high in monounsaturated fats. Also contains small amounts of calcium, iron, vitamin E, potassium and magnesium.

Health Benefits: a study at Pennsylvania State University reveals that adding peanut oil to the regular diet may lower total cholesterol by 10% and "bad" LDL cholesterol by 14%. Monounsaturated fats in peanut oil improve the liver's ability to remove excess cholesterol from the blood so it won't clog your arteries.

—**Safflower Oil:** light and mild; excellent for sautéing and baking. Used mainly in salad oils, shortenings and margarine.

Nutrient Assets: highest in polyunsaturated fats and lowest in saturated fats of all commercial fats and oils.

Health Benefits: a good choice in moderation in a diet to lower cholesterol and reduce heart disease risk.

—**Sesame Oil:** from toasted sesame seeds; used to flavor Chinese and Middle Eastern dishes.

Nutrient Assets: high in poly and monounsaturated fats, contains the natural antioxidant sesamol, and lecithin.

Health Benefits: used in cosmetics as a softener and to soothe troubled skin. Used in TCM to treat constipation, tinnitus and dizziness. A brain food that may help relieve depression. *Note: not recommended if there is diarrhea.*

—**Soy Oil:** a mild, light oil used in dressings and for vegetables or sautéing greens.

Nutrient Assets: high polyunsaturated fats, low in saturated fats, cholesterol-free.

Health Benefits: use in moderation in a healthy diet; soy oil does not retain the cholesterol-lowering or breast cancer preventing effects of soybeans, soy milk, tofu, soy protein or tempeh. *Note: may contain GMOs (genetically modified organisms), a growing health and environmental concern for many consumers.*

—**Sunflower Oil:** delicate - good for stir-frys, salads, dressings, light cooking.

Nutrient Assets: high in polyunsaturated fats, low in saturated fats.

Health Benefits: has a long tradition of use by naturopaths to boost disease resistance and encourage the growth of healthy tissue. May be useful for multiple sclerosis, and to improve endocrine and nervous system health.

—**Walnut Oil:** a robust oil with a distinctive flavor; blend with lighter oils for baking; nice in vinaigrette dressings and other vegetables dishes.

Nutrient Assets: high in polyunsaturated fats.

Health Benefits: a good plant source of heart healthy Omega-3 fatty acids, now proven to help diabetic neuropathy. Toning, hydrating and smoothing properties make walnut oil an excellent addition to anti-wrinkle creams, massage oils and lip balms.

OLIVES: purple black, Greek olives are a good choice for bold spicy flavor anywhere.

Nutrient Assets: contain vitamin A (beta-carotene), iron and calcium. Also have a glycoside, *oleuropein,* for vast antiviral and antimicrobial activity, and the bioflavonoid *quercetin.*

Health Benefits: *oleuropein* is a potent antioxidant and antimicrobial to aid in disease protection. In animal studies, olive leaf helps lower blood pressure and dilates coronary blood vessels for improved blood flow. (For more, see olive leaf under the herbal section of this digest.)

ONION: a bulb root vegetable related to garlic. The most popular vegetable in America next to the potato. Adds flavor to almost any dish.

Nutrient Assets: contains beta carotene, vitamin A, B1, B2 and C. Also offers organosulfur compounds responsible for its sharp flavor and odor.

Health Benefits: reduces blood pressure and asthma attacks. One German study shows drinking onion juice reduces asthma attacks by 50%! Tufts research reveals that yellow or white onion juice can raise heart protective HDL cholesterol 30% over time. Like garlic, onion is a good infection fighter particularly when used regularly in tonic broths. High sulphur in onion is useful for body cleansing, particularly if there is heavy metal toxicity or parasite infection. Decreases blood clotting. When eaten raw, onion even kills the bacteria that causes tooth decay.

ORANGES: the sweet orange is most common. The best oranges are deep orange, heavy and firm with a sweet smell. Avoid oranges with thick, bumpy skin.

Nutrient Assets: ultra-low in sodium and fat, oranges contain 20 antioxidants from the carotenoid family, terpenes, limonoids and flavonoids (natural cancer inhibitors). Oranges are also rich in vitamin C, beta carotene, calcium, magnesium, phosphorus and potassium.

Health Benefits: oranges aid constipation, migraines, epilepsy (in children) and lung cancer. Oranges may prevent cataracts through their high vitamin C. Their vitamin C may also help ward off asthma attacks, bronchitis, breast cancer, atherosclerosis and gum disease. Oranges may boost fertility and healthy sperm count in men. Orange juice may even protect sperm from radiation damage. Oranges alkalize the body and aid digestion.

PAPAYAS: a sweet tropical fruit best known for its high content of papain, a protein-digesting protease enzyme. Hawaiian papayas are best for flavor. Work well with kiwi and mango in tropical fruit salads. Papaya juice is also widely available today.

Nutrient Assets: high in beta carotene, potassium, vitamin C, fiber and papain.

Health Benefits: an anti-inflammatory food specific for arthritic pain and hayfever. A good choice to improve protein digestion, and reduce gas and heartburn problems. Benefit hair, skin, eyes and nails. A good food addition to an overall body detox. Applied topically, the juice has been used with success to reduce freckling.

PASTA: versatile, whole grain, vegetable, low-fat, low calorie, quick and easy to make, compatible with Oriental, Italian, modified macrobiotic, and healthy diets. We use Japanese noodles made from buckwheat (Soba), whole wheat (Udon and Somen), rice (Rice Sticks and Saifun), and combination grain ramens.

Nutrient Assets: low in fat and sodium, high complex carbohydrate Italian pastas include sesame, spinach, artichoke, and soy, in all sorts of shapes and sizes.

Health Benefits: an energizing food for athletes, bodybuilders and those who live stressful, demanding lives. Whole grain pasta stabilizes blood sugar levels for diabetics.

PINE NUTS: from Mediterranean pine cones, they have a sweet, delicate flavor used in appetizers, pestos and stuffing dishes.

Nutrient Assets: high in protein and carbohydrates. Also contains some phosphorous, iron and B complex.

Health Benefits: an excellent protein source for vegetarians.

QUINOA: an ancient Incan supergrain. Light, flavorful, use like rice or millet.

Nutrient Assets: contains complete protein from amino acids (twice the protein of other grains), complex carbohydrates, calcium, iron, phosphorous and vitamin E.

Health Benefits: a food choice for recovering from an illness because it offers high energy carbohydrates, protein for healing and is easy on the digestive system. Gluten-free, it is an acceptable choice for those with candida albicans or who may be sensitive to wheat products. Used traditionally by Peruvian Indians to promote lactation.

RED GRAPES: a seasonal fruit especially good in fruit salads and with low fat cheeses and crackers. Used to make the red wine that many people enjoy with dinner.

Nutrients Assets: a nutraceutical powerhouse high in antioxidant poly-phenols, ellagic acid, resveratrol, tartaric acid and fiber.

Health Benefits: Grapes cool and rehydrate the body — good during summer or for people involved in strenuous sports or exercise. A good cleansing food that benefits the digestive tract, liver, kidneys and blood. Many researchers credit the red grapes used in making wine with the "French Paradox," because Europeans who eat a high fat diet, but drink a lot of red wine still have lower heart disease rates than Americans.

RICE SYRUP: a subtle sweetener, this syrup and malt syrup come in many different consistencies and flavors, easily digestible, with slow, steady energy-producing complex carbohydrates. (For more, see "Sugar & Sweeteners in a Healing Diet" page 91.)

SALMON: today, salmon is farm-raised so we don't have to worry about endangerment as we do with swordfish. Salmon is excellent poached, grilled or lightly smoked.

Nutrient Assets: high omega 3 fatty acids EPA (eicosapentaenoic acid) and DHA (docosahexaenoic acid), vitamin E, calcium, iodine, potassium, magnesium, and zinc.

Health Benefits: a specific for heart health, helps lower cholesterol, and reduces blood pressure and trigylcerides. A libido-nourishing food for women after menopause. Reduces fluid retention. A good choice for brain function and memory enhancement. Because it's high in iodine, salmon 2 to 3 times a week may help enhance thyroid and metabolic balance, too.

SEA SALT: comes from coastal marshes and basins where seawater evaporates naturally.

Nutrient Assets: very high in magnesium; also contains calcium, sulphur, potassium and bromides. Unrefined sea salt is better than salt for health; use in moderation.

Health Benefits: a better choice for health than refined table salt because it is higher in trace minerals and has a better balance of sodium and potassium.

SEEDS: seeds are good sources of protein and minerals. Sesame, sunflower and pumpkin seeds can be used for health benefits in cereal mixes, salads, dips, spreads, grain mixes for pilaf and veggie burgers, and as toppings. Most nuts and seeds are high in fat, but they contain mono or polyunsaturated fats that are actually helpful in lowering cholesterol, and abundance of EFAs to support heart, brain and skin health.

SHALLOTS: small, mild flavored, onion-like bulbs; a member of the allium family.

Nutrient Assets: organosulfur compounds.

Health Benefits: like garlic and onions, shallots can help dissolve blood clots and balance cholesterol, but are milder in action. A gentle immune stimulant that can protect against free radical damage and cancer development.

SOY BEANS: a low fat, nutritive legume.

Nutrient Assets: high in protein and a good source of iron for blood building, soybeans contain the full spectrum of amino acids and are especially high in the amino acid, lysine. Rich in plant hormones (*genistein, diadzein, isoflavonoids and lignans*) that balance estrogen levels in postmenopausal women. Also contain *saponins, isoflavones and phytosterols* for cancer prevention.

Health Benefits: over 50 soy studies show that 25g of soy protein a day can lower cholesterol 10% and reduce heart disease risk by 20%. Soybeans help reduce breast and prostate cancer risk. Eating phytohormone-rich soy foods regularly lengthens the menstrual cycle 2-3 days, reducing excess estrogen surges linked to cancer. Calcium-rich soy foods can reduce hot flashes during menopause, and may help retain bone mass in menopausal women at risk for osteoporosis. But, eating more than 4 large servings a day of soy based foods may disrupt thyroid activity in people who are hypothyroid. Soybeans also contain trypsin inhibitors which create gas and bloating for many people. Cooking soy reduces this effect. Too much soy can also cause the body to excrete important minerals. A little soy within a balanced diet poses no risks.

SOY MILK and SOY CHEESE: soy products that can be used in place of milk and cheese for those who are lactose intolerant or who want to avoid dairy. For more, see "Soy Foods & Cultured Foods for Normalizing Probiotics," on pg. 54.

SPELT: a very low gluten grain related to wheat. A good substitute for wheat and wheat flour in baking.

Nutrient Assets: high in protein and fiber. Also contains iron, potassium, phosphorous, sodium and traces of the B vitamins.

Health Benefits: a good choice for body strengthening in a healing program for those with food allergies (especially gluten sensitivity), Irritable Bowel Syndrome or Candida albicans because it is easily digested and assimilated.

SPINACH: a dark green leafy vegetable ideal for salads, in veggie wraps and cooked in casseroles or by itself.

Nutrient Assets: rich in beneficial essential fatty acids; high in vitamin C, iron, folic acid, beta and other carotenes, lutein and zeaxanthin.

Health Benefits: an intestinal cleanser that helps relieve constipation. A food for the eyes that improves vision and helps reduce risk of macular degeneration 45%. High iron and chlorophyll in spinach are ideal for blood building. An anti-cancer food that may cut risk of lung cancer in half, even in smokers. *Note: overcooking spinach can cause inorganic oxalic acid to form that may lead to calcium deficiency. Just steam cook.*

SPROUTS: delicious, highly nutritious, inexpensive foods. Easy to grow in a sprouting jar or trays at home. Mix different kinds to your own personal taste. Sprouts enhance almost any recipe. Use organic seeds for the best results.

Nutrient Assets: sprouts are a wonderful source of protein in the form of amino acids, chlorophyll, enzymes and plant hormones. They are good sources of vitamins A, C, B, and E, with balanced minerals and trace minerals. Very low in calories.

Health Benefits: sprouts boost energy and reduce stress; are hydrating and enzyme-rich for improved digestion. Sprouts boost immunity and prevent cancer. Used in TCM to tonify the body, accelerate waste release, and reduce inflammation and rheumatism. Should be included in a libido-boosting diet as a source of high quality vitamin E.

My favorite sprouts for healing recipes:

Alfalfa sprouts- use alone as an excellent fresh protein source, or in a sprout mix in salads, with radish, clover and sunflower sprouts, for more crunch and tang.

Mung Bean Sprouts- mild, crunchy sprouts good in salads and stir-fries. Steam slightly first when using raw to enhance the flavor and tenderness.

Radish Sprout- have a tangy, spicy taste with therapeutic, cleansing properties.

Red Clover Sprouts- like light, sweet alfalfa sprouts, they have therapeutic properties, and are delicious as part of a sprout mix in sandwiches and salads.

Sunflower Sprouts- excellent in stir-fries; longer freshness than mung bean sprouts.

STRAWBERRIES: a sweet seasonal berry. In addition to taste enjoyment, strawberries clean your teeth and freshen your breath after a meal.

Nutrient Assets: high in potassium, ellagic acid, vitamin C, folic acid and beta carotene. Also contains traces of the B vitamins and vitamin E.

Health Benefits: Harvard research shows strawberry lovers are 70% less likely to develop cancer (probably as a result of rich, anti-cancer ellagic acid). Especially useful for skin blemishes caused by blood toxicity. A quick source of energy that is easily digested.

SUNCHOKE: (Jerusalem Artichoke) a variety of sunflower with a lumpy brown tuber. Flesh is nutty, sweet and crunchy. Can be eaten raw, in salads or seafood recipes.

Nutrient Assets: low in calories, contains iron, phosphorous, FOS (fructo-oligosaccharides) and B-complex.

Health Benefits: promotes colon health by stimulating growth of friendly intestinal flora. A gentle body balancer.

TAHINI: ground sesame butter; used in healthy candies and cookies, and on toast in place of peanut butter, or as a dairy replacement in soups, dressings or sauces.
> **Nutrient Assets:** low in fat, no cholesterol, rich protein.
> **Health Benefits:** good in a healing program for a creamy flavor without a lot of fat.

TAMARI: a wheat-free soy sauce made by a water extraction of soybeans, grains, water and salt. Add to Asian stir fries, chow mein and chop suey dishes.
> **Nutrient Assets:** lower in sodium and richer in flavor than soy sauce. Bragg's Liquid Aminos, a wonderful energizing protein broth, is also of the tamari family, but unfermented, lower in sodium, and with 8 essential amino acids.
> **Health Benefits:** better than soy sauce in a healing diet because of lower sodium. *Note: read labels. Some tamari has MSG, linked to headaches, visual disturbances and seizures.*

TAPIOCA: a sweet sun-dried starch made by crushing cassava roots with water. The starch is separated, dried, crumbled in a sieve, and tumbled in barrels to form round, gelatin pearls.
> **Nutrient Assets:** a natural thickener in cooking, or a dessert favorite with children.
> **Health Benefits:** easily digested in the elderly and small children.

TEMPEH: a meaty Indonesian fermented soy food with a robust texture and mushroom-like aroma. Offers the texture and richness of meat without health risks.
> **Nutrient Assets:** complete protein and all the essential amino acids.
> **Health Benefits:** tempeh is a pre-digested food (due to enzyme action of the culture process); its nutrients are highly absorbable. (See "Cultured Foods for Probiotics" page 54.)

TOFU: cultured bean curd; a delicious soy food high in protein and B vitamins. (See *Book Two: The Healing Recipes* for a whole chapter of tasty, healthy recipes.)

TOMATOES: a super nutritive vegetable delicious raw, in salads, sandwiches or salsas or in cooked dishes or sauces. To ripen, simply let sit in a cool spot in your kitchen for a few days. (Don't refrigerate fresh tomatoes; you'll spoil their flavor.)
> **Nutrient Assets:** rich in antioxidant lycopene. Cooking tomatoes releases more healing lycopene. Add a little olive oil (lycopene is fat soluble) and for better absorption.
> **Health Benefits:** highly protective against cancers of the prostate, cervix, breast, lungs, mouth and digestive tract. A University of Illinois report shows that women with the highest lycopene levels (in tomatoes) have a fivefold lower risk for developing early signs of cervical cancer than women with low levels. Most recently, a high lycopene diet has been found to cut heart attack risk in half!

TORTILLAS: both whole wheat and corn tortillas make good light nutritious pizza crusts, nachos, and wrappers for Mexican-style sandwiches.
> **Nutrient Assets:** B vitamins, carbohydrates and lignins. Low calories; high in fiber.
> **Health Benefits:** an energy food to combat fatigue and feed the brain. Lignin content may also help inhibit breast cancer.

TRITICALE: a hybrid of wheat and rye berries, with the best properties of both.

Nutrient Assets: lower in gluten and higher in protein than wheat or rye with a better balance of amino acids and more lysine.

Health Benefits: high lysine content helps combat the herpes virus.

TURBINADO SUGAR: refined sugar without all the molasses removed. (See "Sugars & Sweeteners in a Healing Diet" page 96.)

UMEBOSHI PLUMS: pickled Japanese apricots; part of a good macrobiotic diet.

Nutrient Assets: high iron, vitamin C and citric acid.

Health Benefits: alkalizing, bacteria-killing properties relieve indigestion caused by over-eating. Help alleviate nausea from morning sickness. Reduce lactic acid linked to joint inflammation and fatigue. Can be used to help overcome colds and flu. *Note: avoid if you are salt-sensitive.*

VINEGARS: vinegars have been used for 5000 years as healthful flavor enhancers and food preservers. Condiments, relishes or dressings, they help digest heavy foods and high protein meals. The most nutritious vinegars are not overly filtered, and still contain the "mother" mixture of beneficial bacteria and enzymes. They look cloudy.

—**Apple Cider:** a therapeutic vinegar for cleansing and alkalizing, a powerful germkiller. Can ease heartburn and soothe sore throats. Also a good salad vinegar.

—**Brown Rice:** a mild sweet vinegar made from fermented brown rice.

—**Balsamic:** barrel-aged, aromatic, sweet / sour vinegar from balsam tree buds.

—**Herbal:** various herbs steeped in a wine vinegar; best with light salads.

—**Raspberry:** a light, fresh flavor for both vegetables and fruits, and in fish sauces.

—**Ume Plum:** the liquid drawn off from pickled Japanese umeboshi plums and shiso leaves. A good salt and lemon substitute in tart Asian dishes.

WASABI: very hot Japanese powdered horseradish.

Nutrient Assets: high in enzymes.

Health Benefits: a very good choice to help digest a high protein meal or sushi or sashimi. Can help clear mucous congestion.

WATERS: for healing purposes, use distilled, mineral, artesian and sparkling waters. (See "Water is Essential for Healing" page 58.)

WHEAT GERM and WHEAT GERM OIL: the embryo of the wheat berry; high in B vitamins, proteins, vitamin E and iron. It goes rancid quickly; buy nitrogen-flushed packaging and refrigerate.

Nutrient Assets: the oil is primarily a rich vitamin E source; wheat germ contains all the B vitamins, fiber, minerals, plentiful protein and essential fatty acids.

Health Benefits: a powerful body oxygenator. One tablespoon of the oil provides the antioxidant equivalent of an oxygen tent for 30 minutes.

WHEAT, WHEAT FLOUR: the ubiquitous whole grain. Studies from the University of Minnesota reveal the more whole grains a woman eats, the lower her risk for cancer and heart disease! However, wheat and wheat byproducts contain gluten, an allergen for many people that can cause Irritable Bowel symptoms and weight gain.

—**Bulgur:** cracked, toasted wheat berries, quick and easy to cook, nutty and tasty.

—**Whole wheat pastry flour:** a soft, low gluten wheat used mostly for pastries and unleavened baking. Wheat flour still has half the thickening capacity of white flour in cooking, giving you an idea of what it can do in your intestines!

—**Unbleached white flour:** ground wheat berries with the bran and germ removed, but aged naturally with no chemical bleaching or treating agents.

—**High gluten flour:** wheat with the starch removed to concentrate the gluten.

—**Graham flour:** ground hard wheat, coarse in texture with a chewy, nutty taste.

WILD RICE: nutty, brown seeds of a grass; used in grain mixes for stronger flavor.

Nutrient Assets: high in protein, potassium and magnesium; some B vitamins.

Health Benefits: a building food for a recovering body. A good choice for chronic fatigue syndromes, fibromyalgia or any immune compromised disease.

ZEST: the outermost rind of a citrus fruit, used as a flavoring or garnish.

Nutrient Assets: chlorophyll and carotenoids.

Health Benefits: increases digestibility of other foods and boosts energy.

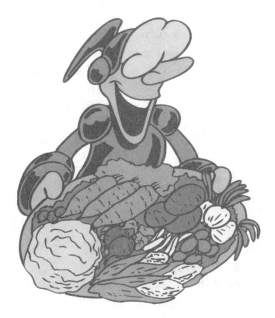

Section 2 - The Herbs

**A complete A to Z glossary of culinary herbs and spices
with major nutrient values and healing benefits.
Use them to enhance your healing results.**

ALFALFA: a clover-like legume with edible leaves, flowering tops, seeds and sprouts. One of the world's richest mineral-source foods, its roots grow as deep as 130 feet into the earth, absorbing and pulling up essential minerals.

Nutrient Assets: at least 19% protein (more than eggs and meat). Has an exceptional amount of trace minerals, fiber, eight of the essential amino acids, and high levels of vitamins K, A and D, magnesium, iron, potassium and zinc. An excellent source of chlorophyll.

Health Benefits: a body cleanser, infection fighter, and natural deodorizer. A good spring tonic that eliminates retained water, and relieves urinary and bowel problems. A natural pain reliever, anti-inflammatory and immune booster. Ideal for normalizing the blood after illness or long courses of prescription drugs. Helpful in withdrawing from drug or alcohol addiction. Effective against arthritis, anemia, intestinal and skin disorders, diabetes, liver problems, even cancer. Today's herbalists use alfalfa to normalize estrogen levels and blood-clotting because of its rich vitamin K.

ALLSPICE: named for its combined tastes of cloves, cinnamon, pepper and juniper berries, allspice is a hot aromatic for cooking and preserving.

Nutrient Assets: carminative volatile oils.

Health Benefits: a good, warming tea for digestive problems, especially for relieving stomach gas (it works almost immediately), and infant colic. To take, just chew an allspice bud, or add $^1/_2$ teasp. to a cup of hot water and drink.

ALOE VERA: a desert lily long used for burns of all kinds and skin care, aloe juice is now widely known for its digestive and soothing laxative properties. Buy aloe juice products that are 100 percent juice with the pulp... just as if you tore a leaf off the plant, squeezed it and drank its juice. Available in many fruit flavors, and in gel caps, aloe vera juice is suitable for children, but not recommended for expecting mothers.

Nutrient Assets: low in calories and fat, high in protein, fiber and minerals like calcium, magnesium, potassium, sodium, iron and copper. Naturally rich in vitamin C, amino acids, mucopolysaccharides and enzymes.

Health Benefits: aloe juice is one of nature's best internal cleansers, detoxifying the stomach, liver, kidneys, spleen and bladder. It helps cleanse the blood and regulate the colon, as well as soothe ulcers and hemorrhoids. Digestive disorders, bladder and kidney infections all respond to treatment with aloe vera juice. Relieves constipation and insomnia, even works as a douche to fight vaginal infections. Reduces arthritis pain and high cholesterol; treats liver disorders and boosts immune response. Aloe vera juice is now undergoing clinical trials as a possible cancer and AIDS treatment. For diabetics, 1 tablespoon of aloe juice for one week can lower blood sugar levels; after two weeks, lowers triglyceride levels. Injections are used for feline leukemia by veterinary hospitals; found to increase survival by up to 70%! Note: when adding aloe vera juice to your diet, start with small doses and work your way up to higher doses. The gel is an antiinflammatory that reduces pain, heals scars and stimulates growth of healthy issue. See "Healing Powerhouses of the Desert," page 108.

ANISE SEED: a member of the carrot family, anise seeds grow wild in many countries and have a licorice-like flavor. Used frequently in cakes, cookies, dressings and soups.

Nutrient Assets: made up of flavonoids like rutin and quercetin, and also contains choline and the volatile oil, anethole.

Health Benefits: used to sweeten breath, as a cough suppressant and digestive aid. Can prevent intestinal cramping and infant colic, and help stimulate production of mother's milk. Anise seeds are expectorant and anti-spasmodic, and are helpful for bronchitis and whooping cough. Mild estrogenic action may even increase libido. Externally, anise seed oil can be applied to help scabies and lice. Chewing anise seed has a history of improving sleep for insomniacs.

ASAFOETIDA: a pungent/bitter spice similar to garlic used in India and the Middle East.

Nutrient Assets: high in volatile oils, resin and gum.

Health Benefits: anti-parasitic and aphrodisiac. Relieves gas, induces sweating to release body toxins, increases the flow of urine, normalizes menstrual flow, and helps remove mucous congestion. Can be used for expelling intestinal parasites and for ailments like weak digestion, asthma, whooping cough and chronic bronchitis.

ASTRAGALUS: a sweet-tasting Asian pea family herb, resembling a tongue depressor. Use in soups made from meats, vegetables or mushrooms.

Nutrient Assets: high in flavonoids, amino acids and trace minerals including selenium. Also contains saponins, and immuno-active polysaccharides.

Health Benefits: key actions are anti-stress, antiviral and immune stimulant, especially for cancer and AIDS where it repairs damaged cells and strengthens the body during recuperation from these diseases. A strong preventative of viral and bacterial invasion in the respiratory system. Diuretic action makes it beneficial in treating those with nephritis or inflammation of the kidneys. Reduces blood pressure, improves circulation and strengthens the heartbeat. Particularly useful for Coxsackie B viral myocarditis, a virus present in the heart tissue which causes severe lesions. *Note: Do not take if you have acute disease, high fever or severe inflammation.*

BARLEY GRASS: A cereal grass which comes from immature barley grains. Can be found in powder or tablet form. I like to add it to juices and as a sprinkle on pet food.

Nutrient Assets: rich in chlorophyll, protein and enzymes. Contains antioxidant beta carotene and vitamin C, B-complex vitamins, calcium and magnesium. Also contains vitamin K and the antioxidant enzyme, superoxide dismutase (SOD).

Health Benefits: a building energy food that strengthens the immune system to fight off colds and flu. Protects against degenerative disease like cancer, heart disease, macular degeneration, even AIDS. Eases ulcers and other gastric ailments by restoring acid-alkaline balance in the body; balances sugar use for hypoglycemia and diabetes. An anti-inflammatory effective for arthritis. Neutralizes heavy metals like mercury, helps clear up skin conditions and aids weight loss. Use in a nutrient-rich daily maintenance drink, and to help dry up mother's milk.

BASIL: a pungent, peppery mint family herb with many of the same medicinal qualities.
Nutrient Assets: mainly volatile oils and tannins.
Health Benefits: use as a tea to soothe stomach distress (1 TB. chopped fresh herb or 1 teasp. dried, in a cup of hot water). A "brain remedy" for mental depression and grief. A basil tea with black peppercorns relieves fevers, colds, headaches and nausea. Ayurvedic medicine uses its antibacterial properties as a specific for acne.

BAY LEAF: an aromatic spice beneficial to the stomach and intestinal tract.
Nutrient Assets: high in volatile oils and essential fatty acids.
Health Benefits: the ancient Greeks dedicated the bay (laurel) tree to their gods of medicine, Apollo and Aesculapius. The Romans believed bay maintained health because bay leaves added to beans (a Roman soldier's staple) prevented gas. Basil tea is effective as a remedy for gas, flatulence and indigestion. Bay oil, made by heating the leaves in olive oil, soothes the pain of fibromyalgia, arthritis, bruises and sprains. *Note: never use basil internally in large amounts.*

BEE POLLEN: collected by bees from male seed flowers, mixed with secretion from the bee, and formed into granules. An effective antidote during allergy season. Two teasp. daily is a usual dose. (For more, see "Healing Powerhouses of the Desert," page 110)
Nutrient Assets: contains every nutrient needed to maintain life. Abundant in enzymes; contains all essential amino acids. Has vitamins galore (vitamins A, C, D, E, K, plus complete B complex, including vitamin B-12, and bioflavonoids.) Contains high minerals.
Health Benefits: a wonderful food for the skin and hair; strengthens the immune system, and counteracts the effects of radiation and chemical toxins. For athletes, bee pollen promotes energy and endurance, accelerates the rate of recovery, and normalizes heart rate and breathing. Quercetin, high in bee pollen, inhibits histamine release, useful for allergies and hay fever. Bee pollen taken during allergy season can often prevent symptoms.

BEE PROPOLIS: a resinous substance gathered by the bees from the leaf buds or the bark of trees like poplar or chestnut. Propolis is aromatic with a mild bitter taste.
Nutrient Assets: made up of resin, balsam, wax, etheric oils and pollen. Rich in B-vitamins and natural antibiotics.
Health Benefits: helps destroy pathogenic bacteria, promoting the immune system's disease-fighting power. Protects against colds, coughs, sore throats, sinusitis, bad breath and gum infections. Enhances the effectiveness of antibiotics like *tetracycline* and *penicillin* by 10 to 100 times. An antibiotic that combats *staph* and *strep* conditions. Protects and stimulates the liver, normalizes cholesterol levels and blood pressure, and improves circulation. Inhibits ulcers, even promotes internal healing when ulcers are already present. Studies show bee propolis helps mend broken bones, speeds cell growth, and heals the skin.

BERGAMOT: an antiseptic and aromatic herb used in aromatherapy and in teas.
Nutrient Assets: high in volatile oils.
Health Benefits: relieves respiratory infections, colds, coughs and nasal congestion. Bergamot contains tannins that control oily skin. Bergamot oil, made by steeping the leaves in sesame oil, is a make-up remover for all skin types, and helps heal eczema, psoriasis and acne. Used in aromatherapy to reduce depression and overeating.

BITTERS: made from the distillation of aromatic herbs, barks, roots and plants, bitters are a liquid used to flavor cocktails, aperitifs or foods.

Nutrient Assets: bitter compounds like *amarogentin* in gentian stimulate the liver and promote the flow of bile.

Health Benefits: used as digestive aids and appetite stimulants through liver detoxification and increased bile flow. Regulate pancreas hormone secretions to balance blood sugar, insulin and glucagon. May help leaky gut syndrome by reversing gut wall damage through the body's own self-healing mechanisms. A short course of herbal bitters regenerates both liver and lymphatic system to enhance immune response against infection. Helps diseases associated with low gastric acidity like rosacea, eczema, asthma and gallbladder disease. Examples of herbal bitters: barberry, boneset, centaury, chamomile, dandelion, gentian, goldenseal, Oregon grape, horehound, mugwort, rue, tansy, wormwood, turmeric, cardamom, lemon peel and yarrow.

BLACK PEPPER: made from crushed, dried, black peppercorns. Use as a spice, an oil, a tea or a compress. Best used in small amounts as a catalyst in nutritional compounds. Too much pepper can cause a hot, burning sensation in the stomach.

Nutrient Assets: *piperine* is the main compound in black pepper. Pepper also keeps vitamin A functioning in the body and safe from destruction.

Health Benefits: good for the nervous system and the spleen. Helpful for chronic indigestion, colon build-up and sinus congestion. A specific against food poisoning. Protects the liver by slowing down enzyme activity that causes toxin build-up. Helpful for poor circulation and fatigue. Helps cool the body by boosting perspiration. A traditional Ayurvedic medicine to enhance the bioactivity of other herbs and to prevent or delay the onset of degenerative disease. Yogis believe black pepper is a perfect food and take a pepper/honey mix daily. Herbalists use pepper's strong oil as an effective aromatherapy treatment for easing withdrawal from nicotine.

BORAGE: tastes and smells like cucumber. Use in salads, like spinach, or to add flavor to iced tea. Long esteemed in European herbal tradition as an herbal salad green, but use caution when preparing foods with fresh borage, it can be toxic.

Nutrient Assets: contains large amounts of potassium, calcium, EFA's, tannins, and vitamin C. Has beta-carotene in abundance, along with B-complex vitamins and choline, iron, magnesium, phosphorus. Borage seed oil contains gamma-linolenic acid, a promising essential fatty especially helpful for skin disorders, female hormone balance and inflammation.

Health Benefits: Helpful in the treatment of depression because it has the power to stimulate the glandular system. Useful for fever because it promotes perspiration. A favorite for fevers and chest colds. In Eastern European countries, borage is chopped with cabbage (two parts cabbage, one part borage) to make a cleansing soup against stomach flu and a "hanging on" cold. Saline content in borage helps flush the kidneys. The fresh herb can be used as an eyewash for inflammation. American herbalists use borage as an important adrenal tonic, not only against stress, but to balance prostaglandin and hormonal activity through its GLA content. An infusion of borage promotes the production of milk in breast-feeding mothers.

CARAWAY: a sweet, acrid herb, frequently added to grain recipes to aid digestion.

Nutrient Assets: contains essential oils, fiber, protein, starches, iron, magnesium, beta carotene and traces of B vitamins.

Health Benefits: chew the seeds, or use in a tea to relieve toothaches, nerves and upset stomach. A few seeds in warm water helps infant colic. Increases mother's milk. Can be used to strengthen the gallbladder and relieve diarrhea. Improves digestion after a fatty meal.

CARDAMON: has a lemon-like flavor and an aroma similar to eucalyptus and pine. Use whole pods for medicinal purposes. Grinding causes them to lose their flavor. Especially good in a stimulating, warming drink like Chai Tea or hot wine.

    Nutrient Assets: mainly volatile oil and starch gum.

    Health Benefits: helps nausea, vomiting and headaches. A favorite Swedish "bitters" herb to stimulate carminative action (digestion and bile production), and relieve flatulence and indigestion quickly. Chewing on the cardamom seeds relieves pain, promotes mental clarity (good for poor memory, fatigue and depression), opens bronchial airways (good for elimination of mucous buildup, sinusitis and coughs), warms the body and even sweetens foul breath.

CAYENNE: referred to as chili powder, paprika, red pepper, bird pepper or African pepper. Use rubber gloves when handling cayenne peppers to avoid skin burning. Take cayenne raw if possible, powdered in tea, or as a poultice. Herbalists consider cayenne to be very therapeutic, especially when taken with food or water rather than in a capsule. (A great deal of its action occurs in the mouth, sending signals through nerve endings to carry fresh blood to wherever it is needed.)

    Nutrient Assets: contains vitamin C and high amounts of vitamin A. Capsaicin in cayenne is responsible for its hot flavor. Also contains salicylates, related to aspirin.

    Health Benefits: aids colds and boosts energy. Has expectorant properties, effective in treating sinus problems. Assists digestion, gastrointestinal and colon problems by stimulating the flow of saliva and gastric juices. Reduces pain, revs up circulation and warms the body. Externally, cayenne treats arthritis, muscle soreness, even shingles. May prevent heart attack. Studies show that cayenne can lower the chance of heart attack by 78% used regularly as a cardiovascular tonic; 20% of those studied no longer had signs of coronary heart disease. (Drops under the tongue were used by traditional herbalists to bring a person out of a heart attack.) Helps arrest hemorrhaging (internal or external) and normalize blood flow. An effective catalyst in delivering therapeutic nutrients in herbal formulations. Increases calorie-burning and thermogenic brown fat activity (1 - 2 teasp. 3 times daily).

CHERVIL: tastes like parsley with a hint of anise. Fresh chopped chervil mixed with a little butter is one of my favorite toppings for a healing mushroom dish.

    Nutrient Assets: high in potassium, vitamin A, chlorophyll.

    Health Benefits: has breath cleansing and gastric soothing qualities.

CHIVES: have a mild, sweet, onion flavor. Chives work best for therapeutic results when used freshly chopped at the last minute to the recipe.

    Nutrient Assets: like all onions, chives contain sulfur, iron and vitamin C.

    Health Benefits: Chinese herbalists recommend raw chives as an antidote for poison and to control excessive bleeding. *Allicin*, a phytochemical in chives (and garlic) helps reduce cholesterol and lower blood pressure. Especially good in appetizers because they stimulate the appetite, promote digestion and serve as a mild laxative.

CHLORELLA: a one-celled green algae. For more, see "Green Superfoods" page 43.

Nutrient Assets: contains 60% protein and at least 19 amino acids (eight of the amino acids necessary for life). Rich in vitamins C, A, B-1, B-2, B-6, B-12, niacin, folic acid, biotin, choline, E and K. Very high in chlorophyll- higher than any other known plant. Plenty of phosphorus, potassium, magnesium, sulfur, iron, calcium, manganese, copper, zinc, iodine and cobalt. Also contains rich amounts of the antioxidant enzyme, SOD (superoxide dismutase).

Health Benefits: supports intestinal health, detoxifying the colon, stimulating peristaltic activity and promoting growth of friendly bacteria. High in lipoic acid for strengthening immune response (increases activity of T- and B-cells). Accelerates wound and ulcer healing, and protects against pollutants and radiation. Reduces arthritis stiffness and lowers blood pressure. Rich nutrient content makes chlorella effective for weight loss, cleansing and maintaining muscle tone during lower food intake. "Controlled Growth Factor" in chlorella provides a substantial increase in sustained energy and immune health.

CILANTRO: fresh coriander leaves, used in Mexican, Chinese and Spanish cooking. The dried herb has almost no flavor. Use cilantro fresh, or substitute parsley.

Nutrient Assets: low in calories and fat. A good source of calcium, magnesium, phosphorous, potassium, sodium and beta carotene. Provides fair amounts of protein, iron, B-1, B-2, B-3 and vitamin C (ascorbic acid).

Health Benefits: has antispasmodic, carminative, diuretic and stomachic properties. Can be used as an herbal digestive aid. Helps purify the blood and strengthen the heart. Useful for gas, indigestion, nausea and vomiting. The leaves may be applied to the skin to relieve burning sensations. A specific in teas to relieve fevers.

CINNAMON: a sweet spice from the bark of the shoot of a tropical evergreen tree.

Nutrient Assets: contains essential oil, tannins, resins, gums, sugar and starch. Also includes: some protein, minerals and vitamins.

Health Benefits: a detoxifier that relieves pain and promotes digestion. Relieves nausea and flatulence, and aids diarrhea. Improves and helps maintain blood sugar control in diabetics. Cinnamon and tumeric, when combined, triple insulin's ability to metabolize glucose. An antibiotic that helps prevent gum disease. Especially strong antibacterial properties against chronic infections like flu, cystitis, bronchitis and colds. Its aroma is reported to be aphrodisiac for men. Has thermogenesis (heat inducing) properties for weight loss. Note: Do not use cinnamon oil during pregnancy — it may be linked to miscarriages.

CLOVES: dried, aromatic flower buds with a pungent, spicy taste. Therapeutically used in herbal formulas to potentiate the action of other herbs.

Nutrient Assets: high volatile oils, plenty of vitamin C; rich in the anti-inflammatory chemical, *eugenol.*

Health Benefits: warms the body, increases circulation, improves digestion, treats flatulence, vomiting and nausea. Aids insulin activity for Type II diabetics. *Eugenol* and *acetyl* in clove oil inhibit blood cell clumping against cardiovascular disease. Directly applied, clove oil is a natural pain reliever for toothaches. A few drops can be used on the gums of teething children to ease pain. Also increases thermogenesis activity and circulation for weight loss.

CORIANDER: see cilantro.

CUMIN: a pungent and spicy culinary herb used in Indian and Middle Eastern dishes. Add $\frac{1}{2}$ to 1 teasp of cumin seeds or ground cumin (careful, cumin has a very strong flavor) to bean dishes to prevent them from causing gas.

Nutrient Assets: high in volatile oils. Contains good potassium and calcium.

Health Benefits: an effective carminative that relieves digestive gas. Use cumin tea while nursing to increase milk flow. (One teasp. of crushed seeds to 1 cup boiling water). A well known anti-inflammatory, new studies show preliminary evidence that cumin also has cancer preventing properties for breast and skin cancers.

DAIKON RADISH: a mild, almost sweet radish used in macrobiotic and Japanese cooking; may be eaten shredded fresh or stir-fried.

Nutrient Assets: low in calories and fat. Contains calcium, magnesium, phosphorus, high potassium, sodium, small traces of B-1, B-2, B-3 and vitamin C.

Health Benefits: daikon is an excellent food diuretic. Daikon helps expel mucous phlegm, cleanse the kidneys and eliminate gallstones. Especially good for hoarseness, clearing the sinuses and alleviating sore throats. Regular intake helps prevent viral infections like the common cold and flu.

DILL WEED: long used as a medicinal herb (even mentioned in the Bible).

Nutrient Assets: mainly volatile oils including D-limonene.

Health Benefits: relieves flatulence and an upset stomach. Increases mother's milk, and relieves breast congestion that occurs during breast-feeding. A small dose given to a colic-y baby will bring gentle relief! Smelling dill weed helps cure hiccups.

ECHINACEA: our Native American pharmacopeia valued echinacea much the same as the Chinese valued ginseng - widely. Introduced into Western culture and medicine in the late 1700s. Add to juices and teas for lymph flushing and immune boosting.

Nutrition Assets: high in cobalt, silicon, zinc, chromium, iron, manganese, selenium and in vitamins C, B-3 and riboflavin.

Health Benefits: increases phagocytic activity of leukocytes (antibodies), stabilizes red blood cell count and stimulates T-Cell formation. Increases levels of properdin that kills infectious microbes. Clears toxins, reduces inflammation, antidotes poison, promotes tissue repair, arrests discharge, dredges the kidneys, promotes skin cleansing, resolves fever and pushes out eruptions. Effective for skin conditions like acne, eczema, psoriasis; for congested lymph gland diseases like chicken pox, ulcers, goiter, strep throat, even cancer and tumors.

EPAZOTE: a pungent, wild herb with a flavor like fresh cilantro. A favorite in Mexican Indian cooking. (Add dried leaves only during the last 15 minutes of cooking.)

Nutrient Assets: high in vitamin C, phosphorous, calcium; traces of the B vitamins.

Health Benefits: the Mayans steeped epazote in milk and sugar to rid their children of intestinal parasites, especially roundworms and hookworms (a constituent, *ascaridol* is a powerful worm expellent). A premier digestive remedy for colic, stomach pains and flatulence. Muscle-relaxing action helps treat spasmodic coughs and asthma.

FENNEL: a sweet-tasting culinary herb and member of the carrot family. Cultivated for culinary use since ancient times.

Nutrient Assets: high in volatile oils, especially *anethole*, an intestinal stimulant.

Health Benefits: has antispasmodic, carminative action that works well with bitter herbs like gentian or cardamom, to support the liver and gallbladder during digestion. Use one teasp. of crushed seeds steeped in boiling water for stomach cramps, gas, colic and to expel mucous. Cool fennel tea is a good, flushing eyewash for conjunctivitis and eyelid inflammation. During nursing, it enriches the quality and quantity of mother's milk and helps prevent colic.

FENUGREEK: widely used by Greeks, Romans and Egyptians for healing cooking.

Nutrient Assets: high in choline, vitamin A, lecithin and a bitter oil.

Health Benefits: removes clogging mucous from the lungs and colon. Actually softens and dissolves masses of accumulated mucous, then helps expel them from the bronchial tubes and lymph system. Take 1 to 2 tsp. steeped in boiling water for 20 minutes. Contains lecithin, a lipotropic (fat-dissolving) substance which helps thin cholesterol and other harmful blood fats.

GARAM MASALA: a medley of cinnamon, cloves, nutmeg and cardamom, garam masala is traditionally used in bean dishes for its flavor and digestive properties.

Health Benefits: A carminative, garam masala lessens discomfort after eating beans. Offers all the health benefits of its spices (cloves, cinnamon, nutmeg and cardamon).

GARLIC: a pungent relative of the onion family highly popular in every culture for cooking and medicinal qualities (used for healing for more than 5000 years — we have written evidence of it from the ancient Egyptians). Use garlic and parsley together in your recipes to neutralize the smell... or simply chew parsley sprigs after eating garlic.

Nutrient Assets: offers a host of immune-boosting, stay well nutrients — vitamins A, C, B, potassium, zinc, iron, selenium, germanium, sulfur, calcium and manganese.

Health Benefits: an *allicin*-containing, universal antibiotic effective against viruses, *staph* and *strep* bacteria. A protective antioxidant, preventing formation of free radicals, boosting immunity and strengthening the body against allergens, heavy metals and pollutants. Balances blood sugar in diabetics. Supports development of beneficial intestinal flora while killing off pathogenic organisms like *H. Pylori*, a bacteria responsible for ulcers. A primary anti-fungal for both internal and external infections. A specific against yeast diseases like *Candida Albicans*. Apply garlic oil directly to fungus-infected areas like nails or athlete's foot to curb fungal growth. Good studies find that garlic lowers cholesterol — by up to 12%. Most people using garlic for cholesterol also say their blood pressure is lower. New studies show garlic's high sulfur may also help prevent colon cancer.

GINGER: an aromatic spice, both fresh and dried ginger have therapeutic properties for digestive and heart problems. Keep fresh ginger on hand without spoilage. Peel fresh roots, chop in the blender, put in a plastic bag, and freeze. Ginger thaws almost immediately. In about 10 minutes, it's ready to use.

Nutrient Assets: contains protein, fiber, calcium, iron, magnesium, phosphorus, potassium, sodium, zinc, manganese, vitamin C, B-complex, vitamin A, and gingerol (an essential oil).

Health Benefits: a premier spice for people with liver or digestive problems, ginger helps prevent nausea and vomiting caused by pregnancy or anesthesia. Acts as a stimulant during recuperation from illness. Aids digestion and assimilation of food, and cleanses the skin, bowels and kidneys. The Japanese actually use ginger to detoxify meat in the intestines. Helps prevent jet lag, motion sickness and vertigo (dizziness). Chewing ginger stimulates saliva flow and soothes sore throats. Stimulates peripheral circulation in cases of bad circulation, chilblains (pain to hands or feet caused by cold) and cramps. Promotes perspiration to lower body temperature during a fever. Normalizes digestive system peristalsis to relieve gas. Gingerol in ginger discourages blood platelet clumping to help prevent a heart attack in the same way that aspirin does, but without the side effects. Destroys influenza viruses and treats chest congestion, diarrhea and nerve diseases. Breaks down inflammatory acids in the joints to relieve the pain of rheumatoid arthritis and osteoarthritis. Has a protective effect on the stomach and liver, stimulating the growth of beneficial lactobacilli while inhibiting pathogenic bacteria. Along with cayenne, ginger contains anti-ulcer constituents and helps lower LDL cholesterol. New research shows that ginger is the world's greatest herbal inhibitor of the 5-LO enzyme, the only food source for prostate cancer cells. Without 5-LO, prostate cancer cells die in 1 to 2 hours.

GINKGO BILOBA: the fifth most widely used herb in the U.S. today, the number one prescription herb in Europe. Called a "living fossil," ginkgo is the oldest tree species in the world, surviving over 200 million years. Well known as the sole tree to survive the Hiroshima bombing. Use ginkgo in "brain drinks" and circulatory stimulants.

Nutrient Assets: calcium, iron, phosphorous, flavonoids including quercetin.

Health Benefits: an anti-aging treasure par excellence, ginkgo is antioxidant, adaptogenic, and gently stimulating. Increases circulation to the brain, heart, sexual organs and extremities making it very useful for Alzheimer's, dementia, heart disease, impotence or low libido, and all vascular disorders. Clinically able to reduce blood clots by disrupting PAF activity (platelet activation factor). Protects brain cells from arterial blockage and is able to cross over the blood brain barrier to significantly increase circulation to the brain. Naturally stimulates release of acetylcholine in the brain, a key neurotransmitter vital to memory. Returns elasticity to blood vessels hardened by cholesterol. Protects against stroke. Supports eye health, protecting against AMD (Age-Related Macular Degeneration) and Diabetic Retinopathy. Improves symptoms of vertigo, dizziness and tinnitus (ringing in the ears). Relieves inner ear problems in children with ADD. Helps inactivate many allergens, making it useful in treating asthma and allergy-related conditions. Safeguards your skin from damaging free radicals and increases circulation for a rosier look; supports hair regrowth. *Note: contraindicated when taking anticoagulants. When taken in extremely high doses, it can cause irritability, diarrhea, headaches and clotting disorders.*

HORNY GOAT WEED: known by the Chinese as Epimedium or Yin Yang Hou, horny goat weed got its notorious name from reports that goats who ate it became more virile, mating much more than other goats. Today, horny goat weed is being rediscovered in the United States for its effect on libido in men and women. The Chinese steep horny goat weed in wine for therapeutic effects. It is also widely available in capsule formulations.

Nutrient Assets: a variety of flavonoids, polysaccharides, sterols and magnaflorine (an alkaloid), some vitamin E, linolenic acid and oleic acid.

Health Benefits: testosterone-like effects help stimulate libido in men and women. Increases sperm production in men and stimulates sensory nerves for enhanced sexual response. Used in Traditional Chinese Medicine to support kidney, joint, liver, back and knee health. Chinese research shows it can inhibit the polio virus and *Staphylococcus aureus*.

HORSERADISH ROOT: a member of the mustard family that adds flavor and bite.
   Nutrient Assets: low fat, high fiber, vitamin C, antibiotic substances and glycosides.
   Health Benefits: a powerful stimulant with strong diuretic and expectorant properties. Relieves sinus congestion immediately, almost violently. (Taken with lemon juice, I have witnessed its decongestant action in this way many times.) Some herbalists believe its strong antiseptic action protects against certain types of cancers, like colon and stomach cancer. A good digestive stimulant, especially for beef, or oily fish like shark. A good ingredient in massage oil because it boosts circulation. Horseradish vinegar can be used for people who want to hide freckles and skin blotches, and as an excellent hair rinse.

KALONJI: small triangular blue-black seeds also called nigella, or black onion seeds, have a distinctive onion flavor. Use kalonji as a substitute for pepper.
   Nutrient Assets: contains protein, fat, calcium, iron, potassium, sodium, vitamin C.
   Health Benefits: has potent antihistamine properties against allergies, colds, bronchitis, fevers, flu, asthma and emphysema. A rich source of anti-cancer sterols. Inhibits tumor growth by preventing tumor cells from entering the bloodstream. Can be used for a variety of ailments - calluses, colic, corns, headaches, jaundice, sclerosis and stomach aches. Helps diarrhea and dysentery (an intestinal infection that causes severe pain, fever and diarrhea).

KUZU (kudzu): a starch similar to arrowroot used as a thickener for sauces and gravies.
   Nutrient Assets: has isoflavones, *daidzin, daidzein, puerarin, arachidic acid* and *B-sitosterol*.
   Health Benefits: strengthens blood vessels and increases circulation, benefitting angina pectoris. Lowers blood pressure and reduces symptoms associated with high blood pressure like headaches, neck stiffness, vertigo and tinnitus. Alkalizes an over-acid body and can relieve hangovers, headaches, and colds and flu. Useful for diabetes and/or hypoglycemia.

LEMON VERBENA: an aromatic shrub especially good in spring cleaning tea blends.
   Nutrient Assets: high in volatile oils and flavonoids.
   Health Benefits: a good tea with licorice or mint to soothe bronchial congestion, break up mucous, and reduce stomach cramps, nausea and palpitations. Use for indigestion and gas after heavy meals. Helps elevate mood in cases of mild depression. A mild, natural antibiotic.

MARJORAM: a mint, with a mild, earthy taste similar to oregano.
   Nutrient Assets: volatile oils, flavonoids, and triterpenoids.
   Health Benefits: used as a purifying herb in ancient times. Carried in a posy pocket to shield ladies from evil smells. Used in love spells to safeguard a lover, worn at weddings to secure happiness, and added to food to strengthen love. Today, it is used as an herbal defense tea to protect against illness during cold season, or to forestall seasickness when taken prior to sea travel. Also a mild pain reliever that may be taken for insomnia, nighttime headaches or menstrual cramps.

MINTS: have light, but potent flavor. All aromatic mints — peppermint, spearmint, orange and lemon mints, even pennyroyal, contain menthol as a main constituent. All mints have breath-and-body freshening qualities. All mints have nervine activity to soothe headaches, tension and anxiety. All mints ease digestion and help control gas, bloating, flatulence and nausea (even morning sickness). Mints seem to boost circulation and increase iron absorption.

Peppermint: a highly aromatic hybrid cousin of spearmint.

Nutrient Assets: menthol, phenolic acids and flavonoids.

Health Benefits: an anti-bacterial for digestive and respiratory problems. The oil can be inhaled for nasal congestion, and amazingly enough, to stop hiccups. The oil is also a specific in colon/bowel cleansing combinations, and to control diarrhea, ulcerative colitis and Crohn's disease. Has anti-viral healing properties, with help against a variety of herpes-type viruses (good news for travelers). The oil can be used topically for itching, ringworm, burns and to repel mosquitos (more good news for travelers). Peppermint promotes body cleansing through mild sweating, and relaxes tight muscles, so it helps insomnia.

Spearmint: may be used like peppermint, but is gentler in its activity.

Nutrient Assets: same as peppermint.

Health Benefits: good for childhood complaints, especially in a digestive enzyme tea, and as a warmer for colds and chills. Effective against indigestion and vomiting.

MUSHROOMS (medicinal): Mushrooms are far more than tasty foods. They are powerful medicine used to combat everything from heart disease and cancer to AIDS.

—**Cordyceps:** a building, restorative mushroom. Also called Caterpillar Fungus.

Nutrient Assets: polysaccharides, protein, fiber, linoleic and oleic acid.

Health Benefits: a tonic that supports liver, endocrine, lung and kidney health. Enhances oxygen uptake to the heart and brain. Has testosterone-like effects, improving libido and sperm count. Reduces fibroid tumors (a specific against ovarian tumors). Stimulates immunity by boosting phagocytosis action and macrophage activity. Increases life-span in animal lymphoma. A wonderful tool for recuperation from surgery, debility, fatigue, anemia or illness.

—**Maitake:** powerful adaptogenic, immune enhancing mushrooms.

Nutrient Assets: polysaccharides a and beta glucan, sterols, unsaturated fatty acids, and an especially promising anti-cancer compound, D-fraction.

Health Benefits: tests by the NCI (National Cancer Institute) reveal that maitake extract can actually prevent HIV from destroying the "helper" T cells of the immune system. Scientists from NCI consider maitake as powerful as the drug AZT, but without the toxic side effects! Tests show maitake inhibits tumor growth by up to 86%. Maitake helps reduce blood pressure and cholesterol levels, and lower blood sugar levels in non-insulin dependent diabetics. May also help CFS, diabetes, hepatitis, HBP, HIV-related infections, and arthritis.

—**Reishi:** an immune stimulating antihistamine and antioxidant, with the effectiveness of a potent adaptogen against degenerative auto immune diseases.

Nutrient Assets: polysaccharides, sterols, triterpenoids, oleic acid.

Health Benefits: specifically stimulates T-cell activity and inhibits replication of the HIV virus. Has strong antitumor properties; take as part of a recovery program from chemotherapy and radiation. Effective for chronic bronchitis, heart palpitations, hypertension, sticky blood and high cholesterol. Modern studies support reishi's ability to combat disorders like ulcers, Alzheimer's disease, insomnia, diabetes, allergic reactions, altitude sickness and edema.

MUSTARD SEED: a pungent spice that offers many medicinal benefits.

Nutrient Assets: a good source of calcium, magnesium, phosphorus, sulphur, potassium, trace minerals and most of the important vitamins.

Health Benefits: stimulates appetite, promotes gastric membranes for digestion; especially helpful in the conversion of cholesterol into bile acid, which helps eliminate excess fats from the body. A valuable thermogenesis source during weight loss — it can keep calorie burning going for up to 3 hours after a meal! Used by herbalists to alleviate PMS symptoms, including fatigue and water retention. Applied topically, it increases blood flow (mustard was a primary "plaster" ingredient in times past to detox the respiratory system). Herbalists use a teasp. of crushed seeds in warm water during a cold or flu as a blood purifier and as a mild laxative to rid the body of infective toxins. Mustard seeds steeped in a carrier oil can stimulate circulation to relieve pain from arthritis. A good detoxifier for cleansing the skin.... brings up circulation to nourish it. *Note: Mustard seed is a valuable aid for narcotic poisoning, as it empties the stomach without depressing system function. Doses over 1 teasp. may have an emetic effect and induce vomiting.*

NUTMEG: a sweet and spicy culinary herb commonly used in Oriental elixirs to warm the stomach and regulate energy flow.

Nutrient Assets: lignins, volatile oil, starch, gum, and myristicin.

Health Benefits: American herbalists use nutmeg as a digestive remedy for nausea, vomiting, indigestion and diarrhea. Try a pinch of nutmeg in warm rice or soy milk before retiring instead of dessert, to aid in weight loss. May improve Crohn's disease. Note: use sparingly especially if you are pregnant (doses about the size of a pea). Large, concentrated doses of pure nutmeg can be toxic and may cause miscarriage.

OLIVE LEAF: a potent antibacterial, antiviral, antifungal, antiparasitic and antioxidant.

Nutrient Assets: oleuropein, an anti-infective member of the iridoid group, flavonoids and antioxidant compounds.

Health Benefits: the <u>extract</u> stimulates the immune system by increasing phagocyte production. Restores energy and boosts stamina. Clinical research shows that olive leaf extract has excellent success against viral, bacterial, fungal, and protozoan infections, especially against herpes I and II, human herpes virus 6 and 7, HIV-AIDS, flu, the common cold, meningitis, Epstein-Barr virus, encephalitis, shingles, chronic fatigue, hepatitis B, pneumonia, tuberculosis, gonorrhea, malaria, severe diarrhea, blood poisoning, and dental, ear, urinary tract and surgical infections. Lab tests done by Upjohn Co. find that olive leaf extract kills 56 pathogens. Tests from East Park Research finds that olive leaf extract treats as many as 120 illnesses.

OREGANO: a favorite culinary spice especially in Italian cuisine, now becoming prized for its volatile oil which has amazing antimicrobial powers.

Nutrient Assets: the oil is rich in flavonoids, two of which, carvacrol and thymol are potent antiseptics.

Health Benefits: the oil contains over 50 compounds with antimicrobial actions that inhibit candida yeast, bacteria, viruses and parasites. The oil is also a powerful antioxidant. Direct contact with oregano essential oil can cause mild burns — avoid irritation by mixing with olive oil. Oregano is sometimes helpful in the treatment of migraine headaches, indigestion, colds and flu. Herbalists recommend it during menses to relieve discomfort.

PAPRIKA: ground sweet chili powder.

Nutrient Assets: high in natural salicylates (like aspirin), a good source of beta carotene, has 3 times as much vitamin C as oranges, contains pain-relieving capsaicin, potassium and quercetin.

Health Benefits: benefits blood and liver disorders. Protects against hypertension and strokes. Normalizes circulation, prevents blood clots, and reduces varicose hemorrhoids and spider veins. Helps stop nosebleeds and warms the body, especially hands and feet. A good choice to help relieve liver congestion. May be effectively applied externally for sprains and bruises. A natural antihistamine helpful for respiratory problems, to thin and expel mucous, and reduce inflammation. A remedy for the common cold, relieving sore throat, mouth sores and coughing. May actually help protect the respiratory system against bronchitis infection. Stops sinus headaches when inhaled. Stimulates metabolism and helps burn body fat and deter cholesterol. Its antiseptic action is a specific for stomach ulcers, even cancerous tumors.

PARSLEY: is a mild, fresh-tasting culinary herb used as a garnish and in detoxifying juice recipes. It is better by far to use it fresh for healing, but is so available and easy to grow, that there is no need to store it.

Nutrient Assets: full of vitamin C, iron and chlorophyll. Parsley is one of the green superfoods, high in vitamin A, B vitamins, potassium and calcium.

Health Benefits: new studies show that parsley extract possesses similar properties to those of calcium channel blockers for high blood pressure and circulatory health. A strong diuretic effective for fluid retention during menstruation. Relieves indigestion and gas, an expectorant for mucous congestion, effective in herbal formulas for intestinal worms. Both Greeks and Romans used parsley's breath freshening properties to mask foul odors (used today in some over-the-counter breath freshening blends). Chaplets of parsley were worn at their banquets to absorb unpleasant wine fumes.

ROSEMARY: one of nature's best antioxidants; a food preserver and water purifier.

Nutrient Assets: rosmarinic acid, volatile oil and flavonoids.

Health Benefits: a specific for memory and problems related to aging. A powerful central nervous system stimulant and a great tonic for the brain. Effective for coughs, sore throat, gum disease, colds and flu. Can prevent cancer-causing chemicals from binding to DNA in the earliest stages of cancer. May be particularly beneficial in the prevention of breast cancer. A strong nervine rich in highly absorbable calcium to counteract depression, and reduce stress and tension. The tea is effective for headaches, neuralgia, tendonitis, rheumatism and muscle pain. A good shampoo to combat premature balding. Promotes liver detoxification by increasing bile flow. Its volatile oils settle an upset stomach, and reduce gas and cramping, especially in women. Useful in a sleep pillow for insomnia caused by hormone imbalances during menopause. Use the oil in a therapeutic bath to soothe aching muscles and ease tension. Rosemary soap is antiseptic and anti-inflammatory for blemishes, dermatitis, and herpes fever blisters. Helps brunettes keep their dark hair beautiful. Simmer 2 to 3 TBS of rosemary sprigs in a small pot of hot water, let cool, and use as a hair rinse to darken and retain original hair color! Use as a natural repellent for fleas, moths and insects.

ROYAL JELLY: the milk-like secretion from the head glands of the queen bee's nurse-workers. The sole food of the queen bee.

    Nutrient Assets: contains every nutrient necessary to support life- a powerhouse of B vitamins, calcium, iron, potassium and silicon. It has enzyme precursors, a sex hormone and all eight essential amino acids.

    Health Benefits: a natural antibiotic that stimulates immune response. Supplies key nutrients for energy and mental alertness, and promotes cell longevity. One of the world's richest sources of pantothenic acid, known to combat stress, fatigue and insomnia. A superb nutrient for healthy skin and hair. Found effective for gland and hormone imbalances that reflect in menstrual and prostate problems. Highly effective for libido boosting in men and women. The highest quality royal jelly products are preserved in their whole, raw, "alive" state, which promotes ready absorption by the body. As little as one drop of pure extract of fresh royal jelly can deliver an adequate daily supply.

SAFFRON: excellent with rice and seafood; used extensively in Ayurvedic cuisine.

    Nutrient Assets: glycoside crocins, carotenoids, and vitamins B-1 and B-2.

    Health Benefits: In Europe, packets of saffron threads were sold as recently as fifty years ago in pharmacies to cure measles, treat period pain and chronic uterine bleeding, and calm indigestion and infant colic. Contains a blood pressure-lowering chemical called crocetin, thought by most researchers to be responsible for the low incidence of heart disease in Spain. Use only a tiny amount: $\frac{1}{2}$ teaspoon of threads is enough for 4 to 8 servings. Never use wooden utensils with saffron unless the wood is polished. Note: Can promote menstruation. May also cause abortion in large quantities. Use only half of the normal amounts during pregnancy.

SAGE: a potent musky herb cultivated as a culinary healer for centuries in Europe.

    Nutrient Assets: high in minerals and volatile oils.

    Health Benefits: sage is a body cleansing spring tonic high in minerals which improves weak digestion and dries up winter mucous excess. Taken to help stop lactation during weaning. A good women's herb with phytoestrogenic properties; a helpful tea for suppressed menses. Can be used in a gargle for sore throats. A sage tea hair rinse returns hair to its original color. Note: Pregnant women and epileptics should avoid sage.

SEA GREENS: "superfoods" of the sea that add an exotic taste to almost any recipe. Very popular in most Asian cuisine.

    Nutrient Assets: ocean plants have superior nutritional content - rich sources of proteins, carbohydrates, minerals, vitamins and algin (binds to and eliminates toxins).

    Health Benefits: good alkalizers which have the ability to detoxify the body of carcinogens, and disease-causing radioactive poisons and heavy metals. Superior body balancers after menopause, used for weight loss, skin tone and texture, and hair and nail regrowth. They support gland health, and successfully help correct thyroid problems. Even pets like sea greens-about 1 tsp. of snipped sea greens for dogs, 1 pinch for cats.

    Most of us are familiar with nori, used to wrap sushi ingredients, but I also like several other sea greens. See my SEA VEGGIE COMBO, a delicious, therapeutic sprinkle to use in place of salt, in *Book Two: The Healing Recipes*. Sea greens you can use in your healing recipes:

Arame: a mild seaweed with high natural sugars, used to flavor sauces and soups.

Bladderwrack: good for iodine therapy; use in healing baths and herb formulas.

Dulse: a delicious red sea veggie; soft and chewy; delicious in soups, stews, salads and sandwiches, or sautéed into chips. Crumble over vegetables, soups and salads; use in seasonings and savory dishes; or take as an effective alkalizing dieting tea.

Hijiki: a popular oriental sea green, with a nutty taste and crisp texture. It is protein and calcium-rich, with absorbable B Complex vitamins.

Kelp: a good salt substitute and high mineral sea vegetable.

Kombu: a delicious iodine-rich sea vegetable with a sweet taste. Just boil until tender and use in soups, snip over salads, or wrap vegetable or rice hors d'oeuvres.

Nori: also known as laver, this sea vegetable is used for sushi wrapping, snipped in soup, or dry roasted for a sweet, nutty taste. High in beta carotene and proteins.

Wakame: best when sun-dried, wakame has a delicate, mild taste, excellent with tofu, miso soup or fish. It is delicious roasted and tossed with a little sesame oil, sesame seeds and mushrooms. Tasty fresh in sushi rolls or sea green salads.

SESAME SEEDS: a favorite seed for salad dressing, entrees, sushi, dips and spreads.

Nutrient Assets: high in calories, EFA's, protein, and B vitamins.

Health Benefits: have a lubricating affect within the digestive tract, so they are a remedy for dry constipation. A handful of sesame seeds are often used by Arab healers for dizziness, tinnitus (ringing-in-the-ears), and blurred vision due to anemia. The seeds stimulate breast-milk for nursing mothers. Sesame seed oil is an excellent skin oil, and a gentle eye make-up remover.

SIBERIAN GINSENG: called the "king of all tonics," Siberian ginseng has been widely researched in Russia; used extensively to treat those exposed to radiation during the Chernobyl accident, and by U.S. astronauts and Russian cosmonauts.

Nutrient Assets: saponins, germanium, glycosides and ginsenosides.

Health Benefits: strengthens, normalizes and regulates all body systems to increase total body energy, and promote longevity and health. Particularly beneficial to the adrenal glands where it supports, counteracts and even prevents the effects of stress. Increases energy on all levels - mental and physical energy, long and short-term energy. Studies show that Siberian ginseng promotes a dramatic increase in total immune cells, especially natural killer cells, to support your immune system against infections. A rich source of germanium which improves oxygen uptake by the body. For deep sea divers, people who work on submarines, and people with respiratory disorders, it can be a lifesaver. Helps support the female system after menopause. Increases the acuity of vision, memory and hearing. Lowers blood sugar levels in non-insulin dependent diabetics. Reduces side effects like nausea, lack of appetite and dizziness from chemotherapy or radiation treatment, and also increases the efficiency of these drugs.

SPIRULINA: a blue-green algae popular in smoothies or sprinkled on foods.

Nutrient Assets: very high in protein; also rich in B vitamins, chlorophyll, beta-carotene, minerals and other trace elements.

Health Benefits: used in natural medicine to lower high cholesterol and boost immune response. A pick-me-up to use for energy without caffeine. Enhances enzyme production and digestion. Helps prevent cancer, especially of the mouth. Accelerates weight loss and improves athletic endurance. Has enough B-12 to help prevent anemia in vegetarians. A Japanese test shows spirulina has anti-viral properties against herpes, HIV, flu, mumps and measles. A good choice for liver disorders and gastric ulcers; also safeguards against heavy metal poisoning.

TARRAGON: an herb related to California sage used to baste chicken, fish or seafood, and in salad dressings, light soups and fresh fruit dishes. Flavor is similar to anise.

Nutrient Assets: high in potassium and volatile oils.

Health Benefits: protects against hypertension and strokes. The tea is used to treat insomnia and hyperactivity in children. The vinegar improves digestion, stimulates the bowels and sweetens breath. Some women use tarragon to promote delayed menstruation. The oil helps stimulate appetite, relieves spasmodic and arthritis pain, swellings and toothaches.

TEAS, Black and Green: all black, green and Oolong teas come from *thea sinensis*, an evergreen shrub that ranges from the Mediterranean to the tropics, and from sea level to 8000 feet. The kind of tea produced is differentiated by the manner in which the leaves are processed. For green tea, the first tender leaves of spring are picked, then partially dried, rolled, steamed and dried with hot air. Oolong tea leaves are allowed to semi-ferment for an hour. Black teas are partially dried, rolled on tile, glass or concrete, and fermented for 3 hours to strengthen aroma and flavor, and reduce bitterness. Black teas are also frequently scented during fermentation with fresh flower blossoms or spices. Tea nomenclature can be confusing. Oolong, black or jasmine teas refer to how the tea was processed (see above). Assam, Darjeeling, Ceylon, etc. refer to the country or region where the tea is grown. Pekoes, orange pekoe, etc. refer to the leaf size. (See "Black and Green Teas" page 67.)

Nutrient Assets: catechins, antioxidant polyphenols (green tea antioxidants are 25 times stronger than vitamin E and a hundred times stronger than vitamin C).

Health Benefits: a new Dutch study shows that drinking black tea may prevent heart disease. The compound EGCG (*epigallocatechin gallate*) in green tea promotes weight loss in animal studies. Both varieties are found to inhibit colon cancer in animal tests. They also increase the activity of antioxidant enzyme superoxide dismutase (SOD). Helps lower high blood sugar, cholesterol and triglycerides. Green tea also shows promise in the fight against rheumatoid arthritis. Japanese studies correlate high green tea consumption to lower rates of stomach, esophageal, lung and breast cancers. New research is also promising for pancreatic cancer. A study by Kaiser Permanente shows drinking just half a cup or more of green or black tea a day boosts a woman's fertility. Green tea helps block cavity-causing bacteria from attaching to teeth. Green tea even helps kill antibiotic resistant *Staphylococcus aureus* in vitro.

THYME: a slightly minty herb used to season seafood, spaghetti, pizza or chili sauce.

Nutrient Assets: volatile oils, thymol and carvacrol, tannins and apigenin.

Health Benefits: an herbal tonic that strengthens the immune system. A good children's remedy for respiratory problems and sluggish digestion. A thyme gargle can be used for sore throat and as a mouthwash for bad breath, tooth decay, and cold sores. A traditional remedy (as a tea) for bed-wetting, nightmares and migraines. Hot thyme chest compresses break up congestion in asthma and bronchitis. The tea is a good eyewash to relieve irritation from chlorinated swimming pools. Thyme paste is a useful antiseptic for fungal and parasitic infections like ringworm, athlete's foot and lice. Internally, it helps candida albicans yeast infections. Mix crushed thyme leaves in a paste with lime juice, onion juice and honey, to treat sores and boils.

TURMERIC: a member of the ginger family with a strong, bitter flavor. Used extensively in Indian cuisine in curries, lentil, rice and meat dishes.

Nutrient Assets: curcuminoids, volatile oil.

Health Benefits: among nature's most potent antioxidants, about five times stronger than vitamin E. Neutralizes free-radical properties of minerals such as iron. Strengthens the cardiovascular system and protects the liver from carcinogens. An effective anti-inflammatory (at about 1,200mg per day); a natural alternative for drugs for rheumatoid arthritis. *Note: use only 1 to 2 teasp. daily to avoid gastrointestinal upset.*

WHEAT GRASS: in the 1960's, Ann Wigmore, founder of Hippocrates Health Institute, referred to her Bible in creating her healing, raw foods programs. She read a verse in Daniel that instructed King Nebuchadnezzar to go into the field and "eat grass as did the oxen." Wigmore found wheatgrass was the most potent and nutritious of the grasses and began the popular movement in the U.S. of wheat grass juicing, enemas and implants for detoxification.

Nutrient Assets: highly nutritious - 15 lbs of wheatgrass has the nutritional value of 350 pounds of vegetables! A rich source of vitamin A, C, B_{12}, fiber, chlorophyll (over 70%), minerals, amino acids (including lysine, leucine, tryptophan, phenylalanine, threonine, valine and leucine). An excellent vegetarian source of protein, laetrile (an anti-cancer compound) and mucopolysaccharides. High in chlorophyll and the antioxidant enzyme, SOD (superoxide dismutase). Wheat grass is NOT a source of the gluten responsible for much of wheat grain allergy today (it's OK for wheat-sensitive people).

Health Benefits: cleanses the blood and gastrointestinal tract. Reduces over-acidity in the blood making it useful for arthritis, rheumatism, candida yeast, chronic fatigue, AIDS and allergies. Normalizes the thyroid gland, beneficial for thyroid-related obesity, fatigue and constipation. High chlorophyll and the fraction P4D1 in wheat grass also protects against radiation exposure damage, and renews cell DNA. Restores energy levels in people with chronic fatigue by improving oxygenation of body tissues. Wheat grass can successfully treat skin ulcers, impetigo or other allergic, itchy skin conditions. A powerful healing tool as a colon implant for colon cancer, bowel toxicity or chronic constipation. High chlorophyll in wheat grass makes it a natural body deodorizer. *Note: large amounts of undiluted wheat grass juice may cause nausea and dizziness. Just add a small "shot" to other fresh vegetable juices.*

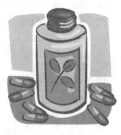

Section 3 - The Nutrients

A complete A to Z glossary of the nutrients in food and herbs
with their primary healing values.
Use it to understand the healing factors you need.

ACIDOPHILUS: a friendly bacteria that lives in the small intestine, acidophilus is a probiotic— a nutrient that improves the environment of the intestinal tract. It has the ability to help synthesize or manufacture all the B vitamins and enzymes in the human body. Food sources: *yogurt, kefir, fortified milk and soy milk, and raw sauerkraut.*

Health Benefits: a natural antibiotic that can kill a variety of pathogens including *candida albicans* and *E. coli.* Beneficial for auto-immune diseases that involve colon toxicity, like rheumatoid arthritis and chronic fatigue syndrome. Treats herpes simplex I and II, acne, mouth ulcers, even high cholesterol. Helps slow cancer growth. Encourages better digestion and friendly flora restoration after drug use. The body naturally produces acidophilus, but it is also available in high quality supplements. Keep below 40°F, but do not freeze. Acidophilus cannot withstand heat of 120°F or higher.

AGAR-AGAR: a vegetarian substitute for gelatin derived from sea algae. Buy it in flakes, and use it like gelatin -1 tablespoon of flakes gels 1 cup of liquid. Let slowly soften in cold water, then slowly simmer to dissolve. Agar-Agar has almost no taste, no calories, and is mostly insoluble fiber that passes through the body undigested.

Health Benefits: increases peristaltic action and relieves constipation. Agar can bond with heavy metals and radioactive toxins in the body, and help eliminate them.

ALANINE: a non-essential amino acid. Food sources: *butternut bark, pumpkin seeds, azuki beans and watermelon seeds.*

Health Benefits: helps maintain blood glucose levels, particularly as an energy storage source for the liver and muscles.

ALLYLIC SULFIDES: organic sulphur compounds found in garlic and onions.

Health Benefits: powerful antioxidant compounds that inhibit bacterial and viral growth including *staphylococcus, streptococcus* and *salmonella,* and provide cardiovascular protection. They also lower cholesterol levels and decrease blood clotting.

ALPHA CAROTENE: see Carotenoids.

ALPHA-LINOLENIC ACID (LNA): an essential fatty acid easily destroyed by heavy processing. Food sources: *walnuts, linseed oil, fish, sea greens, marine algae and eggs.*

Health Benefits: Omega-3 fatty acids, DHA and EPA, synthesized from LNA, support heart health. DHA is the most predominant EFA in brain tissue, and a large part of the retina (it is critical to good eye function). DHA is the most abundant fatty acid in breast milk.

ALPHA TOCOPHEROL (vitamin E): a primary fat soluble isoprenoid antioxidant vitamin which protects healthy cells from free radical destruction. Must be obtained from foods. Food sources: *wheat germ, nut and seed oils, eggs, organ meats, oats and olives.*

Health Benefits: boosts fertility, improves circulation, promotes longevity, prevents blood clots, strengthens capillary walls, and helps our bodies use vitamin A. A good choice to maintain cell membrane health, and healthy skin and hair. Alpha tocopherol is an antioxidant proven in preventing heart disease. See also vitamin E.

AMINO ACIDS: the building blocks of protein in the body — absolutely necessary for the growth, maintenance and repair of our bodies throughout our lives. Protein is composed of, and depends upon the right supply of amino acids. There are 29 of them known, from which over 1600 basic proteins are formed, comprising more than 75% of your body's solid weight of structural, muscle and blood protein cells.

Health Benefits: amino acids are sources of protein energy with a vital role in brain function, acting as neurotransmitters for the central nervous system. They are critical to rapid healing, controlling many antibodies to fight infection, and body chemistry balance. The liver produces about 80% of the amino acids it needs; the remaining 20% must be obtained from our foods. But poor diet, unhealthy habits and environmental pollutants mean that "essential amino acids" (those we need but our bodies can't make), may not be sufficient to produce the "non-essentials" (those formed by metabolism). Increase intake of protein food, or supplement to correct this situation. (Food-source supplements are used more quickly than dietary amino acids.) Specific amino acids produce specific pharmacological effects, and can be used to target specific healing goals. Amino acids work well with other natural healers, like herbs, minerals and antioxidants. The main amino acids are *Alanine, Arginine, Aspartic Acid, Branch Chain Aminos, Carnitine, Cysteine, Cystine, GABA, Glutamic Acid, Glutamine, Glutathione, Glycine, Di-methyl-glycine, Histidine, Inosine, Lysine, Methionine, Ornithine, Phenylalanine, Taurine, Threonine, Tryptophan, Tyrosine. Note: see reference by name in this survey.*

ANTHOCYANIDINS: flavonoids technically called "flavonals." Found in *red wine, grape juice and grapes, bilberries* and *white pine* herb.

Health Benefits: water soluble potent antioxidants that strengthen connective tissue like skin, tendons, ligaments and bone matrix. A very good choice for serious athletes who experience excessive free radical damage to connective tissue regularly.

ARGININE: a semi-essential amino acid, used for hGH and immune response. Rich food sources: *nuts, pumpkin seeds, peanut butter or cheese, and butternut bark.*

Health Benefits: for athletes and body builders, arginine increases muscle tone while decreasing fat. Promotes wound healing, blocks tumor formation and increases sperm motility. Helps lower blood fats and detoxifies ammonia. Curbs appetite and helps metabolize fat for weight loss. Increases nitric oxide (NO) in the body, reducing risk of heart disease like angina and congestive heart failure, and impotence. Take with cranberry or apple juice for best results. *Note: check schizophrenia and herpes virus outbreaks by "starving" them of arginine foods.*

ASCORBIC ACID: see vitamin C.

ASPARTAME: a combination of two amino acids, phenylalanine and aspartic acid, used as an artificial sweetener that is 200 times sweeter than sugar. In major foods like NutraSweet®, Equal® and Diet Coke®, its health side effects increase when used hot or during cooking.

Health Issues: the FDA has received more complaints about adverse reactions to aspartame than any other food ingredient in the agency's history. Aspartame may cause immediate side effects like severe headaches, dizziness, throat swelling and allergic effects. It has been linked to sugar use problems such as PKU seizures, high blood pressure, insomnia, ovarian cancer and brain tumors. May aggravate Parkinson's and Alzheimer's disease, and has been linked to brain damage in fetuses. May lead to methanol toxicity causing blurred or tunnel vision, and perhaps retinal detachment and bleeding. Aspartame can be especially problematic for people with blood sugar disorders because it disrupts the way your body uses insulin and can cause major fluctuations in blood sugar balance. Longterm aspartame toxicity can mimic multiple sclerosis, fibromyalgia and lupus — all diseases found commonly in diet soda drinkers. Healthier alternatives are honey, amazake (a sweet rice drink), molasses, rice syrup, concentrated fruit juices and stevia herb. See "Sugar and Sweeteners," page 97.

ASPARTIC ACID: a non-essential amino acid (a precursor of threonine), abundant in sugar cane and beets; used mainly as a sweetener.

Health Benefits: a neurotransmitter made with ATP that increases resistance to fatigue. Clinically used to counteract depression and in drugs to protect the liver.

B-COMPLEX VITAMINS: essential to almost every aspect of body function.

Health Benefits: assists metabolism of carbohydrates, fats, amino acids and energy production. While the separate B vitamins can and do work for specific problems or deficiencies, take as a whole for broad-spectrum activity. See specific Vitamins.

BETA -1, 3-D-GLUCAN: a complex sugar derived from baker's yeast. Other food sources: *maitake and reishi mushrooms, barley and oats.*

Health Benefits: activates immunity by attaching to immune macrophages that engulf and render invading pathogens harmless. Speeds healing from wounds and reduces inflammation. Also has anti-tumor activity for cancer protection. Especially promising as a preventive for colds, flu, and serious infections like sepsis and pneumonia.

BETA CAROTENE: see Carotenoids listings.

BIOFLAVONOIDS: part of the vitamin C complex. Food sources include: *blueberries, cherries, turmeric, ginger, alfalfa, the white part of the skin of citrus fruits and some herbs.* The best supplementary form is quercetin. The body does not produce its own bioflavonoids; they must be obtained regularly from the diet.

Health Benefits: bioflavs prevent arteries from hardening, and enhance blood vessel, capillary and vein strength. They protect connective tissue integrity, and control bruising, internal bleeding and mouth herpes. They lower cholesterol and stimulate bile production. They are anti-microbial against infections and inflammation. A major study shows that bioflavonoids, combined with enzymes and vitamin C, perform as well as anti-inflammatory drugs in reducing swelling. Bioflavs retard cataract formation, and guard against diabetic retinopathy.

BORON: a mineral which enhances the use of calcium, magnesium, phosphorus and vitamin D in bone formation and structure. Food sources: *vegetables, fruits and nuts.*

Health Benefits: stimulates estrogen production to protect against the onset of osteoporosis. A significant nutritional deterrent to bone loss for athletes.

BROMELAIN: an enzyme derived from pineapple stems.

Health Benefits: popular nutritional therapy widely used to relieve painful menstruation and to treat arthritis. Inhibits blood-platelet aggregation (clotting) without causing excess bleeding. An effective internal sports injury medicine to reduce bruising, relieve pain and swelling, and promote wound healing. May also be used externally, as a paste applied to stings, to deactivate the protein molecules of insect venom. I highly recommend bromelain before and after surgery of all kinds to accelerate healing. See also "Enzymes & Enzyme Therapy," pg. 30.

CALCIUM: the body's most abundant mineral, every cell needs calcium to survive. Food sources: *green vegetables, dairy foods, sea greens, tofu and shellfish.*

Health Benefits: necessary for synthesis of vitamin B-12; uses vitamin D for absorption. Works with phosphorus to build teeth and bones, and with magnesium for cardiovascular health and skeletal strength. Helps blood clotting, lowers blood pressure, prevents muscle cramping, maintains nerve health, deters colon cancer and osteoporosis, controls anxiety and depression, and insures quality rest and sleep. Aluminum-based antacids, aspirin, cortisone, chemotherapy agents, calcium channel blockers and some antibiotics interfere with calcium absorption. Antibiotics and cortico-steroids increase calcium needs. Calcium citrate has the current best record of absorbability.

—**Calcium glucarate:** a natural compound found in *alfalfa sprouts, apples, grapefruits and broccoli.* Best known as a cancer preventive, calcium glucarate (the supplement D-Glucarate derives from calcium glucarate) stimulates glucuronidation, a body cleansing process that helps detoxify carcinogens. Used primarily to prevent cancers of the breast (for high risk women) and lungs in smokers. Also found to lower cholesterol levels in animal tests. Currently being tested as a possible prostate cancer preventive.

CANTHANXANTHIN: see Carotenoids.

CAPRYLIC ACID: a short-chain fatty acid. Occurs naturally as a fatty acid in sweat, in cow's and goat's milk, and in palm and coconut oil.

Health Benefits: an antifungal effective against all candida species, caprylic acid helps restore and maintain a healthy yeast balance. It is not absorbed in the stomach, making it an excellent choice for candida overgrowth.

CARNITINE: an amino acid, vitamin-like nutrient synthesized in the liver and kidney, and found principally in meat (hence the name carnitine).

Health Benefits: carnitine's primary function is to facilitate fat metabolism by transporting long chain fatty-acid molecules into the mitochondria of cells where they are "burned" to produce energy. Enzymatically connects to the fatty acids, enabling them to cross the mitochondria membrane for fat breakdown. There are two forms, D and L-isomers (mirror images of each other) but only L-Carnitine is naturally found in nature and is biologically effective.

Carnitine reduces ischemic heart disease by preventing fatty build-up. It helps prostaglandin metabolism and improves abnormal cholesterol-triglyceride levels. Speeds fat oxidation for weight loss and increases fat use for energy. *Note: High protein weight-loss diets cause ketosis, the accumulation of fat waste ketones in the blood. Uncontrolled, ketosis in this type of weight-loss diet or in diabetes can be life-threatening. Carnitine prevents ketone build up. Consider it if you are on the "zone" protein diet.*

—**Acetyl-L-carnitine** (ALC) is gaining a reputation as a nootropic, a brain nutrient which reduces age-related mental decline. ALC specifically boosts alertness and attention span, improves learning and memory, and boosts eye-hand coordination.

CAROTENOIDS: a major class of antioxidant nutrients used today to combat everything from infections and eye diseases to cancer. More than 600 are identified, but only a small handful have been studied extensively. While each carotenoid reviewed here is a proven health remedy by itself, a combination of carotenoids offers the most protection.

—**Alpha Carotene:** a vitamin A precursor. High food sources: *carrots, pumpkin, and other red/orange and yellow fruits and veggies.*

Health Benefits: although alpha carotene has lower vitamin A activity than beta carotene, it is 38% stronger as an antioxidant and is 10% more protective against cancer of the skin, liver and lungs in animal tests.

—**Astazanthin:** responsible for the pink pigment in the flesh of crustaceans, salmon, scallops, and some types of microalgae.

Health Benefits: astazanthin has 10 times the antioxidant capabilities as beta carotene, and 100 to 500 times the antioxidant capabilities of vitamin E. Able to cross the blood brain barrier, making it promising in natural Alzheimer's, Parkinson's, and ALS treatment.

—**Beta Carotene:** the most well know of the carotenes, beta carotene is a vitamin A precursor, converting to vitamin A in the liver as needed. Food sources: *green leafy vegetables, green pepper, carrots and other orange vegetables, dandelion greens and sea greens.*

Health Benefits: a powerful anti-infective and antioxidant for immune response, anti-tumor immunity protection, early aging and allergy control. Effective protection against environmental pollutants, respiratory diseases and infections. Helps prevent lung cancer.

—**Canthaxanthin:** an antioxidant carotenoid. Food sources: *mushrooms, trout and crustaceans, like crab and mussels.*

Health Benefits: may decrease risk for skin cancer and inhibit other cancer cell growth. Also improves immune response.

—**Cryptoxanthin:** a vitamin A precursor. Food sources: *corn, oranges and paprika, and other red/orange and yellow fruits and veggies.*

Health Benefits: may reduce risk of cervical dysplasia.

—**Lutein and Zeaxanthin:** carotenoid nutrients not converted to vitamin A like beta-carotene, but are potent antioxidants. Food sources: *spinach, kale, most fruits and vegetables.*

Health Benefits: of all the carotenoids, lutein and zeaxanthin lend the most support to the eyes. Lutein and zeaxanthin make up the yellow retinal pigment and appear to specifically protect the macula. A Harvard study reports that people eating the most lutein and zeaxanthin foods are most likely to have healthy retinas and maculae. A new study shows high lutein diets are also protective against colon cancer for men and women.

—**Lycopene:** lycopene gives many foods their reddish color and is a powerful antioxidant. Requires some fat to be absorbed in the body. Food sources: *tomatoes and in smaller quantities in watermelon, guava and pink grapefruit.*

Health Benefits: a promising food medicine against cancer. Men who eat a high lycopene diet cut their risk for prostate cancer by 40%! The International Journal of Cancer reveals that lycopene also protects against cancers of the mouth, pharynx, esophagus, stomach, colon and rectum. A University of Illinois report shows that women with the highest lycopene levels have a fivefold lower risk for developing early signs of cervical cancer. A high lycopene diet may even cut heart attack risk in half!

CATECHIN: the most abundant plant polyphenol. Food sources: *grapes, pomegranates, raspberries, huckleberries, strawberries and green tea.*

Health Benefits: breaks up free radical cell chains of fats, prevents DNA damage, helps block carcinogens, and protects against digestive and respiratory infections. Green tea catechins show excellent antioxidant effects on fatty foods. Antioxidant properties of green tea catechins are 30 times more powerful than vitamin E and 50 times more potent than vitamin C.

CHLORINE: an electrolyte that helps maintain acid/alkaline balance. Good food sources: *seafoods, sea greens and salt.*

Health Benefits: naturally-occurring chlorine stimulates the liver, bile and smooth joint-tendon operation.

CHLOROPHYLL: pigment that plants use for photosynthesis - absorbing the light energy from the sun, and converting it into plant energy. Chlorophyll is in all green plants, but is particularly rich in *green and blue-green algae, wheat grass, parsley, and alfalfa.*

Health Benefits: similar to human blood except that it carries magnesium in its center instead of iron. Eating chlorophyll-rich foods helps our bodies build oxygen-carrying red blood cells. To me, eating green foods is like giving yourself a little transfusion to help treat illness and enhance immunity. Blocks cancer growth, increases resistance to radiation like X-rays, kills harmful bacteria, stimulates tissue regeneration by raising cell oxygen levels, purifies the liver, improves cardiovascular function, and strengthens blood vessel and cell walls. May even be effective against AIDS and HIV.

CHOLINE: a lipotropic, B complex family member, choline works with inositol to emulsify fats. Food sources: *garlic, fenugreek, dandelion and dong quai.*

Health Benefits: a brain nutrient and neurotransmitter that aids memory and learning, and helps retard Alzheimer's disease and neurological disorders. Used as part of a program to overcome alcoholism, liver and kidney disorders. Research shows success in cancer control. Also helps dizziness, lowers cholesterol and supports liver health.

CHROMIUM: an essential trace mineral needed for glucose tolerance and sugar balance. Food sources: *nutritional yeast, clams, honey, grains, liver, corn oil, grapes, raisins.*

Health Benefits: deficiency means high cholesterol, heart trouble, diabetes or hypoglycemia, poor carbohydrate and fat metabolism, and premature aging. Supplementation can reduce blood cholesterol levels, increase HDL cholesterol levels, and diminish atherosclerosis.

Most effective as a biologically active form of GTF (chromium, niacin and glutathione), it helps control diabetes through insulin potentiation. For athletes, chromium is a safe way to convert body fat to muscle. For dieters, chromium curbs appetite as it raises metabolism.

—**Chromium picolinate:** an exceptionally bio-active source of chromium. A combination of chromium and picolinic acid, it is naturally secreted by the liver and kidneys. Picolinic acid is the body's best mineral transporter, combining with elements like iron, zinc and chromium to move them efficiently into the cells. Chromium plays a vital role in sensitizing the body to insulin. Excess body weight in the form of fat impairs insulin sensitivity, making it harder to lose weight. Also helps build muscles without steroid side effects, promotes healthy growth in children, speeds wound healing and decreases proneness to arterial plaque deposits.

CLA (conjugated linoleic acid): an essential fatty acid that plays a role in muscle growth and tone, and nutrient/energy conversion. Food sources: *dairy foods, especially cheese, lamb, sunflower oil and beef.*

Health Benefits: CLA's ability to convert the most energy from the least amount of food makes it popular among athletes for increasing muscle mass and burning fat. Like other fatty acids, CLA contains powerful antioxidants for immune health and shows remarkable results in lowering cholesterol. CLA studies were the first to show that fats can help you lose fat to promote weight loss. CLA especially inhibits body storage of saturated fat by increasing its ability to use fat reserves for energy.

COBALAMIN: see Vitamin B-12. Cyanocobalamin can be made from sugar beet, molasses, or whey.

COBALT: an integral component mineral of vitamin B-12 synthesis. Aids in hemoglobin formation. Food sources: *green leafy vegetables and liver.*

Co-ENZYME-A: a metabolic enzyme critical to both aerobic and anaerobic energy metabolism. Requires pantothenic acid (in grains, legumes and broccoli) to be made.

Health Benefits: critical to fatty acid metabolism so your body maintains normal cholesterol and triglyceride levels. Coenzyme-A starts the manufacture of acetylcholine in the brain and steroid hormones in the adrenal glands. Activates white blood cells for immune response, contributes to hemoglobin formation and helps repair damaged RNA and DNA. By manufacturing important components of connective tissue, like chondroitin sulfate and hyaluronic acid, it helps keep joints flexible. A deficiency means fatty acids cannot be converted into energy.

Co-ENZYME Q-10: an isoprenoid enzyme catalyst in the creation of cellular energy. Food sources: *rice bran, wheat germ, beans, nuts, fish and eggs.*

Health Benefits: supplementation has a long history of effectiveness in immune enhancement, raising cardiac strength against angina, promoting natural weight loss, inhibiting aging and overcoming periodontal disease. Crucial in preventing and treating congestive heart and arterial diseases. Helps reduce high blood pressure without other medication. The newest research at doses of 300mg for breast and prostate cancer protection and treatment is extremely encouraging. Consider supplementing with Co-Q_{10} if you are taking drugs to lower cholesterol because these drugs can deplete Co-Q_{10}. Synergistic in combination with vitamin E.

CREATINE *(methyl guanidine-acetic acid):* made naturally in the human liver, as creatine phosphate. Also found in red meat and fish.

Health Benefits: creatine monohydrate supplements, with more weight of material than any other form, are popular with athletes today who want to gain weight and muscle mass, and increase their stamina. While research shows that using creatine along with an exercise program does increase lean body mass and muscle strength faster, creatine supplementation may cause an electrolyte imbalance. Creatine draws on water from other parts of the body. When using, drink lots of water.

CRYPTOXANTHIN: See Carotenoids listing.

CYSTEINE: a semi-essential antioxidant amino acid. Found in small amounts in onion, carrot, and watermelon seed and fruit.

Health Benefits: works with vitamins C, E and selenium to protect against radiation, cancer carcinogens and free radical damage to skin and arteries. Stimulates immune activity. Helps heal burns, wounds of all kinds, and renders toxic chemicals in the body harmless. Taken with evening primrose oil, cysteine protects the brain from alcohol and tobacco effects (highly effective in preventing hangover). Useful for hair loss, psoriasis, dental plaque prevention and skin dermatitis. Relieves bronchial asthma by breaking up mucous plugs. Take vitamin C in a 3:1 ratio to cysteine for best results.

—**N-acetyl-cysteine, NAC:** an antioxidant amino acid and more stable, bio-available form of L-cysteine. NAC is converted in the body to glutathione, a prime immune T-cell enhancer, especially for people with HIV who have low glutathione. NAC detoxifies from alcohol, heavy metals, X-rays and radiation damage, treats viral diseases, protects the liver, and breaks up pulmonary-bronchial mucus. Note: NAC is a powerful chelator of zinc and copper, capable of removing enough of these minerals from the body to produce deficiencies unless supplies are adequate.

CYSTINE: a semi-essential amino acid, cystine is the oxidized form of cysteine. Food sources: *butternut bark, pumpkin seeds, fenugreek, fennel and green beans.*

Health Benefits: like cysteine, it promotes white blood cell activity and heals burns and wounds. The main constituent of hair, essential to formation of skin. Cystine can sometimes be harmful to the kidneys, and generally should not be used clinically.

DHA *(docosahexaenoic acid):* the most predominant EFA in our brain tissue. Food sources: *sea foods, sea plants and eggs.*

Health Benefits: low levels of DHA are linked to mental problems like depression, memory loss, attention deficit/hyperactivity disorders, hostility, Alzheimer's disease, and senility. Studies show that DHA even protects against Alzheimer's and promotes clearer thinking. DHA can lower blood fats, and normalize high cholesterol and triglyceride levels. An 18-year study published in the journal Pediatrics reveals that breast-fed infants have academic advantage! The determining factor for this effect seems to be the high content of DHA in breast milk!

D-LIMONENE: a nutraceutical found in the rinds and seeds of *citrus fruits and spices like caraway, dill and bergamot.*

Health Benefits: protects against cancer by accelerating liver detoxification. Studies show it inhibits cancer of the stomach, lungs, and breasts. Phase 1 testing on the anti-cancer action of D-Limonene on humans with pancreatic and colorectal cancer is underway at the Charing Cross Hospital in London. Used as a natural solvent and disinfectant in environmentally-friendly household and industrial cleaning supplies.

DLPA, DL-PHENYLALANINE: an amino acid which is safe and generally well tolerated. Food sources: *almonds, fish, poultry, chickpeas and sesame seeds.*

Health Benefits: an effective pain reliever and anti-depressant with an endorphin effect for arthritis, and lower back and cerebro-spinal pain. Increases mental alertness, and improves the symptoms of Parkinson's disease. A normal therapeutic dose is 500-750mg. *Note: avoid DLPA if you have high blood pressure, have psychosis or phenylketonuria, are pregnant, diabetic, or are taking MAO inhibitors.*

ELECTROLYTES: ionized salts in blood, tissue fluids and cells, that transport electrical energy through the body. Electrolytes include sodium, potassium and chlorine.

Health Benefits: essential to cell function and body pH balance, but are easily lost through perspiration, so regular replacement is necessary from drinking electrolytic fluids. When electrolytes are low, we tire easily. When they are adequate, we experience more energy. Electrolyte drinks are very beneficial for athletes and those doing hard physical work. My **Potassium Essence Broth** on pg. 568 is an excellent source of minerals and electrolytes.

ELLAGIC ACID: a phenolic compound. Readily absorbed food sources: *red raspberries, walnuts, grapes, apples, tea and pomegranates.*

Health Benefits: stimulates the natural detoxifying substance glutathione in the body to help eliminate trapped poisons that cause cancer. Ellagic acid is very effective against nicotine-induced lung cancer and skin tumors. Studies with human cells reveal it can reduce cancer occurrence in cell lines exposed to even powerful carcinogens. It possesses anti-viral and anti-bacterial properties that protect against colds and flu.

ENZYMES: vital catalysts required for virtually every body process. See "Enzymes & Enzyme Therapy," page 30.

ESSENTIAL FATTY ACIDS, EFA's: essential fatty acids include linoleic, linolenic and arachidonic acids, necessary for cell membrane function, balanced prostaglandin production and metabolic processes. Food sources: *seafoods, dark green vegetables, flax seed, evening primrose oil, borage seed and black currant seed oil.* See "Fats & Oils," page 74, and CLA, DHA and GLA listings for more.

FIBER: abundant in fruits, vegetables and whole grains, fiber is the part of food which is not digested. Modern American diets consist of refined, processed foods that are stripped of their natural fiber. The dietary fiber consumption of the average American is only one-fifth of what it was one hundred years ago. While the U.S. government recommends 25-30 grams of fiber per day and many doctors recommend 50 to 60 grams per day, the average American eats just 10 grams per day.

Health Benefits: lowers blood cholesterol levels, speeds bowel transit time, stabilizes blood sugar levels, promotes the growth of "friendly" flora, absorbs toxins and promotes easier elimination.

FLUORIDE: a non essential mineral found in trace amounts in the teeth and skeletal system. The difference between calcium fluoride (naturally occurring) and other forms is the higher availability of free fluoride ions in sodium-fluoride, and in fluoride from hydrofluosilicic acid. Found naturally in some water supplies and also added as *hydrofluosilicic acid* from the phosphate fertilizer industries.

Health Issues: new research shows that fluoride is more poisonous than lead, just slightly less poisonous than arsenic. Linked to cancer, Alzheimer's, poor child brain development and nervous system health, and fluorosis (fluoride poisoning of cells that form tooth enamel). Where calcium fluoride occurs naturally in the water, people age before their time, suffer from bone disease, tooth disorders, and premature hardening of the arteries. Disastrous effects are apparent in elderly populations, in people with low calcium-magnesium or vitamin C levels, and people with heart and kidney problems. Postmenopausal women in fluoridated areas are more at risk of fractures. As little as 0.7 parts per million fluoride in water is associated with skeletal fluorosis.

FOS (*fructo-oligosaccharides*): food constituents which encourage the growth of "friendly" bacteria. One gram a day boosts an increase in bifidobacteria by five-fold. Food sources: *Jerusalem artichoke, onions, garlic and asparagus.*

Health Benefits: produces B-vitamins (including B-12) and helps improve the liver's ability to detoxify systemic poisons. Prevents traveler's diarrhea, helps babies digest milk (reducing fecal odor) and fights off harmful bacteria like E. coli. Nourishes friendly intestinal bifidobacteria in the digestive tract while reducing harmful bacteria. Promotes healthy peristalsis and bowel regularity.

GABA, *Gamma-Aminobutyric Acid:* a non-essential amino acid formed from glutamic acid. Some research shows GABA reduces enlarged prostate symptoms by stimulating the release of the hormone prolactin. Used with niacinamide, it is a relaxant.

Health Benefits: useful in treating brain-nerve dysfunctions, like anxiety, depression, nerves, high blood pressure, insomnia, schizophrenia, Parkinson's and Alzheimer's diseases, and ADD in children. GABA acts as a natural tranquilizer, improves libido, and along with glutamine and tyrosine, helps overcome alcohol and drug abuse.

GAMMA ORYZANOL: a substance extracted from rice bran oil used as a medicine in Japan since 1962. A mild anti-inflammatory that may also relieve anxiety.

Health Benefits: acts on the hypothalamus and pituitary gland. Although many bodybuilders believe it increases growth hormone levels, animal studies show it actually inhibits growth hormone secretion as well as prolactin, luteinizing hormone and thyroid-stimulating hormone. Studies show gamma oryzanol reduces menopausal hot flashes, and lowers cholesterol and triglyceride levels. Used successfully in the treatment of Irritable Bowel Syndrome (I.B.S.), gastritis and peptic ulcers.

GENISTEIN: a phytohormone flavonoid constituent of soy.
   Health Benefits: an estrogen balancing substance that relieves hot flashes. Reduces risk of breast, ovarian and prostate cancer, and acts as a natural angiogenesis inhibitor (blocks formation of blood vessels that "feed" cancer) for existing tumors. Animal tests show genistein also slows the progression and growth of colon cancer.

GERMANIUM, *(organic sesquioxide):* an anti-oxidant mineral. Food sources: *chlorella, garlic, onion, tuna, suma, oysters, green tea, reishi mushroom, aloe vera, ginseng, leafy greens.*
   Health Benefits: an anticancer agent, particularly where there is tumor metastasis. An interferon stimulus for immune strength. Facilitates oxygen uptake, detoxifies and blocks free radicals. Effective for viral, bacterial and fungal infections, osteoporosis, arthritis, and heart, blood pressure and respiratory conditions. Studies show success with leukemia, HIV, Epstein-Barr, chronic fatigue, asthma, candida, and brain, lung, pancreatic and lymphatic cancers.

GLA (Gamma Linoleic Acid): an essential fatty acid obtained from evening primrose, black currant, and borage seed oil.
   Health Benefits: a source of energy for the cells, electrical insulation for nerve fibers, a precursor of prostaglandins which regulate hormone and metabolic functions. Aids nerve transmission for M.S., diabetes and muscular dystrophy. GLA significantly reduces tender, swollen joints of rheumatoid arthritis. Helps the body burn fat instead of storing it. Reduces breast tenderness during PMS; relieves menopause symptoms like vaginal dryness; treats schizophrenia and hyperactivity in children; and reduces skin and hair dryness. A Canadian study reveals students taking a high GLA borage oil supplement have lower stress levels, so GLA may be a wonderful tool for resisting "stressed out" reactions. Evening primrose is the best GLA choice for women's hormone balance and skin beauty.

GLUCOSAMINE SULFATE: a *proteoglycan,* or amino sugar that promotes tissue elasticity and cushioning. The supplement is derived from chitin (exoskeleton of shellfish).
   Health Benefits: stimulates manufacture of *glycos-amino-glycans,* important cartilage components that help the body repair eroded cartilage. GS thus stimulates good joint function and joint repair. Glucosamine sulfate is the form used; sulfur takes part in forming cartilage.

GLUTAMIC ACID: a non-essential amino acid; a derivative of glutamine which can be synthesized from ornithine and arginine. Found in: *garlic, basil, Jerusalem artichoke, oat grain and pumpkin seeds.*
   Health Benefits: important for nerve health and sugar-fat metabolism. A prime brain fuel that transports potassium across the blood-brain barrier. Helps correct mental and nerve disorders like epilepsy, muscular dystrophy, mental retardation and severe insulin reactions.

GLUTAMINE: the most abundant amino acid in the body (50% of total amino acids in the body and 60% of amino acids in the muscles). Converts readily into 6-carbon glucose, a prime brain nutrient and energy source. Food sources: *onion, carrot and oranges*; also manufactured by the body.
   Health Benefits: important for athletes because it reduces muscle breakdown relative to the rate of muscle growth. Users report less muscle soreness and longer workout times.

Increases fat burning, reduces cravings for sugar and alcohol, and normalizes insulin production. Vital to proper gastrointestinal health, accelerates recovery from illness and boosts immunity. Supplements rapidly improve memory recall, concentration and alertness. Glutamine helps mental performance in cases of retardation, senility, epileptic seizures and schizophrenia. Also protects against alcohol toxicity, and controls hypoglycemic reactions.

GLUTATHIONE: an amino acid blend of *cysteine, glutamic acid and glycine.* Stimulates prostaglandin metabolism. Food sources: *watermelon, asparagus, avocados, oranges, peaches.*

Health Benefits: an antioxidant that neutralizes radiation toxicity and inhibits free radicals. Assists white blood cells in killing bacteria. A prime immune booster that helps detoxify from heavy metal pollutants, cigarette smoke, alcohol and drug (especially PCP) overload, and from the effects of chemotherapy, X-rays and liver toxins. An anti-aging substance, it works with vitamin E to break down fats linked to atherosclerosis. It protects against stroke, kidney failure and cataract formation. Deficiency symptoms include poor coordination, nervous system problems, tremors and twitching.

GLYCINE: an amino acid which releases growth hormone taken in large doses.

Health Benefits: converts to creatine to retard nerve and muscle degeneration, so therapeutically effective for myasthenia gravis, gout and muscular dystrophy. Animal studies show that it promotes healing after trauma in conjunction with arginine. A key to regulating hypoglycemic sugar drop, especially when taken upon rising.

—**Di-Methyl-Glycine, DMG,** once known as B-15, is a powerful antioxidant and energizer that converts to glycine. Used successfully to improve Down Syndrome and mental retardation, and to curb alcohol addiction cravings. Effective as a control for epileptic seizures, with notable results for atherosclerosis, rheumatic fever, rheumatism, emphysema and liver cirrhosis. Take sublingually before exercise. *Note: Too much DMG disrupts the metabolic chain and causes fatigue. The proper dose produces energy; overdoses do not.*

GLYCYRRHIZIN: a hormone-like saponin primarily found in licorice root.

Health Benefits: effective for normalizing menopausal hormone levels. Helps deter hormone-driven tumors (like those of breast cancer) by its action as a natural estrogen blocker. Glycyrrhizin has anti-viral properties — it is able to slow progression of the HIV virus by inhibiting cell infection and inducing interferon activity for immune response. Glycyrrhizin encourages production of hydrocortisone for anti-inflammatory activity. Like cortisone, but without the side effects, it relieves arthritic and allergy symptoms, including those that accompany candida albicans yeast infections. *Note: excess glycyrrhizin can disrupt the body's sodium and water balance, and may lead to elevated blood pressure.* Using whole licorice root offers inherent protection against this type of reaction. An Italian study shows using whole licorice root extract results in less incidence of side effects and is far safer than using glycyrrhizin alone.

HESPERIDIN: a bioflavonoid present in orange and lemon peel.

Health Benefits: increases capillary strength. Deficiency is linked to nighttime leg cramps, weakness and achiness. Supplements can reduce water retention and edema.

HISTIDINE: a semi-essential amino acid abundant in hemoglobin in adults, essential in infants. Food sources: *fenugreek seeds, pumpkin seeds and butternut bark.*

Health Benefits: needed for good immune response, effective defense against colds, respiratory infections, and for countering allergic reactions. Has strong vasodilating and hypotensive properties for circulatory disorders, anemia and cataracts. Helps prevent anemia; a key to production of both red and white blood cells. Synthesizes glutamic acid, aids copper transport through the joints, and removes heavy metals from tissues, making it successful in treating arthritis. Noticeably raises libido in both sexes. Deficiency may cause hearing loss.

INDOLE 3 CARBINOL: an indole found in cruciferous veggies like broccoli, brussels sprouts and cauliflower, responsible for these vegetables' bitter flavor.

Health Benefits: stimulates natural phase 2 enzymes that eliminate carcinogens before they bind to DNA and cause cancer. New research finds that indole 3 carbinol reduces pain and muscle weakness in 50% of fibromyalgia patients. Regularly used with success for warts on the larynx and genitalia. Powerful medicine for today's women who are bombarded daily with estrogen mimics from the environment and commercial food supply, indole 3 carbinol stimulates estrogen metabolism to control excess estrogen. Reduces breast cancer risk and symptoms of estrogen dominance like weight gain, heavy menstruation and fibrocystic breasts.

INOSINE: a non-essential amino acid.

Health Benefits: stimulates ATP energy and helps provide muscle endurance when the body's glycogen reserves run out. Take with an electrolyte drink before exercise.

INOSITOL: part of the B-complex family, a sugar-like crystalline substance found in the liver, kidney and heart muscle, and in most plants.

Health Benefits: deficiency linked to loss of hair, eye defects and stunted growth.

IODINE: a mineral which exerts antibiotic-like action and also prevents toxicity from radiation. Food sources: *seafoods and sea greens.*

Health Benefits: a key component of good thyroid function and metabolism, necessary for skin, hair and nail health, and for wound healing. White blood cells absorb iodine from the blood and use it in their pathogen killing capacity. Iodine also prevents mucous buildup. Iodine deficiency results in goiter, hypothyroidism, cretinism, confused thinking and PMS. *Sea greens* are my favorite choice for iodine therapy (especially beneficial for menopausal women).

IPRIFLAVONE: synthesized from *isoflavones* (natural plant estrogens) and a new leader in natural osteoporosis treatment.

Health Benefits: studies show ipriflavone inhibits bone cell death and may even increase new bone growth by activating bone building osteoblasts. Three studies from Italy find that 200mg. of ipriflavone three times daily reduces postmenopausal bone loss. *Note: May cause interactions with drugs like theophylline, an asthma drug.*

IRON: a mineral that combines with proteins and copper to produce hemoglobin to carry oxygen through the body. Herbal sources: *alfalfa, bilberry, burdock, catnip, yellow dock root, watercress, sarsaparilla and nettles.*

Health Benefits: iron deficiency means fatigue, muscle weakness and anemia. Strengthens immunity, helps wound healing, and is important for women using contraceptive drugs and during pregnancy. It keeps hair color young, eyes bright, the body strong. However, free, un-bound iron is a strong pro-oxidant, and can be toxic at abnormally high levels. Iron overload is linked to some cancers, heart disease, diabetes, arthritis and gland malfunction. Using herbal or food source iron supplements avoids the problem. Sign of iron overload: orangish skin. Food sources: *molasses, cherries, prunes, leafy greens, poultry, liver, legumes, peas, eggs, fish, whole grains.* Vitamin C-rich foods like tomatoes, citrus and vinegar greatly enhance iron absorption.

ISOPRENOIDS: fat soluble antioxidants that neutralize free radicals by anchoring themselves to fatty membranes, grabbing free radicals attached to the membranes and passing them to other antioxidants. CoQ-10 and vitamin E are isoprenoid antioxidants.

LACTIC ACID: a by-product of the metabolism of glucose and glycogen, present in blood and muscle tissue. Used in cosmetics to exfoliate skin. Food sources: *sour milk, beer, sauerkraut, pickles,* and other foods made by bacterial fermentation.

LACTOBACILLUS: there are several types of lactobacilli, including *L. acidophilus, L. bifidus, L. caucassus,* and *L. bulgaricus.* All are beneficial bacteria that synthesize intestinal tract nutrients, counteract pathogenic microorganisms and maintain intestinal health. Food sources: *yogurt, kefir, miso, tempeh and raw sauerkraut.*
   Health Benefits: skin disorders, chronic candidiasis, irritable bowel syndrome and other intestinal disorders, hepatitis, lupus and heart disease are all associated with a Lactobacillus deficiency. **Note:** *Lactobacillus organisms are readily destroyed by noxious chemicals and drugs, particularly chlorine and antibiotics.* A single long course of antibiotics can destroy most bowel flora, leading to the overgrowth of yeasty pathogenic organisms, like *candida albicans,* which are resistant to antibiotics. Even eating antibiotic-laced meats and dairy products leads to an insidious decline in the number of Lactobacillus organisms in the human body.

LAETRILE (B-17): a nutrient substance derived from apricot seeds discovered in 1950. Contains *cyanide, benzaldehyde and glucose,* and can be toxic at high doses.
   Health Benefits: decade-long studies have been done on laetrile and its effects on cancer cells. The tests are still underway for cancer, and now also include high blood pressure and rheumatism. Even though it has had some success in cancer treatment, laetrile treatment has been banned in the U.S. because of potential toxicity.

LECITHIN: a soy-derived food, used as a natural emulsifier. It may be substituted for $1/3$ of the oil in recipes for a healing diet. A therapeutic food, 2 teasp. added to recipes offer superior phosphatides, choline, inositol, potassium and linoleic acid.
   Health Benefits: a natural emulsifier, (breaks down fat particles), an action essential in controlling cholesterol and triglycerides. Reduces dangerous LDL cholesterol; elevates healthy HDL particles. Helps the brain convert its choline into acetylcholine, vital for memory, Alzheimer's disease protection, mood and muscle control. Improves gallbladder function, eliminates liver spots and helps skin disorders like psoriasis. Helps boost immune resistance to viral infections such as herpes, chronic Epstein Barr virus, multiple sclerosis and AIDS.

LINOLEIC ACID: the most common essential fatty acid in foods like fish and vegetable oils, meat and milk. A healthy body makes GLA (gamma linoleic acid) from linoleic acid if it has sufficient zinc, magnesium and vitamins A, B-6, B-3 and C.

Health Benefits: deficiency results in poor growth, hair loss, skin disorders and slow wound healing. Found in some studies to reduce symptoms of multiple sclerosis.

LIPOIC ACID (*alpha lipoic acid*): a unique antioxidant, both fat and water soluble, able to quench free radicals in both fat and water mediums. High amounts in *nutritional yeast and liver.*

Health Benefits: one of the most powerful liver detoxifiers ever discovered, a potent promoter of glutathione and a chief co-factor in energy metabolism, especially under stress conditions. Increases effectiveness of other antioxidants like vitamins C and E. Shows great promise for heart disease (especially stroke recovery and atherosclerosis), diabetes (approved in Europe for diabetic retinopathy), neuro-degenerative diseases, like Parkinson's and Alzheimer's, inflammatory diseases like arthritis and irritable bowel syndromes, HIV and AIDS, cataracts and heavy-metal toxicity. Helps with appetite control in a natural weight loss program. *Note: lipoic acid is best taken with meals to prolong the delivery and also to prevent a hypoglycemic response.*

LITHIUM: an earth's crust trace mineral used clinically as lithium arginate. Increases brain acetylcholine activity. Food sources: *mineral water, whole grains and seeds.*

Health Benefits: successful in treating manic-depressive disorders, ADD in children, epilepsy, alcoholism, drug withdrawal and migraine headaches. Research shows therapy success with malignant lymphatic growths, arteriosclerosis and chronic hepatitis. Overdoses can cause palpitations and headaches.

LUTEIN: see Carotenoids listings.

LYCOPENE: see Carotenoids.

LYSINE: an essential amino acid found in corn, poultry and avocados.

Health Benefits: a primary treatment for herpes virus; may be used topically or internally. Add high lysine foods if there are recurrent herpes breakouts. Helps rebuild muscle and repair tissue after injury or surgery. Important for calcium uptake for bone growth, and for osteoporosis, reduces calcium loss in the urine. Helps the formation of collagen, hormones and enzymes. Supplements are effective for Parkinson's disease, Alzheimer's and hypothyroidism.

MAGNESIUM: a critical mineral for health. Food sources: *dark green vegetables, seafood, whole grains, dairy foods, nuts, legumes, poultry and hot spices like cayenne.*

Health Benefits: a protector against osteoporosis; critical for a strong skeletal structure. Necessary for good nerve and muscle function, healthy blood vessels, balanced blood pressure and athletic endurance. Important for tooth formation, heart and kidney health, and restful sleep. Counteracts stress, irregular heartbeat, emotional instability and depression. Calms hyperactive children. Magnesium supplements help alcoholism, diabetes and asthma. Deficiency means muscle spasms, cramping, stomach disturbances, sometimes fibromyalgia, and usually accompanying potassium deficiency.

MANGANESE: nourishes brain and nerve centers, aids in sugar and fat metabolism. Food sources: *blueberries, ginger, rice, eggs, green vegetables, legumes, nuts and bananas.*

    Health Benefits: synergistic with calcium in nourishing bones. Also helps eliminate fatigue, nervousness and lower back pain. Reduces seizures in epileptics. Deficiencies result in poor hair and nail growth (white spots on nails), hearing loss, blood pressure disturbances, impotence, latent diabetes, and poor muscle-joint coordination. SOD (*superoxide dismutase*), a powerful free radical quenching enzyme, is solely dependent on manganese for its immune enhancing activity. Tranquilizer drugs deplete manganese.

METHIONINE: an essential amino acid and free radical deactivator. Food sources: *fish, soybeans, eggs, lentils, pumpkin seeds and yogurt.*

    Health Benefits: a major source of organic sulphur for healthy liver activity, lymph and immune health. Protective against chemical allergic reactions. An effective "lipotropic" that keeps fats from accumulating in the liver and arteries, thus keeping high blood pressure and serum cholesterol under control. Effective against toxemia during pregnancy. An important part of treatment for rheumatic fever. Supports healthy skin and nails, and prevents hair loss. Helps remove heavy metals like lead from the body.

MINERALS AND TRACE MINERALS: the building blocks of life, minerals are the most basic of nutrients, the bonding agents between you and food, allowing your body to absorb nutrients. Your body's minerals comprise only about 4% of your body weight, but they are keys to major areas of your health.

    Health Benefits: especially necessary for athletes and people in active sports, you must have minerals to run. Minerals keep your body pH balanced — alkaline instead of acid. They are essential to bone formation and bone health. They regulate the osmosis of cellular fluids, nerve electrical activity and most metabolic functions. They transport oxygen, govern heart rhythm, help you sleep, and keep you emotionally balanced. Trace minerals are only .01% of body weight, but even minute deficiencies in them can cause severe depression, PMS disorders, hyperactivity in children, hypoglycemia and diabetes, nervous stress, high blood pressure, premature aging, memory loss and poor healing. Minerals play a major role in detoxifying cells, and in eliminating acid crystals from the lymphatic system that your immune system relies on to filter and remove any infective organisms.

    Minerals are important. Hardly any of us get enough. Your body doesn't synthesize minerals; they must be regularly obtained from our foods. Today's diet of chemicalized foods inhibits mineral absorption. Minerals from plants and herbs are higher quality and more absorbable than from meat sources. High stress life-styles that rely on tobacco, alcohol, steroids and antibiotics contribute to mineral depletion. Many minerals are no longer even sufficiently present in our fruits and vegetables. They have been leached from the soil by the chemicals and pesticide sprays used in commercial farming. Even if foods show good amounts of minerals they have less than we believe, because measurements were done decades ago when pesticides were not as prolific as they are now. Plant minerals from earth and sea herbs are a reliable way to get mineral benefits. Your body easily uses minerals from herbs like *nettles, yellow dock, alfalfa and watercress* as healing agents and to maintain body nutrient levels. **Minerals can really give your body a boost.** *Note: Electrolyte mineral formulas are superior to colloidal products for maximum absorption. Adding granulated sea greens to your recipes is another great way to take in extra minerals.*

MOLYBDENUM: a metabolic mineral, necessary in mobilizing enzymes. Food sources: *whole grains, brown rice, nutritional yeast and mineral water.*

Health Benefits: new research shows benefits for esophageal cancers and sulfite-induced cancer. Molybdenum amounts are dependent on good soil content.

MSM *(methylsulfonylmethane):* MSM contains 34% sulfur important for hormones, enzymes, antibodies and antioxidants in tissues and body proteins. Food sources: *cruciferous vegetables, fish, garlic, and unpasteurized milk.* Cooking and processing techniques destroy MSM. Supplements, derived from a naturally produced DMSO (dimethyl sulfoxide), provide best benefits.

Health Benefits: contributes to healthy hair and nails, and to skin softness and pliability. Encourages repair of damaged skin by stimulating the production of collagen. Increases circulation and maintains acid-alkaline balance. Boosts both natural detoxification and immune functions by producing antibodies. MSM helps muscle and joint pain, stopping pain impulses before they reach the brain. Patients with degenerative arthritis taking MSM experience an amazing 82% reduction in pain! Relieves constipation, and helps heal burns and scars.

NADH *(nicotinamide adenine dinucleotide):* a potent antioxidant coenzyme involved in the synthesis of ATP that enhances cellular energy in the brain and body. Although NADH is in every living animal and plant cell, the first supplement was derived from yeast in 1993 (the finished product is yeast-free).

Health Benefits: enhances the immune system by its "metabolic burst" step that leads to the destruction of a cytotoxic invader. Also repairs DNA, enhances the two brain neurotransmitters, dopamine and norepinephrine, and has anti-aging potential. Studies promise hope for Alzheimer's and Parkinson's disease, chronic fatigue syndrome and depression. Recommended dosage for energy boosting is 2.5 to 5mg daily.

NUTRITIONAL YEAST: supplement and condiment that has a distinct but pleasant aroma and taste. Nutritional yeast is not the same as candida albicans yeast. One of the best sources of B-complex; rich in selenium, potassium, lecithin, phosphorus, iron, magnesium, copper, chromium and zinc; a very good source of protein, including all the essential amino acids. Rich in nucleic acid—vital for proper cell development.

Health Benefits: improves skin problems like acne because it helps the liver breakdown fats. Its chromium triggers insulin action—good for persons suffering from diabetes. Neutralizes bowel irritation, soothes inflammation and restores normal bowel movements (useful for people suffering from irritable bowel syndrome or constipation). One of the best immune-enhancing supplements in food form. Just 1 to 2 tsp. in a protein drink offer a daily energy lift. (For more, see "Protein in a Healing Diet" page 42.)

OCTACOSANOL: a wheat germ derivative.

Health Benefits: counteracts fatigue and increases oxygen use during exercise and athletic performance. Antioxidant properties help muscular dystrophy and M.S.

OMEGA-3 OILS: for cooking purposes, omega 3 rich flax and olive oil have the best LDL reducing properties. (See "Fats and Oils in a Healing Diet" page 76.)

ORNITHINE: a non-essential amino acid. Food source: *beets, pumpkin seeds, garlic.*

Health Benefits: works with arginine and carnitine to metabolize excess body fat through the liver; with the pituitary gland to promote growth hormone, muscle development, tissue repair, and endurance. Builds immune strength; helps scavenge free radicals.

OXALIC ACID: a component of chard, spinach and beet greens.

Health Benefits: binds to calcium and iron in the body, thus preventing their absorption. To reduce oxalic acid in these foods, lightly cook them until they turn bright green and slightly tender. In addition, consider a Japanese variety of spinach called "Toyo" which is reported to contain less oxalic acid than regular spinach.

PABA, Para-Aminobenzoic Acid: a B Complex family member and component of folic acid. Food sources: *nutritional yeast, eggs, molasses and wheat germ.*

Health Benefits: has sunscreening properties, is effective against sun and other burns, and is used in treating vitiligo, (depigmentation of the skin). Successful with molasses, pantothenic and folic acid in restoring lost hair color. Research shows success against skin cancers caused by UV radiation (lack of ozone-layer protection).

PANTOTHENIC ACID: see vitamin B-5.

PHENYLALANINE: an essential amino acid; a tyrosine precursor that works with vitamin B-6 on the central nervous system.

Health Benefits: acts as an anti-depressant and mood elevator. Successful in treating manic, post-amphetamine, and schizophrenic-type depression (check for allergies first). Aids in learning and memory retention. Relieves menstrual, arthritic and migraine pain. A thyroid stimulant that curbs the appetite by increasing the body's production of CCK. *Contra-indications:* Phenylketonurics (elevated natural phenylalanine levels) should avoid aspartame sweeteners. Pregnant women and those with high blood pressure, skin carcinomas, and diabetes should avoid phenylalanine. Tumors and cancerous melanoma growths have been slowed by reducing dietary intake of tyrosine and phenylalanine. Avoid if blurred vision occurs when using.

PHOSPHATIDYL CHOLINE: a natural component of lecithin (in grains, legumes and egg yolks), phosphatidyl choline is an essential component of cell membranes.

Health Benefits: maintains membrane fluidity, playing a critical role in all membrane metabolic processes. Emulsifying action controls cholesterol and triglyceride levels. Often used to increase the absorption of fat-soluble vitamins and herbs.

PHOSPHATIDYL SERINE, (PS): a brain cell nutrient that rapidly absorbs and readily crosses the blood-brain barrier. Common foods have insignificant amounts of PS, and the body produces only limited amounts. Until recently, concentrated PS was available only as a bovine-derived product with potential safety problems. A new concentrated, safe-source PS is derived from soybeans.

Health Benefits: helps activate and regulate proteins that play major roles in nerve cell functions and nerve impulses. Studies show that PS helps maintain or improve cognitive ability — memory and learning, especially for Alzheimer's victims. Here's how: Phosphatidylserine

(PS) increases acetylcholine, a key neurotransmitter for memory and learning which is usually deficient in Alzheimer's. PS also effectively helps individuals maintain mental fitness, with benefits persisting even for weeks after PS is stopped.

PHOSPHORUS: the second most abundant body mineral. Food sources: eggs, fish, organ meats, dairy foods, legumes, nuts and poultry.
   Health Benefits: needed for skeletal structure, brain oxygen and cell reproduction. Increases muscle performance; decreases muscle fatigue. Antacid abuse depletes phosphorus.

PHYTIC ACID: an antioxidant compound. Food sources: *rye, wheat, rice, lima beans, sesame seeds, peanuts and soybeans.*
   Health Benefits: may prevent colon cancer and enhance immune killer cell activity. Possibly a better antioxidant than vitamin C, because it naturally chelates both iron and zinc to help prevent heart disease.

POLYPHENOLS: plant elements in green tea responsible for health-promoting action.
   Health Benefits: powerful free radical scavengers. In animal studies, polyphenols block formation and growth of cancerous tumors. Skin, lung, stomach and colon tumors respond to treatment with green tea polyphenols. Also help neutralize the effect of dietary carcinogens.

POLYSACCHARIDES: long chains of simple sugars that are used in healing, particularly in stimulating immunity. Food sources with large amounts of polysaccharides: *aloe, green tea, green-lipped mussels, echinacea, astragalus and maitake mushroom.*
   —Mucopolysaccharides: polysaccharides that form chemical bonds with water. An important constituent of connective tissue, binding together the cells to form tissues, and the tissues to form organs. Topically, used to stimulate hair regrowth and stop hair loss. Help boost sperm count and have mild aphrodisiac effects. Mucopolysaccharides, especially as Chondroitin Sulphate A (CSA), are beneficial for prevention and reversal of coronary heart disease. CSA is anti-inflammatory, and anti-stress, used successfully for osteoporosis and accelerating recovery from bone fractures.

POTASSIUM: an electrolyte mineral in body fluids that balances the acid-alkaline system and transmits electrical signals between cells and nerves. Food sources: *fresh fruits, especially kiwis and bananas, potatoes, sea greens, spices like coriander, cumin, basil, parsley, ginger, hot peppers, dill weed, tarragon, paprika and turmeric, lean poultry and fish, dairy foods, legumes, seeds and whole grains.*
   Health Benefits: enhances muscle performance. Works with sodium to regulate the body's water balance, and protects the heart against hypertension and stroke (people who take high blood pressure medication are vulnerable to potassium deficiency). Potassium helps oxygenate the brain for clear thinking and controls allergic reactions. Stress, hypoglycemia, diarrhea and acute anxiety or depression generally result in potassium deficiency. A vegetable potassium broth (page 568) is one of the greatest natural healing tools available for cleansing and restoring body energy.

PROBIOTICS (meaning "for life"): dietary supplements consisting of beneficial microorganisms which have a profound influence on our health.

Health Benefits: When friendly microorganisms are plentiful and flourishing, they inhibit the growth of pathogenic organisms, boost the immune system, manufacture important vitamins (vitamin K and B vitamins - including B-12), improve digestion, combat vaginal yeast infections, maintain the body's vital chemical and hormone balance, and keep our bodies clean and protected from toxins.

PYRIDOXINE: see vitamin B-6.

QUERCETIN: a bioflavonoid cousin of rutin isolated from blue-green algae. Food sources: *red apples, garlic, chlorella and red onions.*
    Health Benefits: controls allergy and asthma reactions, since it suppresses the release and production of the two inflammatory agents that cause asthma and allergy symptoms — histamines and leukotrienes. Also being tested with good results as an anti-viral against herpes, polio and respiratory viruses. A potential natural reverse transcriptase inhibitor for HIV/AIDS. Take quercetin with bromelain for best bioavailability.

RESVERATROL: a natural polyphenol found in grapes and in high amounts in red wine.
    Health Benefits: may help prevent cancer. Clinically, it causes leukemia cancer cells to change back to non-cancerous cells. Resveratrol has antioxidant and anticoagulant properties which protect the heart. Contains mild plant estrogens that protect a woman's heart when she goes through menopause. I regularly recommend a little resveratrol-rich red wine with dinner for heart protection, and to ease digestion and reduce stress. *Note: Has mild estrogenic effects that may aggravate hormone-dependent tumors, or add to high estrogen stores in women already using HRT drugs.*

RIBOFLAVIN: see vitamin B-2.

RIBOSE: a simple sugar found naturally in all body cells, a vital part of the metabolic process for ATP energy, the number one fuel used by cells.
    Health Benefits: people with cardiovascular disease, or athletes who experience diminished heart and muscle nucleotides following high-intensity exercise are good candidates for ribose. Ischemia, when poor blood flow from the heart causes insufficient oxygen to reach the cells, decreases ATP levels by 50 percent or more. Ribose can help the heart rebuild energy. Studies with ribose show that the heart is able to recover 85 percent of its ATP levels within 24 hours. Athletes who experience anoxia (when muscles use oxygen faster than the bloodstream can supply), boost energy recovery with ribose.

SAMe, (S-Adenosyl Methionine): normally produced in the brain from the amino acid methionine. It becomes active methionine in the body by the combining of the amino acid L-methionine with ATP (primary energy molecule). The stable supplement form of SAMe is made by first producing the amino acid L-methionine by a micro-fermentation process followed by an artificial means of zapping it with ATP.
    Health Benefits: widely prescribed in Italy, clinical studies show that SAMe is an effective natural antidepressant. Results in increased levels of serotonin and dopamine, and improved binding of neurotransmitters to receptor sites. Has a quicker onset of action and is

better tolerated than tricyclic antidepressants. Also relieves the pain of osteoarthritis, fibromyalgia and migraine headaches by aiding chemical processes that control pain and inflammation.

The U.S. Arthritis Foundation even states that SAMe "provides pain relief." Helps cirrhosis, hepatitis, cholestasis (blockage of bile ducts), and may prevent liver damage caused by some drugs. May be useful for Alzheimer's disease because its neurotransmitter improvement helps enhance memory centers. Common dosage: 200 to 400mg — therapeutic doses are higher.

Note: SAMe is extremely safe, but people with bipolar (manic) depression should consult a physician. Include B-complex when taking SAMe. When a SAMe molecule loses its methyl group, it breaks down to become homocysteine. Homocysteine is toxic to cells if it builds up. Vitamin B-6, B-12 and folic acid convert homocysteine into the antioxidant glutathione.

SAPONINS: naturally occurring glycosides. Food sources: *legumes (especially soybeans), spinach, tomatoes, potatoes, oats, alfalfa and sea foods are good food sources. Also found in herbs like ginseng, sarsaparilla, licorice and rehmannia.*

Health Benefits: in vivo and in vitro studies show saponins have anticancer effects. Believed to help lower cholesterol, improve immune response and regulate cell proliferation. Believed to have mild hormone-like action in the body.

SELENIUM: a component of glutathione and powerful antioxidant. Food sources: *nutritional yeast, sesame seeds, garlic, tuna, sea foods and sea greens, wheat germ, organ meats, vegetables, nuts and mushrooms.*

Health Benefits: protects the body from free radical damage and heavy metal toxicity. An anticancer substance and immune stimulant, it works with vitamin E to prevent cholesterol accumulation, and protect against heart weakness and degenerative disease. It enhances skin elasticity. Deficiency means aging skin, liver damage, hypothyroidism and often colon cancer.

SILICA, silicon dioxide: a chemical compound of silicon and oxygen, silica comprises a large percent of the earth's crust and mantle, rocks and sand. There is some confusion between silica and silicon. Both are available in health food stores. Silicon is the elemental silicon mineral that is found in man, animals and plants. Silica is generally silicon dioxide, the most abundant silicon compound. Silica gel contains hydrogen, oxygen and silicon, one form of which is an agent used to absorb moisture (as in containers for certain foods and in the bottles of our supplements). Silica gel is derived from quartz crystals. Some silica supplements are water-soluble extracts of the herb horsetail. Others are derived from purified algae. In addition to its benefits for healthy hair, skin and nails, and for calcium absorption in bone formation, silica/silicon maintains flexible arteries and plays a significant role in cardiovascular health.

—Silicon: a mineral responsible for connective tissue growth and health. Prevents arteriosclerosis. Necessary for collagen synthesis. Regenerates body infrastructure, including skeleton, tendons, ligaments, cartilage, connective tissue, skin, hair and nails. Silicon supplements may bring about bone recalcification. Silicon counteracts the effects of aluminum on the body, and is important in the prevention of Alzheimer's disease and osteoporosis. Silicon levels decrease with aging and are needed in larger amounts by the elderly. Food sources: *whole grains, horsetail herb, well water, bottled mineral water and fresh vegetables.*

SODIUM: an electrolyte mineral. Food sources: *celery, seafoods, sea greens, dairy foods.*

Health Benefits: helps regulate kidney and body fluid function. Involved with high blood pressure only when calcium and phosphorous are deficient. An anti-dehydrating agent.

SULFORAPHANE: a sulphur compound in cruciferous vegetables, mustard, horseradish and broccoli sprouts.

Health Benefits: activates phase 2 enzymes (like indole 3 carbinol) that detoxify cancer-causing substances from the body. Induces protective, phase II enzymes, which detoxify carcinogens. Delays onset of cancer, and inhibits size and number of tumors. Reduces breast cancer occurrence by up to 60% in lab animals. Colon cancer risk can be cut in half by eating 2-lbs. of sulforaphane-rich broccoli a week. (Broccoli sprouts are sweet and actually contain 30 to 50 times more sulforaphane as plain old broccoli. But broccoli seeds are often heavily treated with fungicides and pesticides, so organic broccoli sprouts are always the best choice.)

SULPHUR: the "beauty mineral." It is critical to protein absorption. Food sources: *fish, onions, garlic, hot peppers and mustard.*

Health Benefits: improves complexion, hair and nail growth, and collagen synthesis.

SUPER OXIDE DISMUTASE (SOD): an enzyme. Manganese and zinc, in particular, stimulate production of SOD. Food sources: *barley sprouts.*

Health Benefits: prevents damage caused by the toxic oxygen molecule known as superoxide. Many experts do not believe that antioxidant enzyme levels in cells can be increased by taking antioxidant enzymes like SOD orally. Human tests with SOD supplements do not appear to increase the levels of SOD in the blood or tissues.

TAURINE: an amino acid, taurine is a potent anti-seizure nutrient. Found in high concentrations in bile, mother's milk, shark and abalone. Supplements are needed for therapy.

Health Benefits: helps control hyperactivity, nervous system imbalance after drug or alcohol abuse, and epilepsy. Normalizes irregular heartbeat, helps prevent circulatory disorders, hypoglycemia, hypothyroidism, water retention and hypertension. Lowers bad cholesterol.

THIAMINE: see Vitamin B-1.

THREONINE: an essential amino acid important for the formation of collagen, elastin and enamel. Food sources: *basil, oats, ginkgo, and many seeds.*

Health Benefits: works with glycine to help overcome depression, and neurologic dysfunctions like epileptic seizures and M.S.. Works with aspartic acid and methionine as a lipotropic to prevent fatty build-up in the liver. An immune stimulant and thymus enhancer.

TOCOTRIENOLS: compounds related to the vitamin E tocopherols.

Health Benefits: offer potent antioxidant and anti-cancer properties. More effective than tocopherols in decreasing both total and LDL cholesterol levels. Although tocotrienols and tocopherols both offer significant protection against damage to the arterial wall - tocotrienols have a stronger lipid lowering effect. Vitamin E supplements with mixed tocopherols, and the tocotrienols, are the best choice.

TRANSFER FACTORS: molecular messengers of the immune system (specifically immune T lymphocytes) which confer immunity to a pathogen. Naturally present in human blood, but are extracted from cow's colostrum for the supplement form.

Health Benefits: boost immunity. Very promising as part of a natural healing arsenal to fight viral, bacterial, fungal and parasitical illness. May one day treat even serious diseases like antibiotic-resistant "supergerms", cancer, malaria and AIDS.

TRYPTOPHAN: an essential amino acid; a precursor of the neurotransmitter serotonin, involved in mood and metabolism regulation. Food sources: *turkey, oat grain, pumpkin seeds, evening primrose oil and mung beans.*

Health Benefits: a natural, non-addictive tranquilizer for restful sleep. Decreases hyperkinetic aggressive behavior, migraine headaches, and schizophrenia through blood vessel dilation. Counteracts compulsive overeating, smoking and alcohol abuse. An effective anti-depressant. Raises abnormally low blood sugar, and reduces seizures in petit mal epilepsy. Produces natural niacin (nicotinic acid) being tested to counteract the effects of nicotine from cigarettes. It appears in many prescription sleep-aid drugs, and is a safe nutrient sleep aid and relaxant. *Note: At this writing L-Tryptophan supplements are not allowed as over-the-counter nutrients by the FDA.*

—5-HTP (L-5-Hydroxytryptophan): Tryptophan plays a role in the synthesis of serotonin in our bodies. 5-HTP is the step between tryptophan and serotonin. Once tryptophan is taken up into a nerve cell, it is converted into 5-HTP with the help of the enzyme tryptophan hydroxylase. 5-HTP is then converted to serotonin. 5-HTP extracted from a seed, is a supplement to boost serotonin, and is considered to be the native available.

TYROSINE: an amino acid and growth ho... phenylalanine. Food sources: *butternut bark, pumpkin seeds, fenugr...*

Health Benefits: helps the body to build ...ne and thyroid hormones. Rapidly metabolizes as an antioxidant t... as a source of quick energy, especially for the brain. Converts to ...king it a safe therapy for depression, hypertension, and Parkinson ...control drug abuse and aids drug withdrawal. Increases libido and low sex driv... reduce appetite and body fat in a weight loss diet. Produces melanin for skin and hair pigment. *Note: Tumors, cancerous melanomas and manic depression are slowed through dietary reduction of tyrosine and phenylalanine.*

VANADIUM: a mineral cofactor for several enzymes. Food sources: *whole grains, fish, olives, radishes, vegetables, black pepper and dill seeds.*

Health Benefits: deficiency is linked to heart disease, low reproductive ability and infant mortality. Although some studies find that vanadium improves sugar metabolism for non-insulin dependent diabetics, high levels of vanadium can be toxic. Take vanadium in small dosages. 1mg doses of vanadium within a broad spectrum multi-vitamin and mineral formula is a safe choice for a blood sugar stabilizing program.

VINPOCETINE: an extract from the periwinkle plant.

Health Benefits: a "nootropic" brain nutrient that enhances memory by improving brain glucose use, and increasing blood and oxygen to the brain. Boosts brain ATP levels. Vinpocetine is highly effective in formulas for inner ear balance, hearing loss and tinnitus.

VITAMINS: organic micronutrients that act like spark plugs in the body, keeping it "tuned up" and functioning at high performance. You can't live on vitamins; they are not pep pills, substitutes for food, or components of body structure. They stimulate, but do not act as, nutritional fuel. As catalysts, they work on the cellular level, often as co-enzymes, regulating body metabolic processes through enzyme activity, to convert proteins and carbohydrates to tissue and energy. Most vitamins cannot be synthesized by the body, and must be supplied by food or supplement. Excess amounts are excreted in the urine, or stored by the body until needed.

Despite their minute size and amounts in the body, vitamins are absolutely necessary for growth, vitality, resistance to disease, and healthy aging. It is impossible to sustain life without them. Even small deficiencies can endanger the whole body. Unfortunately, it takes months for signs of vitamin deficiencies to appear because the body only slowly uses its supply. Even when your body is "running on empty" in a certain vitamin, problems are hard to pinpoint, because the cells continue to function with decreasing efficiency until they get proper nourishment or suffer irreversible damage.

Vitamin therapy does not produce results overnight. Vitamins fill nutritional gaps at your body's deepest levels. Regenerative changes in biochemistry may require as much time to rebuild as they did to decline. In most cases, after a short period of higher dosage in order to build a good nutrient foundation, a program of moderate amounts over a longer period of time brings about better body balance and results.

Vitamin RDA's were established in the 1950's as a guideline to prevent severe deficiency diseases. But poor dietary habits, over-processed foods and agri-business practices mean that today, we need supplements for adequate nutrition. Not one diet survey shows that Americans take in anywhere near even the basic RDA amounts in their diets. A recent large USDA survey of the daily food intake of 21,500 people over a three day period showed that not a single person got 100% of the RDA nutrients. Only 3% ate the recommended number of servings from the four food groups. Only 12% got the RDA for protein, calcium, iron, magnesium, zinc or vitamins A, C, B_6, B_{12}, B_2, and B_1. The study concluded that long-held dietary habits and ignoring vitamin supplements left much of the American population at nutritional risk.

People most affected by vitamin deficiencies include:
1: Women with excessive menstrual bleeding who may need iron supplements.
2: Pregnant or nursing women who may need extra iron, calcium and folic acid.
3: The elderly, many of whom do not even get two-thirds of the RDA for calcium, iron, vitamin A or C. (Note: The elderly take more than 50% of all drug prescriptions in the U.S.. Since 90 out of the 100 most prescribed drugs interfere with normal nutrient metabolism, many older people don't absorb much of the nutrition that they do eat.)
4: People on medications that interfere with nutrient absorption and digestion.
5: People on weight loss diets with extremely low calorie intake.
6: People at risk for circulatory blockages, and those at risk for osteoporosis.
7: People who have had recent surgery, or suffer from injuries, wounds or burns.
8: People with periodontal disease.
9: Vegetarians, who may not receive enough calcium, iron, zinc or vitamin B_{12}.

Vitamins help us go beyond average health to optimal health.

VITAMIN A: is a fat soluble vitamin, requiring fats, minerals (especially zinc) and enzymes for absorption. Available in both plants and animals, plants contain the beta carotene form while animal sources contain retinol. Food sources: *fish liver oils, seafood, sea greens, dairy foods, yellow fruits and vegetables, leafy greens, yams, sweet potatoes, liver, watermelon, canteloupe, and eggs.*

Health Benefits: counteracts night blindness, weak eyesight, and strengthens the optical system. Supplements lower risk of many types of cancer, particularly lung cancer. Retinoids inhibit malignant transformation, and reverse pre-malignant changes in tissue. An anti-infective that builds immune resistance. Helps develop strong bone cells, a major factor in skin, hair, teeth and gum health. Deficiency results in eye dryness and the inability to tear, night blindness, rough, itchy skin, poor bone growth, weak tooth enamel, chronic diarrhea and frequent respiratory infections. Vitamin A is critical to adrenal and steroid hormone synthesis, and is a key to preventing premature aging. *Note: Avoid high doses of Vitamin A during pregnancy.*

VITAMIN B-1, (Thiamine): known as the "morale vitamin" because of its beneficial effects on the nerves and mental attitude. Food sources: *asparagus, nutritional yeast, brown rice, barley, beans, nuts, seeds, wheat germ, organ meats, salmon and soy foods.*

Health Benefits: promotes proper growth in children, aids carbohydrate utilization for energy and supports the nervous system. Enhances immune response. Helps control motion sickness. Wards off mosquitos and stinging insects. Pregnancy, lactation, diuretics and oral contraceptives require extra thiamine. Smoking, heavy metal pollutants, excess sugar, junk foods, stress and alcohol all deplete thiamine. Deficiency results in insomnia, fatigue, confusion, poor memory and muscle coordination. Food source thiamine is sensitive to heat and chlorine. Avoid washing or cooking thiamine-rich foods in chlorinated water if you suspect you are thiamine deficient. A high sugar diet or too much alcohol increases your thiamine needs.

VITAMIN B-2, (Riboflavin): a vitamin commonly deficient in the U.S. diet. Necessary for energy, and for fat and carbohydrate metabolism. Aids red blood cell development and hormone production. Food sources: *almonds, nutritional yeast, broccoli, leafy veggies, eggs, mushrooms, yogurt, organ meats and caviar.*

Health Benefits: helps prevent cataracts and corneal ulcers, and generally benefits vision. Promotes healthy skin, especially in cases of psoriasis. Helps protect against drug toxicity and environmental chemicals. Pregnancy and lactation, excess dairy and red meat consumption, prolonged stress, sulfa drugs, diuretics and oral contraceptives all require extra riboflavin. Deficiency is associated with alcohol abuse, anemia, hypothyroidism, diabetes, ulcers, cataracts and congenital heart disease.

VITAMIN B-3, (Niacin): an energy production vitamin; for sex hormone synthesis and good digestion, boosts hydrochloric acid in the stomach. Food sources: *almonds, avocados, mushrooms, nutritional yeast, fish, legumes, bananas, whole grains, cheese, eggs, peanuts and sesame seeds.*

Health Benefits: highly effective in improving joint function, strength and endurance if you have osteoarthritis. Lowers cholesterol. A study at Wayne State University reveals niacin combined with chromium can lower blood cholesterol by as much as 30%, and help regulate blood sugar for diabetes and hypoglycemia! Low niacin means dermatitis, headaches, gum disease, often high blood pressure and schizophrenic behavior. Yet since niacin can rapidly stimulate circulation, (a niacin flush is evidence of this), it can act quickly to reverse these disorders.

VITAMIN B-5, (Pantothenic Acid): an antioxidant vitamin vital to proper adrenal activity, Vitamin D and cortisone production, and natural steroid synthesis. Food sources: *nutritional yeast, brown rice, quinoa, mushrooms, avocado, poultry, yams, organ meats, egg yolks, soy products and royal jelly.*

Health Benefits: important in preventing arthritis and high cholesterol. Fights infection by building antibodies, and defends against stress, fatigue and nerve disorders. A key to overcoming postoperative shock and drug side effects after surgery. Inhibits hair color loss. Deficiency results in anemia, fatigue and muscle cramping. Individuals suffering from constant psychological stress have increased need for B-5.

VITAMIN B-6, (Pyridoxine): helps red blood cell regeneration, and protein-carbohydrate metabolism. Food sources: *bananas, nutritional yeast, buckwheat, organ meats, fish, avocados, legumes, poultry, nuts, rice bran, brown rice, wheat bran, sunflower seeds and soy foods.*

Health Benefits: a primary immune stimulant with particular effectiveness against liver cancer. Helps lower high homocysteine levels that threaten heart health. Supplements inhibit histamine release in treating allergies and asthma. Supports all aspects of nerve health including neuropsychiatric disorders, epilepsy and carpal tunnel syndrome. Works as a natural diuretic, especially in premenstrual edema. Controls acne, promotes beautiful skin, relieves morning sickness and is an anti-aging factor. Oral contraceptives, thiazide diuretics, penicillin and alcohol deplete B-6. Deficiency results in anemia, depression, lethargy, nervousness, water retention and skin lesions.

VITAMIN B-7 (Biotin): a member of the B-complex family, necessary for metabolism of amino acids and essential fatty acids, and in forming immune antibodies. Needed for the body to use folacin, B-12 and pantothenic acid. Food sources: *poultry, raspberries, grapefruit, tomatoes, tuna, nutritional yeast, salmon, eggs, organ meats, legumes and nuts.*

Health Benefits: naturally made from yeast, biotin supplements show good results in controlling hair loss, dermatitis, eczema, dandruff and seborrheic scalp problems. Improves glucose tolerance in diabetics. Research shows enhanced immune response for Candida Albicans and CFS. Long term antibiotic courses require extra biotin.

VITAMIN B-9 (Folic Acid): plays a critical role in the synthesis of DNA, enzyme production and blood formation. Food sources: *green leafy vegetables, organ meats, peas, lentils, avocados, beets, asparagus, nutritional yeast, broccoli, fruits, soy foods, chicken, mussels, crabs, brown rice, eggs and whole grains.*

Health Benefits: Essential for division and growth of new cells, it is an excellent supplement during pregnancy (400mcg daily) to guard against spina bifida and neural tube defects. Prevents anemia, helps control leukemia and pernicious anemia; is effective against alcoholism, and some precancerous lesions. Critical in overcoming the immuno-depression state following chemotherapy with MTX. Helps lower high homocysteine levels that tend to thicken the blood; facilitates the conversion of LDL (bad cholesterol) into free radical particles. Lack of folic acid is linked to depression, osteoporosis and atherosclerosis. Aluminum antacids, oral contraceptives, alcohol, long-term antibiotics and anti-inflammatory drugs increase the need for folic acid.

VITAMIN B-12, (Cyano Cobalamin): an anti-inflammatory analgesic that works with calcium for absorption. Food sources: *cheese, poultry, sea greens, yogurt, eggs, organ meats, nutritional yeast, peanuts and fish.*

Health Benefits: critical to DNA synthesis and red blood cell formation; involved in all immune responses. A specific for sulfite-induced asthma. New research shows some success in cancer management, especially in tumor growth, and in lowering homocysteine. Energizes, relieves depression, hangover and poor concentration. Supplied largely from animal foods, B-12 may be deficient for vegetarians, and a deficiency can take five or more years to appear after body stores are depleted. Deficiency results in anemia, nerve degeneration, dizziness, heart palpitations and excess weight loss. Long use of cholesterol drugs, oral contraceptives, anti-inflammatory and anti-convulsant drugs deplete B-12.

VITAMIN C, (Ascorbic Acid): a key to immune strength and health. Food sources: *citrus fruits, green peppers, papaya, tomatoes, kiwi, potatoes, greens, cauliflower and broccoli.*

Health Benefits: protects against cancer, viral and bacterial infections, heart disease, arthritis and allergies. A strong antioxidant against free radical damage. Safeguards against radiation poisoning, heavy metal toxicity, environmental pollutants and early aging. Accelerates healing after surgery, increases infection resistance, and is essential to formation of new collagen tissue. Vitamin C controls alcohol craving, lowers cholesterol, and is a key in treating diabetes, high blood pressure, male infertility, and in suppressing the HIV virus. Helps adrenal and iron insufficiency, especially when the body is under stress. Relieves withdrawal symptoms from drugs, tranquilizers and alcohol. Aspirin, oral contraceptives and smoking deplete C levels. Deficiency results in easy bruising, receding gums, slow healing, fatigue and rough skin. Vitamin C has also been proven clinically to decrease the length and severity of colds.

—Ester C™, a metabolite of vitamin C, biochemically the same as naturally metabolized C in the body. Fat and water soluble, and non-acid. Ester C is absorbed twice as fast into the bloodstream and excreted twice as slowly as ordinary vitamin C.

VITAMIN D: a critical fat soluble " vitamin." Although called a vitamin, D is really a hormone produced in the skin from sunlight. Cholesterol compounds in the skin convert to a vitamin D precursor when exposed to UV radiation. Food sources: *cod liver oil, yogurt, cheese, butter, herring, halibut, salmon, tuna, eggs and liver.*

Health Benefits: works with vitamin A to utilize calcium and phosphorus in building bones and teeth. Twenty minutes a day of early morning sunshine make a real difference to your body's vitamin D stores, especially if you are at risk for osteoporosis or colon cancer. Vitamin D helps in all eye problems including spots, conjunctivitis and glaucoma. Deficiency results in nearsightedness, psoriasis, soft teeth, muscle cramps, slow healing, insomnia, nosebleeds, fast heartbeat and arthritis.

VITAMIN E: a fat soluble antioxidant and immune stimulating vitamin. Food sources: *almonds, leafy greens, seafoods and sea greens, soy, wheat germ, wheat germ oil and organ meats.*

Health Benefits: an effective anticoagulant and vasodilator against blood clots and heart disease. Retards cellular and mental aging, alleviates fatigue and provides tissue oxygen to accelerate healing of wounds and burns. Works with selenium against the effects of aging and cancer by neutralizing free radicals. Beneficial for chronic, so-called incurable diseases like arthritis, lupus, Parkinson's disease and MS. Improves skin tone and texture; helps control alopecia and dandruff. Deficiency results in muscle and nerve degeneration, anemia, skin pigmentation.

VITAMIN K: a fat soluble vitamin necessary for blood clotting; may be taken as a guard against too-easy bleeding. Vitamin K is easy to get in your diet and is stored in the body. Food sources: *seafoods, sea greens, dark leafy greens, liver, molasses, eggs, oats, broccoli, cauliflower, cabbage and sprouts.*

Health Benefits: deficiency occurs from poor nutrient absorption - conditions like celiac disease, intestinal worms or chronic colitis. Antibiotic overload contributes to vitamin K deficiency because these drugs deplete and destroy friendly intestinal flora. Vitamin K reduces excessive menstruation, helps heal broken blood vessels in the eye, aids in arresting bone loss and post-menopausal brittle bones. Vitamin K is an integral part of liver function and is a good source of help for cirrhosis and jaundice.

ZEAXANTHIN: See Carotenoids.

ZINC: a co-factor mineral of SOD to fight free radical damage, essential to the formation of insulin, immune strength, gland, sexual and reproductive health. Food sources: *all sea foods, turkey, many seeds, nutritional yeast, eggs, mushrooms and wheat germ.*

Health Benefits: helps prevent birth defects, enhances sensory perception, accelerates healing. Zinc is a brain food that helps control mental disorders and promotes mental alertness. A high stress life-style depletes zinc, impairing immune response and the ability to heal. People who get little sleep, work a 16-hour day (or more than one job), or those recovering from injury should increase their zinc levels. Zinc picolinate is highly absorbable.

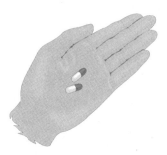

Complete Index

Bibliography

Airola, Paavo, Ph.D. *How To Get Well*. Health Plus, 1974.

American Publishing. *Foods That Heal, Reverse Aging and Extend Your Lifespan*. American Publishing Corp., 1996.

Berdanier, Carolyn. *CRC Desk Reference For Nutrition*. CRC Press, 1998.

"Beware! Healthy Foods Are Falling Prey To Frightening New Trends," Dr. Linda Page's Natural Healing Report, Sept. 1999.

Bragg, Paul C., N.D., Ph.D. & Patricia Bragg, N.D., Ph.D. *Apple Cider Vinegar: Miracle Health System*. Health Science, 1999.

Bragg, Paul C., N.D., Ph.D. & Patricia Bragg, N.D., Ph.D. *Bragg Healthy Lifestyle*. Health Science, 1999.

Bricklin, Mark & Sharon Claessens. *The Natural Healing Cookbook*. Rodale Press, 1981.

Calbom, Cherie & Maureen Keane. *Juicing For Life*. Trillium Health Products, 1992.

Carper, Jean. *The Food Pharmacy*. Bantam Books, 1988.

Carper, Jean. *Food: Your Miracle Medicine*. HarperCollins, 1993.

Cheraskin, E. M.D., D.M.D. et al. *Diet & Disease*. August 1987.

Chevallier, Andrew. *The Encyclopedia of Medicinal Plants*. DK Pub., 1996

Cichoke, Dr. Anthony J. *The Complete Book of Enzyme Therapy*. Avery Pub., 1999.

"Eating Fish Prevents Asthma," First For Women, 10/12/98.

"Eating Fish Reduces Men's Risk of Sudden Cardiac Death," Nutrition Science News, April 1998, Vol. 3, No. 4.

Editors of Prevention Magazine. *The Healing Foods Cookbook*. Rodale Press, 1991.

Ensminger, M.E., Audrey H. Ensminger, James E. Kolande, & John R.K. Robson. *The Concise Encyclopedia of Foods & Nutrition*. CRC Press, 1995.

Enzymatic Therapy - Nutritional Formulas for the Right Body Chemistry.

"Fat-Free Foods: A Health Disaster In The Making," Dr. Linda Page's Natural Healing Report, May 1999.

"Fish Oil May Ease Manic Depression, Study Says, " cnn.com, May 14, 1999.

Garrison, Robert, Jr., M.A., R.Ph. & Elizabeth Somer, M.A., R.D. *The Nutrition Desk Reference.* Keats Pub., 1995.

Gittleman, Ann Louise, M.S., "Parasites In The United States," Let's Live, August 1995.

Gursche, Siegfried, "Healing With Herbal Juices," Alive #134.

Haas, Elson M., M.D. *The Staying Healthy Shopper's Guide.* Celestial Arts, 1999.

Haas, Elson M., M.D. *Staying Healthy With Nutrition.* Celestial Arts, 1992.

Hausman, Patricia & Judith Bell Hurley. *The Healing Foods.* Rodale Press, 1989.

Jacobi, Dana, "Soya, Oh Boya! A Whole New World Of Taste," Better Nutrition, May 1998.

Kirschmann, Gayla J. and John D. Kirschmann. *Nutrition Almanac.* McGraw-Hill, 1996.

Mann, Laura, O.M.D., L.A.c. "Giardia Lamblia: The Cause Of Your Health Problems?" Health World, July/Aug. 1992.

Null, Gary & Steven Null. *How To Get Rid Of The Poisons In Your Body.* Arco Pub, 1984.

Ode, Penelope. *Complete Medicinal Herbal.* DK Pub., 1993.

Onstad, Dianne. *Whole Foods Companion.* Chelsea Green Pub., 1996.

Osborn, Sally, "Does Soy Have a Dark Side?" Natural Health, March 1999.

Page, Linda, N.D., Ph.D. *Healthy Healing 11th Edition: A Guide To Self-Healing For Everyone.* Traditional Wisdom, Inc. 2000, 2001.

Pedersen, Mark. *Nutritional Herbology Volume 1 & Volume 2.* Pederson Pub., 1988, 1990.

"Probiotics For Babies," Herbs For Health, May/June 1999.

"Raw Cultured Vegetables," www.rejuvenative.com.

"Red Wine's Latest Kudos Include Cancer Prevention," The Detroit News, Jan. 10, 1997.

"Seafood," Let's Live, Feb. 1997.

"Should You Be Eating More Protein Or Less?" UC Berkeley Wellness Letter, June 1996.

Teitel, Martin, Ph.D., and Kimberly A. Wilson. *Genetically Engineered Food: Changing The Nature of Nature.* Park Street Press, 1999.

"Tempeh," Natural Health, March 1999.

"The Bittersweet Truth About Sugar and Artificial Sweeteners," Dr. Linda Page's Natural Healing Report, Jan. 1999.

"The Many Health Benefits of Vinegar," Dr. Julian Whitaker's Health & Healing, May 1997.

"Tofu Is A Superfood For the 90s," Let's Live, June 1995.

Trattler, Ross, N.D. D.O. *Better Health Through Natural Healing.* Thorson Publishing, 1985.

Turner, Lisa. *Meals That Heal.* Healing Arts Press, 1996.

Vegetarian Times Magazine - 1988-2001.

"Vinegar For Health," www.freeyellow.com.

Walker, N.W., D. Sci. *Raw Vegetable Juices.* Jove Books, 1987.

"Walnuts Help Lower Cholesterol," Herbs for Health, Sept./Oct. 2000.

Werbach, Melvyn R. *Nutritional Influences on Illness.* Third Line Printing, April 1996.

Whole Foods Magazine - 1989-2001.

"Wine Reduces Death From All Causes By 30%," Feb. 18, 1998, cnn.com.

Wittenberg, Magaret M. *Experiencing Quality: A Shopper's Guide to Whole Foods.* Whole Foods, 1981.

Hundreds of books and articles were reviewed during the writing of this book. Because of space constraints, the editors have chosen to list a representative sampling here.

Product Resources

Where you can get what we recommend.....

The following list is for your convenience and assistance in obtaining further information about the products I recommend in the Cook Book Set. The list is unsolicited by the companies named. Each company has a solid history of testing and corroborative data that is invaluable to me and my staff, as well as empirical confirmation by the stores that carry these products who have shared their experiences with us. We hear from thousands of readers about the products they have used. I consider their information in every one of my books on natural health. I realize there are many other fine companies and products who are not listed here, but you can rely on the companies who are, for their high quality products and good results.

- Alacer Corp., 19631 Pauling, Foothill Ranch, CA 92610, 800-854-0249
- All One, 719 East Haley St., Santa Barbara, CA 93103, 800-235-5727
- Aloe Life International, 4822 Santa Monica Ave. #231, San Diego, CA 92107, 800-414-2563
- Alta Health Products, Inc., 1979 E. Locust Street, Pasadena, CA 91107, 626-796-1047
- America's Finest, Inc., 140 Ethel Road West, Suites S & T, Piscataway, NJ 08854, 800-350-3305
- Anabol Naturals, 1550 Mansfield Street, Santa Cruz, CA 95062, 800-426-2265
- Arise & Shine, P.O. Box 1439, Mt. Shasta, CA 96067, 800-688-2444
- Ark Naturals Products for Pets, 6166 Taylor Road #105, Naples, FL 34109, 800-926-5100
- Barleans Organic Oils, 4936 Lake Terrell Rd., Fern Dale, WA 98248, 800-445-3529
- BD Herbs, 14000 Tomki Road, Redwood Valley, CA 95470, 800-760-3739
- Beehive Botanicals, Route 8, Box 8257, Hayward, WI 54843, 800-233-4483
- BHI (Heel Inc.) 11600 Cochiti Road SE, Albuquerque, NM 33376, 800-621-7644
- Biotec Foods / BioVet, 5152 Bolsa Ave. Suite 101, Huntington Beach, CA 92649, 800-788-1084
- Bodyonics (Pinnacle), 140 Lauman Lane, Hicksville, NY 11801, 800-899-2749
- Boericke & Tafel Inc.,(B & T) 2381 Circadian Way, Santa Rosa, CA 95407, 800-876-9505
- Bragg/Live Food Products, Inc., Box 7, Santa Barbara, CA 93102, 805-968-1028
- CC Pollen Co., 3627 East Indian School Rd., Suite 209, Phoenix, AZ 85018-5126, 800-875-0096
- Champion Nutrition, 2615 Stanwell Dr., Concord, CA 94520, 800-225-4831
- Coenzyme-A Technologies Inc., 12512 Beverly Park Road B1, Lynnwood, WA 98037, 425-438-8586
- Country Life, 28300 B Industrial Blvd., Hayward, CA 94545, 800-645-5768
- Creations Garden, 25269 The Old Road, Suite B, Newhall, CA 91381, 661-254-3222
- Crystal Star Herbal Nutrition, 4069 Wedgeway Court, Earth City, MO 63045, 800-736-6015
- Dancing Paws, 8659 Hayden Place, Culver City, CA 90232, 888-644-7297
- Dr. Diamond/Herpanacine Associates, P.O. Box 544, Ambler, PA 19002, 888-467-4200
- Dr. Goodpet, P.O. Box 4547, Inglewood, CA 90309, 800-222-9932
- EAS, 555 Corporate Circle, Golden, CO 80401, 800-923-4300
- East Park Research, Inc., 2709 Horseshoe Drive, Las Vegas, NV 89120, 800-345-8367 (orders)
- Eidon Products, 9988 Hibert St. #104, San Diego, CA 92131, 800-700-1169
- Enzymatic Therapy, Dept. L, P.O. Box 22310, Green Bay, WI 54305, 800-783-2286
- Enzymedica, 1970 Kings Hwy., Punta Gorda, FL 33980, 888-918-1118
- Earth's Bounty/Matrix Health Products, 9316 Wheatlands Road, Santee, CA 92071, 800-736-5609
- Esteem Products Ltd., 15015 Main St., Suite 204, Bellevue, WA 98007, 800-255-7631
- Ethical Nutrients/Unipro, 971 Calle Negocio, San Clemente, CA 92673, 949-366-0818
- Flint River Ranch, 1243 Columbia Avenue B-6, Riverside, CA 92507-2123, 888-722-4589
- Flora, Inc., 805 East Badger Road, P.O. Box 73, Lynden, WA 98264, 800-446-2110, 604-451-8232

- Futurebiotics, 145 Ricefield Lane, Hauppauge, NY 11788, 800-367-5433
- Gaia Herbs, Inc., 12 Lancaster County Road, Harvard, MA 01451, 800-831-7780
- Golden Pride, 1501 Northpoint Pkwy., Suite 100, West Palm Beach, FL 33407, 561-640-5700
- Green Foods Corp., 320 North Graves Ave., Oxnard, CA 93030 800-777-4430
- Green Kamut Corp., 1542 Seabright Ave., Long Beach, CA 90813, 800-452-6884
- Grifron/Maitake Products, Inc., P.O. Box 1354, Paramus, NJ 07653, 800-747-7418
- Halo-Purely For Pets, Inc. 3438 East Lake Road #14, Palm Harbor, FL 34685, 800-426-4256
- Herbal Answers, Inc., P.O. Box 1110, Saratoga Springs, New York 12866, 888-256-3367
- Health from the Sun/Arkopharma, P.O. Box 179, Newport, NH 03773, 800-447-2249
- Healthy House, P.O. Box 436, Carmel Valley, CA 93924, 888-447-2939
- Heart Foods Company, Inc., 2235 East 38th Street, Minneapolis, MN 55407, 612-724-5266
- Herbal Magic, Inc., P.O. Box 70, Forest Knowlls, CA 94933, 415-488-9488
- Herbal Products & Development, P.O. Box 1084, Aptos, CA 95001, 831-688-8706
- HerbaSway Laboratories,342 Quinnipiac St., Wallingford, CT 06492, 800-672-7322
- Herbs Etc., 1340 Rufina Circle, Santa Fe, NM 87505, 505-471-6488
- Herbs For Life, P.O. Box 40082, Sarasota, FL 34278, 941-362-9255
- Highland Laboratories, P.O. Box 199 110 South Garfield, Mt. Angel, OR 97362, 888-717-4917
- Imperial Elixir, P.O. Box 970, Simi Valley, CA 93062, 800-423-5176
- Jarrow Formulas, 1824 South Robertson Blvd., Los Angeles, CA 90035, 310-204-6936
- Lane Labs, 25 Commerce Drive, Allendale, NJ 07401, 800-526-3005
- MagneLyfe/Encore Technology, Inc., 80 Fifth Ave., Suite 1104, New York, NY 10011, 877-624-6353
- Maine Coast Sea Vegetables, RR1 Box 78, Franklin, Maine 04634, 207-565-2907
- Maitake Products, Inc., P.O. Box 1354, Paramus, NJ 07653, 800-747-7418
- Medicine Wheel, P.O. Box 20037, Sedona, AZ 86341-0037, 800-233-0810
- M.D. Labs, 1719 W. University, Suite 187, Tempe, AZ 85281, 800-255-2690
- Mendocino Sea Vegetable Co., P.O. Box 1265, Mendocino, CA 95460, 707-937-2050
- Metabolic Response, 2633 W. Coast Hwy, Suite B, Newport Beach, CA 92663, 800-948-6296
- Mezotrace Corporation, 415 Wellington St., Winnemucca, NV 89445, 800-843-9989
- Monas Chlorella, 8815 South Decatur Blvd., Las Vegas, NV 89139, 800-275-0343
- Moon Maid Botanicals, 13870 SW 90 Ave., MM104, Miami, FL 33176, 877-253-7853
- Motherlove Herbal Co., P.O. Box 101, Laporte, CO 80535, 970-493-2892
- MRI (Medical Research Institute), 2160 Pacific Ave., Suite 61, San Francisco CA 94115, 888-448-4246
- Natren Inc., 3105 Willow Ln., Westlake Village, CA 91361, 800-992-3323
- Natural Animal Health Products, Inc., 7000 U.S. 1 North, St. Augustine, FL 32095, 800-274-7387
- Natural Balance (Pep Products), 3130 N. Commerce Ct., Castle Rock, CO 80104-8002, 303-688-6633
- Natural Energy Plus, 4630 N. Paseo De Los Cerritos, Tucson, AZ 85745, 888-633-9233
- Natural Labs Corporation (Deva Flowers), P.O. Box 20037, Sedona, AZ 86341-0037, 800-233-0810
- Nature's Apothecary, 6350 Gunpark Drive #500, Boulder, CO 80301, 800-999-7422
- Nature's Path, P.O. Box 7862, Venice, FL 34287, 800-326-5772
- Nature's Plus, 548 Broadhollow Road, Melville, NY 11747-3708, 631-293-0030
- Nature's Secret/Irwin Naturals, 10549 West Jefferson Blvd., Culver City, CA 90232, 310-253-5305
- Nature's Way, 10 Mountain Springs Parkway, Springville, UT 84663, 800-962-8873
- Nelson Bach, Wilmington Technology Park, 100 Research Dr., Wilmington, MA 01887, 800-319-9151
- New Chapter, P.O. Box 1947, Brattleboro, VT 05302, 800-543-7279
- No-Miss Nail Care 6401 E. Rogers Circle Suite 14, Boca Raton, FL 33487, 800-283-1963
- Noni of Beverly Hills, Inc., 16158 Wyancotte Street, Vans Nuys, CA 91406, 310-271-7988
- Nova Homeopathics, 5600 McLeod NE, Suite F, Albuquerque, NM 87109, 800-225-8094
- NOW, 395 S. Glen Ellyn Rd., Bloomingdale, IL 60108, 800-999-8069

- Nutramedix Inc., 212 N. Hwy One, Tequesta, FL 33469, 800-730-3130
- NutriCology /Allergy Research Group, 30806 Santana St., Hayward, CA 94544, 800-545-9960
- Omega Nutrition/Body Ecology, 6515 Aldrich Road, Bellingham, WA 98226, 404-350-8420
- Orthomolecular Specialties, P.O. Box 32232, San Jose, CA 95152-2232, 408-227-9334
- Oshadhi, 1340 G Industrial Ave., Petaluma, CA 94952, 888-674-2344
- Pines International, Inc., 992 East 1400 Road, Lawrence, KS 66044, 800-697-4637
- Planetary Formulas, P.O. Box 533 Soquel, CA 95073, 800-606-6226
- Premier Labs, 27475 Ynez Rd., Suite 305, Temecula, CA 92591, 800-887-5227
- Prime Pharmaceutical, 1535 Yonge St. Suite 200, Toronto, Ontario, Canada M4T 1Z2,800-741-6856
- PureForm, 3240 West Desert Inn Rd., Las Vegas, NV 89103, 888-363-9817
- Quantum, Inc., P.O. Box 2791, Eugene, OR 97402, 800-448-1448
- Rainbow Light, P.O. Box 600, Santa Cruz, CA 95061, 800-635-1233
- Rainforest Remedies, Box 325, Twin Lakes, WI 53181, 800-824-6396
- Real Life Research, Inc., 14631 Best Ave., Norwalk, CA 90650, 800-423-8837
- Rejuvenative Foods, P.O. Box 8464, Santa Cruz, CA 95061, 800-805-7957
- Solaray, Inc., 1104 Country Hills Dr., Suite 300, Ogden, UT 84403, 800-669-8877
- Sonne's Organic Foods, Inc., P.O.Box 2160, Cottonwood, CA 96022, 800-544-8147
- Source Naturals Inc., 23 Janis Way, Scotts Valley, CA 95066, 800-777-5677
- Spectrum Essentials, 133 Copeland St., Petaluma, CA 94952, 707-778-8900
- Springlife Inc., 4630 N. Paseo De Los Cerritos, Tucson, AZ 85745, 888-633-9233
- Sun Wellness, 4025 Spencer St. #104, Torrance, CA 90503, 800-829-2828
- Transformation Enzyme Corporation, 2900 Wilcrest, Suite 220, Houston, TX 77042, 800-777-1474
- Transitions For Health, 621 SW Alder, Suite 900, Portland, OR 97205, 800-888-6814
- Trimedica International, Inc, 1895 South Los Feliz Drive. Tempe AZ 85281-6023, 480-998-1041
- UAS Laboratories, 5610 Rowland Road, Suite 110, Minnetonka, MN 55343, 952-935-1707
- Vibrant Health, 432 Lime Rock Rd., Lakeville, CT 06039, 800-242-1835
- Vitamin Research Products, 3579 Highway 50 East, Carson City, NV 89701, 800-877-2447
- Waddell Creek Organic Bee Pollen, 654 Swanton Road, Davenport, CA 95017
- Wakunaga / Kyolic, 23501 Madero, Mission Viejo, CA 92691, 800-421-2998 / 800-825-7888
- Wisdom of the Ancients, 640 South Perry Lane, Tempe, AZ 85281, 800-899-9908
- Wyndmere Naturals, Inc., 153 Ashley Road, Hopkins, MN 55343, 800-207-8538
- Y.S. Royal Jelly and Organic Bee Farm, RT. 1, Box 91-A, Sheridan IL 60551, 800-654-4593
- Zand Herbal Formulas, P.O. Box 5312, Santa Monica, CA 90409, 360-384-5656
- Zia Natural Skincare, 1337 Evans Ave., San Francisco, CA 94124, 800-334-7546

Special Bonus Recipes For Your Healing Diet

The history of the world would be entirely different if the human diet had been different. Our children are formed from, and become, the nutrients (or poisons) within us. Not only are we what we eat, our children are as well, before and after birth. The secret is knowing how to use foods and herbs (which are foods) to change body chemistry. The latest wonder drugs can't do it. Only foods and herbs can do it.

The cook book set, Cooking for Healthy Healing™ you hold in your hands shows you how to use food as medicine. In *Book One - The Healing Diets*, you've discovered the healing secrets of different foods. Now, learn to make your own food medicines with the recipes in *Book Two - The Healing Recipes!* Each detailed program in this book refers to the easy-to-use recipes in *The Healing Recipes*. There are over 1,000 recipes to choose from in *The Healing Recipes*. In this section, I've listed just a few of the recipes I regularly use in my healing diets. *The Healing Recipes* is filled with many more medicinal recipes designed to help you meet your health goals.

POTASSIUM JUICE

This is the single most effective juice for cleansing, neutralizing acids and rebuilding the body. It is a blood and body tonic that provides rapid energy and system balance.
For one 12-oz. glass:

Juice in a juicer 3 CARROTS, 3 STALKS CELERY, $^1/_2$ BUNCH SPINACH, I TB snipped, dry SEA GREENS, $^1/_2$ BUNCH PARSLEY. —Add I teasp. Bragg's LIQUID AMINOS if desired.

POTASSIUM ESSENCE BROTH

If you don't have a juicer, make a potassium broth in a soup pot. While not as concentrated or pure, it is still an excellent source of energy, minerals and electrolytes.
For a 2 day supply:

Cover with water in a soup pot 3 to 4 CARROTS, 3 STALKS CELERY, $^1/_2$ BUNCH PARSLEY, 2 POTATOES with skins, $^1/_2$ HEAD CABBAGE, I ONION, and $^1/_2$ BUNCH BROCCOLI, 2 TBS snipped, dry SEA GREENS. Simmer covered 30 minutes. Strain and discard solids.
—Add 2 teasp. Bragg's LIQUID AMINOS or I teasp. MISO. Store in the fridge, covered.

DAILY CARROT JUICE CLEANSE

For 2 large drinks:

Juice 4 CARROTS, $^1/_2$ CUCUMBER, 2 STALKS CELERY with leaves, and I TB. chopped DRY DULSE.

PERSONAL BEST V-8 A high nutrient drink for normalizing body balance. A good daily green drink even when you're not cleansing.
For 6 glasses:

Juice 6 to 8 TOMATOES (or 4 cups TOMATO JUICE), 3 to 4 GREEN ONIONS with tops, $^1/_2$ GREEN PEPPER, 2 CARROTS, 2 STALKS CELERY with leaves, $^1/_2$ BUNCH SPINACH, washed, $^1/_2$ bunch PARSLEY, 2 LEMONS, peeled, (or 4 TBS. LEMON JUICE), 1 TB. snipped, dry SEA GREENS (any kind).
—Add 2 teasp. Bragg's LIQUID AMINOS and $^1/_2$ teasp. ground celery seed.

MINERAL RICH ENERGY GREEN
Helps build strong teeth, bones, nails and hair. A good choice for a weight loss cleanse.
For 4 drinks:

Mix up in the blender: $^1/_2$ cup AMAZAKE RICE DRINK, $^1/_2$ cup OATS, 2 TBS. BEE POLLEN GRANULES, 1 packet INSTANT GINSENG TEA GRANULES, 2 Packets BARLEY GRASS OR CHLORELLA GRANULES, 2 TBS. GOTU KOLA HERB, 2 TBS. ALFALFA LEAF, 1 TBS. DANDELION LEAF, 1 TBS. crumbled DULSE, and 1 teasp. VITAMIN C CRYSTALS with BIOFLAVONOIDS.
—Then mix 2 TBS into 2 cups hot water per drink. Let flavors bloom for 5 minutes before drinking. Add 1 tsp. LEMON JUICE or 1 tsp. Bragg's LIQUID AMINOS if desired.

HERB & VEGETABLE IMMUNE ENHANCING BROTH
For 4 cups of broth:

Heat 3 cups homemade VEGETABLE STOCK in a soup pot.
—Add and heat gently: 2 TBS. MISO dissolved in 1 cup WATER, 1 TBS. BREWER'S YEAST FLAKES, 2 TBS. chopped GREEN ONIONS, $^1/_2$ cup TOMATO JUICE and $^1/_2$ teasp. each: dry BASIL, THYME, SAVORY and MARJORAM.

CANCER FIGHTING SOUP *Especially good after chemotherapy. This recipe works for: Immune Breakdown Diseases, Cancerous Tumors*
Makes 12 servings. Use a gallon pot. Store in the fridge for easy re-use.

Fill the soup pot with 4 qts. WATER, 10 ASTRAGALUS STICKS and $^1/_4$ cup PEARL BARLEY.
—Soak 10 dry SHIITAKE MUSHROOMS in $^1/_2$ cup water til soft; then sliver and discard stems. Add mushrooms and soaking water to soup. Simmer 15 minutes.
—Add 1 cup <u>each</u>: diced CARROTS, diced BEETS, diced YAMS, diced BROCCOLI STEMS. Simmer for 30 minutes. Remove from heat. Discard Astragalus pieces.
—Stir in 1 dropperful each: REISHI MUSHROOM extract, SIBERIAN GINSENG extract. Add 1 TB BARLEY GRASS POWDER. Eat hot.

Home Healing Procedures
A reference for healing techniques to accompany your healing diet

Coca's Pulse Test:

Dr. Arthur Coca, an immunologist, discovered that when people eat foods to which they are allergic, there is a dramatic increase in the heartbeat — 20 or more beats a minute above normal. Pulse rate is normally remarkably stable, not affected by digestion or ordinary physical activities or normal emotions. Unless a person is ill or under great stress, pulse rate deviation is probably due to an allergy. By performing COCA'S PULSE TEST one can find and eliminate foods that harm.

1. Take your pulse when you wake in the morning. Using a watch with a second hand, count the number of beats in a 60-second period. A normal pulse reading is 60 to 100 beats per minute.
2. Take your pulse again after eating a suspected allergy food. Wait 20 minutes; take your pulse again. If your pulse rate has increased more than 10 beats per minute, omit the food from your diet.

A 24-Hour Cleanse is an Invaluable Healing Tool

Put this little jewel of a cleanse into action as soon as you realize you aren't feeling well, at the first signs of unexplained low energy, poor skin or congestion. It's one of the best ways I know to recovery quickly from a cold or flu. It's also an easy first step before making a significant diet change. A 24-hour cleanse is a good answer if you need a cleanse, but even a short cleanse seems like too much time.

A 24-hour detox is a juice and herbal tea cleanse that lets you go on with your normal activities, while you "jump start" a healing program. It doesn't have the depth of vegetable juices needed for a major or chronic problem, but it's often enough, is definitely better than no cleanse at all, and it will make a difference in the speed of healing. Even if you're only trying simple, lifestyle changes aimed at better health, a 24 hour cleanse can point you in the right direction.

Is your body showing signs that it needs a twenty four hour cleanse?
—Do you feel "toxic?" Are you tired a lot for no reason?
—Do you feel congested? Do you have the first signs of a cold or flu? (Go right into this cleanse.)
—Is your skin dry or flaky? Is your skin tone sallow? Is your hair dull, dry and brittle?
—Are the soles of your feet or your palms often peeling?
—Do you frequently get mouth herpes? yeast infections? urinary tract infections? allergy reactions?

24-Hour Detox Plan
Drink 8 to 10 glasses of water to hydrate and flush toxins from all cells.

The evening before you begin... have a leafy salad to "sweep" your bowels. Dry brush your skin before retiring to open your pores for the night's cleansing eliminations. Take an herbal laxative.

The next day... the next 24 hours take fresh juices, herbal drinks, water, and a long walk.
—**On rising:** take 2 TBS fresh lemon juice, 1 TB maple syrup and 1 pinch cayenne in water.
—**Breakfast:** juice 1 pear, 2 apples, 4 oranges and 1 grapefruit; or cranberry juice from concentrate.
—**Mid-morning:** have a Zippy Tonic: 1 handful dandelion greens, 3 fresh pineapple rings and 3 radishes; or a cleansing, energizing tea with antioxidants like Crystal Star GREEN TEA CLEANSER™.

—**Lunch:** Focus on chlorophyll-rich foods. Chlorophyll is the most powerful cleansing agent in nature. Juice 4 parsley sprigs or a handful dandelion greens, 3 tomatoes, 1 scallion, $^1/_2$ bell pepper, $^1/_2$ cucumber, 1 lemon wedge; or apple juice with 1 packet chlorella granules dissolved.

—**Mid-afternoon:** a cup of Crystal Star CLEANSING & PURIFYING™ TEA or MEDITATION™ TEA.

—**Dinner:** take a papaya-pineapple juice for enzymes; or this high mineral broth: 7 carrots, 7 celery stalks, beet tops from 1 bunch, 2 potatoes, 1 onion, 4 garlic cloves, 3 zucchini, 1 handful of parsley. Place in a large soup pot, cover with water, bring to a boil and simmer 30 minutes. Discard veggies, then drink broth.

—**Before Bed:** have a cup of mint tea, or I teasp. NUTRITIONAL YEAST BROTH or miso soup.

24-Hour cleanse supplement suggestions:

• **Cleansing boosters:** Crystal Star CLEANSING & PURIFYING™ TEA; Crystal Star LIV-ALIVE™ caps; Nature's Way 5 SYSTEM CLEANSE.

• **Electrolyte boosters for removal of toxic body acids:** Nature's Path TRACE-LYTE .

• **Probiotics:** UAS DDS-PLUS; New Chapter ALL-FLORA.

• **Vitamin C:** Take 1,000mg of vitamin C 3x per day with bioflavonoids.

An overheating bath is a simple, ancient healer

Simple overheating bath therapy can even be effectively practiced in your home, via either a dry sauna or an overheating bath. Both are able to stimulate the body's immune mechanism without the stress of fever-inducing drugs.

How to take an overheating bath:

1) Empty your bladder and colon if possible. Don't eat for two hours before the bath.

2) Get a good thermometer so that you can monitor your bath temperature.

3) Plug the tub's emergency outlet to raise the water to the top of the tub. You must be totally immersed for therapeutic results - with only nose, eyes and mouth left uncovered. Start slowly running water at skin temperature. After 15 minutes raise temperature to 100°F, then in 15 minutes to 103°F. Even though the water temperature is not high, heat cannot escape from your body when you are totally covered, so body temperature will rise to match that of the water, creating a slight healing fever.

4) A therapeutic bath ise about 45 minutes. Any discomfort, sit up in the tub for 5 minutes.

5) Gently massage with a skin brush during the bath to stimulate circulation, bring cleansing blood to the surface of the skin, and relieve the heart from undue pressure.

How to take an enema:

Enemas are potent therapy in any mucous or colon congestion cleansing program. They accelerate release of encrusted colon waste, encourage discharge of parasites, freshen the G.I. tract, and cleanse your body more thoroughly. They are helpful during a healing crisis, or after a serious illness or hospital stay to speed healing. Some headaches and inflammatory skin conditions can be relieved with enemas. Herbal enemas can immediately alkalize the bowel area, help control irritation and inflammation, and provide local healing action for ulcerated tissue.

Herbs for enemas. Use 2 cups very strong tea or solution to 1 qt. of water per enema.

—**Garlic:** helps kill parasites and cleanse harmful bacteria, viruses and mucous. *Blend six garlic cloves in 2 cups cold water and strain. For small children, use 1 clove garlic to 1 pint water.*

—**Catnip:** helps stomach, digestive problems and cramping; also for childhood disease.

—**Pau d' arco:** body chemistry imbalances, as in chronic yeast and fungal infections.

—**Spirulina:** is effective when both blood and bowel are toxic.

—**Aloe vera:** helps heal tissues in cases of hemorrhoids, irritable bowel and diverticulitis.

—**Lemon Juice:** helps rapidly neutralize an acid system, cleanse the colon and bowel.

—**Acidophilus:** helps gas, yeast, and candidiasis infections. Mix 4-oz. powder to 1-qt. water.

—**Coffee enemas:** have become a standard in natural healing for liver and blood related cancers. Use 1 cup of regular strong brewed coffee to 1 qt. water. Also effective for migraines.

How to take a detoxifying, colonic enema:

Place warm enema solution in an enema bag. Hang the bag about 18 inches higher than the body. Attach the colon tube, and lubricate its attachment with vaseline or vitamin E oil. Expel a little water to let out air bubbles. Lying on your left side, slowly insert the attachment about 3 inches into the rectum. Never use force. Rotate attachment gently to ease insertion. Remove kinks in the tubing so liquid will flow freely. Massage loosens old fecal matter. Massage abdomen, or flex and contract stomach muscles to relieve any cramping. When all solution has entered the colon, slowly remove the tube and remain on the left side for 5 minutes. Then move to a knee-chest position with your body weight on your knees and one hand. Use the other hand to massage the lower left side of the abdomen for several minutes. Roll onto your back for 5 minutes; massage up the descending colon, over the transverse colon to the right side and down the ascending colon. Move onto your right side for 5 minutes, to reach each part of the colon. Get up and quickly expel into the toilet. Look for sticky grey-brown mucous, small dark crusty chunks or tough ribbony pieces to be expelled during an enema. These poisonous looking things are toxins interfering with your normal body functions. An enema removes them. Several enemas may be needed until there is no more evidence of these substances.

An herbal "vag pac" can detox the vaginal/urethral area.

A cleansing herbal combination may be used as a vaginal pack by placing it against the cervix, or as a bolus inserted in the vagina. The pack acts as an internal poultice to draw out toxic wastes from the vagina, rectum or urethral areas. A "vag pac" is effective for cysts, benign tumors, polyps and cervical dysplasia. It takes 6 weeks to 6 months for healing, depending on the problem and severity.

How to make a pack:

Formula #1: Mix 1 TB <u>each</u> of the following herbal powders: squaw vine, marshmallow root, slippery elm, goldenseal root, pau d'arco, comfrey root, mullein, yellow dock root, chickweed, acidophilus powder.

Formula #2: Mix 1 TB <u>each</u> of the following herbal powders: cranesbill powder, goldenseal root, red raspberry leaf, white oak bark, echinacea root, myrrh gum powder.

1) Mix the combined, powdered herbs with warmed cocoa butter to form finger-sized suppositories. Place on waxed paper in the refrigerator to chill and harden slightly.

2) Smear a suppository on the end of a cotton tampon and insert; or insert as is, and use a sanitary napkin to catch drainage. Use suppositories at night and rinse out in the morning with white oak bark tea, or yellow dock root tea to rebalance vaginal pH.

3) Repeat for 6 days. Rest for one week. Resume and repeat as needed.

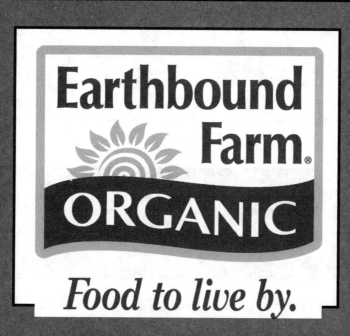
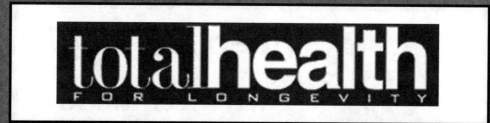

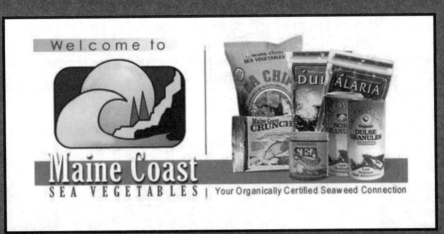
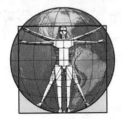

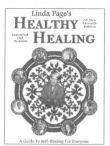

HEALTHY HEALING

by Linda Page, N.D., Ph.D.   *A Guide to Self-Healing for Everyone*

The revised updated 11th edition of the easiest to use, most comprehensive such book on the market includes new sections on health care choices; alternative healing systems and how to use them after surgery, chemotherapy, and radiation; programs for more than 150 ailments and health conditions—including programs for people with special needs; self-diagnosis; foods for a healing diet; the latest home healing products and much more.

COOKING FOR HEALTHY HEALING

by Linda Page, N.D., Ph.D.   *Food is Your Pharmacy*

The Healing Diets - Book One: There are complete nutrient value reference sections for foods, herbs and nutrients, and a complete section dedicated to the importance of organic foods. There are over 90 complete healing diets and programs—from allergies, to childhood disease control, to recovery after radiation and surgery—each detailed program shows how to develop the healing diet and then refers to the easy-to-use recipes in **Cooking For Healthy Healing - The Healing Recipes - Book Two!**

Cooking For Healthy Healing - The Healing Recipes - Book Two contains over 1000 delicious recipes for healing: detoxification and cleansing; healing drinks and tonics; macrobiotic; enzyme rich; low-fat; salads; soups; dairy-free; wheat-free; seafood; mineral-rich; high-fiber; and vegetarian. Each recipe tells you how it can help your health; many provide important nutritional analysis. Much more.

HOW TO BE YOUR OWN HERBAL PHARMACIST

by Linda Page, N.D., Ph.D.   *Expert Herbal Formulations*

There are plenty of books on the market that describe the benefits of specific herbs, but few, if any, show how to combine herbs to address all aspects of specific ailments. This fascinating reference features a "materia medica" on each herb including primary and secondary applications, various part uses, and contraindications; work pages with several herb choices to aid the body in healing itself; examples of how to combine herbs in an effective formula; and suggestions on administering the formula. New to this edition are updated herbal recommendations; an expanded index with more cross referencing; a section about herbal cosmetics; growing pesticide-free herbs and companion planting; and remedies for children and pets.

DETOXIFICATION

by Linda Page, N.D., Ph.D.   *Recharge, Renew and Rejuvenate Your Body, Mind and Spirit*

More than 25 thousand new toxins enter our environment each year. Detoxification and body cleansing is becoming a new commitment for good health. In this complete encyclopedia-guide of detailed instructions for detoxification and cleansing, Dr. Page discusses why body cleansing is so needed in today's world. You'll learn what you can expect when you detox; what a good cleanse really does; how to direct a cleanse for best results. Also included: detailed detox charts for special needs; step by step instructions that guide the reader through every detox program; an extensive "Green Cuisine" recipe section; a Materia Medica herbal directory with over 90 detox herbs; a Glossary of detox terms; a list of detox-spa centers in America and much more.

PLEASE TURN PAGE FOR A COMPLETE LIST OF BOOKS BY LINDA PAGE, N.D., PH.D.

HEALTHY HEALING PUBLICATIONS
Books
(Book availability and prices subject to change.)

HEALTHY HEALING - *Eleventh Edition, A Guide to Self Healing for Everyone* - by Linda Page, N.D., Ph.D. - A 576 page alternative healing reference used by professors, students, health care professionals and private individuals. $32.95 - ISBN 1-884334-89-X
• New - Spiral bound version! $35.95 - ISBN - 1-884334-88-1

COOKING FOR HEALTHY HEALING- *Food Is Your Pharmacy* - by Linda Page, N.D., Ph.D. • **Book One - The Healing Diets** - A 576 page reference work with over 90 healing programs and special sections on nutritional healing. Direct references to recipes in Book Two - The Healing Recipes. $25.95 - ISBN 1-884334-81-4 • **Book Two - The Healing Recipes** - A 552 page reference work with over 1000 healing recipes directly referenced to healing programs in Book One - The Healing Diets. Much more. $25.95 - ISBN 1-884334-82-2

HOW TO BE YOUR OWN HERBAL PHARMACIST - *Herbal Traditions, Expert Formulations* - by Linda Page, N.D., Ph.D. A complete reference guide for herbal formulations and preparations. 256 pages $18.95 - ISBN 1-884334-78-4

DETOXIFICATION - *All You Need to Know to Recharge, Renew and Rejuvenate Your Body, Mind and Spirit!* - by Linda Page, N.D., Ph.D. A complete encyclopedia-guide of detailed instructions for detoxification and cleansing. 264 pages $21.95 - ISBN 1-884334-54-7

PARTY LIGHTS - *Healthy Party Foods & Earthwise Entertaining* - by Linda Page. N.D., Ph.D., and Doug Vanderberg - A party reference book with over 70 parties and more than 500 original recipes you can prepare at home. 358 pages $19.95 - ISBN 1-884334-53-9

THE BODY SMART SYSTEM - *The Complete Guide to Cleansing & Rejuvenation* - by Helene Silver - A complete 21 day regimen and guide that includes diet, relaxation techniques, massage and bath, exercise programs and recipes. 242 pages $19.95 - ISBN 1-884334-60-1

NEW! VHS "UNLEASHING THE HEALING POWER OF HERBS" - Linda Page presents information about herbs in this beautifully produced, educational, hour long video program. $19.95 ISBN 1-884334-95-4

NEW EXPANDED LIBRARY SERIES
by Linda Page, N.D., Ph.D.   ISBN - 1884334 -

14-8 **FATIGUE SYNDROMES 46 pages - $3.95**
64-4 **RENEWING FEMALE BALANCE 48 pages - $4.50**
90-3 **MENOPAUSE & OSTEOPOROSIS 64 pages - $5.95**
36-9 **CANCER 96 pages - $8.95**
15-6 **SEXUALITY 96 pages - $8.95**
66-0 **WEIGHT LOSS** & Cellulite Control **96 pages - $8.95**
67-9 **STRESS & ENERGY** Larger Format **96 pages - $9.95**

THE HEALTHY HEALING LIBRARY SERIES
by Linda Page, N.D., Ph.D.
32 pages, $3.50 each. ISBN - 1884334 -

13-X **REVEALING THE SECRETS OF ANTI-AGING**
47-4 **COLDS, FLU & YOU** - Building Optimum Immunity
34-2 **BOOSTING IMMUNITY WITH POWER PLANTS**
30-X **RENEWING MALE HEALTH & ENERGY**

Continental U.S. shipping info: $4.50 each for books, $1.50 each for Library Series Booklets.

NAME_____ADDRESS_____

CITY_____ STATE_____ZIP_____PHONE_____

☐ Check (Make payable to Healthy Healing)   ☐ Visa   ☐ Mastercard   ☐ American Express   ☐ Discover

CARD #_____EXP. DATE_____SIGNATURE_____

QTY.	BOOK	PRICE	SHIPPING	TOTAL
	CA Residents add 7.25% tax			

Mail to: Healthy Healing Publications, P.O. Box 436, Carmel Valley, CA 93924   **TOTAL** _____
Or, fax your order to: 831-659-4044. Or, Call 1-888-447-2939.
Or order on-line @ www.healthyhealing.com.   Code: CFHH 12/01